# Difficulties in Tracheal Intubation
Second edition

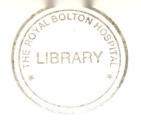

# Difficulties in Tracheal Intubation

## Second Edition

*Edited by*

**Ian Peter Latto** FRCA *and* **Ralph S. Vaughan** FRCA

*Department of Anaesthetics,*
*University Hospital of Wales, Heath Park,*
*Cardiff*

W. B. Saunders Company Ltd
London   Philadelphia   Toronto   Sydney   Tokyo

W.B. Saunders Company Ltd

24–28 Oval Road
London NW1 7DX, UK

The Curtis Center
Independence Square West
Philadelphia, PA 19106–3399, USA

Harcourt Brace & Company
55 Horner Avenue
Toronto, Ontario M8Z 4X6, Canada

Harcourt Brace & Company, Australia
30–52 Smidmore Street
Marrickville, NSW 2204, Australia

Harcourt Brace & Company, Japan
Ichibancho Central Building, 22–1 Ichibancho
Chiyoda-Ku, Tokyo 102, Japan

First edition published 1987

© 1997 W.B. Saunders Company Ltd

This book is printed on acid-free paper

British Library cataloguing in publication data is available
ISBN 0–7020–2116–4

Typeset by Wyvern Limited, Bristol
Printed in Great Britain, Butler and Tanner Ltd, Frome, Somerset

# Contents

# Contributors

**Takashi Asai** MD
*Research Associate, Department of Anaesthesiology, Kansai Medical University, 10–15 Fumizono-cho, Moriguchi City, Osaka, 570 Japan*

**Paul A Clyburn** MB BS, FRCA, MRCP
*Consultant Anaesthetist, University Hospital of Wales Healthcare NHS Trust, Cardiff*

**Nuala M Dunne** MB ChB, FRCA
*Consultant Anaesthetist, University Hospital of Wales Healthcare NHS Trust, Cardiff*

**Stephen G Greenhough** MB ChB, FRCA
*Consultant Anaesthetist, The Manchester Royal Infirmary, Manchester*

**Michael Harmer** MB BS, FRCA
*Senior Lecturer in Anaesthesia, University of Wales College of Medicine, Cardiff*

**Michael Hartley** MB ChB FRCA
*Consultant Anaesthetist, Blackpool Victoria Hospitals NHS Trust, Blackpool*

**Brian Jenkins** MB BS FRCA
*Senior Lecturer in Anaesthesia, University of Wales College of Medicine, Cardiff*

**Ian Peter Latto** MB BS FRCA
*Consultant Anaesthetist, University Hospital of Wales Healthcare NHS Trust, Cardiff*

**Keith R Murrin** MB BCh FRCA
*Consultant Anaesthetist, University Hospital of Wales Healthcare NHS Trust, Cardiff*

**W Shang Ng** MB BCh FRCA
*Consultant Anaesthetist, University Hospital of Wales Healthcare NHS Trust, Cardiff*

**Jeremy Nolan** MB ChB, FRCA
*Consultant in Anaesthesia and Intensive Care, Royal United Hospital, Bath*

**Ralph S Vaughan** MB BS FRCA
*Consultant Anaesthetist, University Hospital of Wales Healthcare NHS Trust, Cardiff*

# Foreword

## Changing times: changing standards

When I started as an anaesthetist (anaesthesiologist) in 1949, it was a sign of professionalism to succeed fairly regularly with tracheal intubation. Today, any failure is unexpected and unacceptable without rigorous explanation. Yet the skills required are not simple and the knowledge-base is extensive.

Two technical advances made tracheal intubation more successful; the wider use of the Macintosh laryngoscope which made laryngoscopy easier and less traumatic, and in 1951, the introduction of suxamethonium allowing prompt and profound muscle relaxation. Thus, the intubation of a normal patient, that is, the vast majority, whether adult or infant, is now always expected to be successful even when performed by non-anaesthetists involved in resuscitation.

In the last two decades, attention has therefore become focused on special problems, such as trauma and the many disease processes, congenital and acquired, which can make intubation difficult. Various solutions to these problems have been devised dependent upon the urgency of the situation. These range from a simple introducer to fibreoptic instrumentation in the premature baby. Therein lies the challenge – to be able to know about and successfully manage, an enormous range of relatively uncommon problems, even in a specialist area such as paediatrics.

As there was no central source of information, my colleagues and I in Cardiff concluded that a book was required which concentrated on the practical problems associated with a clinician's worse nightmare: the inability to intubate in life-threatening circumstances. This proved valuable. In the short period since the first edition, there has been an explosion in knowledge and a tightening of the standards of anticipated success (not uninvolved with our legal colleagues) which has necessitated this update. The many refinements in technical expertise and the expansion of knowledge are reflected in the doubling in size of this book, with eleven new chapters and wide revisions of the ten original chapters.

In recent years a great deal of effort has gone into making it easier to forecast any difficulty, accurately and in advance. In *Predicting a Difficult Intubation*, Dr Vaughan has analysed this new information, some of which is work by him and colleagues in Cardiff, adding his valuable experience and practical advice.

The laryngeal mask airway has had a massive influence on anaesthetic practice and has also saved lives when tracheal intubation has failed. This interest is justly reflected in two chapters – *The Role of the Laryngeal Mask in Patients with Difficult Intubation* and *Difficult Ventilation* by Dr Asai and Dr Latto, and *Difficulty in Insertion of the Laryngeal Mask* by Dr Asai. These will be essential reading for all those involved in anaesthesia, intensive care and resuscitation.

The place of fibreoptic instruments is now established and competence in their use is, or will be, expected of every practitioner. Dr Greenhough and Dr Vaughan illustrate fully the practicalities and consider the training requirements.

Failure to intubate is serious, but persistent oesophageal intubation is mortal. Dr Clyburn deals with the *Detection of Accidental Oesophageal Intubation*. Dr Murrin discusses a related subject *The Legal Implications of Difficult Intubation*. There is no doubt that errors are now judged more harshly. There has been a raising of standards with improved knowledge.

A number of important specialist subjects are introduced; *Paediatric Intubation* by Dr Dunne, *Emergency Airway Access* and *The Combitube* by Dr Jenkins, *Intubation of Patients with Cervical Spine Injuries* by Dr Nolan, and *Difficulties at Tracheal Extubation* by Dr Hartley. All of these have major relevance to special groups – paediatricians, accident and emergency physicians, intensivists, specialist nurses and paramedics. Much of the advice given is difficult to find elsewhere.

Although the authors of the first edition were from Cardiff, the second edition reflects the increase in knowledge of specialists from elsewhere, whose contributions are vitally important. I am proud to have been one of those who started this enterprise to improve safety and save lives. I congratulate my colleagues on this greatly enlarged second edition which has messages to those who work in the developed world and to those in less fortunate circumstances. It reads fluently and is informative. Most important it sets that difficult standard to reach, near 100%. Like boy scouts, we need *to be prepared*. Read on.

**Professor Michael Rosen** CBE Hon LLD
*Executive Officer, World Federation of*
*Societies of Anesthesiology*

# Preface

There have been many advances in the management of tracheal intubation and the airway over the last decade. New equipment has been developed, numerous scientific papers and books have been published and societies devoted to advancing the study of airway management have been established. Thus, in this second edition of *Difficulties in Tracheal Intubation*, we have included eleven new chapters, as well as revising the originals, in an attempt to address current thinking and practice.

The introduction of minimum monitoring standards, particularly pulse oximetry and capnography, has considerably enhanced airway management and consequently, patient safety. It has also enabled anaesthesiologists to become far more aware of physiological changes during the perioperative period.

As the published papers on tracheal intubation and airway management are so numerous, no clinician can be familiar with all current advances. Yet, it is essential that clinicians should be familiar with the most important developments. This book aims to bridge the gap between the mass of published literature and current clinical practice.

For example, the introduction worldwide of the laryngeal mask airway and the increasing use of fibreoptic equipment have greatly increased the options available to the clinician. However, these innovations have tended to reduce the incidence of tracheal intubation and airway management with the traditional facemask.

Prediction of difficult intubation has been extensively, investigated but the unexpected difficult intubation still remains a source of both morbidity and mortality which can result in unfortunate medico-legal consequences. The 'cannot intubate cannot ventilate' scenario has been critically analysed and many algorithms for optimal airway management have been published. There has surprisingly been much less emphasis on the prediction of difficult ventilation.

Clinical practice differs between countries. For example, 'awake intubation' is more commonly undertaken in the United States of America (USA) than in the United Kingdom (UK). Gum elastic bougie assisted intubation is commonly performed in the UK, but the stylet is still used in the USA. Such differences need to be critically analysed.

Furthermore, chapters on intubation and airway management in trauma, neonates, obstetrics and thoracic surgery are included, as well as chapters on extubation and the medico-legal implications of clinical misadventure and mismanagement.

We believe that this edition will be of interest to all those concerned with airway management. In addition, we hope that this book will stimulate discussion and ideas for research leading to enhanced patient safety.

**Ian Peter Latto**
**Ralph S Vaughan**

# Acknowledgements

We wish to thank Mr Adrian Shaw and Mrs Janice Sharp for the art work, and the departments of Medical Illustration at the University Hospital of Wales NHS Trust and Llandough Hospital NHS Trust for the expert photography.

We are indebted to the various editors, authors and publishers for permission to reproduce figures and tables.

Our special thanks go to Mrs M Johnson for her invaluable expertise in producing the manuscript.

We also wish to thank our wives Angela and Marilyn for their considerable patience and assistance during the preparation of this book.

# Anatomy of the Airways

*Ralph S. Vaughan*

The airways, commencing at the mouth and the external nares, terminate at the entrance to the alveoli. Although there may be considerable variation, congenital or acquired, the applied anatomy in an adult will be described and differences in infants and children indicated.

## THE NOSE

The external nares tend to be oval and their shape is used as a guide in selecting an appropriately sized nasotracheal tube. Normally, the adult male accepts a tube of a diameter between 8 and 10 mm ID and the adult female between 5 and 8 mm ID [1]. The distance from the external nares to the carina in male and female averages 32 cm and 27 cm respectively [1].

The respective diameters and lengths are reduced in children and vary depending upon the size of the head and the length of the trachea. There are several working guides [2–5] which can be used to try and calculate the size of the tracheal tube required to intubate a small child.

The external nares open into the nasal cavity, which is divided into two compartments by the nasal septum. Each compartment has a roof, a floor, a medial wall and a lateral wall. Attached to the lateral walls are three overhanging projections, the conchae, covering three meati which are passages draining the paranasal sinuses and naso-lacrimal ducts into the nasal cavities.

The superior and middle conchae arise from the medial aspect of the ethmoid labyrinth while the inferior concha is a separate bone. The medial wall, the nasal septum, is formed from bone and cartilage. In addition, endothelial growths or polypi may project into the cavities between the medial and lateral walls though they may not be visible externally.

The septum is frequently deviated from the mid line so that one nasal cavity is greater in size than the other. If nasal polypi are present, they may cause obstruction and difficulty with instrumentation. It is essential therefore to test the patency of the nasal passages preoperatively in every patient before nasal intubation is contemplated. The floor of the nose slopes upward and backward. However, when the patient is supine, the main part of the floor and its distal portion present a J shape to the anaesthetist with the hook of the J pointing anteriorly (Fig. 1).

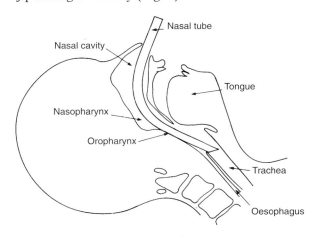

**Figure 1**   Nasal intubation (J shape).

The blood supply to the nasal mucosa is generous in order to warm and humidify the inspired air. Consequently, local anaesthetic agents can be rapidly absorbed and undue trauma can cause considerable bleeding.

The relevant nerve supply to the nose is derived mainly from the maxillary division of the trigeminal nerve with additional nerves from the ophthalmic division. The nerves supplying both medial and lateral walls of the nose are illustrated in Figs 2 and 3. Although these nerves may be blocked separately, the usual method of producing analgesia in the nasal cavities is by spraying with local analgesic solutions or packing the nose with gauze soaked with cocaine and adrenaline.

Posteriorly, the nasal cavity opens into the nasopharynx through the internal nares or the choanae. These are oval in shape and in the same plane as the external nares. In the erect position the nasopharynx is behind the nasal cavities, above the soft palate, and contains the adenoids. The adenoids are a collection of lymphatic tissue situated on the roof and posterior wall of the nasopharynx. When attempting to pass a nasotracheal tube the adenoids may:

- prevent passage
- become dislodged
- obstruct the lumen of the tube

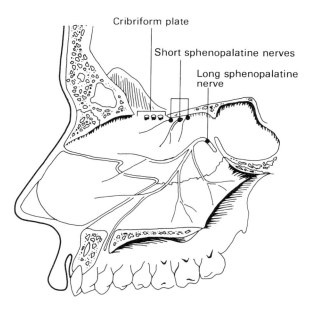

**Figure 2**   Nerve supply to the medial wall of nasal cavity. After Macintosh and Ostlere [6], with kind permission of the authors and publisher.

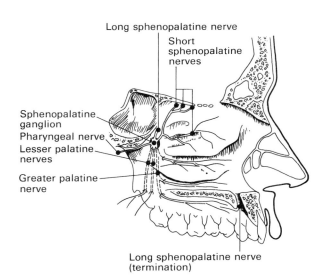

**Figure 3**   Nerve supply to lateral wall of nasal cavity. After Macintosh and Ostlere [6], with kind permission of the authors and publisher.

- be displaced into the larynx
- cause severe haemorrhage

The adenoids atrophy around puberty and their presence in children is a relative contraindication to nasal intubation.

## THE MOUTH

The mouth (Fig. 4) extends from the lips to the oropharyngeal aperture and encloses the vestibule between the teeth, gums and the inside of the cheeks.

The alveolar arches and teeth form the lateral and anterior borders respectively while the oropharyngeal isthmus provides the posterior border. The roof of the oral cavity is formed by the hard and soft palates ending posteriorly in the uvula. Inferiorly, the anterior two-thirds of the tongue and the mucosa on the undersurface forms the floor of the mouth. The tongue is a muscular organ with a large blood supply and is attached to the hyoid bone, styloid process and the back of the mandible. The innervation is derived from the trigeminal, facial, glossopharyngeal, vagus and hypoglossal nerves. However, it is usually the surface of the tongue that is rendered insensitive during awake intubation and is commonly achieved with topically acting local anaesthetic agents.

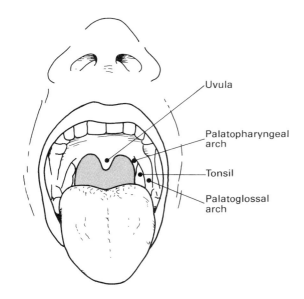

Figure 4   View of mouth open with tongue depressed. After Ellis and Feldman [7], with kind permission of the publisher, Blackwell Scientific Publications.

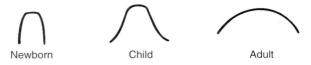

Figure 5   Changes in the shape of the epiglottis with increasing age. From Brown and Fisk [5], with kind permission of the publisher, Blackwell Scientific Publications.

The mucous membrane covering the dorsal surface of the tongue is thickened posteriorly forming three folds. In the mid line the tongue is attached to the epiglottis by the glossoepiglottic fold. Laterally the mucous membrane combines with the pharyngeal mucous membrane to form the pharyngoepiglottic folds. Between these three folds are two similar depressions called the valleculae. The valleculae are important landmarks during laryngoscopy. The tip of the soft palate, the uvula, hangs freely in the mid line and is another important landmark during intubation. Occasionally, however, should the uvula become very swollen, it can cause substantial obstruction to respiration as well as difficulty with nasal and oral intubation.

The oral cavity communicates with the oropharynx through the oropharyngeal isthmus. There are two structures of importance in this area, the tonsils and the tip of the epiglottis. The tonsils are lymphoid tissue and rarely cause difficulty with intubation unless they are considerably enlarged. The tip and the body of the epiglottis come clearly into view during laryngoscopy. These areas are supplied by branches of the trigeminal and glossopharyngeal nerves.

Hence, it is possible to identify a line of structures which can act as landmarks during intubation. The uvula above, the lateral palatopharyngeal arches and the two important inferior areas, the vallecula and the epiglottis. In addition to this imaginary line, three other points must be taken into consideration when attempting to intubate an infant:

- The infant has a relatively large head [5].
- The jaw angle is some 20° greater in the infant – 140° compared with 120° in the young adult.
- The shape of the epiglottis in the newborn is long and thin but, with increasing age, it gradually flattens and widens until it eventually reaches the adult shape (Fig. 5).

## THE PHARYNX

The pharynx extends from the base of the skull down to the sixth cervical vertebra. In shape, it is similar to an ice-cream cone whose walls are mainly derived from the constrictor muscles and fibrous tissue covered by a layer of mucous membrane.

The constrictor muscles are attached above around the base of the skull and below in a wide fan-like manner to the mandible, hyoid bone and the larynx. These muscles sweep around into a common insertion posteriorly, the medial raphe of the pharynx. They support the larynx and oesophagus and are important in the deglutition process. Their nerve supply is mainly derived from the vagus and accessory nerves. Trauma either to the constrictor muscles or to the nerve supply can lead to distortion of the position of the larynx [8].

Anatomically, the pharynx is subdivided into three main parts: the oro- and nasopharyngeal areas dealt with earlier and the laryngopharyngeal area.

### Laryngopharynx

The laryngopharynx lies at C6 level between the tip of the epiglottis and the lower border of the cricoid cartilage. The relations of the laryngopharynx are more easily understood as one tube being pushed into another (Figs 6–8). On either side, two spaces are formed known as the pyriform fossae through which run the right and left superior laryngeal nerves. As the entrance to the larynx slopes downwards and backwards, the aperture of the larynx faces the laryngopharynx while forming its anterior part. The aryepiglottic folds run from the base of the epiglottis into the arytenoid cartilages. The cricoid cartilage forms the posterior inferior border. Finally the muscular cone, which is the pharynx, terminates at the entrance to the oesophagus below and behind the laryngeal opening. It is this area that is seen at the periphery of the anaesthetist's vision when the laryngoscope has been correctly introduced.

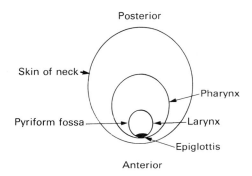

**Figure 6**   Three tube concept of the neck.

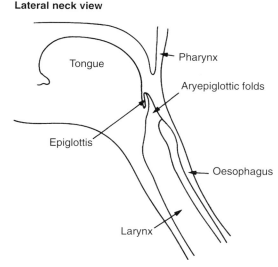

**Figure 7**   Lateral view of key areas of the neck.

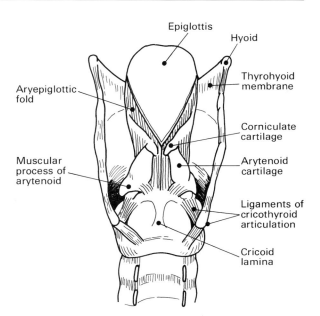

**Figure 8**   The cartilages and ligaments of the larynx seen posteriorly. After Ellis and Feldman [7], with kind permission of the publisher, Blackwell Scientific Publications.

## THE LARYNX

The primary function of the tubular larynx is to act as a sphincter to prevent foreign material entering the respiratory tract. It is secondarily adapted for phonation. In the adult, it extends from the fourth to the sixth cervical vertebrae though in the infant the upper boundary is somewhat higher (between C3 and C4). It has a greater anterior inclination in the infant, so backward pressure on the neck brings the larynx into view, facilitating intubation.

The larynx is constructed mainly from cartilages, ligaments and muscles. It commences at the superior laryngeal opening and terminates below the cricoid cartilage where it is attached to the trachea by the cricotracheal membrane.

### The Cartilages

In the larynx there are single thyroid, cricoid and epiglottic cartilages, and paired arytenoid, corniculate and cuneiform cartilages.

### *The thyroid cartilage*

The thyroid cartilage is the largest cartilage and is attached above and below by ligaments. The anatomy is illustrated in Fig. 9.

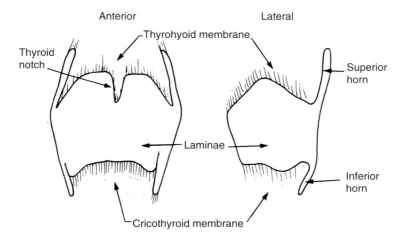

**Figure 9** Anterior and lateral view of the thyroid cartilage with membranes.

The laminae meet anteriorly in the mid line but there is a deficiency anteriorly and superiorly forming the thyroid notch. At the posterior border of each laminae are two projections, the superior and inferior horns.

### The cricoid cartilage

The cricoid cartilage (Fig. 10) is the only complete cartilage in the laryngeal structure. It has been likened to a signet ring with the wider aspect of the ring facing the oropharynx. The front and sides form the arch but posteriorly there is an expansion of the laminae to form two facets which articulate with both thyroid and arytenoid cartilages. This is the narrowest part of the larynx in a child and consequently determines the size of the tracheal tube. Naturally, oedema of the mucosal surface can reduce the airway diameter considerably. In adult life the narrowest part of the larynx is at the level of the vocal cords.

### The arytenoid cartilage

The arytenoid cartilages are pyramidal in shape and are situated on the superior and lateral aspects of the cricoid laminae. The lateral and posterior cricoarytenoid muscles are inserted into two of the three corners of the pyramidal base. The third corner provides the attachment for the vocal ligament. The arytenoid cartilage articulates with the cricoid cartilage forming a synovial joint. This joint may become involved in the general process of rheumatoid arthritis, which could cause hoarseness and some difficulty with intubation.

### The epiglottis

The epiglottis is attached inferiorly to the posterior aspect of the thyroid cartilage by the thyroepiglottic ligament. The anterior surface is free and usually visualized at laryngoscopy. The posterior surface of the epiglottis is attached to

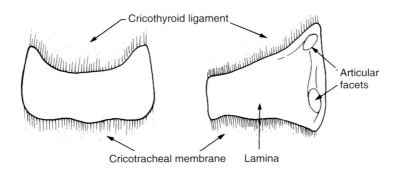

**Figure 10** Anterior and lateral views of cricoid cartilage with membranes. Note signet ring appearance.

the hyoid bone. Despite its shape and position, it is interesting to note that deglutition and phonation can occur if the epiglottis is absent.

The corniculate and cuneiform cartilages are very small and are of little importance in the structure of the larynx.

## The Laryngeal Ligaments (Fig. 11)

The thyrohyoid membrane is one of three extrinsic ligaments and runs between the hyoid bone and the upper border of the thyroid cartilage. It is particularly dense medially, forming the median thyrohyoid ligament. Posteriorly this ligament stretches from the greater horn of the hyoid to the upper horn of the thyroid cartilage. Again, these lateral attachments are very dense, forming the lateral thyrohyoid ligaments. These ligaments provide support for the larynx.

The hyoid bone itself is supported superiorly by the hypoglossus and median constrictor muscles. The superior laryngeal blood vessels and the internal branch of the superior laryngeal nerve pass through this membrane to supply the larynx above the vocal cords.

The intrinsic ligaments form the fibrous surroundings of the small synovial joints of the larynx found between the thyroid, arytenoid and cricoid cartilages. The are not as important as the extrinsic ligaments.

The internal fibrous structures are more important. Superiorly, fibrous tissue connects the base of the epiglottis to the arytenoid cartilages and this free upper surface is termed the aryepiglottic fold. Inferiorly, this fibrous tissue thickens to form the vestibular ligament. The mucous membranes run from the medial edge of the aryepiglottic fold down over these fibrous connections and terminate around the vestibular ligament to form the false cords. Below the false cords there is a thin horizontal recess called the sinus of the larynx. Another membrane, the cricovocal membrane, is attached inferiorly to the cricoid cartilage and runs upwards and forwards to be attached anteriorly to the thyroid cartilage and posteriorly to the vocal process of the arytenoid cartilage. The free

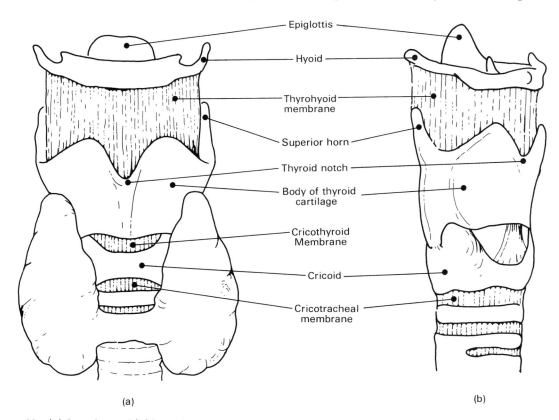

(a)                                      (b)

**Figure 11**   (a) Anterior and (b) lateral view of larynx: note cricothyroid membrane. After Ellis and Feldman [7], with kind permission of the publisher, Blackwell Scientific Publications.

surface, which is also the lower border of the sinus of the larynx, forms the vocal ligament. The vocal ligaments are covered by mucous membranes and become the vocal cords.

The cricovocal membrane is thickened in front and is termed the median cricothyroid ligament. Laterally it is called the lateral cricothyroid ligament.

The muscles of the larynx are also divided into the extrinsic and intrinsic groups. The extrinsic muscles attach the larynx to nearby structures and are responsible for elevation and depression of the larynx. The intrinsic muscles are important during the respiratory cycle, deglutition and phonation. The posterior cricoarytenoid muscle is important as it is the only abductor of the vocal cords. It is the malfunction or non-function of this muscle that can cause problems at intubation and complications following extubation.

The vagus nerve supplies the sensory and motor innervations of the larynx. There are two main branches, namely:

- The superior laryngeal nerve, which divides into two – the small external and the larger internal branches. The former supplies the cricothyroid muscle while the latter passes through the thyrohyoid membrane into the larynx to provide the sensory supply down to the vocal cords.
- The recurrent laryngeal nerves, which have different courses, the left looping around the arch of the aorta while the right loops around the right subclavian artery. Both right and left nerves run upwards in the neck in the groove between the oesophagus and the trachea. They provide sensory fibres below the vocal cords and supply all the muscles of the larynx except the cricothyroid. Damage to either of these main nerves may render the larynx incompetent with a potential for aspiration. Such damage may also present clinically as a hoarse voice.

The main relations of the larynx affecting the anaesthetist are found anteriorly and posteriorly.

The posterior aspect of the larynx faces the oropharynx and the oesophagus. Anything that slips out of the posterior aspect of the laryngeal aperture may end up in the oesophagus. Similarly, fluid or solid matter can enter the larynx from the oesophagus with serious consequences.

Anteriorly, the larynx is related to the superficial fascia and the skin of the neck. The thyroid and cricoid cartilages can be palpated relatively easily through the skin and are important landmarks if a cricothyroid puncture is contemplated. It is between these two cartilages that the anaesthetist places the puncturing needle (Fig. 11).

The larynx, however, is most commonly viewed by anaesthetists during intubation and sometimes at extubation. The anatomy seen under normal circumstances is illustrated (Fig. 12). The space between the relaxed vocal cords is triangular with the greatest distance posteriorly. The apex disappears into the posterior aspect of the epiglottis.

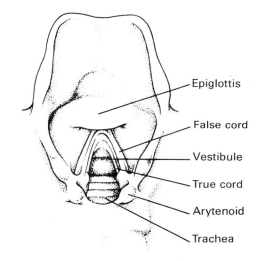

Epiglottis

False cord

Vestibule

True cord

Arytenoid

Trachea

**Figure 12** View of the larynx at laryngoscopy. From Ellis and Feldman [7], with kind permission of the publisher, Blackwell Scientific Publications.

## THE TRACHEA

The trachea commences at the larynx and terminates at the level of the fourth thoracic vertebra where it divides into the two main bronchi. It is approximately 15 cm long, one-third is above and two-thirds below the suprasternal notch. In the newborn the trachea is only 4 cm long, increasing the risks of a tracheal tube entering the right main bronchus. The tracheal architecture consists of a number of horizontal 'C' shaped cartilages which are joined posteriorly by the trachealis muscles. Vertically, these cartilages are joined to each other by fibroelastic tissue. This gives the trachea an appearance similar to that of tyres piled one on top of the other, held together by elastic tissue and both covered by endothelium.

## Relations

Although the trachea is usually a midline structure in the neck, the lower aspect is displaced to the right by the aortic arch (Fig. 13). Above the suprasternal notch, the anterior relations of the trachea are two-fold. The isthmus of the thyroid runs across the trachea at the level of the seventh cervical vertebra. Either side of the isthmus are the thyroid lobes which cover the cricoid cartilage and the anterolateral aspect of the trachea. Both the trachea and thyroid are covered anteriorly by two layers of neck fascia and skin. The oesophagus forms the posterior relationship while the recurrent laryngeal nerves are found running laterally in both tracheo-oesophageal grooves.

At the suprasternal notch the trachea enters the superior mediastinum. Anteriorly, the relations include the inferior thyroid veins, the thymus, the arch of the aorta, the brachiocephalic and left common carotid arteries. The oesophagus continues its close posterior relationship into the thorax. However, as the right recurrent laryngeal nerve loops around the right subclavian artery it is not found in the right intrathoracic tracheo-oesophageal groove.

Laterally on the right side, the trachea has a close relationship with the mediastinal pleura, the azygos vein and the vagus nerve. On the left side, the aortic arch and the major left sided arteries come between the trachea and pleura. The trachea obtains its blood supply from the inferior thyroid arteries and veins. Large lymph nodes are found either side of the tracheobronchial tree and below the carina. These nodes drain along the paratracheal nodes to the deep cervical nodes. The innervation of the trachea is from the recurrent laryngeal branches of the vagus nerve which also carry sympathetic twigs from the middle cervical ganglion. The trachea divides into the right and left main bronchi but the level of this division varies with the respiratory cycle. During full inspiration, the level may be at the sixth thoracic vertebra. In full expiration it will be at the fourth thoracic vertebra. Where the trachea divides into the bronchi, the lowest tracheal cartilage runs beneath thus forcing up that area, called the carina, which, when viewed from above, is similar to the keel of a boat. In addition, the mucous membrane covering the carina gives the sharp appearance normally seen at bronchoscopy (Fig. 14).

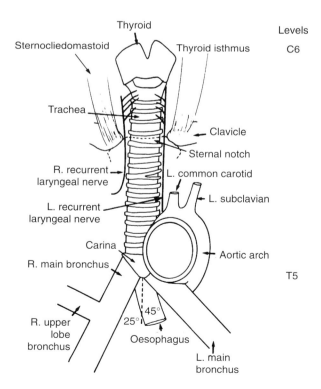

**Figure 13**   Trachea and related structures between levels C6 and T5.

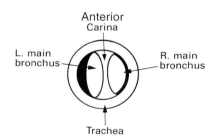

**Figure 14**   The carina.

## Bronchi

The left main bronchus is longer and thinner than the right main bronchus with an overall length of approximately 5 cm (Fig. 15). The right bronchus is wider, shorter and conducts more gases as the right lung has a greater volume. At approximately 2.5 cm from the carina, the right main bronchus divides into the right upper and the communal bronchus of the middle and lower lobes. However, in a small percentage of people, the right upper lobe bronchus originates directly from the lower trachea. Such an abnormal origin could have a considerable bearing on anaesthesia utilizing right sided endobronchial tubes for left side pulmonary surgery.

## Bronchopulmonary segments

There are usually ten bronchopulmonary segments on the right and eight or nine on the left as illustrated below. An excellent way of remembering the names of these segments is based on the APALM [9] mnemonic. The word 'APALM' is written in a vertical direction; it is then rewritten below with the 'P' and the 'M' reversed,

**Right lung**

A-Apical segment
P-Posterior segment  } Right upper lobe
A-Anteior segment
L-Lateral segment  } Right middle lobe
M-Medial segment

A-Apical segment
M-Medial basal segment
A-Anterior basal segment  } Right lower lobe
L-Lateral basal segment
P-Posterior basal segment

**Left lung**

A-Apical segment
P-Posterior segment  } Left upper lobe
A-Anterior segment
S-Superior segment  } Lingula
I-Inferior segment

A-Apical segment
M-No segment
A-Anterior basal segment  } Left lower lobe
L-Lateral basal segment
P-Posterior basal segment

Occasionally, the left apical and posterior segments combine to form a single segment called the apicoposterior segment. The left upper lobe is then divided into an apicoposterior and anterior lobe hence making eight bronchopulmonary segments. In addition, the L/M of the word APALM become the superior and inferior lobes of the lingula.

The bronchi contain five structural layers, which, working from the outside in are:

- The outer coat consisting mainly of fibrous tissue containing plates of supporting cartilage.
- The bronchial muscle which is unstriped and innervated by the autonomic nervous system.
- The elastic tissue layer which runs along the length of the bronchi and has two important functions. Firstly, it acts as the sub-mucous layer and secondly, contributes significantly to the recoil of the air-conducting passages during the respiratory cycle.
- The basement membrane which acts as a support for the mucosal layer.
- The mucosal layer which has been divided into several layers. Essentially, however, the epithelial lining consists of columnar ciliated cells containing secreting goblet cells.

The bronchi are able to change both length and diameter and assist in the removal of small

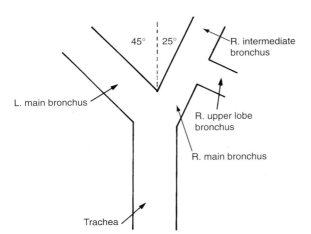

**Figure 15**   Bronchial angles in adults.

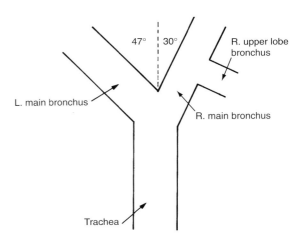

**Figure 16**   Bronchial angles in children.

particles from the bronchial tree. This is achieved by the ciliated columnar cells wafting foreign material trapped in the mucosa towards the trachea forming phlegm which is expelled during coughing.

Anaesthetists in general, and thoracic anaesthetists in particular, should be familiar with the anatomy seen at bronchoscopy as variations can cause difficulty with endobronchial intubation.

Compared with an adult, the level of the carina is higher in infants and also the angles at which the main bronchi divide are different. These differences are illustrated in Figs 15 and 16.

The distal views of bronchial subdivisions are more important to the thoracic surgeon than the anaesthetist: these are illustrated in Figs 17–21.

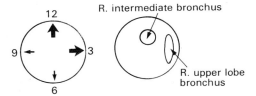

**Figure 17**  Bronchoscopic view at right main bronchus.

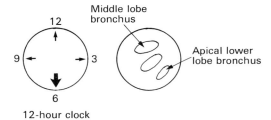

**Figure 18**  Bronchoscopic view after passing right upper lobe orifice.

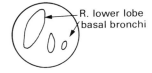

**Figure 19**  Bronchoscopic view at right lower lobe basal bronchi.

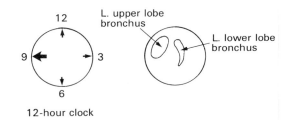

**Figure 20**  Bronchoscopic view at left main bronchus.

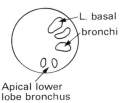

**Figure 21**  Bronchoscopic view at left lower lobe bronchi.

The positions of the major bronchial subdivisions on the clock face are included in the illustrations as a 'learn and remember' guide.

Anaesthetists, especially those who practise thoracic anaesthesia, should be familiar with these subdivisions as they are important in diagnosis, anaesthetic techniques, surgery and ultimately prognosis.

## KEY POINTS

It is essential for the anaesthetist to be aware of the following:

- The anatomy of the airway

- Changes in shape of the epiglottis with age

- Anatomical basis for nerve blocks for awake intubation

- Position of bronchial orifices on a 12-hour clock

- Bronchial anatomy with reference to endobronchial intubation

- Normograms for size and length of tracheal tubes

# REFERENCES

1 Atkinson R. S., Rushman G. B. and Lee J. A. *A Symposium of Anaesthesia*. Bristol: John Wright. 1982; Ch. 13.

2 Morgan G. A. R. and Steward D. J. A pre-formed paediatric orotracheal tube designed based on anatomical measurements. *Canadian Anaesthetists Society Journal* 1982; **29:** 9.

3 Gregory G. A. (ed.) *Pediatric Anesthesia*. Edinburgh: Churchill Livingstone. 1983; Vol. 1, p.10.

4 Jackson Rees G. and Gray T. C. (eds) *Paediatric Anesthesia*. Butterworths. 1981; p. 6.

5 Brown T. C. K. and Fisk G. C. *Anaesthesia for Children*. Oxford: Blackwell Scientific Publications, '1979; Ch.1.

6 Macintosh R. R. and Ostlere M. *Local Anagesia. Head and Neck*. Edinburgh: E. S. Livingstone, 1955.

7 Ellis H. and Feldman S. *Anatomy for Anaesthetists*. Oxford: Blackwell Scientific Publications, 1983.

8 Vaughan R. S. Anaesthesia for open soft tissue injuries of the neck. *Anaesthesia* 1971; **26:** 225.

9 Last R. J. *Anatomy. Regional and Applied*. Section 4. The Thorax. Edinburgh: Churchill Livingstone. 1984.

# APPENDIX

**Table A.1** Endotracheal tube sizes.

| Age (yr) | Tube size* Magill | Int. diam. (mm) | Length (cm) Oral† | Nasal‡ |
|---|---|---|---|---|
| 0–3 months | 00 | 3.0 | 10 | – |
| | 0A | 3.5 | 10–11 | – |
| 3–6 months | 0 | 4.0 | 12 | 15 |
| 6–12 months | 1 | 4.5 | 12 | 15 |
| 2 | 2 | 5.0 | 13 | 16 |
| 3 | 2 | 5.0 | 13 | 16 |
| 4 | 3 | 5.5 | 14 | 17 |
| 5 | 3 | 5.5 | 14 | 17 |
| 6 | 4 | 6.0 | 15 | 18 |
| 7 | 4 | 6.0 | 15 | 18 |
| 8 | 5 | 6.5 | 16 | 19 |
| 9 | 5 | 6.5 | 16 | 19 |
| 10 | 6 | 7.0 | 17 | 20 |
| 11 | 6 | 7.0 | 17 | 20 |
| 12 | 7 | 7.5 | 18 | 21 |
| 13 | 7 | 7.5 | 18 | 21 |
| 14 | 8 | 8.0 | 21 | 24 |
| 15 | 8 | 8.0 | 21 | 24 |
| 16 | 8 | 8.0 | 21 | 24 |
| 17 | 9 | 9.0 | 22 | 25 |
| 18 | 9 | 9.0 | 22 | 25 |
| 20 | 10 | 9.5 | 23 | 26 |
| 22 | 10+ | 10.0+ | 23 | 26 |

$$\text{*Tube size} = \frac{\text{Age (yr)}}{4} + 4.5 \text{ mm}$$

$$\dagger \text{ Oral length} = 12 + \frac{\text{Age (yr)}}{2} \text{ cm}$$

$$\ddagger \text{ Nasal length} = 15 + \frac{\text{Age (yr)}}{2} \text{ cm}$$

(Reproduced with permission from Dunnill RPH and Colvin MP *Clinical and Resuscitative Data*. Oxford: Blackwell Scientific Publications, 1984.)

**Table A.2**

| Tube size (mm) | Age range (yr) | Weight range (kg) | Height range (cm) |
|---|---|---|---|
| 8.0 | 13–15 | 43–62 | 154–164 |
| 7.5 | 10–14 | 31–50 | 144–154 |
| 7.0 | 8–11 | 25–40 | 132–140 |
| 6.5 | 6–9 | 20–30 | 121–133 |
| 6.0 | 4–7 | 18–25 | 144–122 |
| 5.5 | 3–6 | 15–22 | 104–114 |
| 5.0 | 2–4 | 11–17 | 87–104 |
| 4.5 | 0.75–2 | 8–13 | 74–88 |
| 4.0 | 0.5–1.5 | 6–11 | 61–75 |

(Reproduced with permission from Keep PH and Manford MLM. Endotracheal tube sizes for children. *Anaesthesia*. 1974; 29:184. The authors concluded that, of the three variables in children, that is age, weight and height, the most accurate correlation was with height.)

# 2

# Pathophysiological Effects of Tracheal Intubation

*W. Shang Ng*

## INTRODUCTION

Pathophysiological consequences of tracheal intubation are no less important than traumatic and mechanical complications. Many of the body's systems can be affected although the subtle nature of some of the changes means they can remain undetected when only routine monitoring methods are used. Whilst some of these pathological changes may be of little clinical significance to the healthy patient, serious harm can follow when undesirable changes aggravate underlying disease. The possible pathophysiological effects of tracheal intubation are listed in Table 1.

## CARDIOVASCULAR SYSTEM

### Effects of Intubation

Of all the pathophysiological effects of tracheal intubation, the cardiovascular consequences of intubation and their management have attracted the most attention in the literature. When tracheal

**Table 1** Main pathophysiological effects of tracheal intubation.

Cardiovascular system
  Dysrhythmias
  Systemic arterial hypertension

Respiratory system
  Hypoxia
  Hypercarbia
  Increased resistance to respiration
  Laryngeal spasm
  Expiratory spasm of respiratory muscles
  Bronchospasm
  Impaired humidification of inspired gases

Central nervous system
  Increased intracranial tension

Eye
  Increased intraocular tension

Miscellaneous
  Toxic and side effects of topical anaesthetic agents
  Postoperative muscle pains
  Malignant hyperpyrexia
  Increased plasma endorphins

intubation is performed under light general anaesthesia cardiovascular changes occur in response to both laryngoscopy and insertion of the tube. The changes can occur with an easy atraumatic intubation in the absence of coughing, straining, hypoxaemia or hypercarbia.

Observations of acute cardiac dysrhythmias [1] were followed by numerous other reports of cardiac disturbances accompanying tracheal intubation. The reported incidence of dysrhythmias has varied between 0 and 90%; the differences can be attributed to variations in patients, anaesthetic agents, the varying definitions of dysrhythmia and the technique of recording dysrhythmias [2].

These observations of ECG changes were followed by a spate of reports in which investigators noted the marked increase of heart rate and arterial blood pressure associated with intubation [3–15] (Fig. 1).

Early workers soon recognized that reflex cardiovascular disturbances occurred more readily when light anaesthesia was used; deep anaesthesia minimized or eliminated the changes [3,5]. With the introduction of direct and continuous arterial blood pressure measurement in clinical practice confirmation was obtained that changes occurred as soon as laryngeal stimulation commenced and prior to actual intubation [5]. These changes occurred in lightly anaesthetized healthy patients. Both systolic and diastolic pressures rose within 5 s of laryngoscopy, reaching a peak in 1–2 min and returning to prelaryngoscopy levels within 5 min. The average elevation of systolic and diastolic pressures were more than 53 and 34 mmHg respectively. Heart rate increased on average by 23 beats per minute (bpm). Laryngoscopy alone produced a variable response in rate, elevations occurring in only half the cases. No electrocardiographic changes occurred with laryngoscopy alone but extrasystoles and premature ventricular contractions were noted in a small number of patients during intubation. These observations are typical of those described by many other workers.

## Clinical Significance

Transient hypertension and tachycardia are probably of little or no consequence in healthy subjects. Older people (51–80 years) show an exaggerated sympathetic response to intubation, reflected by higher plasma noradrenaline levels and increases of blood pressure which are similar

throughout this age group. On the other hand, the more aged appear more resistant to increases in heart rate [17].

## Patients with hypertension

Hypertensive patients often show an exaggerated increase of blood pressure in response to stress including that induced by laryngoscopy and intubation. Previous drug treatment modifies the

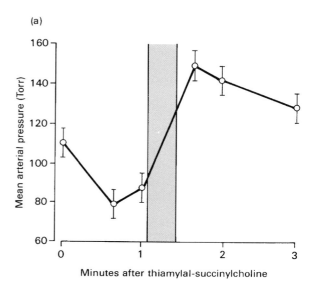

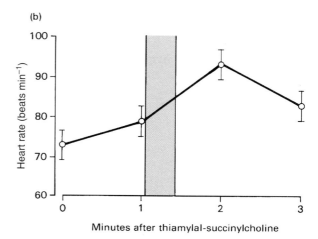

**Figure 1** Changes in arterial blood pressure (a) and heart rate (b) with laryngoscopy and tracheal intubation. Shaded area represents duration of laryngoscopy and tracheal intubation. After Stoelting [16], with kind permission of the International Anesthesia Research Society.

response towards the normal but changes occur even when the individual is taking antihypertensive drugs and is apparently well controlled [13–15]. Increases of mean arterial pressure exceeding 100 mmHg have been described in such patients [13].

A recent study suggests that in patients with only mild to moderate hypertension (diastolic pressure no more than 110 mmHg), the choice of medication to control the pressure preoperatively has no bearing on the magnitude of pressor responses to laryngoscopy and intubation. Surprisingly, no difference could be demonstrated from the changes occurring in untreated subjects [18]. However, this finding has not been confirmed by other workers.

In spite of the very large number of hypertensive patients who undergo surgery, reports of severe circulatory complications following tracheal intubation are rare. It may well be that the changes are so short lived, remaining undetected in most cases, that subsequent cardiovascular sequelae are attributed to other causes. There are many investigators who report ECG evidence of ischaemic changes at intubation occurring in hypertensive patients [19]. However, only two cases of severe complications have been reported in relation to a hypertensive episode following laryngoscopy and intubation. In one case, pulmonary oedema was precipitated and in another (pre-eclamptic) patient a cerebral aneurysm ruptured. Both patients were markedly hypertensive before the start of anaesthesia [20].

### Pregnancy-induced hypertension

This group of patients appear to be at special risk. The marked pressor response to intubation in the hypertensive pregnant patient is well recognized. There is a relationship between cerebral haemorrhage in severe pre-eclamptics and mortality. Severe hypertensive response to tracheal intubation can lead to sudden left ventricular failure and pulmonary oedema [21, 22]. There is also an associated risk of increased intracranial pressure and cerebral haemorrhage. Morbidity and mortality in both mother and child could suffer [24]. While specific reports of complications are few, taking effective measures to prevent significant hypertensive crises in such patients is mandatory.

### Patients with ischaemic heart disease

The balance between oxygen demand and supply is critical in patients with coronary artery disease. Increased blood pressure and heart rate elevate myocardial oxygen demand so circulatory changes at intubation can lead to myocardial ischaemia and infarction [25, 26] as well as depressed left ventricular function [27]. In a large and detailed study of patients who had had a previous myocardial infarction, the incidence of reinfarction after operation was significantly higher in those patients who developed intraoperative hypertension and tachycardia (as well as hypotension). The investigation showed that prompt treatment of haemodynamic aberrations could result in a reduced morbidity and mortality [28].

Several indices of myocardial ischaemia have been suggested (heart rate, rate pressure product, pressure rate ratio), but none appear to be satisfactory. Recommendations of maximum permitted rate pressure product range from 12 000 [29] to 23 000 [30]. The patient's preoperative levels should serve as a useful baseline. In patients with severe coronary artery disease, a tachycardia of more than 110 bpm has been singled out as the main factor in causing myocardial ischaemia during operations [31]. While no absolute confidence can be placed on the value of any of the recommended indices, keeping within the limits proposed and preventing the heart rate from significantly exceeding 100 bpm would seem a wise precaution. Sudden death has followed intubation [11].

### Pathophysiology

Sensory impulses from the root of the tongue, epiglottis and trachea are carried in the vagus nerve. The effector system has been in doubt. An early view was that cardiovascular changes following intubation were produced by a sudden increase of vagal tone [1]. This has not been supported by other workers who found that atropine (3 mg), which is sufficient to block vagal action, did not prevent the pressor response [7]. Later workers have suggested the effector limb to be reflex stimulation of the cardiac accelerator nerves [3, 4]. However, the pressor response is not accompanied by the usual reflex cardiac slowing so this mechanism is unlikely. Another suggested mechanism was that the cardiovascular changes resulted from an overall increase of sympathetic preponderance as a consequence of an increased sympathetic and sympathoadrenal activity [5].

The current view, based on measurements of plasma catecholamine levels, is that stimulation of laryngeal and tracheal tissues at laryngoscopy and intubation cause a reflex increase of both sympathetic and sympathoadrenal activity [32] (Fig. 2).

Significant increase of plasma noradrenaline level was found to parallel elevation of blood pressure at intubation [33]. In addition to confirming this finding, studies by another investigator demonstrated a large increase of plasma adrenaline at intubation, especially when suxamethonium was included in the induction sequence; smaller blood pressure changes followed intubation when pancuronium was used and a smaller increase in adrenaline level occurred [32]. This author suggests that similar levels of increased plasma

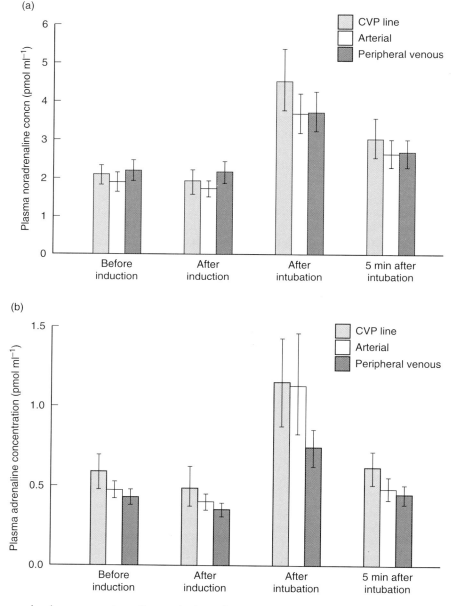

**Figure 2**   Changes in plasma noradrenaline and adrenaline concentrations related to tracheal intubation. Samples taken from three different sites (mean ± SEM; $n$ = 24) Patients are anaesthetized with thiopentone followed by suxamethonium or pancuronium prior to intubation. After Derbyshire [32].

**Table 2**  Methods of preventing or attenuating cardiovascular effects of intubation.

| Technique | Comments |
|---|---|
| **'Deep' Anaesthesia** | |
| Inhalation anaesthesia | Helpful adjunct |
| Propofol | Possible cardiorespiratory depression |
| Opioids | |
| Fentanyl | Effective in high doses |
| Alfentanil | Risk of prolonged respiratory depression |
| | |
| **Topical anaesthesia** | |
| Direct spraying of larynx and trachea | No method reliable |
| Transtracheal spraying | Some techniques involving laryngoscopy provoke |
| Mouthwash and gargle with viscous lignocaine | cardiovascular disturbances |
| Inhalation of nebulized lignocaine | Possible lignocaine toxicity |
| | |
| **Drug prevention of sympathoadrenal responses** | |
| Atropine | Inappropriate |
| Intravenous lignocaine | Not reliable |
| | Possible lignocaine toxicity |
| Peripheral vasodilators | |
| Nitrates by intravenous bolus, by sublingual | Most are effective in preventing pressor effect |
| and buccal spray | but limited or no effect on tachycardia |
| Nitroprusside | |
| Calcium channel blockers | |
| ACE inhibitors | Nicardipine appears to be effective against both |
| Prostaglandins | |
| Ganglion blockers | No effect on tachycardia |
| α-Adrenergic blockers | No effect on tachycardia |
| β-Adrenergic blockers | Only very limited effect on hypertensive response |
| | Esmolol appears to be effective against hypertension |
| | as well |
| Combined α- and β-blockers | Labetalol shown to be effective |
| Magnesium sulphate | Useful in control of hypertension in pregnant hypertensives |
| Precurarization when suxamethonium used | Limited value against hypertensive response |
| **Minimizing mechanical stimulation of the larynx** | |
| Awake intubation | Advantage not proven; said to be less cardiovascular |
| Blind nasal intubation | stimulation |
| Fibreoptic nasotracheal intubation | Cardiovascular effects depend on type of anaesthesia and |
| Fibreoptic oral intubation | route of insertion. Nasal route with patient awake seems |
| | best |
| Laryngeal mask airway (LMA) | Reduced cardiovascular disturbance |
| | Useful when a tracheal tube can be avoided |

adrenaline would occur when intubation was carried out under any light general anaesthetic.

These findings are supported by studies in which intubation was carried out under deep halothane anaesthesia. The pressor response did not materialize and plasma catecholamine levels remained unchanged [34, 35].

Other workers have failed to demonstrate changes in plasma catecholamine levels at intubation following conventional intravenous induction techniques even when a marked pressor response took place [36].

These findings are helpful when selecting drugs to prevent cardiovascular complications of intubation. β-blocking agents alone may inhibit tachycardia and dysrhythmias but an α-blocking drug is needed as well to counter the hypertensive response.

## Prevention of Cardiovascular Effects of Intubation

Numerous methods have been advocated to prevent undesirable cardiovascular disturbances at intubation (Table 2). The efficacy of depth of anaesthesia was recognized early on and deep inhalation anaesthesia has been replaced by intravenous agents, notably fentanyl. Prevention of noxious stimuli by topical anaesthesia applied to the larynx and trachea in a variety of ways remains a popular method used alone or in conjunction with other techniques. Blind nasal and fibreoptic techniques have been used in an attempt to reduce the mechanical stimulation of conventional laryngoscopy. Lastly, a large group of techniques involves intravenous administration of antivagal and antisympathetic drugs to suppress the autonomic effects of intubation.

The large number of techniques suggested to suppress cardiovascular responses reflects the fact that no single method has gained widespread acceptance. Either the reflex is not completely blocked, or the effects are too long lasting or there are undesirable side effects.

Many of the techniques advocated have been investigated in patients with no cardiovascular disease. Caution is therefore advised when applying any method in patients with serious cardiovascular problems. Many are taking cardioactive drugs. Due consideration should be given to these when judging the likely effects of a given technique.

## Deep anaesthesia

### Inhalation anaesthesia

Deep anaesthesia minimizes cardiovascular changes at laryngoscopy and intubation [3, 5, 13]. However, this approach may be inappropriate to patients with severe cardiovascular disease. Other investigators have found that moderately deep anaesthesia such as inhalation of halothane 1% for 5–10 min is not wholly effective in preventing the pressor response [14].

### Propofol

Induction doses of thiopentone do not suppress laryngeal reflexes. Propofol alone, though, appears to do so [40, 41]. No hypertensive response to intubation was found in healthy patients when either propofol alone or propofol with intravenous lignocaine was used in the induction regimen. In another study, both hypertensive and heart rate increases were equally abolished when anaesthesia was induced with a continuous propofol infusion supplemented with a boluses of fentanyl (0.1 or 0.2 mg). This result was independent of whether rigid or fibreoptic laryngoscopy was employed [42].

### Fentanyl (conventional dose)

Moderate doses of fentanyl to supplement thiopen-

tone induction can minimize the cardiovascular effects of intubation in healthy adults [43, 44]. In one study involving patients with no cardiovascular disease [44] a dose of 6 µg kg$^{-1}$ was sufficient to abolish both pressor and heart rate changes. Indeed, the blood pressure fell gradually to 18% below base levels. A smaller dose of 2 µg kg$^{-1}$ prevented any significant change of heart rate and the systolic pressure never rose by more than 20 mmHg.

The fall of pressure with the 6 µg kg$^{-1}$ dose was of no clinical concern in these healthy patients but it is possible that much greater falls could occur in the more labile hypertensive subject.

Several mechanisms could be at play to account for the way in which fentanyl attenuates the pressor response to intubation. The analgesic effect could block the nociceptive stimuli of intubation, centrally mediated depression of sympathetic tone [45], and activation of vagal tone. The stable heart rate with fentanyl, even in the lower dose, would seem to put the technique at an advantage over other regimens in which control of the heart rate is more difficult than control of the pressure. The mode of action again possibly includes fentanyl's analgesic effect but also results from parasympathetic activity in the presence of sympathoadrenal stimulation by laryngoscopy and intubation [46]; lastly, fentanyl is known to cause bradycardia [47–49].

The main disadvantage of using fentanyl in this way, especially if the 6 µg kg$^{-1}$ dose is used, is the increased risk of postoperative respiratory depression especially after short procedures. If this danger is appreciated the technique would seem to be a useful one in patients with significant cardiovascular disease. Similar results were found in another investigation [44] in which nitrous oxide and fentanyl (4 µg kg$^{-1}$) were used prior to intubation in patients with minimal cardiovascular disease. With this drug regimen heart rate, arterial systolic and mean pressure and cardiac output were all significantly reduced, peripheral vascular resistance remaining unchanged. However, tracheal intubation aided by suxamethonium did not result in any further alteration of these cardiovascular parameters.

### Fentanyl (high dose)

Low dose fentanyl following conventional thiopentone induction or when used in conjunction with nitrous oxide, satisfactorily attenuates circulatory responses to tracheal intubation in normal subjects as well as those with minimal circulatory disease. It is uncertain whether these regimens would be equally effective in patients with serious cardiovascular disease. A higher dose of fentanyl was used in a series of cases undergoing mitral valve replacement [50]. Prior to administration of suxamethonium and intubation, fentanyl (8–15 μg kg$^{-1}$) was given in sufficient dosage to produce loss of responsiveness to verbal commands and pinprick stimulation. The average dose administered was 660 μg, equivalent to a dose of 11 μg kg$^{-1}$. Apart from diazepam, no other drugs were used. Respiration was invariably depressed and necessitated manual assistance. Injection of suxamethonium, laryngoscopy and intubation produced no significant alteration of cardiovascular variables. Similar results were found in an investigation in the definite 'at risk' group of patients – those undergoing coronary artery surgery [51]. The average dose of fentanyl needed to induce loss of consciousness was 18 μg kg$^{-1}$. A further infusion of fentanyl to make a total of 50 μg kg$^{-1}$ was administered before suxamethonium was given and intubation accomplished. No significant changes occurred either in arterial blood pressure or heart rate. This finding contrasts sharply with the lack of protection from cardiovascular changes at intubation conferred by morphine. Morphine was commonly used as the main anaesthetic agent in patients undergoing cardiac surgery in doses ranging between 1 and 3 mg kg$^{-1}$, supposedly equipotent with the fentanyl dosages described above. However, with the morphine regimen, heart rate and blood pressure are consistently elevated even when used in conjunction with other anaesthetic agents [52–54]. Equipotency with fentanyl may apply to analgesia but it has been suggested that fentanyl is more than 100 times as potent as morphine in the suppression of laryngotracheal reflexes [37].

The main disadvantage of these higher dose regimens of fentanyl is the significant increase of postoperative respiratory depression. Prolonged respiratory depression ranged from 2 to 8 h [51] to 8 to 12 h [52]. Furthermore, as fentanyl is administered in such large doses spontaneous respiration rapidly diminishes so that assisted respiration with a facemask becomes necessary. Difficulty may result if the rigid chest wall syndrome develops and gastric distension may also be produced. The method does not appear to be suitable for those patients with a full stomach.

## Alfentanil

Alfentanil has been shown to reduce the cardiovascular changes of intubation with the advantage over fentanyl of a shorter duration of action so that undue postoperative respiratory depression is avoided [54].

A dose of 15 μg kg$^{-1}$ (equivalent to 4–5 μg kg$^{-1}$ of fentanyl) prevents the pressor response but a higher dose of 30 μg kg$^{-1}$ is needed to prevent increases of heart rate as well. No cardiac dysrhythmias were observed in patients treated with alfentanil.

In healthy patients, when suxamethonium facilitated intubation is carried out, much larger doses of alfentanil were required to block cardiovascular responses. These doses of the order of 75 μg kg$^{-1}$ result in substantial total doses [55]. These doses may lead to a significant incidence of postoperative respiratory depression and chest wall rigidity. Such dose levels can also cause profound hypotension and bradycardia in patients receiving concurrent β-adrenergic blockers.

## Topical anaesthesia

### Direct spray with topical anaesthesia

Spraying of the larynx and trachea with lignocaine 4% was commonly practised to prevent coughing and cardiovascular responses to intubation although reports on the efficacy of the technique vary. Most workers have found the technique to have no effect on the magnitude of blood pressure and heart rate increases although these changes were more transient when a spray had been used [56]. The undesirable effects of the laryngoscopy thus appear to largely cancel out the value of topical anaesthesia [9,57,58].

Plasma levels of lignocaine due to absorption from the mucous membrane probably never reach therapeutic concentrations sufficient to suppress ventricular dysrhythmias [59].

Care should be exercised when spraying the larynx in children. Severe bradycardia occurs in many healthy children in the 6–7 year age group. Routine preoperative intramuscular atropine or glycopyrrolate does not prevent the changes although intravenous administration of either drug is effective in controlling the bradycardia. In a comparable adult group, bradycardia was not observed [60].

### Transtracheal spraying

Transtracheal injection of lignocaine (2 ml of 4%) has been used to prevent circulatory responses to intubation [61]. Injection was performed 3 min after induction of anaesthesia with thiopentone and halothane. Suxamethonium preceded intubation. The treated patients were largely protected from the pressor response to intubation whereas 72% of a control group had a rise of mean arterial pressure averaging 65 mmHg lasting for 1–5 min. No significant heart rate or rhythm changes occurred in treated and untreated patients.

However, in the treated cases a transient hypertension (mean rise of 78 mmHg lasting for 10–60 s) always followed the tracheal injection itself. In one patient suffering from hypertension blood pressure rose with tracheal injection from 185 to 280 mmHg systolic.

Whilst there is some benefit in reducing the pressor response to intubation because of the hypertension produced by transtracheal injection there would seem to be little indication to administer topical anaesthesia in this way.

### Mouthwash and gargle with viscous lignocaine

In order to avoid the stimulation of laryngoscopy, topical anaesthesia has been attempted by mouthwash and gargling with viscous lignocaine. This method has been used in normal [58] and coronary artery surgery patients [57]. Two 12.5 ml doses of 2% viscous lignocaine were given 10 min prior to induction of anaesthesia: the patient was in the sitting position. Any residual lignocaine was swallowed. In both studies the pressor response was attenuated but no effect on the heart rate was noted. Another study has shown that the haemodynamic disturbance produced by the stimulating effect of gargling with viscous lignocaine exceeds that produced by spraying [58].

### Inhalation of nebulized lignocaine

This method is another attempt to arrest the cardiovascular responses to instrumentation in the laryngeal area [62]. In the sitting position the patient inhales between 6 and 8 ml of a mixture of one-third 2% viscous lignocaine and two-thirds 4% aqueous lignocaine. The viscous lignocaine is added to increase the droplet size in order to enhance drop out in the upper airways. The solution is nebulized with a Bird™ nebulizer modified to ensure coarser droplet size to improve drop out in the upper airways. Compared with a control group, nebulized lignocaine treatment significantly reduced but did not abolish all the changes due to laryngoscopy. Blood pressure rose on average by 10% compared with a 56% rise in the

control group and heart rate increased by 16% compared with a 38% rise in the control group. No dysrhythmias occurred in those inhaling the aerosol compared with an incidence of 40% in controls. However, the changes following intubation were not as well suppressed, probably because the mist did not effectively anaesthetize the trachea.

The elimination of dysrhythmias can be accounted for partly by systemic absorption of the lignocaine which was found to reach over 2 µg ml$^{-1}$ in some patients in this study; 2–5 µg ml$^{-1}$ is sufficient to treat premature ventricular contractions [63]. Systemic absorption of lignocaine could also contribute to dampening of the reflex response to laryngoscopy since intravenous lignocaine is known to obtund the cough reflex [64].

Although the method appears effective, the technique requires a co-operative patient. The technique is unsuitable in patients with a full stomach and those who are hypersensitive to local anaesthetics.

A commercially available metered dose of lignocaine spray has been used to give patients inhalations of local anaesthetic [58]. With the patient supine the tongue and pharynx were sprayed with 10 doses of lignocaine 10% (Xylocain 10 mg dose, Astra, Sweden). Subsequently, 10 doses were sprayed into the mouth whilst the patient was taking deep breaths. Some patients complained of the bitter taste but generally accepted the technique.

Moderate attenuation of the pressor response to laryngoscopy and intubation was obtained but the aerosol was ineffective in suppressing tachycardia.

## Drug prevention of sympathoadrenal responses

### Atropine

Following the suggestion that circulatory responses to intubation could be mediated by 'vasovagal' pathways, the use of large doses of atropine sufficient to block vagal transmission was studied [7].

Atropine (3 mg) was given intravenously prior to intubation in healthy subjects. The customary increase in blood pressure was prevented. There was no further increase in heart rate but this was already significantly elevated following the injection of atropine. Some of the patients developed transient cardiac dysrhythmias. In another study, conventional doses of atropine appeared to be potentially harmful [65]. Atropine (0.6 mg) was given either intramuscularly 30 min preoperatively or intravenously 5 min before induction to patients free of cardiovascular disease. Compared with patients who received only normal saline, atropine was associated with significantly greater increases of heart rate and incidence of dysrhythmias at intubation. The greatest increase in heart rate and the incidence and severity of the abnormal rhythms were seen in patients given intravenous atropine. Neither atropine regimens had any influence on the typical hypertension produced by intubation. There seems no basis, therefore, for using atropine to prevent cardiovascular responses to intubation. Indeed the enhanced pulse rate could increase the danger of intubation in patients at risk. When an antisialogogue is essential in such patients, glycopyrrolate is preferable to atropine [66].

### Intravenous lignocaine

Intravenous lignocaine has been found by several workers to be effective in reducing cardiovascular responses to intubation [67–69]. The usual dose of 1.5 mg kg$^{-1}$ given prior to induction and laryngoscopy results in only minimal increases in blood pressure and heart rate and an absence of dysrhythmias. Lower doses of intravenous lignocaine, in the order of 0.7 mg kg$^{-1}$, are ineffective and some studies suggest that intravenous lignocaine is less reliable than inhalation of nebulized lignocaine [62].

There is some controversy as to whether the beneficial effect of topically applied lignocaine is due to systemic absorption with its subsequent depressant effect on the circulatory system. In most cases plasma concentrations are unlikely to reach therapeutic levels. Even the intravenous lignocaine technique, which results in levels approaching the therapeutic level needed to suppress dysrhythmias, is not sufficient to produce suppression of the typical blood pressure and heart rate increases seen at intubation [70]. It is likely that some of the beneficial effects of intravenous lignocaine are due to a direct action of the drug on the mucous membrane of the airways.

Intravenous lignocaine (1 mg kg$^{-1}$) administered 2 min before tracheal extubation prevents coughing, blood pressure and heart rate changes during and after removal of the tube. This technique has been recommended in patients with ischaemic heart disease [71]. However, other workers have noted the need to use larger doses (2 mg kg$^{-1}$) to produce suppression of coughing at extubation.

Although intravenous lignocaine appears to be fairly reliable in its suppression of cardiovascular responses to intubation, caution should be exercised when substantial doses are administered to patients with a serious cardiovascular disease for fear of producing excessive depression.

### Peripheral vasodilators

Many vasodilators can attenuate the pressor response but, as a class, the vasodilators are not very effective in controlling tachycardia. In practice, they can be difficult to titrate accurately and inadvertent hypotension may follow. With the lack of comparative studies with other agents, it is not possible to indicate a clear place for these drugs in controlling cardiovascular responses to intubation.

***Nitrates*** Nitroglycerine has been used in severe pregnancy-induced hypertension (arterial blood pressure exceeding 160/110). In one study, before induction, the preoperative mean arterial pressure was lowered by 20% with an infusion of nitroglycerine (200 μg ml$^{-1}$). This regimen was successful in controlling the pressor response to intubation following the rapid sequence technique [72]. There was no effect on the increased heart rate. Nitroglycerine has some advantages in these at-risk patients in that the drug is easily controlled, so avoiding undesirable hypotension. However, particular caution should be exercised in using nitrates in such patients because some may have increased intracranial pressure or signs of cerebral oedema.

Intranasal nitrogycerine [73] is a simple method of gaining some control of blood pressure at intubation. Topical nitroglycerine ointment has also been found effective in healthy patients [74]. Topical nitroglycerine can, however, produce tachycardia. Good attenuation of the hypertensive response to intubation as well as to subsequent median sternotomy in patients undergoing cardiac surgery was obtained with topical nitroglycerine applied 1 h before induction of anaesthesia. Topical nitroglycerine 2% was applied over an area of 10 cm by 5 cm on the forehead. There was no useful reduction of heart rate [75].

Isosorbide dinitrate has been used in several forms. Intravenous injection of a bolus dose of 80 μg kg$^{-1}$ had little effect on blood pressure and none at all on the increased heart rate [76].

The relative safety of isosorbide dinitrate buccal

spray is reflected by its widespread use for self administration in patients suffering from angina. This safety makes it attractive as an agent for controlling cardiovascular responses to intubation. When administered between 90 and 150 s (better response with the longer time interval) prior to intubation, hypertension is usefully attenuated in healthy patients but no effect on the tachycardia is seen. The addition of a β-blocker is recommended when the technique is used in patients with myocardial ischaemia or intracranial aneurysms [77].

**Nitroprusside** Sodium nitroprusside, used in a dose of 1–2 $\mu g$ $kg^{-1}$ administered by rapid intravenous injection about 15 s before laryngoscopy, attenuates but does not fully prevent, the pressor response [16]. The timing of injection is made so that its peak effect coincides with the maximum hypertensive effect of intubation. The technique does not prevent the increased heart rate.

**Calcium channel blocker** Calcium channel blocking drugs that are used in the treatment of hypertension (dihydropyridines) act mainly by reducing afterload and could be expected to influence the pressor response to intubation although not the tachycardia.

Nifedipine has been used in patients with pregnancy-induced hypertension in sublingual doses of 10 mg or 20 mg before undergoing Caesarean section under general anaesthesia. The hypertensive response is well attenuated but heart rates tended to rise when compared with a control group [78].

Verapamil in intravenous doses of 0.05 mg $kg^{-1}$ or 0.1 mg $kg^{-1}$ administered 45 s before starting laryngoscopy attenuated the systolic blood pressure increases, but failed to control the tachycardia [79,80].

The negative inotropic effect of verapamil is undesirable in subjects with poor left venticular function. Rhythm problems may follow its negative chronotropic effect in patients with abnormal conduction systems [81].

Nicardipine is a new dihydropyridine derivative. It produces an immediate and short acting reduction of blood pressure without provoking adverse effects such as hypotension, conduction problems or myocardial depression. It showed consistent improvement in coronary blood flow and oxygen delivery to ischaemic myocardial areas. Nicardipine in a dose of 30 $\mu g$ $kg^{-1}$ administered

intravenously after the induction of anaesthesia can suppress the rise of mean arterial pressure associated with intubation in both hypertensive and normotensive patients. Increases in heart rate are even better controlled in hypertensive patients compared with normotensive subjects. Nicardipine has therefore been recommended as an effective drug in controlling the effects of intubation in patients with cardiovascular disease [82].

**ACE inhibitors** Angiotensin converting enzyme (ACE) inhibitors have a role in the management of hypertensive disease. Captopril doses of 12.5 or 25 mg administered sublingually 25 min before induction and intubation in healthy patients have been shown to attenuate the pressor response but appears ineffective in controlling increased heart rate. Unpredictable hypotension has been a feature in treated patients [83]. An ACE inhibitor (ramipril) given the night before operation followed by a further dose repeated 2 h before induction gave some attenuation of the hypertensive response and tachycardia after intubation in healthy patients [84].

**Prostaglandins** Prostaglandin E1 can be effective in controlling the sympathetic response to intubation [85].

**Ganglion blockers** Trimetaphan has been used for treating hypertensive emergencies and in the technique of controlled hypotension in the perioperative period. Trimetaphan was effective in controlling the pressor response to intubation when an infusion of trimetaphan 1 mg $min^{-1}$ was administered for 3–9 min prior to intubation [86]. In a recent study, the more practical technique of administering a bolus of trimetaphan 0.05 mg $kg^{-1}$ or 0.1 mg $kg^{-1}$ given 1.75 min prior to intubation was also successful in attenuating the hypertensive response. However, the reduction of pressure was most marked when patients were in the sitting position and least when in the supine position [87].

In neither study was control of increased heart rate obtained. Indeed, ganglion blockers can produce tachycardia.

### Adrenergic blocking agents

*α-Adrenergic blockers* Phentolamine has peripheral α-adrenergic blocking actions. In doses of

5 mg given intravenously, phentolamine has been shown to effectively block both heart rate and pressor response to intubation [7]. Surprisingly, no fall of blood pressure occurred in healthy subjects anaesthetized and lying supine. A 5 mg dose of phentolamine is substantial and normally causes a rapid fall of blood pressure. Caution should therefore be used when administering this drug in patients with unstable cardiovascular systems.

The value of centrally acting α-adrenergic antagonists has also been investigated. In two separate studies in patients undergoing coronary artery bypass graft operations, oral clonidine was given the night before operation [88] or 90 min before intubation [89,90]. With both techniques, a marked reduction in the amount of fentanyl required to suppress the sympathetic cardiovascular responses to laryngoscopy was noted.

In both regimens it appears that clonidine decreased central sympathetic outflow, resulting in some attenuation of the circulatory effects of intubation. However, because of the time required for absorption before tracheal intubation can proceed, the possibility of drug interaction and the prolonged action would appear to make clonidine an unsuitable choice.

*β-Adrenergic blockers* Many authorities have advocated the use of β-adrenergic blocking agents to inhibit the reflex sympathoadrenal discharges following intubation [15, 91, 92]. There is unanimity in the recommendation that patients receiving β-blockers preoperatively in the treatment of their cardiovascular disease should continue to do so up to the time of surgery [93–97]. Patients with coronary artery disease are protected to some extent from the circulatory effects of intubation when preoperative β-receptor antagonists are not stopped compared with similar patients in whom therapy has been discontinued. Of equal importance is the finding by these workers that continuation of β-blockade does not lead to adverse haemodynamic function during anaesthesia in patients with coronary artery disease. Whilst β-blockers should therefore be continued, techniques that are of proven value in attenuating undesirable consequences of intubation should always be used in such patients [98].

The use of intravenously administered β-blocking agents prior to the induction of anaesthesia in patients not previously taking these drugs

is controversial. Their use must be based on the careful assessment of all the relevant details of the patient's condition. The use of β-blockers to attenuate the pressor response to intubation led to circulatory collapse and cardiac arrest in a 80 kg patient who was probably hypovolaemic [99]. The drug employed was practolol (12 mg injected over 4 min) preceded by atropine (0.9 mg). This latter dose of atropine produced an increase in heart rate from 88 to 157 bpm but fell to 112 bpm after practolol administration.

β-Blockers have proved useful in reducing the heart rate and incidence of dysrhythmias but not the pressor response to rapid (crash) intubation sequence (induction agent with suxamethonium followed by immediate intubation). Both acebutolol (0.5 mg kg$^{-1}$) and propranolol (0.04 mg kg$^{-1}$), which represent subclinical doses, proved effective [100].

Esmolol is a new ultra short acting cardioselective β-blocker. The advantage of esmolol is its short duration of action (elimination half-life of 9 min), which permits rapid titration to a desired level of β-blockade. Similarly, cessation of esmolol infusion rapidly terminates β-blockade. The drug does not cause clinically significant cardiovascular depression.

Esmolol in doses of 150–200 mg given intravenously before induction and intubation reliably limits the undesirable haemodynamic effects of intubation when compared with other established techniques [101] (Fig. 3). When esmolol was given by intravenous infusion over a 12-min period (500 μg kg$^{-1}$ for 4 min and then 300 μg kg$^{-1}$ for 8 min) before induction and intubation, good prevention of postintubation increases of heart rate was obtained. Control of hypertension was less marked [102]. Other workers noted poorer control of the hypertensive response compared with pulse rate [103]. The possibility of combining an intravenous esmolol infusion with a peripheral vasodilator to overcome this deficiency has been suggested [102].

*Combined α and β blockers* β-Adrenergic blockers alone are unlikely to suppress fully the hypertensive response to laryngoscopy, since this is a predominantly α-adrenegic response. Furthermore, drugs are relatively contraindicated in patients with any form of bronchospastic pulmonary disease.

A more rational approach is to use drugs with

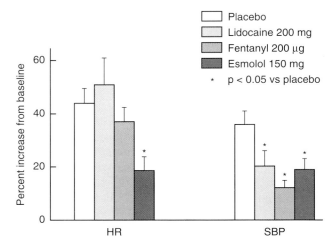

**Figure 3**   Effect of esmolol, fentanyl, lidocaine (lignocaine) and placebo on changes in heart rate (HR) and systolic blood pressure (SBP) at tracheal intubation. After Helfman [101].

combined α- and β-blocking properties. Labetalol is a combined α-1 and nonselective β-adrenergic blocking drug. The drug was effective in controlling both the increased blood pressure and tachycardia after intubation when doses ranging from 0.25 to 0.75 mg kg$^{-1}$ were administered 5 min prior to induction of anaesthesia. Attenuation of cardiovascular changes occurred in a dose-dependent fashion [104].

In a study involving pregnant women suffering from pregnancy-induced hypertension about to undergo Caesarean section, labetalol was given before induction as a bolus of 20 mg followed by further 10 mg increments up to a total of 1 mg kg$^{-1}$. This regimen also proved effective in suppressing cardiovascular changes [105]. On the other hand, other workers have failed to demonstrate an effect on postintubation hypertension when the smaller dose of 10 mg labetalol was administered [106].

***Magnesium sulphate*** Magnesium sulphate has been in use for many years in obstetric practice in the treatment of pre-eclampsia. In addition to its action as an 'anticonvulsant', it produces peripheral vasodilatation and depression of heart rate.

Magnesium sulphate was comparable to alfentanil in preventing pressor responses to intubation in patients suffering from moderate to severe gestational proteinuric hypertension [37]. While alfentanil was better at controlling heart rate, it was more likely to depress foetal respiration. This did not occur with magnesium sulphate. A combination of alfentanil and magnesium sulphate pro-

duced better control of arterial pressure and heart rate than magnesium sulphate alone [107].

The mechanism of action of magnesium sulphate in attenuating cardiovascular effects of intubation is probably multifactorial. It inhibits the release of catecholamines at the time of intubation, it is an α-adrenergic antagonist and has direct vasodilator properties [38]. Alfentanil acts primarily on depression of catecholamines by central depression [39]; doses of 10 μg kg$^{-1}$ appear to produce satisfactory cardiovascular control without giving undue reduction of arterial pressure.

**Pretreatment with nondepolarizing muscle relaxants when suxamethonium is used**

This is commonly practised to prevent some of the undesirable side effects of suxamethonium, such as muscle fasciculation. Pretreatment has also been shown to have some stabilizing effect on cardiac rhythm during intubation [108].

In this study, patients free of cardiorespiratory disease were premedicated with pethidine and atropine and induced with thiopentone. The cardiovascular effects at intubation were compared in groups receiving either d-tubocurarine (0.05 mg kg$^{-1}$), alcuronium (0.03 mg kg$^{-1}$), pancuronium (0.008 mg kg$^{-1}$) or no pretreatment at all.

Whilst the systolic and diastolic pressures increased in all patients following intubation, the tubocurarine treated patients showed only small increases. Attenuation was least with pancuronium, which exhibited no improvement from the control group in which blood pressure rose by more than

50 mmHg. The alcuronium group was intermediate in reducing pressure increases. Heart rate increased in all groups and was maximal immediately after intubation except in the alcuronium group, where the greatest rise occurred rather later. There was no difference between the groups, the rises lying between 20 and 30 bpm. Comparison of heart rate changes in the control group was difficult to assess because many of the patients in the control group had high starting pulse rates. Some changes in cardiac rhythm occurred at the time of laryngoscopy and intubation, the highest incidence occurring in the pancuronium group and the lowest in the alcuronium patients.

The beneficial effect of reducing blood pressure changes found with d-tubocurarine, and to a lesser extent with alcuronium, is mirrored by their ability to abolish muscle fasciculations produced by suxamethonium whereas pancuronium pretreatment prevented fasciculation in less than half of the subjects and was correspondingly less successful in protecting against blood pressure elevations.

Thus, when using suxamethonium to aid intubation it is useful to know that pretreatment with d-tubocurarine (and alcuronium) reduce blood pressure changes but it should be remembered that supplementary measures are needed to guarantee effective control of blood pressure changes in high risk cases.

## Avoidance of mechanical stimulation of the larynx

### Awake intubation
This technique does not appear to confer any advantage over general anaesthesia. However, neither does it produce more adverse circulatory response when skilfully carried out in healthy subjects [109]. These 'awake' patients were, in fact, sedated with intravenous diazepam, fentanyl and lignocaine (1.5 mg kg$^{-1}$) administered over a 20-minute period whilst topical anaesthesia was applied. Both oral and blind nasal techniques were employed.

### Blind nasal intubation
Another approach to minimize stretching of the tissues of the laryngopharynx with a rigid laryngoscope is to insert the tracheal tube by blind nasal intubation. This technique successfully avoided hypertension and tachycardia in four patients undergoing dental surgery, although in two of the

patients, previous laryngoscopy had produced a marked pressor response [14]. However, these patients were anaesthetized with nitrous oxide with 10% carbon dioxide and intubation was successful at the first attempt. The lack of circulatory changes is surprising in view of the use of carbon dioxide.

The Augustine Guide™ is a new device aimed at facilitating blind oral intubation in the management of the difficult airway [110, 111]. However, when tested against intubation aided by conventional laryngoscope in patients with no airway problem, the blind technique was associated with significantly lower levels of serum noradrenaline. However, this finding was not reflected in any difference in the pressor and heart rate changes compared with those when intubation was laryngoscope aided. Blind oral intubation with the Augustine Guide took longer to perform than intubation with a laryngoscope [112].

### Awake fibreoptic nasotracheal intubation
Pressure on the laryngeal tissues precipitates cardiovascular reflexes. Pressures of up to 2.5 kg have been recorded in routine laryngoscopy and up to 4 kg in difficult intubations [113]. One study set out to see whether avoiding laryngoscopy with a rigid laryngoscope and the use of suxamethonium would reduce cardiovascular effects [114]. Patients were sedated with a mixture of diazepam and fentanyl after premedication with combinations of diazepam, opiates and atropine. Sedation was taken to the point at which the patient could still obey commands. Before laryngoscopy was started topical anaesthesia was secured. Between 1 and 1.5 ml of cocaine (6%) was applied to the nasal passage using cotton-tipped swabs. Anaesthesia of the larynx and trachea was achieved by transtracheal injection of 3 ml of lignocaine (4%). These steps would leave out the oropharynx and posterior portion of the tongue. A well-lubricated nasal tube was passed over the fibreoptic scope when the latter has been successfully inserted. The average changes in the group of 200 subjects appeared very satisfactory. Even during application of topical anaesthesia no significant change of mean arterial pressure occurred. The greatest increase of mean pressure was a modest 10 mmHg above the baseline when the tube passed through the nasal passage. Although alterations in heart rate occurred progressively through the whole process the changes

were again modest. The maximum rise of 14 beats per minute occurred when the tube entered the trachea. However, in 32% of cases mean arterial pressure rose by more than 20 mmHg and by more than 30 mmHg in 11% of patients. Heart rate increased by more than 20 beats per minute in 30% of cases and more than 30 beats per minute in 12% of patients. More than half the patients coughed, some severely, when transtracheal puncture was carried out. Half the patients were aware of the intubation process although only a few found it very unpleasant.

Fibreoptic assisted tracheal intubation through the nasal route with an awake patient in whom topical anaesthesia has been applied, therefore, appears to produce less cardiovascular stimulation than oral intubation using conventional laryngoscopy. Other workers have confirmed these findings [115, 116] while other investigators found no difference between the two techniques [117].

However, if awake fibreoptic nasal intubation is less disturbing to the cardiovascular system, then it would support the finding that blind nasal intubation causes no significant increases in heart rate or blood pressure [14]. Skill is of course needed in fibreoptic techniques and awake intubation is not always appropriate in patients with severe cardiovascular disturbance.

On the other hand, when general anaesthesia is used, fibreoptic assisted intubation through the nasal route produces less pressor response than with the conventional Macintosh laryngoscope, but results in greater and more sustained tachycardia [118].

When the oral route is employed, under general anaesthesia, tracheal intubation using a fibreoptic laryngoscope results in even greater pressor and more sustained heart rate increases than those seen with conventional laryngoscopy However, these undesirable effects can be reduced by including fentanyl as one of the induction agents [118, 119]. Continuous propofol infusion supplemented with fentanyl can be effective in eliminating all cardiovascular responses, whatever form of laryngoscopy is used.

Although the fibreoptic laryngoscope may produce less mechanical stimulation on the tissues of the anterior pharynx, so producing less sympathetic response, intubation using the fibreoptic laryngoscope tends to take much longer than with conventional laryngoscopy. Increasing the time of stimulation has been shown to result in increased

pressor effect. It is possible that the beneficial effect of less pharyngeal stimulation with the fibrescope is outweighed by the increased time that it takes to complete intubation successfully [120].

### Laryngoscope design

Traditional teaching suggests that straight bladed (e.g. Magill or Forreger) laryngoscopes produce a greater change in heart rate and rhythm than the Macintosh type. The straight blade is inserted posterior to the epiglottis, an area innervated by the superior laryngeal nerve, which is a branch of the vagus nerve. The Macintosh blade, on the other hand, is positioned in front of the epiglottis which is supplied by the glossopharyngeal nerve. Contrary to this teaching, some studies showed that the Macintosh blade produced a greater effect on heart rate than the straight blade [8, 9]. However not all these patients were fully anaesthetized and some were suffering from pulmonary tuberculosis.

In fact, when healthy subjects were fully anaesthetized prior to intubation, no difference in cardiovascular response could be demonstrated between the patients intubated with a straight laryngoscope blade and those intubated with a curved blade [114].

### Laryngeal mask airway (LMA)

While the laryngeal mask airway can in no way be a substitute for a tracheal tube, it is used in a number of situations where a tracheal tube would have been indicated hitherto.

Several studies have shown beneficial effects on cardiovascular reflexes with the LMA when compared with laryngoscopy and tracheal intubation [121–123]. In healthy subjects, elevation of the systolic blood pressure has been found to be significantly less with the LMA. Changes in the heart rate were similar, although the increase appears to persist for longer in the tracheal intubation group (Fig. 4). To what extent these findings can be applied to patients with severe cardiovascular disease is not certain. However, when a LMA is an appropriate means of airway management, it is probably a better choice than conventional intubation in those patients at risk from adverse cardiovascular effects.

## *Effects of extubation*

In comparison with the effects of intubation, problems associated with tracheal extubation have received very little attention [124]. Since extubation is usually carried out during light planes of anaesthesia, it is not surprising that similar effects to those seen at intubation occur. Increases in blood pressure and heart rate have been demonstrated in a high proportion of ASA grade I and II patients [125, 126]. Similar pressor and heart rate changes following tracheal extubation have also been seen in studies of patients who have undergone a period of postoperative ventilation following coronary artery surgery [127].

Disturbances of pathophysiogolgy at the time of extubation appears to be a potentially fruitful field of study.

## RESPIRATORY SYSTEM

### Hypoxaemia and Hypercarbia

There are two ways in which undesirable effects on respiration may complicate tracheal intubation. Firstly, whatever technique is used, impairment of blood gas exchange will result from hypoventilation, apnoea, respiratory obstruction or expiratory muscle spasm. Secondly, when muscle relaxants are used to facilitate intubation, a period of hypoventilation leading to apnoea normally occurs. If ventilation is not artificially maintained a further period of apnoea occurs before intubation is completed, and connection to a breathing system and inflation of the lungs have taken place. The time interval between injection of the induction agent and laryngoscopy has been reported to be $124 \pm 10$ s and the time from laryngoscopy to intubation $43 \pm 6$ s [128]. The further time interval between intubation and inflation of the lungs does not appear to have been studied. All these times may be considerably prolonged when intubation is difficult or if the operator is inexperienced.

(a)

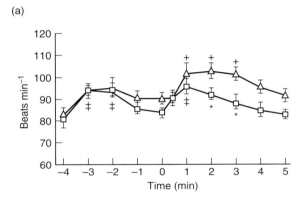

(b)

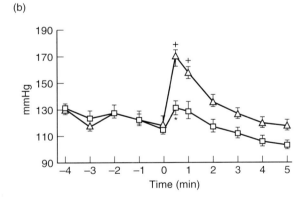

(c)

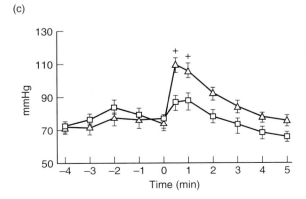

**Figure 4**   Comparison of cardiovascular responses to the insertion of the laryngeal mask airway and laryngoscopy and intubation. Anaesthesia was induced with thiopentone and maintained with enflurane in nitrous oxide and oxygen; muscle relaxation was produced by vecuronium. Reproduced from Wilson *et al* [234].
(a) Heart rate expressed as mean (SEM). Differences where $p < 0.05$ are illustrated as follows: * = between groups at that time; + = within group 1 (tracheal tube) compared with T = 0; ‡ = within group 2 (LMA) compared with T = 0. △ = tracheal intubation group; ☐ = LMA group.
(b) Systolic arterial pressure expressed as mean (SEM). Differences where $p < 0.005$ are illustrated as follows: * = between groups at that time; + = within group 1 compared with T = 0. △ tracheal intubation group; ☐ LMA group.
(c) Diastolic arterial pressure expressed as mean (SEM). + = $p < 0.05$ within group 1 compared with T = 0. △ = tracheal intubation group; ☐ = LMA group.

## Fall of arterial oxygen saturation

When oxygen is not administered prior to induction and paralysis secured with suxamethonium, arterial oxygen saturation falls rapidly to a mean value of about 75% in 1 min after administration of these drugs [129, 130]. The introduction of routine pulse oximetry has confirmed the high incidence of hypoxaemia (oxygen saturation less than 90%), even in healthy patients when no preoxygenation is administered. Some become hypoxaemic as soon as 10 s after the onset of apnoea that frequently follows administration of an intravenous induction agent [131]. The danger of hypoxaemia during laryngoscopy has long been recognized and the need to elevate the arterial oxygen by denitrogenation prior to induction has been advocated by many authorities [129, 130, 132–138]. Pulse oximetry studies during induction and tracheal intubation reinforce the value of preoxygenation in all patients receiving general anaesthesia [139].

Clinical practice varies. Some anaesthetists do not routinely administer oxygen, whilst others employ one of a variety of techniques:

- Preoxygenation with a facemask with tidal breaths over a period varying between 2 and 10 min.
- Preoxygenation with a facemask with three or four vital capacity breaths over a period of 30 s.
- Combination of (1) and (2).
- Manual inflation of the lungs with oxygen after the onset of hypoventilation or apnoea following induction.
- Both preoxygenation and post induction oxygenation

### Preoxygenation with tidal breaths (Fig. 5)
Several recommendations have been made as to the duration of preoxygenation, varying between 2 and 10 min [140]. The reasons for these differing recommendations are not wholly clear. Normal subjects breathing 100% oxygen achieve over 98% denitrogenation after 7 min [141]. Different times would therefore be advocated depending on the degree of denitrogenation thought advisable. However, reducing the alveolar nitrogen concentration to 4% is a satisfactory level to aim for and gives 5–6 min of apnoea without hypoxaemia [140]. The difference in oxygen store in the lungs when completely denitrogenated and at 4% levels of nitrogen is very small, 2.53 and 2.65 L respectively.

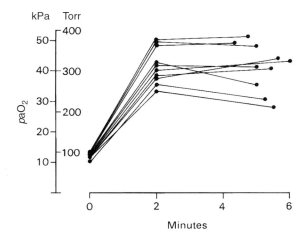

**Figure 5**   Preoxygenation with tidal breaths and changes on $paCO_2$ during induction and intubation. Preoxygenation started at time 0, thiopentone at 2 min; termination of intubation is represented by the last point on each graph. After Gabrielson and Valentin [143], with kind permission of the editor of *Acta Anaesthesiologica Scandinavica*.

Another reason for the various times recommended is that studies have involved the use of different breathing systems. Circuits using low fresh gas flows take longer to complete denitrogenation of the lungs. Most studies, though, show that rapid nitrogen washout is easily accomplished with non-rebreathing systems [140].

Three minutes of breathing has been recommended with the Magill (Mapleson A) system using an 8 l oxygen flow rate [140]. One minute of oxygen breathing with a Magill system using a 10 L gas flow gives 3 min of apnoea time before the arterial oxygen saturation falls more than 6% [142]. When a circle system is used with a 5 L oxygen flow, an adequate level of denitrogenation is reached within 5 min [128]. However, these times are based on administration of oxygen with leak-proof facemasks, a proviso not always achieved in clinical practice because of inadequate technique or awkward facial anatomy. When there is a leak, preoxygenation may be far from satisfactory and desaturation of arterial blood exceeding 10% can easily occur at intubation [142]. Even when a close fit is achieved the recommendations may be inadequate in certain types of patient (see below).

A recent study found that 11% of routine surgical patients could not be satisfactorily preoxygenated, due largely to a poorly fitting facemask. Of those patients who could be preoxygenated,

23% required more than 3 min (some up to 6 min), though it was not possible to identify these patients in advance. For this reason the authors recommend the routine monitoring of end tidal oxygen to determine when a satisfactory end point has been reached [144].

**Preoxygenation with vital capacity breaths** (Fig. 6)
An alternative to the traditional tidal breathing method involves the subject taking four voluntary maximal deep breaths of 100% oxygen over a period of 30 s. This yields a similar level of oxygenation to 5 min of tidal breathing of oxygen. Very deep inhalations lead to more rapid denitrogenation of the inspiratory reserve volume and the functional residual capacity than the shallower tidal breathing. It would appear that this technique would require a non-breathing system with a large reservoir bag and a large fresh gas flow rate. Nevertheless, satisfactory results are obtained with a circle system employing a 5 l fresh gas flow. Similarly satisfactory oxygenation has been obtained using a Magill (Mapleson A) system with a fresh gas flow rate of 8 l. The patient is encouraged to inhale slowly so that the reservoir bag does not completely collapse [142].

**Oxygenation after induction**
This technique is commonly practised in routine intubations and is even used when patients have been adequately preoxygenated, during the period while awaiting full paralysis and satisfactory intubating conditions. The technique is invariably used when non-depolarizing muscle relaxants have been administered and where the onset of full action is delayed for at least 2 min. When preoxygenation is adequate, post induction hyperventilation and oxygenation is superfluous in most patients. However, the presence of oxygen in the respiratory passages slows down the fall of arterial oxygen tension even in the absence of ventilation [130]. This adds a safety margin in those intubations that prove to be unexpectedly prolonged. Most anaesthetists employ oxygenation after induction routinely in elective cases where easy intubation is anticipated.

Oxygen administration after induction is thought to be significantly less effective than preoxygenation because the volume of manual inflation is limited by the volume of the reservoir bag. Functional residual capacity is less under anaesthesia and only the inspiratory reserve volume is used [141]. On the other hand, workers elsewhere could demonstrate no difference between arterial oxygen levels 3 min after induction with either the post induction oxygenation or preoxygenation technique [128]. However, post induction oxygenation was found to be less effective than four deep breaths of oxygen before induction in that arterial oxygen tension was lower at the moment of laryngoscopy than in preoxygenated patients, although in neither group did

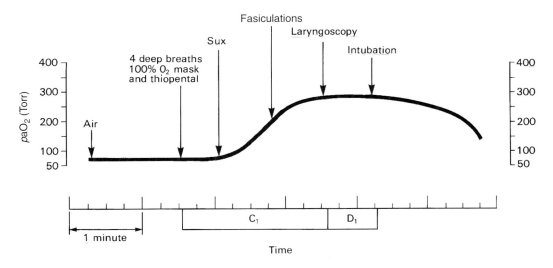

**Figure 6** Preoxygenation with deep breaths and changes in $paO_2$ during induction and intubation. $C_1$ = time from induction of anaesthesia to end of laryngoscopy; $D_1$ = time from laryngoscopy to end of intubation. After Gold and Muravchick [128], with kind permission of the International Anesthesia Research Society.

hypoxaemia ensue [128]. Occasionally a patient may refuse preoxygenation (fear of facemask) and the anaesthetist may have to rely on post induction oxygenation. This can provide adequate cover if intubation is not delayed. Patients at risk should be encouraged to change their minds and perhaps an alternative technique not involving a tight-fitting facemask may be more acceptable (see below).

### Preoxygenation and post induction oxygen administration

When preoxygenation has been carried out with either tidal breathing or deep breaths, further oxygenation after induction does not significantly increase oxygen stores. However, where preoxygenation has been less than perfect, it offers an additional reserve of available oxygen and is of value in patients at risk. In patients who have potentially full stomachs, extra care is needed to ensure adequate preoxygeneration as inflation of the lungs after induction is contraindicated.

Anaesthetists recognize that patient acceptance of a tight-fitting mask may be an obstacle to effective preoxygenation. Various techniques have been tried to improve patients' tolerance of the preoxygenation regimen.

A lightweight plastic disposable oxygen mask (Hudson Oxygen Therapy Co.) has been found to be more acceptable than a tight-fitting rubber mask. Satisfactory preoxygenation can be achieved after 3 min of tidal breathing while a high oxygen flow rate (48 l min$^{-1}$) is delivered through small bore tubing to the plastic mask by continuous pressure on the oxygen flush button on the anaesthetic machine. However, the authors did not feel confident enough to recommend the method in patients at risk [145].

Although the Bain and Magill breathing circuits are not the most efficient ones for securing good preoxygenation, they are the most commonly available in the anaesthetic induction room. If used in the conventional tidal breathing technique, these circuits permit rebreathing and therefore less effective oxygen wash-in. Very good oxygenation wash-in can be achieved with the Bain circuit if the patient is instructed to take deep breaths in a slow fashion whilst the oxygen flush is kept in the on position. The reservoir bag is first filled with 100% oxygen and is kept full during the deep breath. At the end of inspiration, signalled by maximum movement of the chest and abdomen, the oxygen flush is released to allow easier expira-

tion. The cycle is repeated. Using this technique, four or five such breaths produce oxygen wash-in comparable to tidal breathing for 3 min with the Bain, while six breaths in this manner consistently exceeded the level of oxygen wash-in with the tidal technique. However, good mask fit is always important whichever method is used [146].

While the regimen described above appears to be satisfactory for most patients, greater attention is necessary in obese and pregnant patients. Other groups at risk are those with deficient oxygen carrying capacity, poor lung function, patients with full stomachs and those in whom difficult intubation is likely. Lastly, alteration of lung function in elderly patients can alter the efficacy of different preoxygenation techniques.

### Obese patients

In these patients lung volume is decreased in the supine anaesthetized state [147] so arterial saturation falls more rapidly during apnoea. Careful preoxygenation is therefore obligatory.

### Pregnant women

In these patients lung volume is again small and in labour oxygen consumption is high so that arterial oxygen tension falls more rapidly during apnoea than in nonpregnant women [138]. Maternal oxygen tension has been observed to fall below 100 mmHg following intubation [148]. The pregnant woman is particularly at risk during intubation for emergency operations whilst in labour. Supplementation of preoxygenation by manual inflation after induction is usually avoided to reduce the chance of regurgitation. Three minutes of preoxygenation or four deep breaths of oxygen over 30 s before induction have both been shown to provide adequate maternal and fetal oxygenation at Caesarean section [149]. However, additional preoxygenation in excess of these minimum recommendations for routine operations is probably an advantage [142].

### Poor lung function

Complete denitrogenation in these patients takes longer because of the larger functional residual capacity, small vital capacity and poor alveolar mixing which impairs oxygen wash-in. In one study, complete filling of the lungs with oxygen took nearly 3 min in normal subjects while in those with moderate or serious lung disease complete filling took over 4 min and 7 min respectively. However, there was not much difference in the time required to reach 90% filling of the lungs: 1 min in normal subjects against up to 1.5 min in the diseased groups [150].

Relatively routine periods of preoxygenation can, therefore, produce adequate saturation of the blood with oxygen in patients with pulmonary pathology. However, when lung volume is reduced by disease, absolute oxygen content is smaller and this limits the maximum time during which arterial oxygen levels remain adequate during intubation. In practice in patients with serious lung disease, a longer period of preoxygenation is probably beneficial to complete denitrogenation and this should be supplemented by post induction oxygenation to increase the safety margin.

### Patients with full stomachs or anticipated difficult intubation

In both these groups careful preoxygenation is essential since manual inflation after induction cannot be safely carried out in those with full stomachs and may be difficult in those with anatomical problems. Prolonged intubation may also be a feature of the latter type of patient.

### Aged patients

The efficiency of various techniques of preoxygenation have been evaluated mainly in young subjects. Yet, an increasing proportion of patients presenting for surgery are elderly.

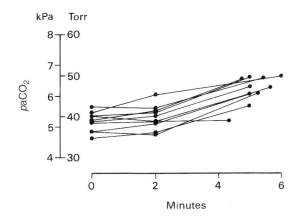

**Figure 7**  Changes in $paCO_2$ during anaesthesia and tracheal intubation. Thiopentone at 2 min; termination of intubation is represented by the last point on each graph. After Gabrielson and Valentin [143], with kind permission of the editor of *Acta Anaesthesiologica Scandinavica*.

Studies have been carried out on the implications of the differing physiology of respiration in the older patient on preoxygenation techniques [151]. It seems that the decreased basal oxygen consumption in the older subject (>60 years) does not compensate for the less efficient uptake of oxygen in the elderly. The main factor of increasing closing volume with age results in less efficient denitrogenation during preoxygenation while breathing at normal tidal volumes.

However, elderly patients may not be able to achieve vital capacity breath in the supine position. Four 'deep breaths' in these patients does not produce such a wide safety margin (apnoea time) as does 2–4 min of the tidal breathing technique [151, 152].

### *Elevation of arterial carbon dioxide tension* (see Fig. 7)

The rate at which the arterial carbon dioxide tension rises in apnoea has been investigated by numerous workers and has been reviewed [153]. In a study conducted by that reviewer, eight lightly anaesthetized subjects were subjected to apnoeic oxygenation for periods of up to 53 min. In six of these individuals arterial $pCO_2$ levels reached between 130 and 160 mmHg. The mean average rise of carbon dioxide tension was 3 mmHg per min (range 2.7–4.9 mmHg). Onset of ventricular dysrhythmias terminated the period of apnoea in two patients. In more recent studies, involving elderly patients with serious cardiac disease, the rate of rise of carbon dioxide tension in one group below the age of 60 was 2.2 mmHg and 3.5 mmHg per min in another group over 60. The period measured was that between induction, which included administration of a muscle relaxant, and intubation. Although respiration decreased rapidly after induction, true apnoea was not present for the entire time interval [143].

Interestingly enough, in one study when intubation was preceded by a 'slow' inhalation induction using cyclopropane and ether until the patient was sufficiently relaxed to intubate, carbon dioxide levels rose rapidly and markedly from the onset of anaesthesia until intubation. The average rise was 15 mmHg (range 7–35 mmHg). Depression of respiration caused by the inhalation induction agent was responsible. This technique, which is sometimes used in the poor risk patient, is therefore less safe than might be thought [134].

In most cases the small increase of arterial $CO_2$ tension is unlikely to be of any clinical significance when the conventional intravenous induction and muscle relaxant technique precedes intubation. Hyperventilation during the period of preoxygenation reduces this potential danger further in those patients with pre-existing elevations of arterial $CO_2$ tension. Furthermore, unless contraindicated by complications such as a full stomach, manual ventilation whilst awaiting optimum intubating conditions is a further safeguard in those patients in whom intubation is likely to be prolonged.

## Resistance to Breathing

Tracheal intubation bypasses the upper airways which normally contribute about one-third of the total airway resistance when spontaneously breathing through the mouth. The tracheal tube does, however, substitute its own mechanical resistance to spontaneous respiration. The length and radius of the commonly used adult tracheal tube is more likely to result in turbulent than linear air flow. This turbulent flow is increased if there are sharp angulations in the tube and its connections. However, the most important factor remains the radius of the cross-section of the tube, as resistance is proportional to the fourth power of the radius.

Recent work suggests that tracheal intubation imposes a further resistance to respiration in the airways distal to the tube [154]. Significant increases of airway resistance, up to 210%, were reported in awake healthy subjects. Intubation was preceded by topical anaesthesia only. Reflex bronchoconstriction reduced by irritation of the airway by the tube was thought to be the cause. These findings suggest that increased bronchoconstriction might result if adequate general anaesthesia is not deep enough or if topical anaesthesia to the trachea is not used.

Patients with chronic obstructive pulmonary disease showed an enhanced response to tracheal irritation by demonstrating an even greater increase in airway resistance.

## Changes in Functional Residual Capacity (FRC)

Tracheal intubation bypasses the glottis. This can cause a reduction of functional residual capacity that may predispose to atelectasis. In infants, where FRC is quite close to residual volume (at about 15–20% of total lung capacity), a tracheal tube can be associated with both a reduced FRC and impaired oxygenation [155]. In adults, the FRC typically occurs between 35 and 40% of total lung capacity, which greatly exceeds residual volume. There appears to be no significant change in FRC in adults after intubation [156]. In patients with obstructive airways disease, FRC may actually increase [157].

## Impairment of Humidification

The normal warming and humidifying of inspired gases is lost when the upper airways are bypassed by a tracheal tube. Any humidifying of dry medical gases falls entirely to the lower respiratory tract. Earlier workers showed that inhalation of dry gases is harmful to the normal function of the respiratory mucous membrane [158] and this has been confirmed by more recent studies. Inhalation of dry gases produces drying of the mucous membrane and damages the ciliated cells so that ciliary movement virtually ceases in the tracheobronchial tree extending as far as the pulmonary alveoli [159, 160]. These changes have been correlated with an increase in postoperative pulmonary complications, notably when exposure to dry gases exceeds 1 h. Conversely, complications can be reduced if gases are adequately humidified [160].

Longer term inhalation of dry gases through a tracheal tube leads to fibrous exudation and crusting of the mucous membranes of the trachea and larger bronchi. All these changes can be effectively prevented by adequate humidification of inspired gases.

## Fibreoptic Tracheal Intubation

Tracheal intubation using a fibreoptic laryngoscope undoubtedly takes longer than with conventional laryngoscopy, even in patients who have no severe intubation problems. This is true of both experienced operators and inexperienced personnel (with whom the time can be markedly prolonged) [161].

Not surprisingly, fibreoptic intubation under general anaesthesia poses severe problems of maintaining an adequate level of anaesthesia while preventing hypoxaemia, carbon dioxide retention and cardiovascular depression. In one study in which patients spontaneously breathed a deep halothane in nitrous oxide/oxygen mixture, there were significant falls of blood pressure and heart rate. However, of most concern was the high incidence of hypoxaemia. In one-third of patients, saturation fell below 90%, and in several patients below 80%. These complications were largely related to the inadequacies of the anaesthetic technique and its application (for instance preoxygenation was not performed) and not to the actual insertion of the fibreoptic laryngoscope itself. However, the experience of these authors is an object lesson in the difficulties involved when the patient remains breathing spontaneously (see Table 3).

In contrast, some workers have reported good results when fibreoptic intubation is carried out with the patient anaesthetized and apnoeic following administration of a muscle relaxant. When fibreoptic intubation was achieved in 1 min, oxygen saturation never fell below 98% in one series [163] and never below 96% in another study where the time taken fell between 1 and 3

min [164]. In these cases the highest level of $CO_2$ reached was 5.3 kPa. However, in another series where intubation took up to 3 min, oxygen saturation fell rapidly 1 min after starting. In three-quarters of the patients, oxygen saturation fell below 90% and in 20% of patients this fell to below 80%. These authors recommended that controlled ventilation be used during apnoeic fibreoptic intubation for at least a part of the procedure. The method of intermittent ventilation guided by monitoring the pulse oximeter can successfully prevent any significant hypoxaemia, even during more prolonged attempts at intubation such as occur during training sessions [161].

Controlled ventilation through an oral airway when the patient is anaesthetized and apnoeic is described as being satisfactory for nasal fibreoptic intubation. Propofol anaesthesia permits 100% oxygen to be used as the inflating gas. When fibreoptic intubation is carried out through the oral route, oxygen can be inflated through a nasal airway [166].

## INTRACRANIAL CHANGES

Hypoxia, hypercarbia and respiratory obstruction associated with increased venous pressure can all increase brain volume. This effect is sometimes easily seen in the cerebral congestion and swelling of the brain in intracranial operations. These changes are accompanied by elevations of cerebrospinal fluid pressure which reflects intracranial tension. Changes in cerebrospinal fluid pressure have been demonstrated at laryngoscopy and tracheal intubation [167]. Similar observations have been described by other workers (Fig. 8). The rise of intracranial tension can be as much as 10 mmHg [168] although most other authors found changes of a lesser degree [169–173]. Some studies have reported rises of as much as 50 mmHg [171] and 100 mmHg [168]. However, these workers used agents that are usually avoided in other studies in this field. In the first, suxamethonium was used to assist tracheal intubation. In the other study, methohexitone was used as an induction agent.

Increases of intracranial pressure have been related to a number of factors that could be associated with tracheal intubation: the use of succinylcholine [174], increased arterial blood

**Table 3** Fibreoptic tracheal intubation under general anaesthesia with spontaneous respiration. The lowest oxygen saturation ($SpO_2$) is given, together with the reason for the desaturation and the timing in 18 patients out of 60 who developed $SpO_2 < 90\%$ during the intubation sequence. No patient received preoxygenation. After Smith et al. [162].

| Lowest $SpO_2$ | Reason for desaturation | Timing of desaturation |
|---|---|---|
| 89% | Hypoventilation | After induction |
| 89% | Obstruction | Airway insertion |
| 18% | Coughing | Airway insertion |
| 85% | Hypoventilation | After induction |
| 89% | Hypoventilation | After induction |
| 89% | Cardiac depression | Bradycardia |
| 76% | Coughing | Lignocaine to cords |
| 88% | Coughing | Lignocaine to cords |
| 81% | Hypoventilation | After induction |
| 77% | Coughing | Lignocaine to cords |
| 88% | Shunting | Tracheal tube in right main bronchus |
| 88% | Cardiac depression | Bradycardia |
| 89% | Coughing | Lignocaine to cords |
| 74% | Airway obstruction | Airway insertion |
| 47% | Coughing | Lignocaine to cords |
| 89% | Cardiac depression | Bradycardia |
| 89% | Hypoventilation | After induction |
| 88% | Bronchospasm | After intubation |

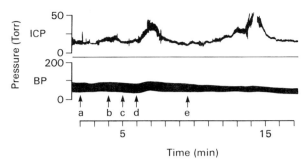

**Figure 8**   Changes in intracranial tension with induction of anaesthesia, laryngoscopy and intubation in patients with pre-existing raised intracranial pressure. a, b = increments of thiopentone; c = suxamethonium; d = laryngoscopy and intubation; e = halothane on. After Shapiro *et al.* [169], with kind permission of the editor and J. B. Lippincott Co., publishers of *Anesthesiology*.

pressure [167, 173] and increased venous pressure [173, 175] (Fig. 9).

Of equal importance to changes in intracranial pressure produced at the time of intubation are the changes in cerebral blood flow that can result. Cerebral perfusion pressure is the difference between mean arterial blood pressure and intracranial pressure. While an increase in arterial pressure may mitigate the effect of an increase in intracranial pressure, by the same token, a fall of blood pressure would aggravate an increase in brain tension and lead to a reduction of cerebral perfusion. Even more subtle changes may take place. If cerebral blood flow is marginally adequate in a patient with cerebrovascular disease a rise of venous pressure could lead to cerebral insufficiency, especially if the arterial blood pressure were to fall at the same time. In some situations an intracerebral 'steal' can occur: when local brain disease is associated with local acidosis, and therefore a state of maximal local vasodilation already exists, cerebral vasodilation due to any cause could increase blood flow to normal brain tissue at the expense of the diseased area.

Limited and transient increases of intracranial tension and alterations of cerebral blood flow are unlikely to be of any clinical significance in the healthy. However, such changes may be of crucial importance in patients with pre-existing raised intracranial pressure, due to a tumour or other space occupying lesions, in whom increases of intracranial pressure are much more marked [169,

171]. These increases produce pressure gradients across intracranial compartments which can lead to dangerous brain shifts [169], precipitate cerebral oedema, or impair an already inadequate cerebral blood flow.

Whilst numerous factors can contribute to alterations in intracranial pressure, intubation itself, drugs used to facilitate intubation and the consequent physiological changes have all been incriminated. These are listed below:

- laryngoscopy and intubation;
- suxamethonium;
- hypercarbia and hypoxia;
- elevated venous pressure produced by coughing and straining;
- inhalation anaesthetic agents and ketamine.

### Laryngoscopy and intubation

When these manoeuvres are performed faultlessly the change of intracranial pressure can be very slight, even in patients with pre-existing raised intracranial tension with papilloedema. Even packing the pharynx produced no alteration [173].

However, laryngoscopy and intubation can produce a rise in arterial blood pressure. In healthy patients, if other contributing factors are kept within the normal range, cerebral blood flow does not alter greatly between systolic blood pressures of 60–150 mmHg over a whole range of intracranial pressures [170]. However, it has been suggested that the acute hypertension seen at laryngoscopy can induce rapid cerebral swelling in patients with a brain tumour or acute cerebrovascular disease [176]. In patients with pre-existing raised intracranial tension, a further large rise in pressure may result from the raised arterial pressure. Cerebral perfusion pressure is aided by this hypertension but, on the other hand, the raised intracranial pressure can lead to undesirable brain shifts. So while the arterial pressure should be controlled it should not be allowed to fall excessively thus compromising cerebral perfusion [169, 170].

### Suxamethonium

The use of suxamethonium is a common factor in many studies in which patients exhibited elevations of intracranial pressure [169, 172]. Indeed, the greatest changes in intracranial tension with intubation occurred in those series where suxamethonium was employed with increases of up to 100 mmHg reported [168, 171]. Elevation of brain tension was much smaller in those series where intubation was facilitated by non-depolarizing relaxants. Pancuronium and tubocurarine gave rise to smaller changes compared with suxamethonium [170, 173]. However, the anaesthetic techniques were not always comparable in individual cases. Patients receiving non-depolarizing relaxants still showed a marked rise in intracranial pressure [173]. Why suxamethonium should be associated with raised intracranial pressure is not entirely clear. Administration of suxamethonium without subsequent intubation produces elevation of spinal fluid pressure in healthy subjects and this has been attributed to increased cerebral blood flow [174]. Others have suggested that the raised pressure is related to muscle fasciculations, the direct action of the drug, or because the period of hyperventilation before intubation is shorter than when non-depolarizing relaxants are used. In the latter cases the longer period of hyperventilation produces a lower level of carbon dioxide which can restore defective autoregulation of the cerebral circulation [177].

## Hypercarbia and hypoxia

The depressed respiration and apnoea associated with induction of anaesthesia and the use of muscle relaxants preceding intubation must result in a fall of oxygen tension and a rise of carbon dioxide level which are of clinical importance when intubation is not carried out immediately. Hypoxia can be reliably prevented by preoxygenation but the increase of carbon dioxide tension goes on until ventilation is resumed. Hypercarbia results in increased cerebral blood flow. It has been shown that for every 1 mmHg elevation of arterial $PCO_2$ over the range between 20 and 60 mmHg, cerebral blood flow increases by 1 ml $min^{-1}$ per 100 g brain tissue [178]. Normal cerebral blood flow is 44 ml $min^{-1}$ per 100 g brain tissue. However, in a well-conducted intubation any small rise in $PCO_2$ is unlikely to contribute significantly to raising intracranial tension [172]. On the other hand, when intubation is prolonged the increase of intracranial pressure can be significant [170]. In one report, intracranial pressure rose above 27 mmHg when the level of carbon dioxide rose by 8.2 mmHg to reach a level of only 39 mmHg at the time of intubation [173].

Hyperventilation immediately after induction is commonly practised not only to prevent hypercarbia but deliberately to reduce $PCO_2$ as a protective measure. The maximum decrease in cerebral blood flow can be obtained by reducing carbon dioxide levels to the range 10–20 mmHg [179], but this results in extreme cerebral vasoconstriction and possible cerebral hypoxaemia. Therefore levels between 30 and 35 mmHg should be aimed for [170]. Another advantage of hyperventilation before intubation is that the low $PCO_2$ may protect against the increased cerebral blood flow as a consequence of the acute elevation of arterial blood pressure that occurs with laryngoscopy and intubation; hypocarbia possibly restores defective autoregulation of cerebral blood flow [177].

Hypoxia has a marked effect on cerebral blood flow. A fall in inspired oxygen concentration of 10% results in an increased cerebral blood flow of 30% [180]. Cerebral oedema is a well recognized complication of severe hypoxaemia.

## Elevated venous pressure due to coughing and straining

Coughing and straining increase intracranial pressure substantially. In one study in patients with intracranial pathology, where induction and intubation were carried out with great care, only one patient showed a marked increase in intracranial tension and this was due to straining on the tube; the intracranial pressure rose by 13 mmHg [173].

An abrupt increase of venous pressure, especially if associated with a fall of arterial pressure, may further compromise cerebral blood flow.

## Inhalation anaesthetics and ketamine

Adequate depth of anaesthesia is desirable before attempting laryngoscopy because it helps to prevent the arterial hypertension that follows intubation. Unfortunately, most volatile halogenated agents produce cerebral vasodilatation which can lead to increased intracranial tension. This can be marked with pre-existing elevated intracranial pressure [181, 182]. Ketamine is also a cerebral vasodilator and has the same danger in patients at risk [180]. Enflurane and isoflurane are the exceptions in that they do not increase intracranial pressure. Inhaling enflurane at concentrations between 0.85 and 3.2% has no effect on cerebral blood flow [170].

Agents that are advisable for induction of

anaesthesia in high risk patients prior to intubation are those which are potentially vasoconstricting, such as thiopentone [183] and a combination of fentanyl and droperidol.

### Other methods

Other suggestions include the administration of thiopentone or trimetaphan immediately before intubation [184], and pretreatment with β-blocking agents [185] or lignocaine [186].

One study involving patients undergoing intracranial surgery found that the technique of giving a second dose of thiopentone was effective in preventing a rise of intracranial tension in most patients [187]. Thiopentone 5 mg kg$^{-1}$ was given followed by muscle relaxant. Three minutes later a second dose of thiopentone 2.5 mg kg$^{-1}$ was administered over 30 s to prevent undue hypotension. Laryngoscopy followed 30 s later and respiration was controlled throughout. However, the authors were doubtful if the technique could be recommended in patients who had already suffered a subarachnoid haemorrhage from an aneurysm for fear of precipitating bleeding, since thiopentone did not prevent a rise of blood pressure at intubation. On the other hand, in other patients, where thiopentone produced a fall of arterial pressure and intracranial tension remained unchanged, there was the risk of underperfusion of compromised tissues.

Elevation of intracerebral pressure in patients can be successfully minimized by employing a very careful technique in intubating patients at risk [170,173]. Helpful measures include the use of liberal amounts of intravenous induction agent; the use of long acting non-depolarizing muscle relaxants, rather than suxamethonium; and awaiting full muscle relaxation before laryngoscopy and intubation.

## THE EYE – INCREASED INTRAOCULAR TENSION

There are several ways in which tracheal intubation may result in an undesirable elevation of intraocular pressure (Table 4). Whatever anaesthetic technique is employed, insertion of the tube itself may increase the tension. The use of suxamethonium to facilitate intubation is a well-demonstrated cause of increased intraocular pressure. During the process of intubation, tension will be grossly

**Table 4**  Causes of raised intraocular tension during tracheal intubation.

| |
|---|
| Increased venous pressure |
|    Coughing |
|    Straining |
|    Respiratory obstruction |
| Suxamethonium |
| Hypoxaemia |
| Hypercarbia |

increased by coughing, straining or any obstruction to venous return. Furthermore, any hypoxia and hypercarbia may increase eye tension.

### Laryngoscopy and Intubation

There appear to be no report on the effects of laryngoscopy alone on ocular pressure. Laryngoscopy and tracheal intubation may produce an increase of intraocular pressure in adults and children. The increased tension follows the same time course as the elevation of arterial pressure [122]. Passage of a tracheal tube may produce a reflex rise of intraocular tension even in the absence of coughing and straining and, even when intubation is preceded by topical analgesia applied to the airways.

### Suxamethonium (see Fig. 9)

Since the original report [190] that suxamethonium raised the intraocular pressure in conscious volunteers as well as in anaesthetized subjects, numerous investigators have studied this relationship. The original findings [191] were soon confirmed by many other workers [192–194]. The normal intraocular tension lies between 15 and 20 mmHg [195]. An average rise of 7.8 mmHg after suxamethonium occurred in one series [191]. In some cases the tension rose by up to 15 mmHg. In another series rises of up to 30 mmHg occurred with an average rise of 19 mmHg. Similar rises were found by other workers in the 1960s [196, 197] as well as by recent workers [198, 199]. Suxamethonium administered by intravenous drip in adults likewise produced elevation of intraocular tension in about half the patients. Increases were also found in infants and small children in whom intramuscular suxamethonium with hyaluronidase was administered [197]. No

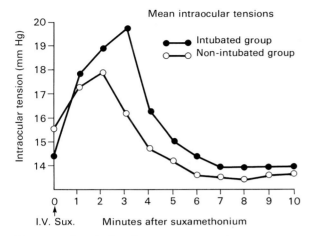

**Figure 9**   Graph showing mean pre- and post-suxamethonium intraocular tensions in intubated and non-intubated patients. Arrow marked 'I.V. Sux' indicates time of administration of suxamethonium. After Pandey *et al.* [201].

elevation of intraocular tension occurred if suxamethonium was injected in patients moderately deeply anaesthetized [191, 200]. Glaucomatous patients do not seem to be at a greater risk than normal patients [194].

### Suxamethonium followed by intubation

Much of the literature on suxamethonium and intraocular tension relates to the effects of the drug itself, measurements being made prior to passage of the tracheal tube. However, some investigators have shown that the elevation of ocular pressure following suxamethonium was further increased when intubation followed [192]. The time course of intraocular hypertension produced by suxamethonium has been studied in patients devoid of systemic or ophthalmic disease [201]. The peak action occurred 2–4 min after suxamethonium was given and had subsided by 6 min. Tropical anaesthesia with lignocaine (4%) was applied to the larynx and trachea before intubation. Tracheal intubation produced a further significant rise but this had vanished within 1 min (Fig. 9). The increase of pressure was usually below 10 mmHg rising by 13 mmHg in one case. In none of these patients did the pressure exceed the upper level of the normal range.

Other studies [198, 199] show a similar pattern of change of intraocular tension. Intubation after suxamethonium produced a further significant

peak of pressure in over half the patients in one series and in 80% in another series. However, elevation of eye tension never exceeded 10 mmHg. Again in all these patients, topical analgesia preceded intubation.

Other workers [196] failed to show a further rise of eye pressure when a tube was inserted in patients who had received suxamethonium.

How suxamethonium increases intraocular tension remains uncertain. Fasciculation and contracture of the external ocular muscles is an important factor [191, 193] but elevation of tension still occurs when the extraocular muscles are cut [197]. Another mechanism may be a vascular one, transient dilatation of the choroidal blood vessels [202].

Several specific techniques to reduce or prevent the elevation of ocular tension created by suxamethonium have been advocated.

### Pretreatment with non-depolarizing muscle relaxants

Drugs that prevent fasciculation might be expected to be at least partly effective. Unfortunately, the evidence is conflicting.

Many workers have found these drugs effective. Hexafluorenium has been effectively employed [203]. Gallamine (20 mg) or d-tubocurarine (3 mg) given 3 min prior to suxamethonium was successful in both normal and glaucomatous eyes [204, 205]. In these studies, however, intubation was not carried out.

Other workers have found opposing results. Ocular tension rose in spite of pretreatment with d-tubocurarine in one study [206] whilst others found the effect of pretreatment to be inconsistent albeit with very small rises of tension [207].

Recent studies [198, 199] compared the effect on intraocular pressure between control groups and groups pretreated with gallamine (20 mg), d-tubocurarine (3 mg), and pancuronium (1 mg). No significant difference was found between any of the groups as regards the incidence or severity of elevated intraocular pressure.

### Suxamethonium self taming

Pretreatment with small sub-paralysing doses of suxamethonium prior to administration of the main bolus of the drug reduces muscle fasciculation. However, a small dose of suxamethonium can itself produce elevation of intraocular tension and furthermore does not prevent the usual rise of eye tension associated with full doses of suxamethonium. This technique, therefore, offers no solution to the problem in the patient where the integrity of the eye is lost or threatened [208].

## Methods of Minimizing Elevation of Intraocular Pressure Associated with Intubation

### High doses of non-depolarizing muscle relaxants

An alternative to suxamethonium in the rapid sequence intubation technique has constantly been sought for emergency eye surgery. Self taming cannot be relied upon to inhibit elevation of intraocular pressure when suxamethonium is used [209]. High doses of the newer muscle relaxants have been investigated. Vecuronium in a dose of 0.2 mg kg$^{-1}$ can produce good intubating conditions in a mean time of 45 s (120 s in some subjects) from loss of eyelash reflex to intubation. Vecuronium in a dose of 0.25 mg kg$^{-1}$ can produce satisfactory relaxation within 60 s for emergency intubation, a period comparable to suxamethonium in unpremedicated patients [210] and 0.2 mg kg$^{-1}$ will produce satisfactory intubating conditions in opiate premedicated patients. Conditions are excellent in 60% of patients and adequate in the remainder [211].

These workers showed that while intraocular pressure increased in one-third of cases intubated with their vecuronium regimen, the rise was modest (mean 3.3 mm; 5 mm being the worst). The increase in pressure waned within minutes, whereas elevation of the intraocular tension with suxamethonium may be prolonged. Vecuronium reduces intraocular pressure and it has been advocated as the relaxant of choice in penetrating eye injuries requiring emergency tracheal intubation and general anaesthesia. However, the large doses needed to achieve a fast enough onset may result in long and unpredictable paralysis.

Administration of vecuronium before injection of the induction agent has been suggested as a means of achieving excellent relaxation for tracheal intubation without the prolonged onset time (compared with suxamethonium). The patient is warned of the weakness that develops after the relaxant has been given. When hand grip is lost, the intravenous induction agent is injected and intubation can proceed almost immediately [212]. Atracurium in doses comparable to those in the high dose vecuronium technique produces equal relaxation but is accompanied by marked and possibly undesirable cardiovascular depression [213]. High dose pancuronium has also been tested but prolongation of paralysis may be excessive [214]. High dose d-tubocurarine does reduce intraocular pressure, but even in increased dosage the onset time is too long [215]. Furthermore, the resultant hypotension and bradycardia may be undesirable.

The recommendation to use high dose vecuronium has been challenged by the introduction of rocuronium (see below) which, when used in high doses, has an onset time to excellent or good intubating conditions of half that of vecuronium [216].

### Alternatives to suxamethonium

Rocuronium is a newer steroidal non-depolarizing muscle relaxant related chemically to vecuronium. It has minimal effects on intraocular pressure. It has a much shorter duration of action but, in particular, the onset time is significantly shorter. Compared with suxamethonium 1 mg kg$^{-1}$, rocuronium 0.6 mg kg$^{-1}$ produced similar mean times to intubating conditions [217, 218]. Increasing the dose of rocuronium to between 0.9 and 1.2 mg kg$^{-1}$ shortened the onset time to equal that of suxamethonium [219].

Because of its fast onset time and minimum changes in intraocular tension, rocuronium would appear to be an ideal substitute for suxamethonium in emergency surgery for penetrating eye injuries where a rapid sequence technique is indicated (Fig. 10). Giving the drug before administering the induction agent, as with vecuronium, would further reduce the time to intubation [220]. One study found only a small improvement in intubating conditions when rocuronium preceded intravenous thiopentone induction. Better results were seen when propofol was substituted for thiopentone [221].

### High doses of induction agent

All the commonly used intravenous anaesthetic agents, volatile inhaled anaesthetics and narcotic analgesics tend to lower intraocular tension. For instance, large doses of intravenous induction agent and atracurium 0.6–0.8 mg kg$^{-1}$ provide excellent conditions with minimal changes in intraocular pressure [222].

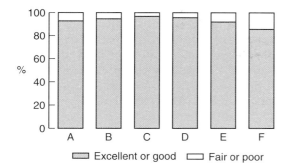

*Group A*: rocuronium followed by thiopental 5 mg kg⁻¹ and intubation at 90 s.

*Group B*: as in Group A but intubation at 60 s.

*Group C*: thiopental 5 mg kg⁻¹ followed by suxamethonium and intubation at 90 s.

*Group D*: as in Group C but intubation at 60 s.

*Group E*: thiopental 5 mg kg⁻¹ followed by rocuronium and intubation at 90 s.

*Group F*: as in Group E but intubation at 60 s.

**Figure 10**   Comparison of suxamethonium and rocuronium for rapid sequence induction of anaesthesia. After Connolly *et al.* [221].

Ketamine is possibly the exception, although the changes are small [222].

## Propofol

When propofol rather than thiopentone is used as the induction agent, the elevation of intraocular pressure with intubation is less [223]. Propofol is even more protective of increases in intraocular tension in patients suffering from glaucoma [224]. Similarly, propofol is superior to etomidate [225].

### Laryngeal mask airway

Changes in intraocular pressure are significantly less when a laryngeal mask airway (LMA) is inserted compared with conventional tracheal intubation [121, 123, 225]. In one study the greatest rise of tension occurred at extubation. This was 2.3 mmHg with the LMA but 14.5 mm with a tracheal tube [121]. Another investigation was performed in children of ages 1–7 years. In contrast to the marked increases of blood pressure, heart rate and intraocular pressure seen when a tracheal tube was inserted, the LMA under a similar anaesthetic regimen produced no changes at all [122] (Fig. 11).

The combination of propofol induction followed by the insertion of an LMA appeared to be a highly satisfactory technique for introcular surgery in patients with glaucoma. Compared with the tracheal tube, no adverse changes of intraocular pressure occurred [224]. However, careful screening is required to eliminate patients with contraindications to the use of a laryngeal mask. Furthermore, the method should only be used by those with good experience in insertion and ventilation with the LMA.

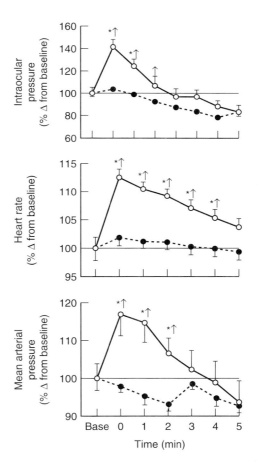

**Figure 11**   Comparison of percentage changes (%△) in intraocular pressure, heart rate and mean arterial pressure over baseline (Base) values (100%) after the insertion of a laryngeal mask airway (●) or tracheal tube (○). Time zero is the time of insertion of the airway device. Error bars are ± SEM. *$p < 0.05$ compared with baseline values. ↑$p < 0.05$ compared with laryngeal mask group. After Watcha [122].

## β-Blocking agents

The use of β-adrenergic blocking agents is based on the suggestion that increases of introcular tension are mediated by β-adrenergic pathways [226]. Pretreatment with propranolol may limit the rise of intraocular tension, but it is uncertain whether this is achieved primarily or secondary to the drug's effect on lowering blood pressure and heart rate or some other mechanism. Cardiovascular depression may be a serious consequence in some patients.

Topical β-blocking agents have been used successfully in the treatment of glaucoma. However, pretreatment with the β-blocking topical timolol ophthalmic solution was ineffective in preventing intraocular tension changes when tracheal intubation followed a standard thiopentone and suxamethonium rapid induction regimen [227].

## Topical analgesia of larynx and trachea

Surface analgesia is effective in reducing the further increase of pressure from suxamethonium which intubation imposes [192, 196, 228].

## Acetazolamide (Diamox)

This carbonic anhydrase inhibitor has been advocated to prevent elevation of intraocular tension [229] but needs further evaluation [202].

## Haemodynamic Changes

### Arterial blood pressure

Tracheal intubation often results in marked elevation of arterial blood pressure. Fortunately, these changes are relatively unimportant since any rise of arterial blood pressure leads to displacement of aqueous humour from the anterior chamber and blood from the choroidal vessels [230]. It has been shown [202] that in normal eyes intraocular pressure remains constant over a fairly wide range of normal blood pressures, but once mean arterial pressure falls to below 90 mmHg then intraocular tension also falls.

### Venous pressure

If the stimulation of intubation results in an increased venous pressure, such as is produced by cough or straining or respiratory obstruction, then this is transmitted immediately to the globe [191].

The choriocapillaries distend and back pressure is produced on the aqueous veins draining the canal of Schlemm. The highest elevations of intraocular pressure measured have occurred in venous obstruction produced by coughing [228], although they returned to normal levels very quickly after relief of venous obstruction. Respiration obstruction may increase intravenous tension by up to 60% whilst a slight cough may elevate the pressure.

## Hypoxaemia and Hypercarbia

Hypoxaemia and hypercarbia may easily arise during intubation especially when apnoea is produced by muscle relaxants. In dogs, hypoventilation elevates the intraocular tension and 5% carbon dioxide added to the inspired mixture produces a marked rise. The ocular pressure can be lowered by hyperventilation [230]. Similar changes have been found in man [202]. Hypoxaemia may also tend to elevate intraocular tension [230].

## Conclusion

Suxamethonium greatly facilitates tracheal intubation and it should not necessarily be withheld in ophthalmic surgical cases because of its tendency to produce only modest increases of intraocular tension. In any case, increases vanish within minutes, which is a sufficient interval between induction and incision of the eye. However, in elective surgery, the eye which has been affected by chronic glaucoma is equally at risk from undue elevation of intraocular tension. Based on ophthlamic studies of the eye in advanced glaucoma, it appears that the intraocular tension should be kept below 20 mmHg to avoid loss of central vision [224]. Suxamethonium is best avoided in these cases and intubation can be carried out with a combination of an adequate induction agent and non-depolarizing muscle relaxant.

An LMA may offer an appropriate alternative to tracheal intubation in those cases where intraocular pressure changes are undesirable, e.g. when diagnostic measurements of intraocular pressure are being made.

Suxamethonium alone should not be used for the first time while the eye has been opened and is definitely contraindicated in penetrating eye injuries. Unfortunately, it is in these very cases that suxamethonium is indicated to facilitate intubation when the patient has a full stomach. Pretreatment with non-depolarizing relaxants has been shown to be unreliable in preventing a rise of pressure. Nevertheless, the sequence of pretreatment with d-tubocurarine or gallamine before induction of anaesthesia with adequate barbiturate dosage and suxamethonium prior to intubation, has not been associated with a single published report of loss of intraocular contents. The safety of this method in emergency surgery for penetrating eye injury is supported by extensive practical experience [231]. Some of the newer non-depolarizing relaxants may well offer an alternative to suxamethonium.

## MISCELLANEOUS EFFECTS

Many other undesirable pathophysiological consequences could be indirectly attributed to tracheal intubation. The use of suxamethonium is associated with a host of unwanted effects that include postoperative muscle pain, elevation of serum potassium level and malignant hyperpyrexia. Detailed examination of these subjects is dealt with in other texts.

Unusual physiological effects of tracheal intubation continue to be reported. A recent study indicates that plasma β-endorphin level is activated by intubation. Release of endorphins is thought to play a part in the endocrine response to surgical stress. Since endorphin release can be prevented by topical anaesthesia to the airways or deeper levels of anaesthesia, it suggests that ascending neurological pathways exist analogous to those that mediate cardiovascular responses to tracheal intubation [232].

## KEY POINTS

- The enormous range of ways of inhibiting the undesirable cardiovascular effects of tracheal intubation is a manifestation of the unreliability and ineffectiveness of most of them.

- In patients who are at risk:
  - Preoperative control of blood pressure and heart rate is as important as any technique used intraoperatively.
  - An adequate level of anaesthetic, supplemented by carefully selected adjuvant drugs, can minimize the harmful effects of intubation.
  - Appropriate haemodynamic monitoring at induction is obligatory.
  - Topical anaesthetic agents used alone are not reliable.
  - Where relevant it is worth considering using a laryngeal mask airway rather than a tracheal tube.

- Routine pulse oximetry and routine oxygenation before induction of anaesthesia have undoubtedly reduced the incidence and severity of hypoxaemia associated with tracheal intubation.

- The prevention of undesirable increases of intracranial and intraocular pressure is based on providing an adequate level of anaesthesia and the avoidance of suxamethonium where possible.

- Some of the newer non-depolarizing muscle relaxants may be regarded as a satisfactory substitute for suxamethonium.

- Where feasible, inserting a laryngeal mask airway rather than a tracheal tube can be advantageous in avoiding elevation of intraocular tension.

## REFERENCES

1  Reid L. C. and Brace D. E. Irritation of the respiratory tract and its reflex effect on the heart. *Surgery, Gynecology and Obstetrics* 1940; **70**: 157.

2  Katz R. L. and Bigger J. T. Cardiac arrhythmias during anesthesia and operation. *Anesthesiology* 1970; **33:** 193.

3  Burstein C. L., LoPinto F. J. and Newman W. Electrocardiographic studies during endotracheal intubation. I. Effects during usual routine technics. *Anesthesiology*, 1950; **11:** 224.

4  Burstein C. L., Woloshin G. and Newman W. Electrocardiographic studies during endotracheal intubation. II. Effects during general anaesthesia and intravenous procaine. *Anesthesiology* 1950; **11:** 229.

5  King B. D., Harris L. C., Greifenstein F. E, Elder J. D. and Dripps R. D. Reflex circulatory responses to direct laryngoscopy and tracheal intubation performed during general anesthesia. *Anesthesiology* 1951; **12:** 556.

6  Noble M. J. and Derrick W. S. Changes in electrocardiogram during endotracheal intubation and induction of anaesthesia. *Canadian Anaesthetists Society Journal* 1950; **6:** 276.

7  DeVault M., Greifenstein F. E. and Harris L. C. Circulatory responses to endotracheal intubation in light general anesthesia – the effect of atropine and phentolamine. *Anesthesiology* 1960; **21:** 360.

8  Wycoff C. C. Endotracheal intubation: effects on blood pressure and pulse rate. *Anesthesiology* 1960; **21:** 153.

9  Takeshima K., Noda K. and Higaki M. Cardiovascular response to rapid anesthesia induction and endotracheal intubation. *Anesthesia and Analgesia* 1964; **43:** 201.

10  Sagarminaga J. and Wynands J. E. Atropine and electrical activity of the heart during induction of anaesthesia in children. *Canadian Anaesthetists Society Journal* 1963; **10:** 328.

11  Gibbs J. M. The effects of endotracheal intubation on cardiac rate and rhythm. *New Zealand Medical Journal* 1967; **66:** 465.

12  Dottori O., Lof B., Axelson and Ygge H. Heart rate and arterial blood pressure during different forms of induction of anaesthesia in patients with mitral stenosis and constrictive pericarditis. *British Journal of Anaesthesia* 1970; **42:** 849.

13  Forbes A. M. and Dally F. G. Acute hypertension during induction of anaesthesia and endotracheal intubation in normotensive man. *British Journal of Anaesthesia* 1970; **42:** 618.

14  Prys-Roberts C., Greene L. T., Meloche R. and Foex P. Studies of anaesthesia in relation to hypertension. 11 Haemodynamic consequences of induction and endotracheal intubation. *British Journal of Anaesthesia* 1971; **43:** 531.

15  Prys-Roberts, C., Foex P., Biro G. P. and Roberts J. G. Studies of anaesthesia in relation to hypertension. V: Adrenergic beta-receptor blockade. *British Journal of Anaesthesia* 1973; **45:** 671.

16  Stoelting R. K. Attenuation of blood pressure response to laryngoscopy and tracheal intubation with sodium nitroprusside. *Anesthesia and Analgesia* 1979; **58:** 116.

17  Bullington J., Mouton Perry S. M., Rigby J. *et al.* The effect of advancing age on the sympathetic response to laryngoscopy and tracheal intubation. *Anesthesia and Analgesia* 1989; **68:** 603.

18  Sear J. W., Jewkes C. and Foex P. Does the choice of antihypertensive therapy influence haemodynamic responses to induction, laryngoscopy and intubation? *British Journal of Anaesthesia* 1994; **73:** 303.

19  Bedford R. F. and Feinstein B. Hospital admission blood pressure: a predictor of hypertension following endotracheal intubation. *Anesthesia and Analgesia* 1980; **59:** 367.

20  Fox E. J., Sklar G. S., Hill C. H., Villanueva R. and King B. D. Complications related to the pressor response to endotracheal intubation. *Anesthesiology* 1977; **47:** 524.

21  Fox E. J., Sklar G. S., Hill C. H., Villaneuva R. and King B. D. Complications related to the pressor response to endotracheal intubation. *Anesthesiology* 1977; **47:** 525.

22  Hodgkinson R., Hussain F. J. and Hayashi R. H. Systemic and pulmonary blood pressure during caesarean section in parturients with gestational hypertension. *Canadian Anaesthetists Society Journal* 1980; **27:** 389.

24  Lawes E. G., Downing J. W., Duncan *et al.* Fentanyl-droperidol supplementation of rapid sequence induction in the presence of severe pregnancy-induced and pregnacy-aggravated hypertension. *British Journal of Anaesthesia* 1987; **59:** 138.

25  Roy L. W., Edelist G. and Gilbert B. Myocardial ischemia during non-cardiac surgical procedures in patients with coronary artery disease. *Anesthesiology* 1979; **51:** 393.

26  Prys-Roberts C. and Meloch R. Management of anesthesia in patients with hypertension or ischemic heart disease. *International Anesthesiology Clinics* 1980; **18:** 181.

27  Barash P. G., Kopriva C. J. and Giles R. W. *et al.* Global ventricular function and intubation: Radionuclear profiles. *Anesthesiology* 1980; **53:** S-109.

28  Rao T. L. K., Jacobs K. H. and El-Etr A. A. Reinfarction following anesthesia in patients with myocardial infarction. *Anesthesiology* 1983; **59:** 499.

29  Kaplan J. A. (ed.) *Hemodynamic Monitoring in Cardiac Anesthesia.* New York: Grune and Stratton. 1979, 109.

30  Cokkinos D. V. and Voridis E. M. Constancy of rate-pressure product in pacing induced angina pectoris. *British Heart Journal* 1975; **38:** 39.

31  Slogoff S. and Keats A. S. Randomized trial of primary anesthetic agents on outcome of coronary artery bypass operations. *Anesthesiology* 1989; **70:** 179.

32  Derbyshire D. R., Chmielewski A., Fell D., Vater M., Achola K. and Smith G. Plasma catecholamine response to tracheal intubation. *British Journal of Anaesthesia* 1983; **55:** 855.

33  Russell W. J., Morris R. G., Frewin D. B. and Drew S. E. Changes in plasma catecholamine concentrations during endotracheal intubation. *British Journal of Anaesthesia* 1981; **53:** 837.

34  Stanley T. H., Berman L., Green O. and Robertson D. Plasma catecholamine and cortisol responses to fentanyl-oxygen anesthesia for coronary artery operations. *Anesthesiology* 1980; **53:** 250.

35  Hoar P. F., Nelson N. T., Mangano D. I., Bainton C. R. and Hickey R. F. Adrenergic responses to morphine diazepam anesthesia for myocardial revascularization. *Anesthesia and Analgesia* 1981; **60:** 406.

36  Zsigmond E. K. and Kumar S. M. Endotracheal intubation and catecholamines after anesthesia induction. *Proceedings of the 7th World Congress of Anaesthesiologists*, Amsterdam: Excerpta Medica. 1980, 447.

37  Allen R. W., James M. F. M. and Uys P. C. Attenuation of the pressor response to tracheal intubation in hypertensive proteinuric pregnant patients by lignocaine, alfentanil and magnesium. *British Journal of Anaesthesia* 1991; **66:** 223.

38  James M. F. M., Beer R. E. and Essex J. D. Intravenous magnesium sulfate inhibits catecholamine release associated with tracheal intubation. *Anesthesia and Analgesia* 1989; **68:** 772.

39  Crawford D. C., Fell D., Achola K. J. and Smith G. Effects of alfentanil on the pressor and catecholamine responses to tracheal intubation. *British Journal of Anaesthesia* 1987; **59:** 707.

40  McKeating K., Bali I. M. and Dundee J. W. The effects of thiopentone and propofol on upper airway integrity. *Anaesthesia* 1988; **43:** 638.

41  Keaveny J. P. and Knell P. J. Intubation under induction doses of propofol. *Anaesthesia* 1988; **43** (Suppl.): 80.

42  Schaefer H.-G. and Marsch S. C. U. Comparison of orthodox with fibreoptic orotracheal intubation under total I.V. anaesthesia. *British Journal of Anaesthesia* 1991; **66:** 608.

43  Bennett G. M. and Stanley T. H. Human cardiovascular responses to endotracheal intubation during morphine-$N_2O$ and fentanyl-$N_2O$ anesthesia. *Anesthesiology* 1980; **52:** 520.

44  Kautto U-M. Attenuation of the circulatory response to laryngoscopy and intubation by fentanyl. *Acta Anaesthesiologica Scandinavica* 1982; **26:** 217.

45  Laubie M., Schmitt H., Canellas J., Roquebert J. and Demichel P. Centrally mediated bradycardia and hypotension induced by narcotic analgesics: dextromoramide and fentanyl. *European Journal of Pharmacology* 1974; **21:** 66.

46  Tomori Z. and Widdicombe J. G. Muscular bronchomotor and cardiovascular reflexes elicited by mechanical stimulation of the respiratory tract. *Journal of Physiology* 1969; **200:** 25.

47  Tammisto T., Takki S. and Toikka P. A comparison of the circulatory effects in man of the analgesics fentanyl, pentazocine and pethidine. *British Journal of Anaesthesia* 1970; **42:** 317.

48  Graves C. L., Downs N. H. and Browne, A. B. Cardiovascular effects of minimal quantities of Innovar, fentanyl and droperidol in man. *Anesthesia and Analgesia* 1975; **54:** 15.

49  Reitan J. A., Stengert K. B., Wymore M. L. and Martucci B. W. Central vagal control of fentanyl-induced bradycardia during halothane anaesthesia. *Anesthesia and Analgesia* 1978; **57:** 31.

50  Stanley T. H. and Webster L. R. Anesthetic requirements and cardiovascular effects of fentanyl-oxygen and fentanyl-diazepam-oxygen anesthesia in man. *Anesthesia and Analgesia* 1978; **57:** 411.

51  Lunn J. K., Stanley T. H., Eisele J., Webster L. and Woodward A. High dose fentanyl anesthesia for coronary artery surgery: plasma fentanyl concentrations and influence of nitrous oxide on cardiovascular responses. *Anesthesia and Analgesia* 1979; **58:** 390.

52  Arens J. F., Benbow B. P. and Ochsner J. L. Morphine anesthesia for aorto-coronary bypass procedures. *Anesthesia and Analgesia* 1972; **51:** 901.

53  Kistner J. R., Miller E. D., Lake C. L. *et al*. Indices of myocardial oxygenation during coronary revascularization in man with morphine versus halothane anesthesia. *Anesthesiology* 1979; **50:** 324.

54  Black T. E., Kay B. and Healy T. E. J. Reducing the haemodynamic responses to laryngoscopy and intubation. A comparison of alfentanil with fentanyl. *Anaesthesia* 1984; **39:** 883.

55  Scheinin B., Scheinin M., Vuorinen J. and Lindgren L. Alfentanil obtunds the cardiovascular and sympathoadrenal responses to suxamethonium-facilitated laryngoscopy and intubation. *British Journal of Anaesthesia* 1989; **62:** 385

56  Stoelting R. K. and Peterson C. Circulatory changes during anesthetic induction: impact of d-tubocurarine pretreatment, thiamylal, succinylcholine, laryngoscopy and tracheal lidocaine. *Anesthesia and Analgesia* 1976; **55:** 77.

57  Stoelting R. K. Circulatory changes during direct laryngoscopy and tracheal intubation: Influence of duration of laryngoscopy with or without prior lidocaine. *Anesthesiology* 1977; **47:** 381.

58  Kautto U-M. and Heinonen J. Attenuation of circulatory response laryngoscopy and tracheal intubation: a comparison of two methods of topical anaesthesia. *Acta Anaesthesiologica Scandinavica* 1982; **26**: 599.

59  Rosenberg P. H., Heinonen J. and Takasari M. Lidocaine concentration in blood after topical anesthesia of the upper respiratory tract. *Acta Anaesthesiologica Scandinavica* 1980; **24**: 125.

60  Mirakhur R. K. Bradycardia with laryngeal spraying in children. *Acta Anaesthesiologica Scandinavica* 1982; **26**: 130.

61  Ward R. J., Allen G. D., Deveny L. J. and Green H. D. Halothane and the cardiovascular response to endotracheal intubation. *Anesthesia and Analgesia* 1965; **44**: 248.

62  Abou-Madi M., Keszler H. and Yacoub O. A method for prevention of cardiovascular reactions to laryngoscopy and intubation. *Canadian Anaesthetists Society Journal* 1975; **22**: 316.

63  Gianelly R., von der Groeben J. O., Spivack A. P. *et al.* Effects of lidocaine on ventricular arrhythmias in patients with coronary artery disease. *New England Journal of Medicine* 1967; **277**: 1215.

64  Bromage R. and Robson J. Concentrations of lignocaine in the blood after intravenous, intramuscular, epidural and endotracheal administration. *Anaesthesia* 1961; **16**: 461.

65  Fassoulaki A. and Kaniaris P. Does atropine premedication affect the cardiovascular response to laryngoscopy and intubation? *British Journal of Anaesthesia* 1982; **54**: 1065.

66  Sawhney S. and Dhar C. L. Pressor response to laryngoscopy and endotracheal intubation: effect of anticholinergic premedication. *Journal of Anaesthesiology and Clinical Pharmacology* 1994; **10**: 95.

67  Denlinger J. K., Ellison N. and Ominsky A. J. Effects of intratracheal lidocaine on circulatory responses to tracheal intubation. *Anesthesiology* 1974; **41**: 409.

68  Abou-Madi M. N., Keszler H. and Yacoub J. M. Cardiovascular reactions to laryngoscopy and tracheal intubation following small and large intravenous doses of lidocaine. *Canadian Anaesthetists Society Journal* 1977; **24**: 12.

69  Hamill J. F., Bedford R. F., Weaver D. C. and Colohan A. R. Lidocaine before endotracheal intubation: intravenous or laryngotracheal. *Anesthesiology* 1981; **55**: 578.

70  Thomas D. V. Intratracheal lidocaine – local anesthesia or direct cardiac effect? *Anesthesiology* 1975; **42**: 517.

71  Bidwai A. V., Bidwai V. A., Rogers C. R. and Stanley T. H. Blood pressure and pulse-rate responses to endotracheal extubation with and without prior injection of lidocaine. *Anesthesiology* 1979; **51**: 171.

72  Hood D. D., Dewan D. M., Francis M. J. III, Floyd H. M. and Bogard T. D. The use of nitroglycerin in preventing the hypertensive response to tracheal intubation in severe pre-eclampsia. *Anesthesiology* 1985; **63**: 329.

73  Elkayam U. and Aronow W. S. Glyceryl trinitrate (nitroglycerine) ointment and isosorbide dinitrate: a review of their pharmacological properties and therapeutic use. *Drugs* 1982; **23**: 165.

74  Kamra S., Wig J. and Sapru R. P. Topical nitroglycerine. A safeguard against pressor responses to tracheal intubation. *Anaesthesia* 1986; **41**: 1087.

75  Mahajan R. P., Ramachandran R., Saxena N. Topical nitroglycerine prevents the pressor response to tracheal intubation and sternotomy in patients undergoing coronary artery bypass graft surgery. *British Journal of Anaesthesia* 1993; **48**: 297.

76  Hatano Y., Imai R., Komatsu K. and Mori K. Intravenous administration of isosorbide dinitrate attenuates the pressor response to laryngoscopy and tracheal intubation. *Acta Anaesthesiologica Scandinavica* 1989; **33**: 214.

77  Bijoria K., Wig J., Bajaj A. and Sapru R. P. Isosorbide dinitrate spray. Attenuation of cardiovascular responses to laryngoscopy and intubation. *Anaesthesia* 1992; **47**: 523.

78  Kumar N., Batra Y. K., Bala I. and Gopalan S. Nifedipine attenuates the hypertensive response to tracheal intubation in pregnancy-induced hypertension. *Canadian Journal of Anaesthesia-Journal Canadien d'Anesthesie* 1993; **40**: 329.

79  Yaku H., Mikawa K., Maekawa N. and Obara H. Effects of verapamil on the cardiovascular responses to tracheal intubation. *British Journal of Anaesthesia* 1992; **68**: 85.

80  Nishikawa T. and Namiki A. Attenuation of the pressor response to laryngoscopy and tracheal intubation with intravenous verapamil. *Acta Anaesthesiologica Scandinavica* 1989; **33**: 232.

81  Singh B. N. and Roche A. H. G. Effects of intravenous verapamil on hemodynamics in patients with heart disease. *American Heart Journal* 1977; **94**: 593.

82  Omote K., Kirita A., Namiki A. and Iwasaki H. Effects of nicardipine on the circulatory responses to tracheal intubation in normotensive and hypertensive patients. *Anaesthesia* 1992; **47**: 24.

83  McCarthy G. J., Hainsworth M., Lindsay K., Wright J. M. and Brown T. A. Pressor response to tracheal intubation after sublingual captopril. *Anaesthesia* 1990; **45**: 243.

84  Bottcher M., Behrens K., Moller E. A. *et al.* ACE inhibitor premedication attenuates sympathetic responses during surgery. *British Journal of Anaesthesia* 1994; **72**: 633.

85  Mikawa K., Ikegaki J., Maekawa N. *et al.* Effects of

prostaglandin E1 on the cardiovascular response to tracheal intubation. *Journal of Clinical Anaesthesia* 1990; **2**: 420.

86  Siedlecki J. Disturbances in the function of cadiovascular system in patients following endotracheal intubation and attempts of their prevention by pharmacological blockade of sympathetic system. *Anaesthesia, Resuscitation and Intensive Care Therapy* 1975; **3**: 107.

87  Saitoh N., Mikawa K., Kitamura S. *et al.* Effects of trimetaphan on the cardiovascular response to tracheal intubation. *British Journal of Anaesthesia* 1991; **66**: 340.

88  Orko R., Pouttu J., Ghignone M. *et al.* Effect of clonidine on haemodynamic responses to endotracheal inubation and on gastric acidity. *Acta Anaesthesiologica Scandinavica* 1987; **31**: 325.

89  Ghigone M., Quintin L., Duke P. C. *et al.* Effects of clonidine on narcotic requirements and hemodynamic response during induction of fentanyl anesthesia and endotracheal intubation. *Canadian Journal of Anaesthesiology* 1986; **64**: 36.

90  Batra Y. K., Indu B. and Puri G. D. Attenuation of pulse rate and blood pressure response to laryngoscopy and tracheal intubation by clonidine. *International Journal of Clinical Pharmacology and Therapeutic Toxicology* 1988; **26**: 360.

91  Siedlecki J. Disturbances in the function of cardiovascular system in patients following endotracheal intubation and attempts of their prevention by pharmacological blockade of sympathetic system. *Anaesthesia and Intensive Care* 1975; **3**: 107.

92  Greenbaum R., Cooper R., Hulme A. and Mackintosh J. P. In: *Recent Advances in Anesthesiology and Resuscitation*. The effect of induction of anaesthesia on intracranial pressure. Amsterdam: Excerpta Medica. 1975; 794.

93  Kaplan J. A., Dunbar R. W. Bland J. W., Sumpter R. and Jones E. L. Propranolol and cardiac surgery: a problem for the anesthesiologist? *Anesthesia and Analgesia* 1975; **54**: 571.

94  Kaplan J. A. and Dunbar R. W. Propranolol and surgical anesthesia. *Anesthesia and Analgesia* 1976; **55**: 1.

95  Kopriva C. J., Brown A. C. D. and Pappas G. Hemodynamics during general anesthesia in patients receiving propranolol. *Anesthesiology* 1978; **48**: 28.

96  Slogoff S., Keats A. S. and Ott E. Preoperative propranolol therapy and aortocoronary by pass operation. *Journal of the American Medical Association* 1978; **240**: 1487.

97  Prys-Roberts C. Beta-receptor blockade and tracheal intubation. *Anaesthesia* 1981; **36**: 803.

98  McCammon R. L., Hilgenberg J. C. and Stoelting R. K. Effect of propranolol on circulatory responses to induction of diazepam-nitrous oxide anesthesia and to endotracheal intubation. *Anesthesia and Analgesia* 1981; **60**: 579.

99  Farnon D. and Curran J. Beta-receptor blockade and tracheal intubation. *Anaesthesia* 1981; **36**: 803.

100  Takahashi T., Sakai T., Nakajo N. *et al.* Clinical use of acebutolol (beta blocking agent) during induction of anesthesia accompanied with crash intubation technique. *Japanese Journal of Anesthesiology* 1978; **27**: 37.

101  Helfman S. M., Gold M. I., DeLisser E. A. and Herrington C. A. Which drug prevents tachycardia and hypertension associated with tracheal intubation: lidocaine, fentanyl, or esmolol. *Anesthesia and Analgesia* 1991; **72**: 482

102  Liu P. L., Gatt S., Gugino L. D. *et al.* Esmolol for control of increases in heart rate and blood pressure during tracheal intubation after thiopentone and succinylcholine. *Canadian Anaesthetists Society Journal* 1986; **33**: 556.

103  Oxorn D., Knox J. W. D. and Hill J. Bolus dose of esmolol for the prevention of perioperative hypertension and tachycardia. *Canadian Journal of Anaesthesia* 1990; **37**: 206.

104  Leslie J. B., Kalayjian R. W., McLoughlin T. M., Plachetka J. R. Attenuation of the hemodynamic responses to endotracheal intubation with preinduction intravenous labetalol. *Journal of Clinical Anesthesia* 1989; **1**: 194.

105  Ramanathan J., Sibai B. M., Mabie W. C. *et al.* The use of labetalol for attenuation of the hypertensive response to endotracheal intubation in preeclampsia. *American Journal of Obstetrics and Gynecology* 1988; **159**: 650.

106  Inada E., Cullen D. J., Nemeskal A. R. and Teplick R. Effect of labetalol or lidocaine on the hemodynamic response to intubation: a controlled randomized double-blind study. *Journal of Clinical Anesthesia* 1989; **1**: 207.

107  Ashton W. B., James M. F. M., Janicki P. and Uys P. C. Attenuation of the pressor response to tracheal intubation by magnesium sulphate with and without alfentanil in hypertensive proteinuric patients undergoing caesarean section. *British Journal of Anaesthesia* 1991; **67**: 741.

108  Karhunen U., Heinoen J. and Tammisto T. The effects of tubocurarine and alcuronium on suxamethonium induced changes in cardiac rate and rhythm. *Acta Anaesthesiologica Scandinavica* 1972; **16**: 3.

109  Long U. S., Zebrowski M. E. and Graney W. F. Awake vs. anesthetized intubation: a comparison of hemodynamic responses. *Anesthesiology* 1982; **57**: A30.

110  Carr R. J. and Belani K. G. Clinical assessment of the Augustine Guide (tm) for endotracheal intubation. *Anesthesia and Analgesia* 1993; **76**: S 37.

111  Krafft P., Fitzgerald R. D., Pernerstorfer T. *et al.* A

new device for blind oral intubation in routine and difficult airway management. *European Journal of Anaesthesiology* 1994; **11:** 207.

112 Pernerstorfer T., Krafft P., Fitzgerald R. D. *et al.* Stress response to tracheal intubation: direct laryngoscopy compared with blind oral intubation. *Anaesthesia* 1995; **50:** 17.

113 Scheck P. A. E. Measurements of the pressure of the laryngoscope during tracheal intubation. *Anaesthesia* 1982; **37:** 370.

114 Cozanitis D. A., Nuuttila K., Merrett J. D. and Kala R. Influence of laryngoscope design on heart rate and rhythm changes during intubation. *Canadian Anaesthetists Society Journal* 1984; **31:** 155.

115 Hawkyard S., Morrison A., Doyle L., Croton R. and Wake P. Fibreoptic intubation: attenuating the hypertensive response to laryngoscopy and intubation. *British Journal of Anaesthesia* 1989; **63:** 624P.

116 Hawkyard S. J., Morrison A., Doyle L. A., Croton R. S. and Wake P. N. Attenuating the hypertensive response to laryngoscopy and endotracheal intubation using awake fibreoptic intubation. *Acta Anaesthesiologica Scandinavica* 1992; **36:** 10.

117 Schrader S., Ovassapian A., Dykes M. H. and Avram M. Cardiovascular changes during awake rigid and fiberoptic laryngoscopy. *Anesthesiology* 1987; **67:** A28.

118 Smith J. E., Mackenzie A. A., Sanghera S. S. and Scott-Knight V. C. E. Cardiovascular effects of fibrescope-guided nasotracheal intubation. *Anaesthesia* 1989; **44:** 907.

119 Finfer S. R., MacKenzie S. I. P., Saddler J. M. and Watkins T. G. L. Cardiovascular responses to tracheal intubation: A comparison of direct laryngoscopy and fibreoptic intubation. *Anaesthesia and Intensive Care* 1989; **17:** 44.

120 Smith J. E., King M. J., Yanny H. F. *et al.* Effect of fentanyl on the circulatory responses to orotracheal fibreoptic intubation. *Anaesthesia* 1992; **47:** 20.

121 Lamb K., James M. F. M. and Janicki P. K. The laryngeal mask airway for intra-ocular surgery: effects on intra ocular pressure and stress responses *British Journal of Anaesthesia* 1992; **69:** 143.

122 Watcha M. F., White P. F., Tychsen L. and Stevens J. L. Comparative effects of laryngeal mask airway and endotracheal tube insertion on intraocular pressure in children. *Anesthesia and Analgesia* 1992; **75:** 355.

123 Braude N., Clements E. A. F., Hodges U. M. *et al.* The pressor response and laryngeal mask insertion. *Anaesthesia* 1989; **44:** 551.

124 Hartley M. and Vaughan R. S. Problems associated with tracheal extubation. *British Journal of Anaesthesia* 1993; **71:** 561.

125 Edde R. R. Cardiovascular responses to extubation. *Anesthesiology* 1979; **51:** S195,

126 Dyson A., Isaac P. A., Pennant J. H., Giesecke A. H., Lipton J. M. Esmolol attenuates cardiovascular responses to extubation. *Anesthesia and Analgesia* 1990; **71:** 675.

127 Wolner E. C., Usubiaga L. J., Jacoby R. M. and Hill G. E. Cardiovascular effects of extubation. *Anesthesiology* 1979; **51:** S194.

128 Gold M. I. and Muravchick S. Arterial oxygenation during laryngoscopy and intubation. *Anesthesia and Analgesia* 1981; **60:** 316.

129 Weitzner S. W., King B. D. and Ikezono E. The rate of arterial oxygen desaturation during apnea. *Anesthesiology* 1959; **20:** 624.

130 Heller M. L. and Watson T. R. Polarographic study of arterial oxygenation during apnea in man. *New England Journal of Medicine* 1961; **264:** 326.

131 Thorpe C. M. and Gauntlett I. S. Arterial oxygen saturation during induction of anaesthesia. *Anaesthesia* 1990; **45:** 1012.

132 Hamilton W. K. and Eastwood D. W. A study of denitrogenation with some inhalation anesthetic systems. *Anesthesiology* 1955; **16:** 861.

133 Dillon J. B. and Darsi M. L. Oxygen for acute respiratory depression due to administration of thiopental sodium. *Journal of the American Medical Association* 1955; **159:** 1114.

134 Lachman R. J., Long J. H. and Krumperman L. W. The changes in blood gases associated with various methods of induction for endotracheal anesthesia. *Anesthesiology* 1955; **16:** 29.

135 Bartlett R. G. Jr., Brubach H. F. and Specht H. Demonstration of aventilatory mass flow during ventilation and apnoea in man. *Journal of Applied Physiology* 1959; **14:** 97.

136 Downes J. I., Wilson J. F. and Goodson D. Apnea, suction and hyperventilation: effect on arterial oxygen saturation. *Anesthesiology* 1961; **22:** 29.

137 Heller M. L., Watson T. R. and Imredy D. S. Apneic oxygenation in man: polarographic arterial oxygen tension study. *Anesthesiology* 1964; **22:** 25.

138 Archer G. W. Jr. and Marx G. F. Arterial oxygen tension during apnoea in parturient women. *British Journal of Anaesthesia* 1974; **46:** 358.

139 Kung M. C., Hung C. T., Ng K. P. *et al.* Arterial desaturation during induction in healthy adults: should preoxygenation be a routine? *Anaesthesia and Intensive Care* 1991; **19:** 192.

140 Berthoud M., Read D. H. and Norman J. Preoxygenation – how long? *Anaesthesia* 1982; **38:** 96.

141 Fowler W. S. and Comroe J. H. Lung function studies. I. The rate of increase of arterial oxygen saturation during the inhalation of 100% $O_2$. *Journal of Clinical Investigation* 1948; **27:** 327.

142 Drummond G. B. and Park G. R. Arterial oxygen

saturation before intubation of the trachea. *British Journal of Anaesthesia* 1984; **56:** 987.

143 Gabrielsen J. and Valentin N. Routine induction of anaesthesia with thiopental and suxamethonium: apnoea without ventilation? *Acta Anaesthesiologica Scandinavica* 1982; **26:** 59.

144 Machlin H. A., Myles P. S., Berry C. B. *et al.* End-tidal oxygen measurement compared with patient factor assessment for determining preoxygenation time. *Anaesthesia and Intensive Care* 1993; **21:** 409.

145 Ooi R., Pattison J., Joshi P. *et al.* Pre-oxygenation: the Hudson mask as an alternative technique. *Anaesthesia* 1992; **47:** 974.

146 Rooney, M. J. Pre-oxygenation: a comparison of two techniques using a Bain system. *Anaesthesia* 1993; **49:** 629.

147 Don H. F., Wahba W. M. and Craig D. B. Airway closure, gas trapping and the functional residual capacity during anesthesia. *Anesthesiology* 1972; **36:** 533.

148 Marx G. F. and Mateo C. V Effects of different oxygen concentrations during general anaesthesia for elective caesarean section. *Canadian Anaesthetists Society Journal* 1971; **18:** 587.

149 Norris M. C. and Dewan D. M. Preoxygenation for caesarean section: a comparison of two techniques. *Anesthesiology* 1984; **61:** A400.

150 Braun U. and Hudjetz W. The duration of preoxygenation in patients with normal and impaired pulmonary function. *Anaesthetist* 1980; **29:** 125.

151 McCarthy G., Elliott P., Mirakhur R. K. and McLoughlin C. A comparison of different pre-oxygenation techniques in the elderly. *Anaesthesia* 1991; **46:** 824.

152 Valentine S. J., Marjot R. and Monk C. R. Preoxygenation in the elderly: a comparison of the four-maximal-breath and three-minute techniques. *Anesthesia and Analgesia* 1990; **71:** 516.

153 Frumin M. J., Epstein R. M. and Cohen G. Apneic oxygenation in man. *Anesthesiology* 1959; **20:** 789.

154 Gal T. J. and Suratt P. M. Resistance to breathing in healthy subjects following endotracheal intubation under topical anesthesia. *Anesthesia and Analgesia* 1980; **59:** 270.

155 Berman L. S., Fox W. W. and Raphaely R. Optimum levels of CPAP for tracheal extubation of newborn infants. *Journal of Pediatrics* 1976; **89:** 109

156 Gal T. J. How does tracheal intubation alter respiratory mechanics? *Problems in Anesthesia* 1988; **2:** 191.

157 Matsushima Y., Jones R. L., King E. G. *et al.* Alterations in pulmonary mechanics and gas exchange during routine fiberoptic bronchoscopy. *Chest* 1984; **86:** 184.

158 Burton J. D. K. Effects of dry anesthetic gases on the respiratory mucous membrane. *Lancet* 1962; **i:** 235.

159 Marfia S., Donahoe P. K. and Hendren W. H. Effect of dry and humidified gases on the respiratory epithelium in rabbits. *Journal of Pediatric Surgery* 1975; **10:** 583.

160 Chalon J., Patel C., Mahgul A. *et al.* Humidity and the anesthetized patient. *Anesthesiology* 1979; **50:** 195.

161 Hartley M., Morris S. and Vaughan R. S. Teaching fibreoptic intubation. Effect of alfentanil on the haemodynamic response. *Anaesthesia* 1994; **49:** 335.

162 Smith M., Calder I., Crockard A. *et al.* Oxygen saturation and cardiovascular changes during fibreoptic intubation under general anaesthesia. *Anaesthesia* 1992; **47:** 158.

163 Finfer S. R., MacKenzie S. I. P., Saddler J. M. and Watkins T. G. L. Cardiovascular responses to tracheal intubation: a comparison of direct laryngoscopy and fibreoptic intubation. *Anaesthesia and Intensive Care* 1989; **17:** 48.

164 Schaefer H.-G., Marsch S. C. U. and Staender S. Fibreoptic intubation under general anaesthesia need not be associated with hypoxia and hypotension. *Anaesthesia* 1992; **47:** 812.

165 Marian F., Spiss C. K., Heismayr M. and Draxler V. Uberwachung der fiberoptischen intubation mittels nicht invasiver pulseoxometrie. *Anaesthetist* 1985; **34:** 630.

166 Calder I., Smith M., Nichol M. *et al.* Fibreoptic intubation under general anaesthesia need not be associated with hypoxia and hypotension. *Anaesthesia* 1992; **47:** 812.

167 Stephen C. R., Woodhall B., Golden J. B., Martin R. and Nowill W. K. The influence of anesthetic drugs and techniques on intracranial tension *Anesthesiology* 1954; **15:** 365.

168 Greenbaum R., Cooper R., Hulme A. and Mackintosh I. P. The effect of induction of anaesthesia on intracranial pressure. In: *Recent Advances in Anaesthesiology and Resuscitation* (ed. A. Arias). Amsterdam: Excerpta Medica. 1990: 794.

169 Shapiro H. M., Wyte S. R., Harris A. B. and Galindo A. Acute intraoperative intracranial hypertension in neurosurgical patients. *Anesthesiology* 1972; **37:** 399.

170 McLeskey C. H., Cullen B. F., Kennedy R. D. and Galindo A. Control of cerebral perfusion pressure during induction of anesthesia in high risk neurosurgical patients. *Anesthesia and Analgesia* 1974; **53:** 985.

171 Misfeldt B. B., Jorgensen P. B. and Rishoj M. The effect of nitrous oxide and halothane upon the intracranial pressure in hypocapnic patients with intracranial disorders. *British Journal of Anaesthesia* 1974; **46:** 853.

172 Burney R. G. and Winn R. Increased cerebrospinal fluid pressure during laryngoscopy and intubation

for induction of anesthesia. *Anesthesia and Analgesia* 1975; **54:** 687.

173 Moss E., Powell D., Gibson R. M. and McDowall D. G. Effects of tracheal intubation on intracranial pressure following induction of anaesthesia with thiopentone or althesin in patients undergoing neurosurgery. *British Journal of Anaesthesia* 1978; **50:** 353.

174 Halldin M. and Wahlin A. Effect of succinylcholine on the intraspinal fluid pressure. *Acta Anaesthesiologica Scandinavica* 1959; **3:** 155.

175 Hunter A. R. Present position of anaesthesia for neurosurgery. *Proceedings of the Royal Society of Medicine* 1952; **45:** 427.

176 Alexander S. C. and Lassen N. A. Cerebral circulatory response to acute brain disease. *Anesthesiology* 1970; **32:** 60.

177 Paulson O. B., Olesen J. and Christensen M. S. Restoration of autoregulation of cerebral blood flow by hypocapnia. *Neurology* 1972; **22:** 286.

178 Kety S. S., Shenkin H. and Schmidt C. F. The effects of increased intracranial pressure on cerebral circulatory function in man. *Journal of Clinical Investigation* 1948; **27:** 493.

179 Wollman H., Alexander S. C., Cohen P. J. *et al.* Cerebral circulation during general anesthesia and hyperventilation in man. *Anesthesiology* 1965; **26:** 329.

180 Atkinson R. S., Rushman G. B. and Lee J. A. *A Synopsis of Anaesthesia*, 9th edn. Bristol: John Wright. 1982: 420.

181 Christensen M. S., Hoedt-Rasmussen K. and Lassen N. A. Cerebral vasodilatation by halothane anaesthesia in man and its potentiation by hypotension and hypercarbia. *British Journal of Anaesthesia* 1967; **39:** 927.

182 McDowall D. G., Jennett W. B. and Barker J. The effect of halothane anaesthesia on cerebral perfusion and metabolism and on intracranial pressure. *Progress in Brain Research* 1968; **28:** 83.

183 Pierce E. C., Lambertsen C. J., Deutsch S., Chase P. E., Linde H. W., Dripps R. D. *et al.* Cerebral circulation and metabolism during thiopental anesthesia and hyperventilation in man. *Journal of Clinical Investigation* 1962; **41:** 1664.

184 Shapiro H. M. and Aidinis S. J. Neurosurgical Anesthesia. *Surgical Clinics of North America* 1975; **55:** 913.

185 Greenbaum R. Anaesthesia for intracranial surgery. *British Journal of Anaesthesia* 1976; **48:** 773

186 Bedford R. F., Winn H. R., Tyson G. *et al.* Lidocaine prevents increased intracranial pressure after endotracheal intubation; In *Intracranial Pressure IV* (ed. K. Shulman) Berlin: Springer-Verlag. 1980: 595.

187 Unni V. K. N., Johnston R. A., Young S. A. and McBride R. J. Prevention of intracranial hyperten-

sion during laryngoscopy and endotracheal intubation. Use of a second dose of thiopentone. *British Journal of Anaesthesia* 1984; **56:** 1219.

190 Hofmann H., Holzer H., Bock J. and Spath F. Die Wirkung von Muskelrelantien auf den introklaren Druck. *Klinische Monatsblatten Augenheilkunde (Stuttgart)* 1953; **123:** 1.

191 Lincoff H. A., Breinin G. M. and DeVoe A. G. Effect of succinylcholine on extraocular muscles. *American Journal of Ophthalmology* 1957; **43:** 440.

192 Wynands J. E. and Crowell D. E. Intraocular tension in association with succinylcholine and endotracheal intubation: a preliminary report. *Canadian Anaesthetists Society Journal* 1960; **7:** 39.

193 Dillon J. B., Sabawala P., Taylor D. B. and Gunter R. Action of succinylcholine on extraocular muscles and intraocular pressure. *Anesthesiology* 1957; **18:** 44.

194 Taylor T. H., Mulcahy M. and Nightingale D. A. Suxamethonium chloride in intraocular surgery. *British Journal of Anaesthesia* 1968; **40:** 113.

195 Duke-Elder S. *Glaucoma, a Symposium* 1st edn. Oxford: Blackwell Scientific Publications, 1955: 309.

196 Goldsmith E. Succinylcholine and gallamine as muscle relaxants in relation to intraocular tension. *Anesthesia and Analgesia* 1967; **46:** 557.

197 Craythorne N. W. B., Rottenstein H. S. and Dripps R. D. The effects of succinylcholine on intraocular pressure in adults, infants and children during general anaesthesia. *Anesthesiology* 1960: **59:** 63.

198 Bowen D. J., McGrand J. C. and Hamilton A. G. Intraocular pressures after suxamethonium and endotracheal intubation. *Anaesthesia* 1978; **33:** 518.

199 Bowen D. J., McGrand J. C. and Palmer R. J. Intraocular pressures after suxamethonium and endotracheal intubation in patients pretreated with pancuronium. *British Journal of Anaesthesia* 1976; **48:** 1201.

200 Macri F. J. and Grimes P. A. The effects of succinylcholine on intraocular pressure. *American Journal of Ophthalmology* 1957; **44:** 221.

201 Pandey K., Badola R. P. and Kumar S. Time course of intraocular hypertension produced by suxamethonium. *British Journal of Anaesthesia* 1972; **44:** 191.

202 Adams A. K. and Barnett K. C. Anaesthesia and intraocular pressure. *Anaesthesia* 1966; **21:** 202.

203 Sobel A. M. Hexafluorenium, succinylcholine and intraocular tension. *Anesthesia and Analgesia* 1962; **41:** 399.

204 Miller R. D., Way W. L. and Hickey R. F. Inhibition of succinylcholine-induced increased intraocular pressure by non-depolarising muscle relaxants. *Anesthesiology* 1968; **29:** 123.

205 Dickman P., Goecke M and Wiemars K

Beeinflussung der intraocularen Drucksteigerung nach Succinylcholin durch depolarisationshemmende Relaxantien. *Anaesthetist* 1969; **18**: 370.

206 Wahlin A. Clinical and experimental studies on effects of succinylcholine. *Acta Anaesthesiologica Scandinavica* 1960; **5** (Suppl): 1.

207 Smith R. B. and Leano N. Intraocular pressure following pancuronium. *Canadian Anaesthetists Society Journal* 1973; **20**: 742.

208 Meyers E. F., Singer P. and Otto A. A controlled study of the effect of succinylcholine self-taming on intraocular pressure. *Anesthesiology* 1980; **53**: 72.

209 Murphy D. F. Anesthesia and introcular pressure. *Anesthesia and Analgesia* 1985; **64**: 520.

210 Lennon R. L., Olson R. A. and Gronert G. A. Atracurium or vecuronium for rapid sequence endotracheal intubation. *Anesthesiology* 1986; **64**: 510.

211 Abbott M. A. The control of intra-ocular pressure during the induction of anaesthesia for emergency eye surgery. A high-dose vecuronium technique. *Anaesthesia* 1987; **42**: 1008.

212 Mirakhur R. K., Shepherd W. F. I. and Elliott P. Intraocular pressure changes during rapid-sequence induction of anaesthesia. Comparison of propofol and thiopentone in combination with vecuronium. *British Journal of Anaesthesia* 1988; **60**: 379.

213 Scott R. P. F., Savarese J. J. and Basta S. J. *et al.* Clinical pharmaclgogy of atracurium given in high dose. *British Journal of Anaesthesia* 1986; **58**: 834.

214 Brown E. M. and Krishnaprasad D. and Smiler B. G. Pancuronium for rapid induction technique for tracheal intubation. *Canadian Anaesthetists Society Journal* 1979; **26**: 489.

215 Al-Abrak M. H. and Samuel J. R. Effects of general anaesthesia on the intraocular pressure in man. Comparison of tubocurarine and pancuronium in nitrous oxide and oxygen. *British Journal of Ophthalmology* 1974; **58**: 806.

216 Robertson E. N., Hull J. M., Verbeek A. M. and Booij L. H. D. J. A comparison of rocuronium and vecuronium: the pharmacodynamic, cardiovascular and intra-ocular effects. *European Journal of Anaesthesiology* 1994; **11** (Suppl. 9): 116.

217 Fuhringer F. K., Khueni-Brady K. S., Killer J. and Mitterschiffthaler G. Evaluation of the endotracheal intubating conditions of rocuronium (ORG 9426) and succinylcholine in outpatient surgery. *Anesthesia and Analgesia* 1992; **75**: 37.

218 Cooper R., Mirakhur R. K., Clarke R. S. J. and Boules Z. Comparison of intubating conditions after administration of ORG 9426 (rocuronium) and suxamethonium. *British Journal of Anaesthesia* 1992; **69**: 269.

219 Magorian T., Flannery K. B. and Miller R. D. Comparison of rocuronium, succinylcholine and vecuronium for rapid-sequence induction of anesthesia in adult patients. *Anesthesiology* 1993; **79**: 913.

220 Mirakhur R. K. Safety aspects of non-depolarizing neuromuscular blocking agents with special reference to rocuronium bromide. *European Journal of Anaesthesiology* 1994; **11** (Suppl. 9): 133.

221 Connolly F. M., Loan P. B., Mirakhur R. K. and McCoy E. P. Comparison of succinylcholine and rocuronium for rapid sequence induction of anesthesia. *Anesthesiology* 1994; **81** (Suppl. 3A): A1072.

222 Badrinath S. K., Vazeery A., McCarthy R. J. and Ivanovich A. D. The effect of different methods of inducing anesthesia on intraocular pressure. *Anesthesiology* 1986; **65**: 431.

223 Mirakhur R. K., Elliott P., Shepherd W. F. I. and Archer D. B. Intra-ocular pressure changes during induction of anaesthesia and tracheal intubation. A comparison of thiopentone and propofol followed by vecuronium. *Anaesthesia* 1988; **43** (Suppl): 54.

224 Barclay K., Wall T., Wareham K. and Asai T. Intra-ocular pressure changes in patients with glaucoma. Comparison between the laryngeal mask airway and tracheal tube. *Anaesthesia* 1994; **49**: 159.

225 Holden R., Morsman C. D. G., Butler J. *et al.* Intra-ocular pressure changes using the laryngeal mask airway and tracheal tube. *Anaesthesia* 1991; **46**: 922.

226 Cook J. H., Feneck R. O. and Smith M. B. Effect of pretreatment with propranolol on intra-ocular pressure changes during induction of anaesthesia. *European Journal of Anaesthesiology* 1986; **3**: 449.

227 Bricker S. R. W., McGaillard J. N., Mercer N. P. *et al.* Effects of timolol ophthalmic solution on the intra-ocular pressure rise induced by suxamethonium and tracheal intubation. *Anaesthesia* 1992; **47**: 163.

228 Bain W. E. S. and Maurice D. M. Physiological variations in the intraocular pressure. *Transactions of the Ophthalmological Society UK* 1959; **79**: 249.

229 Carballo A. S. Succinylcholine and acetazolamide (Diamox) in anaesthesia for ocular surgery. *Canadian Anaesthetists Society Journal* 1965; **12**: 486.

230 Duncalf D. and Weitzner S. W. The influence of ventilation and hypercapnia on intraocular pressure during anesthesia. *Anesthesia and Analgesia* 1963; **42**: 232.

231 Libonati M. M., Leahy J. J. and Ellison N. The use of succinylcholine in open eye surgery. *Anesthesiology* 1986; **62**: 637.

232 Lehtinen A.-M., Hovorka J., Leppaluoto J. Vuolteenaho O. and Widholm O. Effect of intratracheal lignocaine, halothane and thiopentone on changes in plasma beta-endorphin immunoreactivity in response to tracheal intubation. *British Journal of Anaesthesia* 1984; **56**: 247.

233 Kaufman L. General anaesthesia in ophthalmol-
    ogy. *Proceedings of the Royal Society of Medicine*
    1967; **60:** 1280.

234 Wilson G., Fell D., Robinson S. L. and Smith G.
    Cardiovascular responses to insertion of the laryn-
    geal mask. *Anaesthesia* 1992; **47:** 300.

# 3

# The Cuff

*Peter Latto*

## FUNCTIONS OF THE CUFF

The inflatable cuff has two main functions. It should seal the airway thus preventing aspiration of pharyngeal contents into the trachea and it should ensure that there are no leaks past the cuff during positive pressure ventilation. At the same time the pressure exerted by the inflated cuff on the trachea should not be so high that capillary circulation is compromised. A 'high' cuff pressure prevents aspiration into the trachea and ventilatory leaks but can result in tracheal damage; a 'low' cuff pressure minimizes tracheal damage but may result in aspiration past the cuff. The ability to meet these conflicting requirements depends both on the design and the management of the cuff. The early thick-walled rubber cuffs frequently caused major trauma when used for more than a few hours. Modern plastic cuffs with thin walls and high volume, low pressure characteristics can, if properly managed, provide an adequate seal without significant tracheal damage. However, there is room for improvement both in cuff design and the accurate control of cuff pressures.

Early tracheal tubes did not have cuffs and a throat pack was used to prevent aspiration and to ensure relatively leak-free positive pressure ventilation. Young children are commonly managed with uncuffed tubes but this can result in a high incidence of silent aspiration. Ten out of 13 such children who were being ventilated showed evidence of silent tracheal aspiration 10 min after dye had been placed on the back of the tongue [1].

## HISTORY

The development of cuffed tubes is closely linked with the development of tracheal tubes and the associated anaesthetic techniques [2].

In 1871, Friedrich Trendelenburg described a tube which was inserted into the trachea through a tracheostomy [3] (Fig. 1). The tube had a small, thick-walled, low volume, inflatable rubber cuff which made a watertight contact with the tracheal wall. This tube was widely used for clinical anaesthesia during the last three decades of the nineteenth century [2]. In 1880, William Macewen, a Glasgow surgeon, sought an alternative to Trendelenburg's tracheostomy tube and described the use of a tracheal tube passed blindly through the mouth [4]. This tube was used to relieve airway obstruction as well as for anaesthesia and was introduced in conscious patients without the use of local anaesthesia. The technique employed manual palpation in the throat. A finger depressed the epiglottis onto the tongue and the tube was guided over the back of the finger into the larynx. A sponge was then placed at the upper end of the larynx to prevent aspiration of blood. In 1893, Eisenmenger in Vienna described the first tracheal tube with an inflatable high volume cuff [5]. A large pilot balloon signalled the tension in the cuff and intracuff pressure could be limited. In 1910, Dorrance described a tube with an inflatable cuff similar to those in use today (Fig. 2). In 1921, Rowbotham and Magill reported their experience with tracheal anaesthesia using to-and-fro breathing through uncuffed rubber tubes in managing cases for head and neck surgery [6]. In 1930, Magill published a description of his experience with blind nasal intubation using uncuffed curved soft rubber catheters [7]. The pharynx was packed with gauze both to reduce the risk of aspiration past the uncuffed catheter and to help obtain a gas-tight fit.

In 1928, Guedel and Waters described a cuffed tracheal tube designed for closed circuit intratracheal administration of anaesthesia using a carbon dioxide absorption technique [8]. This tube was similar to the earlier cuffed tube described by Dorrance [9]. It had a thin rubber cuff, 1½ inches (3.8 cm) long and with a diameter of ⅝ of an inch (1.6 cm) when the rubber was just starting to stretch. The cuff was cemented to the tube. When deflated, the rubber cuff lay in folds close to the catheter wall. They showed the effectiveness of the cuff in preventing aspiration in a dog anaesthetized with ethylene which survived total immersion in water for 1 h. The cuffed tube was then tested in two patients whose mouths and noses were filled with water. Only a very small drop in the level of the water was observed at the end of 5 min [8]. In 1943, Macintosh described a tube with a self inflating cuff designed by Mushin

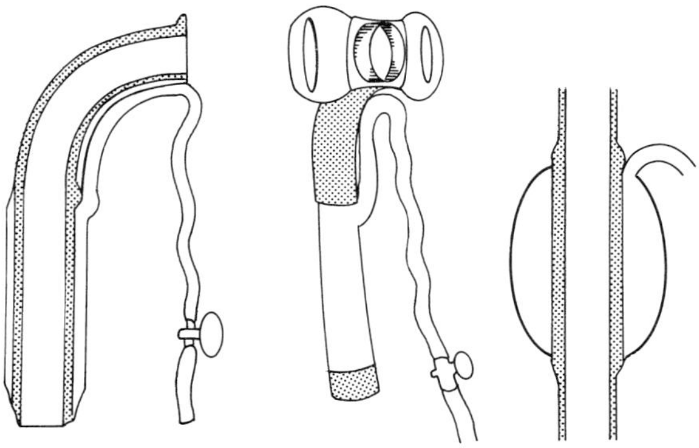

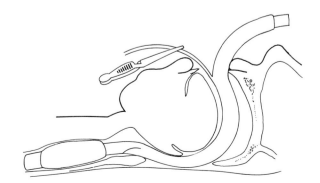

**Figure 1**  Trendelenburg's cuff catheter, which was inserted through a tracheostomy. After Trendelenburg [3].

**Figure 2**  Dorrance's cuffed catheter with cuff inflated. After Dorrance [9].

[10] (Fig. 3). This cuff facilitated controlled ventilation for thoracic anaesthesia. Holes were cut in the tube underneath the cuff. The cuff thus inflated only on inspiration. The holes, however, sometimes became blocked by plugs of mucus.

Although the first cuffed tracheal tube had been described in 1893, non-cuffed tubes were more commonly used until the 1950s. In 1952, during the polio epidemic in Copenhagen, cuffed tubes were used [11, 12]. After that experience it became standard clinical practice to use cuffed tubes during anaesthesia. The use of plain tubes is now largely restricted to children and neonates.

Early tubes were made of red rubber with rigid thick-walled cuffs and high cuff and tracheal wall pressures were required to effect a seal. When these cuffed tubes were left *in situ* for long periods it soon became apparent that major complications could result from the high pressure exerted on the tracheal wall. Increased understanding of cuff-related tracheal pathology has led to improved design of cuffs and techniques for limiting intracuff pressure.

An important development was the introduction of disposable plastic tubes which have largely displaced rubber tubes. Several reasons support this trend. The high pressure on the tracheal wall that can occur with the use of rubber cuffs is undesirable. The cuffs of red rubber tubes frequently inflate eccentrically; this results in the tip being pushed against the tracheal wall, introducing the risk of distal tracheal erosion. Rubber can release toxins and irritants resulting in allergic reactions especially when used long-term. There is also the potential hazard of cross infection associated with repeated sterilization. Finally, rubber deteriorates on repeated autoclaves.

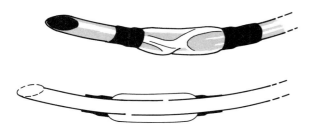

**Figure 3**   Self inflating cuff described by Macintosh in 1943. Redrawn from Macintosh [10], with kind permission of the author and the *British Medical Journal.*

Manufacturers are continually improving and refining the design of plastic cuffs. There has been a move towards high volume, low pressure cuffs for long-term use. One design objective here is to eliminate wrinkles which can occur in these sometimes bulky cuffs. It is important to recognize, however, that any cuff, even a so-called low pressure cuff, can be overfilled *in vivo* resulting in high intracuff and tracheal wall pressures. Even 'ideal' cuffs require careful management.

## POSITION OF THE CUFF AND THE TIP OF THE TRACHEAL TUBE

Malposition of a tracheal tube can result in an increase both in morbidity and mortality, especially in those patients in respiratory failure [13]. The position of the cuff and tube tip are therefore often identified with a chest X-ray in patients in the intensive care unit. In critically ill patients endobronchial intubation is particularly harmful; the potential for intubation of the right main bronchus is clearly increased if long uncut tubes are used. An alternative, less commonly used method, is to assess the position of the tip of the tube in relation to the carina with a fibreoptic laryngoscope [14].

Such precautions are not usually taken to confirm the proper placement of a tube during general anaesthesia. The cuff is usually seen passing through the cords at intubation and can then easily be placed in the required position. In one study it was shown that the distance from the cricothyroid membrane to the carina was approximately 11 cm and from the vocal cords to the cricothyroid membrane was 1 cm [15]. The tracheal tube measured 5.5 cm from the proximal end of the cuff to the tip. Thus, if the proximal end of the cuff was placed 1 cm below the cords, the tip of the tube was approximately 5 cm from the carina.

On rare occasions, however, the tube is not seen passing through the cords after induction of anaesthesia and there is doubt about the length of tube in the trachea. Under these circumstances a chest radiograph enables the position of the tube to be determined accurately. It is important to auscultate the chest to confirm that there is bilateral air entry and that the tip of the tube is not in the right main bronchus; it is well known however, that this technique can be misleading [16]. Difficulty may be encountered in patients with limited chest movement or quiet breath sounds. In these circumstances it is important also to listen over the trachea and left hypogastrium. A case was reported in which intubation of the right main bronchus, resulting in massive atelectasis, did not give rise to cyanosis, tachycardia or other changes in vital signs during general anaesthesia [16].

Fluid can accumulate in the trachea above the cuff of a tube. Pharyngeal suction may not remove this fluid and aspiration may occur when the cuff is deflated. To prevent this it has been recommended that the inflated cuff be withdrawn until resistance is felt, which signals that the upper end of the cuff is impinging on the lower surface of the vocal cords [17]. The patient is extubated in a 10° head down position and aspiration is performed through the tube before removal. In the United States, where the use of uncut disposable tracheal tubes is routine, in some centres it is common practice to withdraw the tube to the cords. If the upper end of the cuff impinges on the vocal cords however, pressure damage could result. On occasions part of the cuff may be positioned above the cords. This is most likely to occur when the cords cannot be seen at intubation and the tube is too short.

A number of alternative methods are available for checking the position of the tube in the trachea. The trachea can be palpated between the suprasternal notch and the cricoid cartilage and the distension of the trachea may be felt when the cuff is rapidly inflated [15]; alternatively, the filled pilot balloon can be lightly palpated and an increase in pressure should be detected in the balloon on applying pressure over the trachea at the site of the cuff [18]. A less desirable method of tube placement in adults is to deliberately intubate the right main bronchus and then to withdraw the tube 1–2 cm above the position at which bilateral air sounds are first heard [19]. An electromagnetic sensing device has also been described but this is not commercially available [20]. This allows detection of a foil marker band fixed into the tracheal tube at the level of the proximal cuff junction. The accuracy of the technique was confirmed by comparing assumed placement with this method with the position of the tube assessed on a chest radiograph.

It is important to remember that the cuff and tip of a tube may move both in adults and children if the neck is flexed or extended [21]. Tracheal tube movement can therefore result in inadvertent endobronchial intubation on neck flexion and extubation on neck extension. With nasotracheal tubes in adults, an average of 1.5 cm movement towards the carina occurred with neck flexion and 1.5 cm away from the carina with neck extension. The maximum movement observed away from the carina was 3.5 cm and towards the carina was 2.9 cm. Such movements of the cuff may also result in trauma to the tracheal epithelium. To minimize the risk both of extubation and accidental endobronchial intubation associated with head movement it has been recommended that the cuff should be placed in the middle third of the trachea [21].

In normal practice for the adult, the tube is cut to an appropriate length and the cuff is placed under direct vision 1–2 cm below the cords. If the tube is not seen passing through the cords other techniques may be required.

## CUFF INFLATION

It is common clinical practice to inflate the cuff slowly until no leak is audible while applying positive pressure to the airway. It has been recommended that the pressure in large volume cuffs should be measured during inflation with an in line pressure gauge [22]. This should help to keep the cuff pressure within safe limits. However, it is not always possible with high volume cuffs to determine accurately the exact seal point. It has been suggested that it would be more practical to inflate large volume cuffs to a fixed pressure of 25–30 cm regardless of the cuff volume [23]. It is always essential to avoid overfilling the cuff. If the cuff is inflated by an impatient and unskilled assistant, then it is common for the cuff to be inflated well past the seal point, with resulting high pressures on the tracheal mucosa. Care and time should be taken during cuff inflation which should preferably be undertaken by the anaesthetist.

## TRACHEAL WALL PRESSURES: METHOD OF MEASUREMENT

Many methods have been described for measuring the lateral pressure exerted by the cuff on the tracheal wall. No single method is entirely satisfactory [24]. Indirect methods have been described for calculating the pressure exerted by tracheal cuffs on the tracheal wall [25, 26, 27], although some of the assumptions made in the calculations have been questioned [28]. In an *in vitro* study Cross [28] stated that

$$P_{ic} = P_{tw} + P_{f(d \cdot s)}$$

where $P_{ic}$ = intracuff pressure, $P_{tw}$ = tracheal wall pressure and $P_{f(d \cdot s)}$ = a pressure which is a function of the cuff diameter ($d$) and the stiffness of the cuff material ($s$). Therefore, if the cuff pressure is monitored, the pressure on the tracheal wall will always be less than or equal to this easily measured value. If $P_{f(d \cdot s)}$ is very low, then pressure in the cuff approximates to the pressure on the tracheal wall.

Another *in vitro* method [29] involved inflating the cuff with a measured volume of air and measuring the cuff pressure ($P_1$); the cuff pressure was then measured in a model trachea when the cuff was inflated with the same volume of air ($P_2$). The pressure exerted on the model tracheal wall ($P$) was calculated from the formula:

$$P = P_2 - P_1$$

However, in a more detailed study of tracheal pressure *in vitro* with both high and low volume cuffs, it was shown that this formula was not always correct [27]. There was a large difference between the measured tracheal wall pressure and the calculated tracheal wall pressure in some instances.

For direct measurement, transducers have been implanted in a model trachea, in the tracheal wall in animals and in the excised human trachea [24, 30, 31]. Pressures on the trachea have also been measured *in vivo* with small balloons lying between the cuff of the tube and the tracheal wall [32, 33]. The mean pressure on the anterior tracheal wall at seal volume of the cuff (leak-free ventilation) was 38 mmHg (range 24–68 mmHg) in 11 patients [32]. Latex-armoured tracheal tubes were used. In another five patients the mean pressure was found to be 40.8 mmHg on the anterior tracheal wall and 27.2 mmHg on the posterior tracheal wall. Thus, in the normal head position the pressure on the anterior tracheal wall is greater than that on the posterior tracheal wall. This is because the posterior membranous tracheal wall is more distensible than the cartilaginous anterolateral portion. In the same study, three patients were positioned with the head extended and the mean anterior and posterior wall pressures were 51 and 59 mmHg respectively;

thus the difference in pressure was reduced and even reversed in some patients. In this position the vertebral column gives extra support to the posterior trachea. The pressures exerted on the tracheal wall increased as patients recovered consciousness, possibly due to increased muscle tone. The higher anterior tracheal wall pressure explains why cuff-related tracheal damage is most severe over the anterior trachea [34].

A number of authors have studied the pressure exerted on the tracheal wall with different tracheal tubes [24, 27, 31, 33]. A wide range of tracheal pressures have been reported with different tubes and slightly different experimental designs. Lateral tracheal pressures at airway seal varied with different tubes from 26 to 240 mmHg [24] in a model trachea, from 15 to 160 mmHg [33] in another model trachea (Fig. 4) and from 30 to 205 mmHg [31] in a dog. It is clear therefore that the design of the cuff is of paramount importance in limiting the pressure exerted on the tracheal wall. Cuff management is also important because

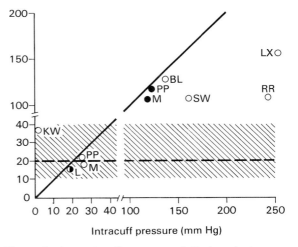

**Figure 4** Lateral wall pressure plotted against intracuff pressure during *in vitro* evaluation of tracheal tubes. Dashed line represents mean capillary pressure and shaded area theoretical limits of venous capillary pressure. ○ Tubes at seal-point pressure. ● Tubes inflated 5 ml beyond seal point. ◑ Lanz tubes at seal point and over inflated by 20 and 40 ml. BL = Portex blue line; PP = Portex profile; M = Mallinckrodt; L = Lanz; KW = Kamen-Wilkinson; RR = Red rubber; LX = Armoured latex; SW = Soft way. Modified from Leigh and Maynard [33], with kind permission of the authors and the *British Medical Journal*.

inflation with as little as 1 ml of air after the seal point can result in potentially damaging increases in lateral wall pressure [24] (Fig. 5).

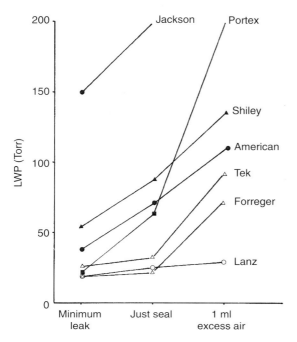

**Figure 5**   Lateral tracheal wall pressure with different tracheostomy tubes and three different inflation points. From Wu *et al.* [24], with kind permission of the authors and the publishers. © 1973 The Williams & Wilkins Co., Baltimore.

## INTRALARYNGEAL PRESSURE EXERTED BY TRACHEAL TUBES

Although major emphasis has been placed on tracheal trauma caused by the cuff, the tube can exert considerable pressure on the larynx that can result in severe pathology [35]. Prolonged intubation can give rise to a varying amount of posterior glottic stenosis [36, 37]. Indeed the commonest cause of such stenosis is prolonged intubation [36]. The pressure exerted by tubes on the posterior glottis was quantified in dogs [35]. In three dogs, pressures of 75–400 mmHg (often grossly in excess of capillary perfusion pressure) were exerted on the posterolateral portion of the larynx. Both the area of pressure and the extent of trauma is greater with a large diameter tube. It has therefore been recommended that the smallest tube compatible with acceptable ventila-

tion should be used to minimize trauma to the posterolateral larynx [32, 38].

The conventional tube exerts forces on the airway due to its elastic recoil which can result in tracheal and laryngeal trauma [39] (Fig. 6). Such damage can be limited by the use of oral or nasal Lindholm tubes which conform to the lateral contours of the airway [40–44]. Preliminary results with these tubes in a multicentre intensive care study indicate less severe lesions in the posterior subglottic and cuff areas during prolonged intubation [45].

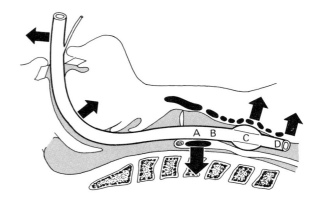

**Figure 6**   Forces on airway. Arrows indicate forces acting to restore an elastic tracheal tube to its original shape when inserted into the patient's airway. A = Inner posterior part of larynx; B = cricoid ring level which constitutes narrowest part of the airway; C = cuff site; D = tube tip. From Lindholm [39], with kind permission of the author and the editor of *Lackartidningen*.

## CONTROL OF TRACHEAL WALL PRESSURE FOR LONG-TERM INTUBATION

In two patients on artificial ventilation, one with a Lanz tube and one with a red rubber tube, both inflated to the seal point, the pressures on the tracheal wall were 17 and 87 mmHg with intracuff pressures of 19 and 225 mmHg respectively [33]. A Lanz tube has a pressure regulating mechanism which prevents both excessive rise and fall in cuff and tracheal wall pressures (Figs 7a and b). This mechanism clearly must be used with a cuff capable of effecting a seal at the pressure fixed by the regulator. The pressures exerted on the tracheal wall by the cuffs were measured with a small balloon inserted between the cuff and the tracheal wall [33]. It was suggested that the use of the Lanz tube should be obligatory for all patients requiring long-term ventilation. Furthermore, although similar control of wall pressure was thought desirable during routine (short duration) anaesthesia, financial constraints would clearly restrict the use of Lanz tubes on such a large scale. Measurements *in vitro* using eight different commonly used tubes showed that only three tubes (Lanz, Portex Profile and Mallinckrodt) were able to effect a seal with lateral wall pressures of less than 30 mmHg [33] (Fig. 4).

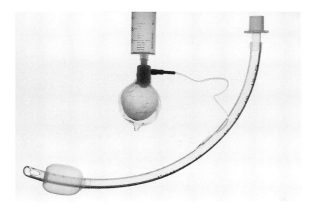

(a)

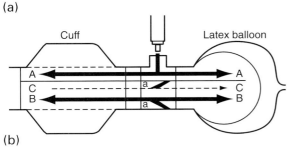

(b)

**Figure 7** **(a)** Lanz tube with cuff and balloon inflated. **(b)** The Lanz tube valve. A: A syringe is inserted into the Lanz valve and approximately 30 ml air is injected. The syringe is then removed. A cuff pressure not exceeding 25 mmHg is automatically provided. B: The valve system automatically keeps the cuff pressure below 25 mmHg for the duration of intubation. C: A special valve mechanism (a) regulates the speed of pressure release from the cuff to the latex balloon. The thin latex balloon expands and contracts within the operating range with no change in internal pressure. If the tracheal cuff pressure exceeds the balloon pressure, the balloon expands and controls the cuff pressure. If the cuff pressure falls, the balloon contracts forcing volume into the cuff maintaining a low pressure seal.

In four of these types of tubes the lateral wall pressures at the seal point were greater than 100 mmHg including one in which the pressure was approximately 160 mmHg.

## LONG-TERM INTUBATION PRACTICE IN THE UNITED KINGDOM

A postal questionnaire was used to determine the long-term intubation practice of members of the Intensive Care Society in the UK [46]. A mixture of tracheal cuffs had been in use; approximately 60% high volume, 25% intermediate volume and 10% low volume cuffs. The cuffs were generally inflated to no leak ventilation; cuff pressures were measured in only 17% of cases. The general policy of different units was to leave tubes *in situ* for periods ranging from less than 3 to more than 21 days before doing a tracheostomy. In 50% of cases, a tracheostomy was done between 7 and 14 days. With proper control of cuff pressures and improved design of cuffs and tube shape the safety of long-term oral or nasotracheal intubation should be increased.

## RATIO OF CUFF AND TRACHEAL DIAMETERS AND TRACHEAL WALL PRESSURE

An *in vitro* study was performed with a number of different makes of tubes and cuff sizes in an artificial trachea built with an elastic posterior wall to simulate the human trachea [47]. Residual volumes (RVs) were first obtained from cuff pressure volume graphs (Fig. 8). There were large differences between residual volumes of different makes of tubes and a trend towards an increase in volume with increased tube size. Residual volumes ranged from 1.8 to 27.3 ml. The seal volumes (SV = the volume preventing aspiration of water), the cuff pressures at SV, and the wall pressures were then measured in the model trachea. For tubes with a sealing volume/residual volume ratio (SV/RV) of 1 and over the ratio correlated with the wall pressures at seal point (Fig. 9). Thirty-seven per cent of tubes with an SV/RV ratio of one or less achieved a water-tight seal at wall pressures of less than 35 mmHg. It is likely that the higher wall pressures (up to 52 mmHg) required to effect a seal in the other tubes with a SV/RV ratio less than one resulted from the extra pressure required

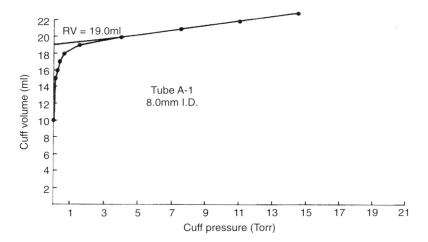

**Figure 8**   Graphic extrapolation method for determining the residual volume of a cuff. From Tonnesen *et al.* [47], with kind permission of the authors, the editor of *Anesthesiology* and the publishers, J. B. Lippincott Co.

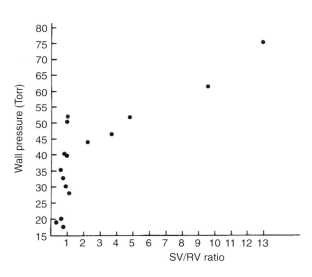

**Figure 9**   Relationship between sealing volume/residual volume ratio and wall pressure at which a water tight seal was effected. Each point represents the mean value of nine or ten tubes for each brand and size. From Tonnesen *et al.* [47], with kind permission of the authors, the editor of *Anesthesiology*, and the publishers, J. B. Lippincott Co.

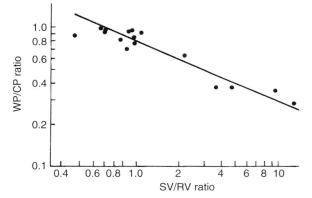

**Figure 10**   Relationship (log vs log) between the seal volume/residual volume ratio and the wall pressure/cuff pressure ratio. The lower the SV/RV ratio the more closely the cuff pressure represents wall pressure. From Tonnesen *et al.* [47], with kind permission of the authors, the editor of *Anesthesiology*, and the publishers, J. B. Lippincott Co.

to obliterate wrinkles formed in the large volume cuffs. In tubes with SV/RV ratio less than 1, wall pressure and cuff pressure was very nearly identical (Fig. 10). In tubes with a SV/RV ratio greater than 1 however the cuff pressure was greater than the wall pressure. The wall pressure was greater with a small volume than a large volume cuff. It

was concluded that the cuff should effect a seal before being filled to residual volume. A residual volume of more than 12 ml was required to effect a seal at low wall pressure in the model tested.

In clinical circumstances, measurement of cuff pressure was considered valuable because cuff pressure always exceeded wall pressure. If a seal can be effected at a cuff pressure of 25 mmHg or less, then the risk of serious tracheal damage is minimized [22, 48]. Cuff and wall pressure difference increased as the residual volume of the cuff became smaller. The final pressure on the tracheal wall at the seal point was always higher with low rather than with high volume cuffs.

## CUFF STIFFNESS AND TRACHEAL WALL PRESSURE

Low pressure high volume cuffs have compliant walls and can adapt to the tracheal contour without deforming the shape of the trachea [49] (Fig. 11). In contrast, stiff-walled low volume cuffs deform the normal tracheal contours. Consequently, such cuffs exert more pressure on the tracheal walls [31]. As the cuff is inflated, it first touches the trachea at the narrowest point at that level. The areas in contact are subject to increasing pressure as the cuff is inflated. Cuff compliance is particularly important if the trachea constricts or becomes more rigid *in vivo* under autonomic control [50].

In 1969, when rigid cuffs were used routinely, Geffin and Pontoppidan attempted to minimize tracheal distortion and damage by prestretching cuffs in a warm water bath with 20–30 ml air [51]. This effectively converted the early low volume into high volume cuffs. Following the introduction of the technique in the respiratory unit, no patient developed respiratory obstruction following extubation. Tracheal stenosis and respiratory obstruc-

tion were not uncommon, however, before introduction of the manoeuvre. With improvements in cuff design prestretching of cuffs is no longer required.

## PRESSURE AND TRACHEAL BLOOD FLOW

The blood flow in the mucosa of the rabbit's trachea has been investigated using isotope labelled microspheres before and after insertion of a high volume cuffed tracheal tube [48]. The resting blood flow was 0.3 ml $min^{-1}$ $g^{-1}$ tissue which is about 60% of cerebral blood flow. Insertion of a tracheal tube with the cuff deflated surprisingly increased blood flow to approximately 10 times the control value (Fig. 12). This was thought to be due to release of histamine-like substances which decreased arteriolar tone. If the cuff of the tube was then inflated there was a linear decrease in blood flow so that there was virtually no flow at a cuff pressure of 80–120 mmHg (approximately arterial pressure). Nordin and his colleagues believed that pressure gradients exist and that initially, as the cuff is inflated, the flow to the mucosa over the cartilages is decreased and there is reactive hyperaemia between the cartilages [48]. The initial decrease in mucosal flow resulted from this phenomenon and there was a later flow reduction in the areas between the cartilages. With an

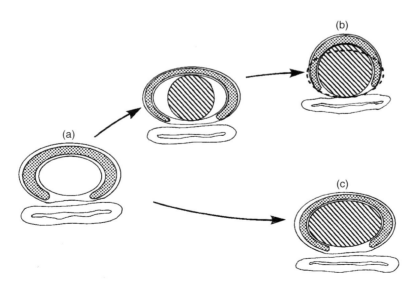

**Figure 11**   The trachea and the cuff. (a) Normal trachea and oesophagus. (b) High pressure cuff distorts the trachea and makes the tracheal contour the same as the shape of the cuff. (c) Soft low pressure cuff conforms to the normal tracheal lumen. From Cooper and Grillo [49], with kind permission of the editor of *Chest*.

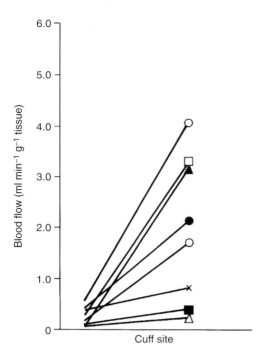

**Figure 12**  Change in mucosal blood flow from the resting condition to the condition after insertion of the tracheal tube (with fixed cardiac output) but with no inflation of the cuff. (The symbols refer to individual animals.) From Nordin *et al.* [48], with kind permission of the editor of *Acta Anaesthesiologica Scandinavica.*

ideal large diameter cuff the capillary perfusion decreases at pressures above 30 mmHg but does not cease until the tracheal pressure is much greater. A theoretical analysis indicated that a large volume cuff might exert pressure more evenly over the mucosa so minimizing the effect on the cartilage [48]. A rigid low volume cuff should exert pressure mainly over the cartilages with early reduction of blood flow. It was therefore recommended that the cuff should be inflated to a pressure not exceeding 30 cm $H_2O$.

Dobrin and Canfield investigated tracheal blood flow in the dog by measuring changes in tracheal temperature with a number of tracheal tubes with different characteristics and with varying cuff and wall pressures [31]. Cuff pressure was increased gradually resulting in a rise in measured wall pressure and a drop in tracheal temperature. When inflated to obtain a seal, compliant cuffs reduced the calculated blood flow to 98% of control while stiff cuffs reduced the flow to 20–40% of control. Stiff cuffs exerted a greater pressure on

the mucosa than compliant cuffs. Further work showed that the blood flow was reduced more in the superficial mucosal layers rather than in the deeper tracheal structures.

In a later study, Seegobin and van Hasselt used an endoscopic photographic technique to assess tracheal mucosal blood flow during intubation with large volume cuffed tubes [22]. The mucosa in contact with the cuff was examined for changes in colour which gave an indication of alteration in blood flow. At cuff pressures of 30 cm $H_2O$, impairment of mucosal flow could be observed over the anterior tracheal cartilages. Total obstruction of blood flow over the tracheal rings and over the stretched posterior muscular wall was observed at cuff pressures of 50 cm $H_2O$. It was recommended that the cuff should be inflated to a pressure not exceeding 30 cm $H_2O$. Mehta however pointed out that the intracuff pressures measured in the above experiments in large volume cuffs did not necessarily accurately reflect the pressure exerted on the tracheal wall [52]. The pressure exerted on the tracheal wall only equals the intracuff pressure with large volume, low pressure cuffs provided there is no tension in the wall of the cuff [53].

## TRACHEAL PATHOLOGY AND CUFF PRESSURE

The effect of cuff pressures on the trachea was investigated in the rabbit by Nordin [54] who concluded that the severity of tracheal pathology was influenced by the product of the duration of intubation and the lateral wall pressure. However, pressure was more important in causing damage than time. At a wall pressure of 20 mmHg, superficial but non-progressive mucosal damage resulted within 15 min. At a higher pressure of 50 mmHg, changes were noted within 15 min with partial denuding of the basement membrane. At 100 mmHg after 4 h there was damage almost down to the cartilage accompanied by bacterial invasion. This study emphasized the importance of limiting the pressure exerted on the tracheal wall. If the lateral wall pressure is limited to 20 mmHg then the trachea can tolerate long-term intubation with a cuffed tube. Experiments in pigs demonstrated that intubation for 4.5 h caused variable damage to the ciliated epithelium which could result in obstruction to mucus transport

[55]. It was not possible, however, to demonstrate a correlation between the extent of tracheal damage and the tendency to mucus arrest. In dogs following intubation for 2 h, ciliary regeneration could be seen 2 days after extubation and was nearly complete by 7 days [56].

## METHODS OF DECREASING TRACHEAL TRAUMA

Major complications were common following long-term ventilation with the rubber cuffs used before the introduction of plastics. Improvements in cuff design and management have been used to try to reduce the incidence of cuff related complications [26, 51, 57–70] (Table 1). These methods have been designed to limit the magnitude or the duration of the pressure applied to the tracheal mucosa. With a number of the early methods there was an increased risk of aspiration of pharyngeal contents and these are now rarely used.

The introduction of plastic tubes has enabled manufacturers to produce cuffs with improved characteristics; these allow a seal to be achieved at cuff pressures that do not jeopardize capillary circulation in the tracheal wall. Thin-walled,

**Table 1**  Cuff management techniques and cuff design.

| *Management techniques* | |
| --- | --- |
| Intermittent cuff deflation [57] | With modern high volume cuffs the tracheal wall pressure exerted does not restrict capillary blood flow thus rendering obsolete the practice of regular cuff deflation used with high pressure cuffs |
| Allowing small leaks around the cuff [58,59] | Still frequently used during long-term ventilation. There is a risk of aspiration of pharyngeal contents with this method. |
| Intermittent cuff inflation with equipment attached to the ventilator [60–64] | This equipment is cumbersome and the technique allows aspiration during expiration unless PEEP is applied. It was introduced to prevent complications developing with long-term tracheostomy tubes |
| Intermittent measurement of cuff pressures and adjustment of pressures as required | Simple but requires an appropriate measuring system. Should be routine clinical practice |
| Cuff with pressure control balloon which is used in place of the normal pilot balloon (the Lanz tube) [26] | This mechanism prevents both rises and falls in cuff pressure. The final cuff pressure depends on the compliance of the large pilot balloon which is connected in series with the cuff |
| Fill cuff with gas of the same composition as that inspired during general anaesthesia | |
| Fill cuff with liquid to prevent diffusion of gas into the cuff | See 'Nitrous oxide diffusion into cuffs', p.64 |
| Use of devices to prevent rises in cuff pressure above set value | |
| *Design* | |
| Self inflating cuffs [65–67] | These cuffs exerted a lateral tracheal wall pressure the same as airway pressure during inspiration. During expiration, there is an increased risk of aspiration |
| Prestretching of cuffs [51] | This effectively converted early high pressure low volume cuffs into high volume low pressure cuffs with much lower intracuff pressures providing a seal |
| Kamen Wilkinson polyurethane foam cuff [68] | The pressure inside this self inflating cuff is equal to atmospheric pressure and the cuff exerts a very low pressure on the tracheal wall |
| High volume low pressure cuff [69] | The cuff and tracheal wall pressures should be identical if the cuff is carefully selected |

high volume, low pressure cuffs usually enable a tracheal seal to be obtained without any stretching of the cuff. The intracuff pressure will thus be equal to the pressure exerted on the tracheal mucosa. Careful monitoring and control of the cuff pressure is still indicated to prevent both increases and decreases in cuff pressure.

A system which automatically controls the cuff pressure, such as occurs with the Lanz tube, should be used. The introduction of the Lanz tube resulted in a tenfold decrease in the incidence of major tracheal complications and a significant decrease in deaths due to such sequelae during long-term ventilation [70]. These authors found that 25% of their intensive care patients required ventilation for more than 1 week and 10% required ventilation for more than 2 weeks [71]. A reliable system of control of cuff pressure is mandatory during such long-term ventilation.

Methods have also been described to limit the pressure increase due to diffusion of nitrous oxide into the cuff during general anaesthesia (see p. 64). This can result in a large increase in pressure but anaesthesia is usually of relatively short duration and this is therefore less important than the problems related to high cuff pressure in intensive care units.

## DECREASE IN CUFF PRESSURE WITH TIME

In contrast to the numerous reports of increases in cuff pressure during general anaesthesia, there is very little information available on decrease in cuff pressures during long-term ventilation. Jacobsen and Greenbaum, however, investigated the decrease in pressure in both high residual volume, low pressure and low residual volume, high pressure cuffs with time [72]. A wide range of initial cuff pressures occurred with high and low volume cuffs (Table 2). Cuff pressures decreased with time but no correlation was found between the magnitude of the decrease and time. The decrease in pressure was thought to result both from diffusion of gas and slow movement ('creeping') of the plastic in the cuff. The movement was speeded up by warm moist conditions in the trachea and transient increases in intracuff pressure [72]. The 'creeping' mimics the prestretching of cuffs advocated by Geffin and Pontoppidan [51]. It seems likely that the movement of the plastic occurs within the first few hours and after this the decrease in pressure is

**Table 2** Decrease in cuff pressure and time. From Jacobsen and Greenbaum [72].

|  | Initial cuff pressure (mmHg) | Terminal cuff pressure (mmHg) | Time (h) |
|---|---|---|---|
| Low residual volume, high pressure cuffs | 110 | 60 | 17 |
|  | 95 | 75 | 6 |
|  | 30 | 20 | 10 |
|  | 65 | 25 | 30 |
|  | 30 | 20 | 6 |
| High residual volume, low pressure cuffs | 23 | 15 | 6 |
|  | 20 | 5 | 12 |
|  | 20 | 5 | 9 |
|  | 34 | 20 | 6 |
|  | 15 | 5 | 10 |
|  | 45 | 28 | 10 |
|  | 20 | 20 | 6 |
|  | 16 | 10 | 6 |

due to diffusion of gases through the cuff. The movement of the plastic results in an increase in cuff volume and a decrease in pressure [73]. Of course, a leak from an improperly applied occluding device or leaking three-way taps will also reduce cuff pressure. A decrease in cuff pressure may result in aspiration of pharyngeal contents [74] or even inadequate ventilation.

## DYNAMIC CUFF PRESSURE CHANGES

The effect of ventilation on low and high pressure cuffs has been investigated both *in vitro* and *in vivo* [75]. The effect of ventilation on cuff pressure is less important in high (Fig. 13) than low pressure cuffs (Figs 14 and 15). Small changes in pressure in a high volume cuff seen on the trace (Fig. 15) are due to cardiac displacement; the intratracheal inflation pressure is transmitted to the cuff during inspiration. These dynamic changes show that it is not necessary for the cuff pressure to be above the inflation pressure to maintain a seal. In a spontaneously breathing patient, the cuff pressure changed in a negative direction on inspiration and in a positive direction on expiration.

Transient large increases in cuff pressure were measured during coughing [72] (Fig. 16). These frequently occurred following the stimulus of tracheal suction. The open tube prevents a large increase in intrathoracic pressure, thus precluding this as the causative mechanism. It was suggested that during a cough, the trachea changes in shape

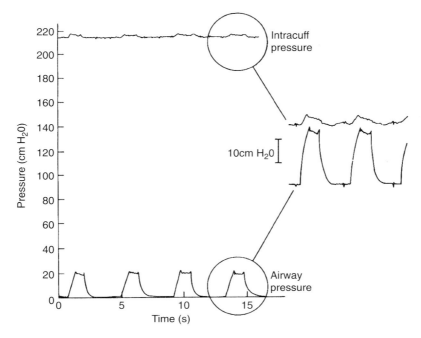

**Figure 13**   Variation of intracuff and airway pressure for the low volume cuff in a patient. From Crawley and Cross [75], with kind permission of the authors and Academic Press, publishers of *Anaesthesia*.

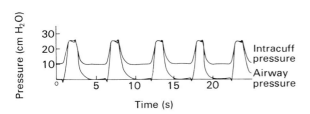

**Figure 14**   Variation of intracuff and airway pressure for the high volume cuff in a model trachea. After Crawley and Cross [75], with kind permission of the authors and Academic Press, publishers of *Anaesthesia*.

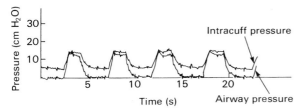

**Figure 15**   Variation of intracuff and airway pressure for a high volume cuff in a patient. The small superimposed changes in pressure are due to cardiac displacement. After Crawley and Cross [75], with kind permission of the authors and Academic Press, publishers of *Anaesthesia*.

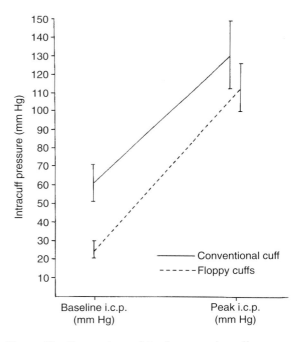

**Figure 16**   Comparison of the increase in cuff pressure with coughing. (Bars represent SEM.) From Jacobsen and Greenbaum [72].

and constricts the cuff of the tube. Cuff pressure with low pressure cuffs increased from 24 to 110 mmHg during coughing and with high pressure cuffs from 61 to 129 mmHg. There was no relationship between the cough force and peak cuff pressure. Such high pressures could theoretically, at least, cause collapse of the tube or cuff herniation. The pressure on the tracheal wall exerted by the cuff has also been shown to rise temporarily during vibration and 'bagging' physiotherapy [76] (Figs 17 and 18). It also rises when a patient 'fights the ventilator' (Fig. 19). Therefore, if this is prolonged, potential damage to the mucosa could result.

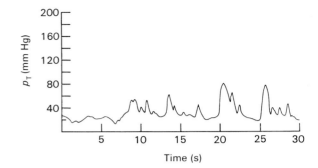

**Figure 19**   The effect of 'fighting the ventilator' on tracheal wall pressure. After Mackenzie *et al.* [76].

In 1974, it was first demonstrated *in vitro* that nitrous oxide diffused into the cuffs of tracheal tubes with consequent increase in cuff volumes [78, 79]. In 1975, it was shown that both pressure and volume increase occurred *in vivo* [80]. The rise in pressure varied with different makes of tubes. The increase ranged from 1.35 to 5 times the initial pressure. It was suggested that these pressure changes could be limited by increasing the thickness of the cuff and that diffusion occurred less rapidly through latex rubber than through polyvinyl chloride. Cuff volumes increased by 42–89% over a test period of approximately 2 h. Analysis of cuff contents showed that 76–88% of the volume changes were due to nitrous oxide diffusion and 2–10% due to diffusion of oxygen. Less than 5% of the pressure increase *in vivo* occurred as a result of warming the air in the cuff from room to body temperature. It was suggested that these changes would be less *in vivo* than *in vitro* because only the cuff area below the tracheal wall would be exposed for diffusion. Thin-walled, high volume, low pressure cuffs have a large portion of the cuff in contact with the tracheal wall, which also acts as an area for diffusion. This area is about 10 times that of the cuff not in contact with the trachea [81].

Cuff pressure and volume changes can be almost eliminated by filling the cuff with the same gas as that inspired [82]. When low pressure cuffs were filled with room air, however, pressures increased by approximately two times the control when breathing either 60% nitrous oxide in oxygen or 98% oxygen and 2% ethrane. Volume and pressure changes following nitrous oxide anaesthesia were similar with both low and high pressure cuffs. It was recommended that cuffs should routinely be filled with gas of the same

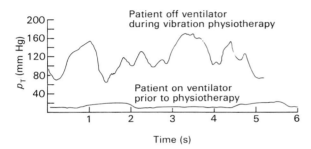

**Figure 17**   Comparison of pressures on the tracheal wall during IPPV and vibration physiotherapy. After Mackenzie *et al.* [76].

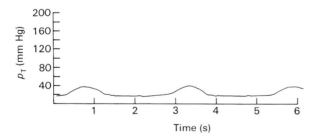

**Figure 18**   The effect of 'bagging' on tracheal wall pressure. After Mackenzie *et al.* [76].

## NITROUS OXIDE DIFFUSION INTO CUFFS

It was shown as early as 1965 that gas-filled spaces in the body will expand during general anaesthesia when nitrous oxide is inspired [77]. When a 75% nitrous oxide concentration was inspired, intestinal gas volumes increased 100–200% in 4 h and the volumes of a pneumothorax increased by 200–300% in 2 h. The increase was influenced by the blood gas solubility and blood flow.

composition as that of the inspired mixture. It is interesting that these increases can not be prevented by breathing oxygen.

A linear increase in pressure occurred over the first 3 h in air-filled high volume low pressure and small volume cuffs during nitrous oxide anaesthesia [83]. This effectively converts a low pressure to a high pressure cuff. These changes were prevented by filling the cuff with gas of the same composition as that inspired or saline (Fig. 20). It was recommended that the cuff pressure should be measured even when the cuff is filled with the same gas as the inspired mixture. If the cuff residual volume is low the filling volume at which the cuff pressure remains low is limited. The volume pressure relationships of one large and one small cuff were demonstrated *in vitro* by Revenas and Lindholm (Fig. 21) [83].

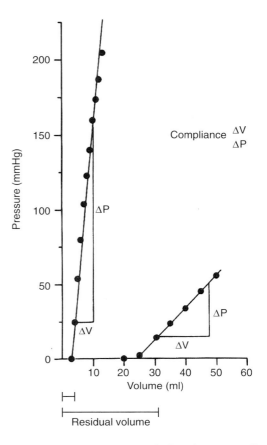

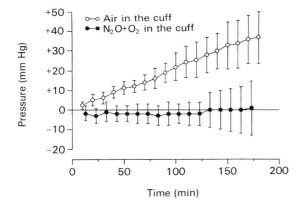

**Figure 20** Pressure changes as a function of time using the large volume cuff during nitrous oxide–oxygen anaesthesia (70–30%). The cuff was filled with air or the nitrous oxide/oxygen mixture. Mean and 95% confidence interval. After Revenas and Lindholm [83], with kind permission of the editor of *Acta Anaesthesiologica Scandinavica*.

**Figure 21** Volume-pressure relations in one small and one large volume cuff tested *in vitro*. From Revenas and Lindholm [83], with kind permission of the editor of *Acta Anaesthesiologica Scandinavica*.

A number of different tubes were investigated both for cuff volume changes with time after being exposed to nitrous oxide *in vitro* and also for the physical characteristics of the cuffs [84]. The rate of nitrous oxide transfer varied inversely with cuff thickness and directly with the partial pressure of nitrous oxide. Cuff thickness ranged from 0.033 to 0.55 mm. Diffusion rates also varied with cuffs of the same composition but different densities, as well as with cuffs of different compositions. Most cuffs were made of polyvinyl chloride. The factors influencing the volume of gas diffusing into a cuff were defined in the following equation by Mehta [85]:

$$V = \frac{KAT\,(P_1 - P_2)}{X}$$

where $V$ = volume of gas diffusing into the cuff, $A$ = area available for diffusion, $T$ = time available, $X$ = thickness of the membranes, $P_1 - P_2$ = difference in pressure of the gas on the two sides of the membranes, and $K$ is a constant which depends on diffusion and solubility characteristics.

Permeability is also affected by the nature of the permeating gas and the physical characteristics of the cuff material.

The use of large diameter, thin-walled cuffs was recommended by Bernhard and his colleagues [84]. However, a thin cuff wall facilitates nitrous oxide transfer and cuff pressures during anaesthesia should therefore be adjusted at 30 min intervals [84] or be used with pressure regulating devices [85–89].

A later simple cuff pressure regulator working on the principle of a tube immersed in water was also shown to be effective in clinical practice [88]. In a group of patients with high volume, low pressure cuffs a large increase in cuff pressure due to nitrous oxide diffusion was demonstrated during anaesthesia (Fig. 22). Any significant rise in pressure was prevented by the use of the 'Tracheal Tube Cuff Pressure Stabilizer'. An electropneumatic device, the Cardiff Cuff Controller, will prevent both rises and falls in cuff pressure [89]. Major changes in cuff pressure due to diffusion of nitrous oxide have also been demonstrated during cardiopulmonary bypass [90].

In conclusion, the increases in cuff pressures and volumes due to diffusion of nitrous oxide are well documented. Clear recommendations have been made that cuff pressures should be

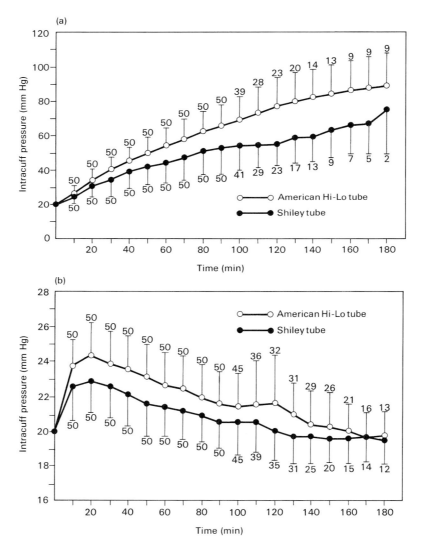

**Figure 22**   Intraoperative changes in intracuff pressure of two types of tracheal tubes when the intracuff pressure was not controlled (a) and when it was controlled (b) by the 'Tracheal tube cuff pressure stabilizer'. Intracuff pressure started at 20 mmHg in all tubes. Vertical bars indicate standard deviation of the mean. Number of tubes is shown at the end of each vertical bar. After Kim [88] with kind permission of the International Anesthesia Research Society.

**Table 3**  Techniques to reduce the effect, or limit the diffusion, of nitrous oxide into the cuff.

| | |
|---|---|
| Fill the cuff with the same mixture as that inspired | Easily done but mixture needs to be changed if inspired mixture changes [82] |
| Fill the cuff with saline | Easily done and no further adjustments required [83] |
| Fill the cuff with air | Measure cuff pressure regularly and adjust as required |
| Fill cuff with air and use devices which limit rises in cuff pressure | • Use pressure release valve [87]<br>• Use 'Tracheal Tube Cuff Pressure Stabilizer' [88]<br>• Use Lanz tube with pressure-limiting balloon [86]<br>• Use electropneumatic control system [89] |
| Kamen Wilkinson Tube with foam cuff | This cuff is self inflating and the cuff can be left open to the atmosphere |
| Brandt Tube with large pilot balloon | The pilot balloon has a larger volume and higher compliance than the cuff. When nitrous oxide diffuses into the system the increase in cuff pressure is therefore limited to safe levels [97] |
| Use of a weight-loaded (2 nickels = 10 g) disposable Concord/Portex Pulsator epidural syringe held in a vertical position and connected to the cuff inflation port | This system is found to reduce reliably the TT cuff pressures both *in vitro* and *in vivo* to values between 10 and 30 cm $H_2O$. When nitrous oxide diffusion into the system is expected, venting of the cuff should be undertaken at regular intervals [98] |

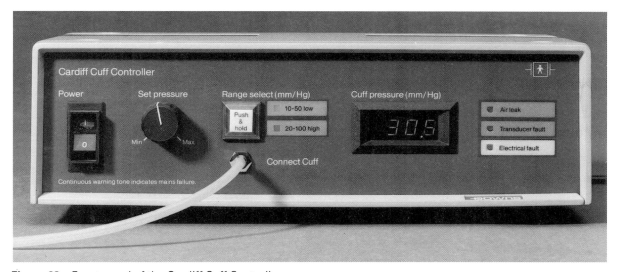

**Figure 23**  Front panel of the Cardiff Cuff Controller.

measured during clinical anaesthesia and appropriate measures taken to prevent an undue rise (Table 3).

## THE CARDIFF CUFF CONTROLLER

This is an electropneumatic device that will prevent both rises and falls in cuff pressures [89].★ It can inflate the cuff to the desired pressure and then maintain that pressure at a constant level as long as required. This should therefore minimize the harmful effects of under- and over-inflation of the cuff and could be of particular benefit to patients receiving long-term ventilatory support.

The Cardiff Cuff Controller is shown in Fig. 23. A schematic diagram of the device is shown in

---

★ Downs Surgical Ltd, Parkway Close, Parkway Industrial Estate, Sheffield, S9 4WJ, UK. Tel: 01742 730346.

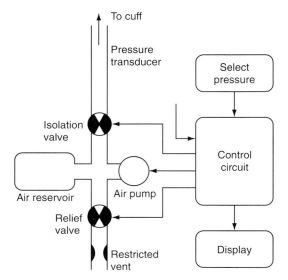

**Figure 24**   Schematic diagram of the Cardiff Cuff Controller. From Morris and Latto [89].

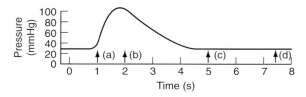

**Figure 25**   Control of cuff pressure by the instrument. (a) Compression of the cuff. (b) Operation of a solenoid valve after 1 s. (c) Release of compression. (d) Cuff restored to original volume. From Morris and Latto [89].

Fig. 24. The reservoir of approximately 150 cm$^3$ helps to stabilize the system. The effect of compressing a cuff *in vitro* is shown in Fig. 25.

It has been shown that gross overinflation resulted when a 10 ml syringe was used to inflate the cuffs of Portex Blue Line disposable tracheal tubes [91]. This problem can be minimized by accurate display of the cuff pressure during inflation. It was shown that the Cardiff Cuff Controller accurately maintained cuff pressures at the desired level for a wide range of surgical times and for different surgical procedures [91]. A later study showed that overinflation also resulted when Portex tubes with higher volume profile cuffs were inflated with 10 ml syringes [92]. It is perhaps surprising that the Cardiff Cuff Controller is not more widely used in clinical practice.

## CONTROL AND MEASUREMENT OF CUFF PRESSURE IN CLINICAL PRACTICE

It is clear that in the UK very few anaesthetists either measure or control the pressure in the cuffs of tracheal tubes. Financial constraints mean that purchase of expensive devices such as the 'Cardiff Cuff Controller' come very low on the list of purchasing priorities. Since the virtual disappearance of red rubber tubes for long-term ventilation there appears to be a reduction in the incidence of major complications related to intubation.

The situation seems to be much better in Sweden [93]. The intracuff pressure was monitored continuously in 57.1% of teaching hospitals and in 25.5% of non-teaching hospitals. In a further 25.5% of non-teaching hospitals and 14.2% of teaching hospitals these pressures were measured, but only intermittently. About 90% of hospitals cuffs were inflated with a volume of gas which provided 'no leak ventilation'. The cuff was inflated to a predetermined pressure in only a small number of hospitals. Most hospitals used air to inflate the cuff but 42.9% of teaching hospitals and 13.8% of other hospitals used the appropriate anaesthetic gas mixture.

In intensive care practice, 85% of hospitals monitored intracuff pressure as a routine and in over 70% of units the cuff was inflated to no-leak ventilation [94]. High residual volume, low pressure cuffs were used routinely in all hospitals. It was stressed that while it is possible to seal the airway with very low cuff pressures, such pressures do not necessarily protect against aspiration [95]. It is safest to maintain an intracuff pressure during expiration of between 2.5 and 3 kPa [96].

## ASPIRATION

'Silent' regurgitation of stomach contents into the pharynx with tracheal intubation during anaesthesia has been reported in 22 out of 152 patients (14.5%) [99] and 58 of 472 patients (12.3%) [100]. Upper abdominal surgery, the prone position or artificial ventilation were all associated with an increased incidence of regurgitation. Therefore, the risk of aspiration is decreased by frequent oropharyngeal suction to prevent the accumulation of fluid in the pharynx [101]. Pharyngeal contents can accumulate in the trachea above the cuff of a tracheal tube. To minimize the volume collecting in the trachea, it has been recommended that the cuff should be placed just beyond the vocal cords and, after cuff inflation, the tube should be withdrawn until resistance is met [17]. At extubation, patients should be placed in a 10° head down in the lateral position and suction applied to the tube.

Speaking tracheostomy tubes (Vocalaid tubes from Portex) have a channel just above the cuff. This channel is normally used for insufflation of oxygen to enable the patient to phonate but can be used for aspiration of secretions which collect above the cuff. We have noted sometimes when these tubes are used in the intensive care unit that quite large volumes of fluid can be aspirated through the oxygen channel. In patients with such large volumes of pharyngeal secretions, aspiration will certainly occur if the cuff is not properly inflated. It has been shown that aspiration past the cuff of tracheostomy tubes can result in fever and pulmonary complications [102]. Aspiration of these secretions through the oxygen channel can result in daily volumes as high as 600 ml being collected with rapid improvement in pulmonary

complications. Thus a cuff protects against massive aspiration but not necessarily against repeated small volumes in patients with laryngeal dysfunction.

Aspiration past tracheal tubes has been studied *in vivo* with dye placed in the mouth [103, 104]. Aspiration of dye occurred in 56% of intensive care patients with low volume, high pressure cuffs and 20% of patients with high volume, low pressure cuffs [104]. However, there were no data on cuff pressures. In patients with a tracheostomy using a high volume, low pressure cuff aspiration occurred in about 16% of patients [105]. Unrecognized aspiration has been suggested as one of the causes of postoperative pulmonary complications; 16% of 300 unselected patients undergoing anaesthesia had evidence of dye aspiration postoperatively [106].

A prospective investigation has been performed to determine the cuff pressure required to prevent aspiration with different cuffs *in vivo* [103]. Evans Blue dye was placed in the pharynx and afterwards the respiratory tract was inspected for evidence of soiling. Aspiration occurred when cuff pressures were kept at 20 cm $H_2O$ but not at 25 cm $H_2O$ or above with both Lanz and Hi-Lo cuffs. Aspiration however did occur even at a cuff pressure of 25–27 cm $H_2O$ with the thicker walled Portex tubes (Tables 4 and 5).

Folds or wrinkles (Fig. 26) can occur in high volume cuffs when the circumference of the cuff is greater than that of the trachea [107]. The

**Table 4** Tube and cuff types, intracuff pressures and incidences of aspiration. From Bernhard *et al.* [103], with kind permission of the authors, the editor of *Anesthesiology*, and the publishers, J. B. Lippincott Co.

| Tube | Cuff size | Intracuff pressure (cm $H_2O$) | Tracheal aspiration of dye (% of cases) |
|---|---|---|---|
| Lanz | Large | 20 | 38.5 |
| American/ NCC Hi-Lo | Large | 20 | 38.5 |
| Lanz | Large | 25 | 0 |
| American/ NCC Hi-Lo | Large | 25 | 0 |
| Lanz | Large | 27–34 | 0 |
| American/ NCC Hi-Lo | Large | Minimal occluding volume (25–27) | 0 |
| Portex Blue Line | Large | Minimal occluding volume (25–27) | 35.3 |
| Rusch Red Rubber | Small | Minimal occluding volume (approx 250) | 0 |

**Table 5** Cuff physical characteristics, intracuff pressures and incidences of aspiration. From Bernhard *et al.* [103], with kind permission of the authors, the editor of *Anesthesiology*, and the publishers, J. B. Lippincott Co.

| Tube | Cuff diameter (mm)±s.d. | Cuff thickness (mm)±s.d. | Intracuff pressure (cm $H_2O$) | Aspiration |
|---|---|---|---|---|
| American Hi-Lo | 33.28±0.76 | 0.044±0.005 | 25 | No |
| Lanz | 30.07±0.63 | 0.104±0.007 | 27–34 | No |
| Portex Blue Line | 28.75±1.63 | 0.25±0.029 | Minimal occluding volume (25–27) | Yes |
| Rusch | 14.52±0.44 | 0.537±0.029 | Minimal occluding volume (±250) | No |

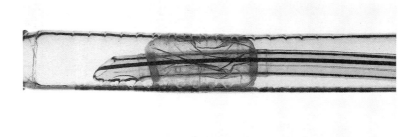

**Figure 26**    Large volume cuff inflated in a model trachea to demonstrate the formation of wrinkles in the cuff.

magnitude of aspiration of liquid past the wrinkles depends on three main factors [96]. These are the viscosity of the liquid, the hydrostatic pressure of the liquid above the cuff and the number and size of the folds or wrinkles. With stiff thick walled cuffs, the wrinkles become collapsed less easily than with thin walled cuffs. Higher cuff pressures are therefore required to prevent leaks with such high volume cuffs particularly where the cuff wall is thicker and less pliable. Aspiration has been reported in two spontaneously breathing patients [107, 108] past properly inflated large volume cuffs and one of the patients died from hypoxia [108]. In the other patient, aspiration was controlled by inserting a low volume high pressure cuffed tube. The extent of aspiration may be accentuated in a spontaneously breathing patient if a subatmospheric pressure is generated distal to the cuff. A thin-walled, high volume cuff is required to fit the tracheal contours at a low inflation pressure without forming wrinkles. Such a cuff would have a diameter when just inflated which is approximately the same as that of the trachea.

*In vitro* tests with three different types of tubes showed that in all instances irrespective of wrinkle formation, leaks could be eliminated by increasing intracuff pressures to high levels [107]. However, aspiration should be prevented with low cuff and tracheal wall pressures so as to decrease the risk of tracheal trauma. Leaks could be minimized when the cuff diameter was approximately the same as the tracheal diameter and wrinkles were not formed [107]. However, in the short term and in high risk situations such as in spontaneously breathing patients, the cuff can be temporarily overinflated to decrease the risk of aspiration [109]. Tests with two types of tubes showed that

the cuff pressures required to produce leak-free ventilation were greater than that at which aspiration occurred in a model trachea with 2 cm $H_2O$ above the cuff [95] (Table 6). The peak airway pressure was fixed at 1.96 kPa. The two tubes had the same cuff thickness but the circumference and stiffness of the Portex cuff was greater than that of the Searle cuff.

The incidence of minor aspiration of pharyngeal contents in clinical practice is not easy to determine and will be influenced by the volume of pharyngeal contents, posture, cuff pressure and design characteristics of the cuff. There may be a difference between the viscosity of aqueous dye and pharyngeal secretions. Thus, the clinical incidence of aspiration past the cuff at a given pressure may not correlate with the expected incidence from *in vitro* tests.

In conclusion, aspiration can be prevented by overinflating the cuff. The cuff is often overinflated during short-term intubation for surgery and serious complications are not normally evident. For the longer term it is important to control cuff pressures accurately.

## THE CUFF AND OTHER FACTORS AND POSTOPERATIVE SORE THROAT

A sore throat after intubation usually lasts for only a few days and is considered a minor unavoidable complication of general anaesthesia [110]. Severe pain elsewhere, following major surgery, often ensures that the less severe pain in the throat is largely ignored. After minor surgery however, a sore throat may be the main cause of postoperative discomfort. This complication occurs more commonly in women than men [111].

**Table 6**  Mean cuff diameters (in 10 cuffs) and aspiration in two types of tubes with the same cuff thickness. Tubes were tested in a model trachea connected to a model lung. From Mehta [95], with kind permission of the editor of *Annals of the Royal College of Surgeons of England.*

| Tube | Wall thickness (mm) | Circumference and (diameter) at residual volume (mm) | Residual volume (ml) | Cuff diameter/ tracheal diameter | Mean cuff pressure to produce leak free ventilation (kPa)* | Mean cuff pressure at which aspiration started to occur (kPa)* |
|------|------|------|------|------|------|------|
| Portex Profile | 0.125 | 93.6 (29.8) | 13.05 | 1.49 | 4.16 | 2.93 (with two tubes aspiration occurred at 5.98) |
| Searle Sensiv | 0.125 | 69.9 (22.2) | 6.9 | 1.11 | 1.06 (in no case higher than 1.47) | 0.54 (in no case higher than 1.08) |

* 1 kPa = 10.2 cm H$_2$O

The incidence of sore throat after general anaesthesia administered by mask varies from 15% [112] to 22% [113, 114] and is generally short lasting and of minor severity [111–121]. These studies have tried to isolate and examine individual contributing causes. In some areas, however, such as the effect of local anaesthetics on the cuff, the evidence is conflicting. The cause of sore throats associated with mask anaesthesia has been attributed to inspiring unhumidified gas with consequent drying of the mucous membranes of the pharynx and trachea. A bolus of succinylcholine administered during mask anaesthesia however resulted in 68.2% incidence of sore throat [122]. The incidence in a control group not receiving succinylcholine was 9.5%. The severity of sore throat correlated with the degree of postoperative myalgia. Atropine, oropharyngeal airway, laryngoscopy and pharyngeal suction were avoided in that study.

The incidence of sore throat after short-term tracheal intubation varies from 6.6% [115] to 90% [112]. A figure widely quoted in the literature is 60% [123]. This is, however, higher than the average values of 30–40% [111–121]. It is not always possible to determine whether a sore throat results from the presence of a tube in the trachea or from the trauma of the intubation [118]. The incidence of sore throat is higher in patients intubated with uncuffed tubes compared with those intubated with cuffed tubes [112].

The use of cuffs with low tracheal contact areas [112–114, 119] reduces the incidence of sore throat. It also seems sensible to adjust cuff pressures intermittently to avoid major pressure rises due to diffusion of nitrous oxide into the cuff [111, 119]. Lubricants are applied routinely to tubes in most centres as an aid to easy and atraumatic intubation. There is conflicting evidence, however, on the use of local anaesthetic lubricants on the incidence of sore throat [110, 114, 119]. Recent evidence [119] suggests that lubrication of the tube with water-soluble jelly, lignocaine ointment or lignocaine jelly does not influence the incidence of sore throat [119].

It is clear that the cuff-related causes only partly influence the incidence of postoperative sore throat (Table 7). However, reducing cuff contact area, intracuff pressure control and improved tube design [121] should all decrease the incidence of this annoying complication. Papers continue to be published investigating single factors which might influence the incidence of sore throat following intubation. It is often shown that changing one factor results in a marked decrease in the incidence of this complication. Since many different causal factors have been described, it does not seem very likely that there is any simple way of totally eliminating this sometimes distressing problem.

**Table 7** Factors which may influence the incidence of postoperative sore throat.

Trauma at intubation to:
    Tonsillar pillars
    Pharynx
    Tongue
    Larynx
    Trachea

Use of stylet

Ryle's tube

Coughing on intubation or extubation

Blind pharyngeal suction

Use of pharyngeal pack

Cuff not deflated at extubation

Tube characteristics
    Pharyngeal contour tubes [41]
    Cuff
        material
        cuff to tracheal contact area
        wrinkles on the cuff
        cuff to tracheal wall pressure

Control of cuff pressures

Control of nitrous oxide diffusion into cuff

Uncuffed compared with cuffed tubes

High compared with low pressure cuffs

Effect of lubricants and local anaesthetics

Method of investigation
    Direct questioning
    Indirect questioning

## CUFF DESIGN RECOMMENDATIONS

Different recommendations have been made regarding the optimal size of large volume cuffs relative to the tracheal size. Mehta recommended that the cuff diameter should be at least one and a half times the tracheal diameter [23]. It is well recognized, however, that wrinkles can form with large volume cuffs. The number and size of these are influenced by the cuff – tracheal circumference ratio, cuff thickness, cuff composition and by the intracuff pressure. Other recommendations are that the cuff circumference and diameter at residual volume should be close to those of the trachea [40, 95]. This should minimize wrinkle formation. At the same time the intracuff pressure should approximate to the tracheal wall pressure. Small volume, high pressure cuffs are undesirable as they produce high minimum sealing pressures

and increase the potential for tracheal trauma. Seegobin and van Hasselt recommended that the residual volume of the ideal tracheal tube should be slightly less than the diameter of the trachea [124]. They recommended that there should be a 10% increase in cuff diameter over the inflation pressure range of 20–30 cm $H_2O$. This should avoid cuff infoldings and allow a seal to be reached at a pressure that does not compromise tracheal mucosal blood flow.

The cuff material should be strong and tear resistant but thin, soft, pliable and flexible. This should ensure a low pressure seal and minimize the size of any wrinkles formed. It should be biologically compatible and not allow diffusion of anaesthetic gases [95]. Early low volume cuffs had large tracheal contact areas; a later recommendation is that a smaller cuff tracheal contact area should be used. Pear shaped or tapered cuffs were thought to be preferable to cylindrical cuffs [95].

## INFLATION OF THE CUFF OF THE LARYNGEAL MASK AIRWAY (LMA)

The pressure exerted on the tracheal mucosa by the cuff of tracheal tube has been widely investigated. The pressure exerted by the LMA cuff on the pharyngeal mucosa has been investigated using similar methodology [125]. The cuff pressure was first measured when the cuff was inflated in free space $P$ (air). The pressure in the cuff was then measured when this cuff was in the pharynx $P$ (pharynx). The pressure exerted on the pharyngeal mucosa $P$ (mucosa) was then calculated from the following formula

$$P \text{ (mucosa)} = P \text{ (pharynx)} - P \text{ (air)}.$$

The cuff pressure rose during anaesthesia if the cuff was inflated with room air. A 20% rise in cuff pressure was noted after 30 min of nitrous oxide anaesthesia. It has been shown, however, that this method may underestimate the pressure exerted on the pharyngeal mucosa [126].

Others have shown that the diffusion across the cuff of nitrous oxide and carbon dioxide was more rapid than the diffusion of nitrogen and oxygen [127]. It was stressed that as the pharynx is distensible the effect of an increase in cuff pressure on the pharyngeal capillary perfusion may be difficult to predict. The effect of an increase in cuff pressure is therefore likely to be of less significance in the distensible pharynx than in the rigid trachea.

If cuffs were inflated with the 'normal' injection volumes, the residual volumes of the cuffs were exceeded [128]. The intracuff pressures *in vivo* were in the range 103–251 mmHg. It was calculated that the pressure on the pharyngeal mucosa exceeded the capillary perfusion pressure. It would appear, therefore, to be important to control cuff inflation and to minimize pressure effects on the mucosa. It is striking, however, that despite these results, the number of significant traumatic complications recorded is very very small.

## CONTROLLING THE INCREASE IN PRESSURE IN THE CUFF OF THE LMA

The same methods that are used to control the pressure in the cuff of the tracheal tube can be used to control the pressure in the cuff of the LMA. It is important to prevent undue rises in cuff pressure. Falls in pressure may be of less significance because the laryngeal mask is not designed to effect a tracheal seal.

The methods that can be used to minimize the effect of diffusion of nitrous oxide into the cuff of the LMA have been compared [127]. The cuff can be filled with the nitrous oxide mixture used for the anaesthetic or the cuff can be filled with water. Pressure relief valves can be used. The Cardiff Cuff Controller would keep the cuff pressure at a predetermined level [89]. Lastly, the pressure can be monitored and the cuff can be deflated if required. This last method was recommended for its simplicity. It was recommended that this technique should be considered in any procedure lasting more than 30 min. The manufacturers also recommend that the cuff pressure should be monitored 'to avoid postoperative throat discomfort' [129].

It has been recommended that cuff pressures should be kept below 30 mmHg. However, this does not appear to be compatible with the manufacturer's recommendations on inflation volumes [126]. Size 3 and 4 laryngeal masks are often inflated with 20 and 30 ml of air, respectively [130], but these maximum volumes can result in excessive cuff pressures and may not be required to produce a seal. Asai and Morris concluded that the cuff should only be inflated with an adequate volume of air [130]. This is often much less than the maximum recommended volumes. The cuff pressure should be monitored and controlled. If the cuff is inflated with fluid, the laryngeal mask airway should not be used again.

## TRAUMA CAUSED BY THE CUFF OF THE LMA

There has been one report of pharyngeal trauma following the repeated use of an LMA [131]. In another case paralysis of the right hypoglossal nerve occurred following 3 h of anaesthesia [132]. Complete recovery followed after 1 week of treatment with steriods and vitamin $B_{12}$. It was suggested that the hypoglossal nerve had been compressed between the cuff of the mask and the hyoid bone (fig. 27). This lesion occurred on the dependent side. The hyoid bone was pushed towards the pharynx by a pillow placed under the head and neck on the right side.

Pharyngeal trauma may be attenuated by pharyngeal accommodation and distension during cuff inflation. In addition there is a reduction in pharyngeal muscle tone associated with general anaesthesia [133]. The incidence of sore throat is lower after use of the laryngeal mask than after tracheal intubation. The incidence ranged from 7 to 12% in three studies [134–136]. A complaint of a 'dry throat' was noted in 36% of patients in one of these three studies [136]. The pressure exerted by the cuff of the tracheal tube causes a significant incidence of tracheal pathology.

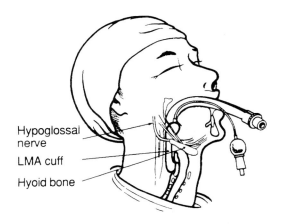

Hypoglossal nerve

LMA cuff

Hyoid bone

**Figure 27** The hypoglossal nerve and the LMA: the hypoglossal nerve passes just behind the greater cornu of the hyoid bone. The distended LMA cuff compressed the hypoglossal nerve against the hyoid bone. With permission from Nagai *et al.* [132].

The absence of significant numbers of problems associated with the cuff of the LMA is a tribute to the design of the device.

## SUMMARY

Improvements in cuff design and management can confidently be expected in the future. This should enable long-term intubation to be accomplished with increased safety.

---

### KEY POINTS

- Disposable plastic tubes are now used in preference to the older red rubber tubes.

- Measurement and control of cuff pressures is carried out in only a minority of cases.

- Despite this, the incidence of major complications appears to be less than when red rubber tubes were more commonly used.

- The cause of sore throat after tracheal intubation is multifactorial. Therefore the incidence by is unlikely to be altered by changing a single aetiological factor.

- The incidence of cuff-related trauma after use of the LMA appears to be remarkably low. This is partly because, in contrast to the tracheal tube, long-term use of the LMA is most unusual.

- Clinicians should aim to measure and control cuff pressures in all cases. This is particularly important in long-term tracheal intubation.

---

## REFERENCES

1 Browning D. H. and Graves S. A. Incidence of aspiration with endotracheal tubes in children. *Journal of Paediatrics* 1983; **102**: 582.

2 Waters R. M., Rovenstine E. A. and Guedel A. E. Endotracheal anaesthesia and its historical development. *Anesthesia and Analgesia* 1933; **12**: 196.

3 Trendelenburg F. Beitrage zur den operationen au den Luftwegen Tamponade der Trachea. *Arch J Klin Chir* 1871; **12**: 121.

4 Macewen W. Clinical observations on the introduction of tracheal tubes by the mouth instead of performing tracheotomy or laryngotomy. *British Medical Journal* 1880; **2**: 122, 163.

5 Eisenmenger V. Zur Tamponade des Larynx nach Prof Maydl. *Wiener Medizinische Wochenschrift* 1893; **43**: 199.

6 Rowbotham E. S. and Magill I. W. Anaesthetics in plastic surgery of the face and jaws. *Proceedings of the Royal Society of Medicine* 1921; **14**: 17.

7 Magill I. W. Technique in endotracheal anaesthesia. *British Medical Journal* 1930; **2**: 817.

8 Guedel A. E. and Waters R. M. A new intratracheal catheter. *Anesthesia and Analgesia* 1928; **7**: 238.

9 Dorrance G. M. On the treatment of traumatic injuries of the lungs and pleurae: with the presentation of a new intratracheal tube for use in artificial respiration. *Surgery, Gynecology and Obstetrics* 1910; **2**: 160.

10 Macintosh R. R. Self-inflating cuff for endotracheal tubes. *British Medical Journal* 1943; **2**: 234.

11 Ibsen B. The anaesthetist's viewpoint on the treatment of respiratory complications in poliomyelitis during the epidemic in Copenhagen. *Proceedings of the Royal Society of Medicine* 1952; **47**: 72.

12 Lassen H. C. A. A preliminary report on the 1952 epidemic of poliomyelitis in Copenhagen. With special reference to the treatment of acute respiratory insufficiency. *Lancet* 1953; **i**: 37.

13 Zwillich C. W., Pierson D. J., Creagh C. E. *et al.* Complications of assisted ventilation. *American Journal of Medicine* 1974; **57**: 161.

14 Whitehouse A. C. and Klock L. E. Evaluation of endotracheal tube position with the fibreopticintubation laryngoscope. *Chest* 1975; **68**: 848.

15 Chander S. and Feldman E. Correct placement of endotracheal tubes. *New York State Journal of Medicine* 1979; **79**: 1843.

16 Hamilton W. K. and Stevens W. C. Malpositioning of endotracheal catheters. *Journal of the American Medical Association* 1966; **198**: 1113.

17 Mehta S. The risk of aspiration in the presence of cuffed endotracheal tubes. *British Journal of Anaesthesia* 1972; **44**: 601.

18 Triner L. A simple maneuver to verify proper positioning of an endotracheal tube. *Anesthesiology* 1982; **57**: 548.

19 Wallace C. T. and Cooke J. E. A new method for positioning endotracheal tubes. *Anesthesiology* 1976; **44**: 272.

20 Cullen D. J., Newbower R. S. and Gemer R. A new method for positioning endotracheal tubes. *Anesthesiology* 1975; **43**: 596.

21 Conrady P. A., Goodman L. R., Lainge F. and Singer M. M. Nasotracheal tube mobility with flexion and hyperextension of the neck. *Critical Care Medicine* 1973; **1**: 117.

22 Seegobin R. D. and Van Hasselt, G. L. Endotracheal cuff pressure and tracheal mucosal blood flow: endoscopic study of effects of four large volume cuffs. *British Medical Journal* 1984; **288:** 965.

23 Mehta S. Endotracheal cuff pressure. *British Medical Journal* 1984; **288:** 1763.

24 Wu W.-H., Lim I.-T., Simpson F. A. and Turndorf H. Pressure dynamics of endotracheal and tracheostomy cuffs. Use of a tracheal model to evaluate performance. *Critical Care Medicine* 1973; **1:** 197.

25 Dobrin P. B., Goldberg E. M. and Canfield T. R. The endotracheal cuff. A comparative study. *Anesthesia and Analgesia* 1974; **53:** 456.

26 McGinnis G. E., Shively J. G., Patterson R. L. and Magovern G. J. An engineering analysis of intratracheal tube cuffs. *Anesthesia and Analgesia* 1971; **50:** 557.

27 Black A. M. S. and Seegobin R. D. Pressure on endotracheal tube cuffs. *Anesthesia* 1981; **36:** 498.

28 Cross E. D. Recent developments in tracheal cuffs. *Resuscitation* 1973; **2:** 77.

29 Mackenzie C. F., Klose S. and Browne D. R. G. (1976) A study of inflatable cuffs on endotracheal tubes. Pressures exerted on the trachea. *British Journal of Anaesthesia* **48:** 105.

30 Carrol R., Hedden M. and Safar P. Intratracheal cuffs. Performance characteristics. *Anesthesiology* 1969; **31:** 275.

31 Dobrin P. and Canfield T. Cuffed endotracheal tubes: mucosal pressures and tracheal wall blood flow. *American Journal of Surgery* 1977; **133:** 562.

32 Knowlson G. T. G. and Bassett H. F. M. The pressures exerted on the trachea by endotracheal inflatable cuffs. *British Journal of Anaesthesia* 1970; **42:** 834.

33 Leigh J. M. and Manard J. P. Pressure on the tracheal mucosa from cuffed tubes. *British Medical Journal* 1979; **1:** 1173.

34 Cooper J. D. and Grillo H. C. Experimental production and prevention of injury due to cuffed tracheal tubes. *Surgery, Gynecology and Obstetrics* 1969; **129:** 1235.

35 Weymuller E. A., Bishop M. J., Fink B. R., Hibbard A. W. and Spelman F. A. Quantification of intralaryngeal pressure exerted by endotracheal tubes. *Annals of Otology, Rhinology and Laryngology* 1983; **92:** 444.

36 Olson N. R. and Bogdasarian R. S. Posterior glottic laryngeal stenosis. *Otalaryngological Head and Neck Surgery* 1980; **88:** 765.

37 Keane W. M., Denneny J. C., Rowe L. D. and Atkins J. P. Complications of intubation. *Annals of Otology, Rhinology and Laryngology* 1983; **91:** 584.

38 Stenqvist O., Sonander H. and Nilsson K. Small endotracheal tubes. Ventilator and intratracheal pressures during controlled ventilation. *British Journal of Anaesthesia* 1979; **51:** 375.

39 Lindholm C. E. Den iatrogent fororsakade trakealstenosens etiologi. *Lakartidningen* 1977; **74:** 2344.

40 Lindholm C. E. and Carroll R. G. Evaluation of tube deformation pressure *in vitro*. *Critical Care Medicine* 1975; **2:** 196.

41 Lindholm C. E. Experience with a new orotracheal tube. *Acta Otolaryngology (Stockholm)* 1973; **75:** 389.

42 Lindholm C. E. and Grenvik A. Flexible fibreoptic bronchoscopy and intubation in intensive care. In: McLedingham I. (ed.) *Recent Advances in Intensive Therapy*. Edinburgh: Churchill Livingstone. 1977; 55.

43 Alexopoulos C., Larsson S. G. and Lindholm C. E. Anatomical shape of the airway. *Acta Anaesthesiologica Scandinavica* 1983; **27:** 185.

44 Alexopoulos C., Larsson S. G. and Lindholm C. E. The anatomical shape of the airway after orotracheal intubation. *Acta Anaesthesiologica Scandinavica* 1983; **27:** 331.

45 Lindholm C. E. and Grenvik A. Tracheal tube and cuff problems. *International Anaesthesiology Clinics* 1982; **20:** 103.

46 Pippin L. K., Short D. H. and Bowes J. B. Longterm tracheal intubation practice in the United Kingdom. *Anaesthesia* 1983; **38:** 791.

47 Tonnesen A. S., Vereen L. and Arens J. F. Endotracheal tube cuff residual volume and lateral wall pressure in a model trachea. *Anesthesiology* 1981; **55:** 680.

48 Nordin U., Lindholm C.-E. and Wolgast M. Blood flow in the rabbit tracheal mucosa under normal conditions and under the influence of tracheal intubation. *Acta Anaesthesiologica Scandinavica* 1977; **21:** 81.

49 Cooper J. D. and Grillo H. C. Analysis of problems related to cuffs on intratracheal tubes. *Chest* 1972; **62:** 21S.

50 Palombini B. and Coburn R. F. Control of the compressibility of the canine trachea. *Respiratory Physiology* 1972; **15:** 365.

51 Geffin B. and Pontoppidan H. Reduction of tracheal damage by the prestretching of inflatable cuffs. *Anesthesiology* 1969; **31:** 462.

52 Mehta S. Endotracheal cuff pressure. *British Medical Journal* 1984; **288:** 1763.

53 Carroll R. G., McGinniss G. E. and Grenvik A. Performance characteristics of tracheal cuffs. *International Anesthesiology Clinics* 1974; **12:** 111.

54 Nordin U. The trachea and cuff induced tracheal injury. An experimental study on causative factors and prevention. *Acta Otolaryngology* 1976; **345:** 1.

55 Alexopoulos B., Jannson B. and Lindholm C.-E. Mucus transport and surface damage after endotracheal intubation and tracheostomy. An experi-

mental study in pigs. *Acta Anaesthesiology Scandinavica* 1984; **28:** 68.

56 Klainer A. S., Turndorf H., Wu W.-H., Maewal H., Allender P. Surface alterations due to endotracheal intubation. *American Journal of Medicine* 1975; **58:** 674.

57 Andrews M. J. and Pearson F. G. Incidence and pathogenesis of tracheal injury following cuffed tube tracheostomy with assisted ventilation. *Annals of Surgery* 1971; **173:** 249.

58 Hardy K. L., Fettel B. E. and Shiley D. P. New tracheostomy tube. *Annals of Thoracic Surgery* 1970; **10:** 58.

59 Gibson P. Aetiology and repair of tracheal stenosis following tracheostomy and intermittent positive pressure respiration. *Thorax* 1967; **22:** 1.

60 Crosby W. M. Automatic intermittent inflation of tracheostomy-tube cuff. *Lancet* 1964; **ii:** 509.

61 Kirby R. R., Robison E. J. and Schulz J. Intermittent cuff inflation during prolonged positive pressure ventilation. *Anesthesiology* 1970; **32:** 364.

62 Rainer W. G. and Sanchez M. Tracheal cuff inflation: synchronous timed with inspiration. *Annals of Thoracic Surgery* 1970; **9:** 384.

63 Arens J. F., Ochsner J. L. and Gee G. Volume limited intermittent cuff inflation for long term respiratory assistance. *Journal of Thoracic and Cardiovascular Surgergy* 1969; **58:** 837.

64 Nordin U. and Lyttkens L. New self-adjusting cuff for tracheal tubes. *Acta Otolaryngol (Stockholm)* 1976; **82:** 455.

65 Benveniste D. Endotracheal and tracheostomy tubes with self-inflating cuff. *Acta Anaesthesiologica Scandinavica* 1967; **11:** 85.

66 Abouav J. and Finley T. N. Self-inflating parachute cuff. A new tracheostomy and endotracheal cuff. *American Journal of Surgery* 1976; **125:** 657.

67 Jackson R. R. and Rokowski W. J. A disposable endotracheal tube with self-inflating cuff. *Archives of Surgery* 1967; **94:** 160.

68 Kamen J. M. and Wilkinson C. J. A new low-pressure cuff for endotracheal tubes. *Anesthesiology* 1971; **34:** 482.

69 Lomholt N. A new tracheostomy tube. *Acta Anaesthesiologica Scandinavica* 1967; **11:** 311.

70 Lewis F. R., Schlobohm R. M. and Thomas A. N. Prevention of complications from prolonged tracheal intubation. *American Journal of Surgery* 1978; **135:** 452.

71 Lewis F. R., Blaisdell F. W. and Schlobohm R. M. Incidence and outcome of post-traumatic respiratory failure. *Archives of Surgery* 1977; **112:** 436.

72 Jacobsen L. and Greenbaum R. A study of intracuff pressure measurements, trends and behaviour in patients during prolonged periods of tracheal intubation. *British Journal of Anaesthesia* 1981; **53:** 97.

73 Hill D. W. *Physics Applied to Anaesthesia* 3rd edn. Butterworths: London. 1976; p. 226.

74 Bernhard W. N., Cottrell J. E., Sivakumaran C., Patel K., Yost L. and Turndorf H. Adjustment of intracuff pressure to prevent aspiration. *Anaesthesiology* 1979; **50:** 363.

75 Crawley B. E. and Cross D. E. Tracheal cuffs. A review and dynamic pressure study. *Anaesthesia* 1975; **30:** 4.

76 Mackenzie C. F., Klose S. and Browne D. R. G. A study of inflatable cuffs on endotracheal tubes. *British Journal of Anaesthesia* 1976; **48:** 105.

77 Eger E. I. and Saidman L. J. Hazards of nitrous oxide anesthesia in bowel obstruction and pneumothorax. *Anesthesiology* 1965; **26:** 61.

78 Stanley T. H. Effects of anesthetic gases on endotracheal tube cuff gas volumes. *Anesthesia and Analgesia* 1974; **53:** 480.

79 Stanley T. H., Kawamura R. and Graves C. Effects of nitrous oxide on volume and pressure of endotracheal tube cuffs. *Anesthesiology* 1974; **41:** 256.

80 Stanley T. H. Nitrous oxide and pressures and volumes of high and low-pressure endotracheal tube cuffs in intubated patients. *Anesthesiology* 1975; **42:** 637.

81 Brandt L. Nitrous oxide in oxygen and tracheal tube cuff volumes. *British Journal of Anaesthesia* 1982; **54:** 1238.

82 Stanley T. H., Liu W-S. Tracheostomy and endotracheal tube cuff volume and pressure changes during thoracic operations. *Annals of Thoracic Surgery* 1975; **20:** 144.

83 Revenas B. and Lindholm C-E. Pressure and volume changes in tracheal tube cuffs during anaesthesia. *Acta Anaesthesiologica Scandinavica* 1976; **20:** 321.

84 Bernhard W. N., Yost L., Turndorf H., Cottrell J. E. and Paegle R. D. Physical characteristics of and rates of nitrous oxide diffusion into tracheal tube cuffs. *Anesthesiology* 1978; **48:** 413.

85 Mehta S. Effects of nitrous oxide and oxygen on tracheal tube cuff gas volumes. *British Journal of Anaesthesia* 1981; **53:** 1227.

86 Magovern G. J., Shiveley J. G, Fecht D. and Thevoz F. The clinical and experimental evaluation of a controlled pressure intratracheal cuff. *Journal of Thoracic and Cardiovascular Surgery* 1972; **64:** 747.

87 Stanley T. H., Foote J. L. and Liu W-S. A simple pressure relief valve to prevent increases in endotracheal tube cuff pressure and volume in intubated patients. *Anesthesiology* 1975; **43:** 478.

88 Kim J–M. The tracheal tube cuff pressure stabilizer and its clinical evaluation. *Anesthesia and Analgesia* 1980; **59:** 291.

89 Morris G. and Latto I. P. An electropneumatic instrument for measuring and controlling the pressures in the cuffs of tracheal tubes: 'The Cardiff

Cuff Controller'. *Journal of Medical Engineering and Technology* 1985; **9**: 229.

90  Ikeda S. and Schweiss J. F. Tracheal tube cuff volume changes during extracorporeal circulation. *Canadian Anaesthetists Society Journal* 1980; **27**: 453.

91  Willis B. A., Latto I. P. and Dyson A. Tracheal tube cuff pressure. The clinical use of the Cardiff Cuff Controller. *Anaesthesia* 1988; **43**: 312.

92  Willis B. A. and Latto I. P. Profile-cuffed tracheal tubes and the Cardiff Cuff Controller. *Anaesthesia* 1989; **44**: 524.

93  Mehta S. and Mickiewicz M. Work practices relating to intubation in operating rooms in Sweden. *Acta Anaesthesiologica Scandinavica* 1986; **30**: 480.

94  Mehta S. and Mickiewicz M. Work practices relating to intubation and associated procedures in intensive care units in Sweden. *Acta Anaesthesiologica Scandinavica* 1986; **30**: 637.

95  Mehta S. Performance of low-pressure cuffs. An experimental evaluation. *Annals of the Royal College of Surgeons of England* 1982; **64**: 54.

96  Mehta S. Safe lateral wall cuff pressure to prevent aspiration. *Annals of the Royal College of Surgeons of England* 1984; **66**: 426.

97  Brandt L., Muller-Spath R. and Moussa R. G. *Reduction of Nitrous Oxide Induced Endotracheal Tube-cuff Pressure Rise during Anaesthesia with the 'Rediffusion System'.* Germany: Mallinckrodt Scientific Edition Booklet, 2nd edn. Mallinckrodt GmbH division, Hennef. 1990.

98  Resnikoff E. and Katz J. A. A modified epidural syringe as an endotracheal tube cuff pressure-controlling device. *Anesthesia and Analgesia* 1990; **70**: 208.

99  Turndorf H., Rodis I. D. and Clark T. S. 'Silent' regurgitation during general anesthesia. *Anesthesia and Analgesia* 1974; **53**: 700.

100  Blitt C. D., Gutman H. L., Cohen D. D., Weisman H. and Dillon J. B. 'Silent' regurgitation and aspiration during general anaesthesia. *Anesthesia and Analgesia* 1970; **49**: 707.

101  Macrae W. and Wallace P. Aspiration around high-volume low pressure endotracheal cuff. *British Medical Journal* 1981; **283**: 1220.

102  Shahvari M. B. G., Kigin C. M. and Zimmerman J. E. Speaking tracheostomy tube modified for swallowing dysfunction and chronic aspiration. *Anesthesiology* 1977; **44**: 290.

103  Bernhard W. N., Cottrell J. E., Sivakumaran C., Patel K., Yost L and Turndorf H. Adjustment of intracuff pressure to prevent aspiration. *Anesthesiology* 1979; **50**: 363.

104  Spray S. B., Zuidema G. D. and Cameron J. L. Aspiration pneumonia. Incidence of aspiration with endotracheal tubes. *American Journal of Surgery* 1976; **131**: 701.

105  Bone D. K., Davies J. L., Zuidema G. D. and Cameron J. L. Aspiration pneumonia. Prevention of aspiration in patients with tracheostomies. *Annals of Thoracic Surgery* 1974; **18**: 30.

106  Cameron J. L. and Zuidema G. D. Aspiration pneumonia. Magnitude and frequency of the problem. *Journal of the American Medical Association* 1972; **219**: 1194.

107  Pavlin E. G., Van Nimwegan D. and Hornbein T. F. Failure of a high-compliance low-pressure cuff to prevent aspiration. *Anesthesiology* 1975; **42**: 216.

108  Routh G., Hanning C. D. and McLedingham I. Pressure on the tracheal mucosa from cuffed tubes. *British Medical Journal* 1979; **1**: 1425.

109  Egatinski J. Overinflating low-pressure cuffs to prevent aspiration. *Anesthesiology* 1975; **42**: 114.

110  Riding J. E. Minor complications of general anaesthesia. *British Journal of Anaesthesia* 1975; **47**: 91.

111  Saanivaara L. and Grahne B. Clinical study on an endotracheal tube with a high-residual volume, low pressure cuff. *Acta Anaesthesiologica Scandinavica* 1981; **25**: 89.

112  Loeser E. A., Stanley T. L., Jordan W. and Machin R. Postoperative sore throat: influence of tracheal cuff lubrication versus cuff design. *Canadian Anaesthetists Society Journal* 1980; **27**: 156.

113  Loeser E. A., Orr D. L., Bennett G. M. and Stanley T. H. Endotracheal tube cuff design and post operative sore throat. *Anesthesiology* 1976; **45**: 684.

114  Loeser E. A., Bennett G. M., Orr D. L. and Stanley T. H. Reduction of postoperative sore throat with new endotracheal tube cuffs. *Anesthesiology* 1980; **52**: 257.

115  Lund L. O. and Daos F. G. Effects on postoperative sore throats of two analgesic agents and lubricants used with endotracheal tubes. *Anesthesiology* 1965; **26**: 681.

116  Stanley T. H. Nitrous oxide and pressures and volume of high- and low-pressure endotracheal tube cuffs in intubated patients. *Anesthesiology* 1965; **42**: 637.

117  Loeser E. A., Machin R., Colley J., Orr D., Bennett G. M. and Stanley T. H. Postoperative sore throat – importance of endotracheal tube conformity versus cuff design. *Anesthesiology* 1978; **49**: 430.

118  Stenqvist O. and Nilsson K. Postoperative sore throat related to tracheal tube cuff design. *Canadian Anaesthetists Society Journal* 1982; **29**: 384.

119  Jensen P. J., Hommelgaard P., Sondergaard P. and Erikson S. Sore throat after operation: influence of tracheal intubation, intracuff pressure and type of cuff. *British Journal of Anaesthesia* 1982; **54**: 453.

120  Stock C. and Downs J. B. Lubrication of tracheal tubes to prevent sore throat from intubation. *Anesthesiology* 1982; **57**: 418.

121 Alexopoulos C. and Lindholm C. E. Airway complaints and laryngeal pathology after intubation with an anatomically shaped tube. *Acta Anaesthesiologica Scandinavica* 1983; **27:** 339.

122 Capan L. M., Bruce D. L., Patel K. P. and Turndorf H. Succinylcholine induced postoperative sore throat. *Anesthesia and Analgesia* 1983; **62:** 245.

123 Wylie W. D. and Churchill-Davidson H. C. Examination of the respiratory tract and tracheal intubation. In: *A Practice of Anaesthesia, Anesthesia and Analgesia* 3rd edn. Chicago: Year Book Medical Publishers. 1964; 368–371.

124 Seegoblin R. D. and van Hassett G. L. Aspiration beyond endotracheal cuffs. *Canadian Anaesthetists Society Journal* 1986; **33:** 2730.

125 O'Kelly S. M., Heath K. J. and Lawes E. G. A study of laryngeal mask inflation. Pressures exerted on the pharynx. *Anaesthesia* 1993; **48:** 1075.

126 Marjot R. Laryngeal mask cuff pressures. *Anaesthesia* 1994; **49:** 447.

127 Lumb A. B. and Wrigley M. W. The effect of nitrous oxide on laryngeal mask pressure. *In vitro* and *in vivo* studies. *Anaesthesia* 1992; **47:** 320.

128 Brain A. I. J. The intavent laryngeal mask. Instruction manual, 2nd edn. Windsor: Colgate Medical Ltd, 1991.

129 Asai T. and Morris S. Inflation of the cuff of the laryngeal mask. *Anaesthesia* 1995; **49:** 1098.

130 Marjot R. Trauma to the posterior pharyngeal wall casused by a laryngeal mask airway. *Anaesthesia* 1991; **46:** 589.

131 Nagai K., Sakuramoto C. and Goto F. Unilateral hypoglossal nerve paralysis following the use of the laryngeal mask airway. *Anaesthesia* 1994; **49:** 603.

132 Nandi P. R., Charlesworth C. H., Taylor S. J., Nunn J. F. and Dore C. J. Effect of general anaesthesia on the pharynx. *British Journal of Anaesthesia* 1991; **66:** 157.

133 Alexander C. A. and Leach A. B. Incidence of sore throats with laryngeal masks. *Anaesthesia* 1991; **46:** 791.

134 Sarma V. J. The use of the laryngeal mask airway in spontaneously breathing patients. *Acta Anaesthesiologica Scandinavica* 1990; **34:** 669.

135 Maltby J. R., Loken R. G. and Watson N. C. The laryngeal mask airway: clinical appraisal in 250 patients. *Anaesthesia* 1990; **37:** 509.

136 Marjot R. Pessure exerted by the laryngeal mask airway cuff upon the pharyngeal mucosa. *British Journal of Anaesthesia* 1993; **70:** 25.

# 4

# Predicting a Difficult Intubation

*Ralph S. Vaughan*

---

**Clinical history**

**Clinical examination**
    Mouth opening
    Jaw movement
    Inspection of the back of the mouth
    Cervical spinal movements

**Measurements**
    Patil distance
    Wilson risk score
    Distance between the mandible and the hyoid
    bone
    Savva distance

**Radiological investigations**

**Combination of tests**

**Pregnancy**

**Response to predicted difficulty**

**Predicting a difficult airway**

**Key points**

**References**

---

When a laryngoscope is correctly placed in a normal patient who is properly positioned, the axes of the oral cavity, the pharynx and the trachea tend to come into a straight line (Fig. 1). Such a line generally allows the easy passage of a tracheal tube. In order to achieve such an easy intubation, certain anatomical features must be present. These are:

- a normal temporomandibular joint;
- normal forward movement of the mandible and tongue;
- normal anatomy at the back of the mouth;
- normal flexion of the neck;
- normal movement of the occiput on the atlas.

Predicting a potential normal or abnormal intubation, therefore depends on a combination of the history, clinical examination, additional measurements and occasionally, radiology [1].

## CLINICAL HISTORY

It is important to ask all patients if they have received a general anaesthetic in the past. The majority of patients will respond positively and further questioning will indicate that there had been no difficulties. However, on very rare occa-sions, a different response will be obtained. The patient may:

- recall that an anaesthetist had said that there had been some difficulty with the airway.
- produce written information from an anaesthetist with regard to the difficulty that occurred. The details may also be recorded in the case notes.
- carry some form of bracelet which warns of the difficulty. Such information should always be noted, as failure to take cognizance of these warnings could lead to dire consequences, particularly for the patient.

## CLINICAL EXAMINATION

Any gross malformation of the upper airway anatomy should be immediately apparent. Thereafter, the examination of the upper airway is orientated towards the anatomical features associated with a normal laryngoscopy.

### Mouth Opening

Most patients, when they open their mouth fully, should be able to place their three middle fingers

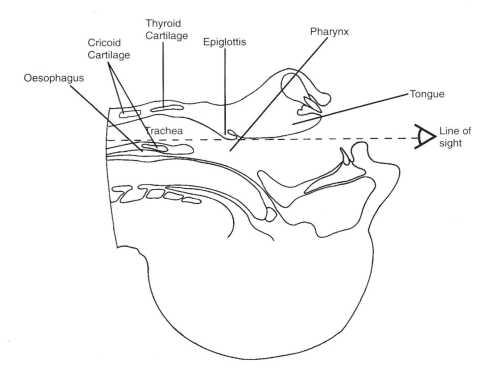

**Figure 1**   Drawing the normal axes of the oral cavity, pharynx and trachea.

between the upper and lower teeth. This distance can vary between 4 and 6 cm. This usually means that the movement of the temporomandibular joint is normal.

## Jaw Movement

Most people should be able to move their lower teeth in front of their upper teeth. There are three possible end positions [2].

- The lower teeth can be protruded more anteriorly than the upper teeth. This could be called position A.
- The lower teeth can close against the upper teeth but cannot move any further forward. This can be called position B.
- The lower teeth cannot reach the closed position (i.e. position B). This could be called position C.

If the patient has buck teeth, it is extremely difficult to obtain position A and this often makes subsequent laryngoscopic demonstration of the cords much more difficult.

## Inspection of the Back of the Mouth

During this examination, it is recommended that the examiner sits immediately opposite the patient. If the patient is in a bed and unable to sit up, the anaesthetist looks directly down at the patient. The patient is asked to open the mouth as wide as possible and, at the same time, protrude the tongue as far as possible. This examination, introduced by Mallampati *et al.* [3], extended by Samsoon and Young [4], and modified by Frerk [5], can be divided into four grades, as illustrated (Fig. 2). In general, the higher the grade, the greater the possible difficulty with intubation.

## Cervical Spinal Movements

Cervical spinal movements [6] can be divided into two separate components.

### *General cervical movement*

This is easily observed by asking the patient to flex and extend the head to the maximum range which

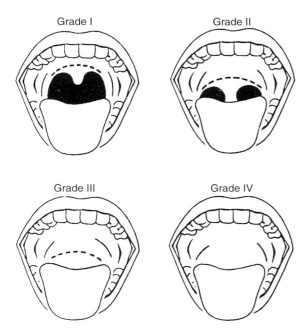

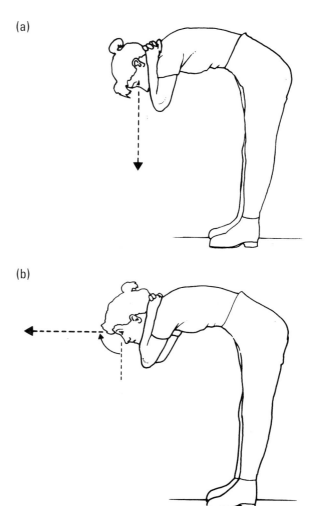

behind the neck and then elevate the head as far forward anteriorly as possible, the normal movement should be around 90° (Fig. 3). If the angle is less than 90°, there is increasing difficulty with laryngoscopy. Furthermore, a recent paper by Calder *et al.* [8] has highlighted this increased difficulty in patients with cervical spine disease.

The combination of these five clinical investigations can indicate potential difficulty in airway management. If these examinations are within the normal limits, intubation is usually easily accomplished.

(a)

(b)

**Figure 2** Junction of hard and soft palate (- - -). Views seen at back of the oral cavity with the mouth open as far as possible and the tongue fully protruded. After Frerk. Predicting difficult intubation. *Anaesthesia* 1991; **46**: 1005.

is usually greater than 90°. Flexion of the cervical vertebrae is important as it is one of the components which produce the classical intubation position of 'sniffing the morning air'. The side to side movement of the cervical spine does not seem to be a contributory factor in a difficult airway.

### *Specific atlanto-occipital movement*

The second, and more important component of the 'sniffing the morning air' position, is the movement of the occiput on the atlas. Clinically, this is not easy to elicit. A warning sign has been described by Delilkan [7]. It involves placing the index finger of each hand, one underneath the chin and one under the inferior occipital prominence with the patient's head in the neutral position. The patient is asked to fully extend the head on the neck. If the finger under the chin is seen to be higher than the other, there would appear to be no difficulty with intubation. If the level of both fingers remains the same or the chin finger remains lower than the other, increased difficulty is predicted. In addition, if one asks the patient to flex the neck as fully as possible, place both hands

**Figure 3** Specific atlanto-occipital movement. (a) Eyes looking at the floor with the neck held by the hands. (b) Eyes into horizontal position with the neck still held by the hands.

## MEASUREMENTS

There have been several measurements made over several years which have contributed to the prediction of a difficult airway.

## Patil Distance

The distance between superior and anterior aspects of the thyroid cartilage and the tip of the mandible has been measured [9] (Fig. 4). It has been found that the normal distance is above 6 cm and any distance greater than this length is usually associated with easy laryngoscopy. Any distances below 6 cm are associated with increasing degrees of difficulties.

## Wilson Risk Score

Wilson and colleagues [10], following a study involving 1500 patients, were able to construct a scoring system based on five variables (Table 1). These variables were: weight, head and neck movement, jaw movement, mandibular recession and the presence of buck teeth. These variables were arbitrarily awarded a score of 0 for normal patients, which could increase through 1 and 2 with increasing abnormalities. The greater the difficulty with each individual part, the higher the score awarded. At the end of the examination the total score was deduced with a maximum of 10. In particular, any risk score above 4 was associated with very low false positive rates.

**Table 1** The Wilson 'risk score'.

| Risk factor | Risk level | Normal | Difficult | P |
|---|---|---|---|---|
| Weight | 0 | 533(95%) | 45(90%) | |
| | 1 | 27(5%) | 3(6%) | 0.05 |
| | 2 | 1(0.2%) | 2(4%) | |
| Head and neck movement | 0 | 297(91%) | 27(54%) | |
| | 1 | 21(6%) | 11(22%) | 0.001 |
| | 2 | 8(3%) | 12(24%) | |
| Jaw movement | 0 | 457(92%) | 19(38%) | |
| | 1 | 36(7%) | 17(34%) | 0.001 |
| | 2 | 2(0.4%) | 14(28%) | |
| Receding mandible | 0 | 506(97%) | 29(58%) | |
| | 1 | 16(3%) | 16(32%) | 0.001 |
| | 2 | 1(0.2%) | 5(10%) | |
| Buck teeth | 0 | 504(96%) | 32(64%) | |
| | 1 | 18(3%) | 12(24%) | 0.001 |
| | 2 | 2(0.4%) | 6(12%) | |

## Distance between the Mandible and the Hyoid Bone

Chou and Wu examined X-ray evidence in a small number of patients who had been difficult to laryngoscope. They found that the vertical distance between the mandible and the hyoid bone was substantially longer [11].

## Savva Distance

Recently, Savva [2] has looked at the methods that have been used to predict a difficult intubation. He also measured the distances between the sternum and the tip of the jaw – the sterno mental distance – when the patient's head was fully extended on the neck with the mouth closed (Fig. 4). In his series, he noted that a distance of less than 12.5 cm was associated with the difficulty found in 14 out of 17 patients. It is suggested that measuring this distance may be

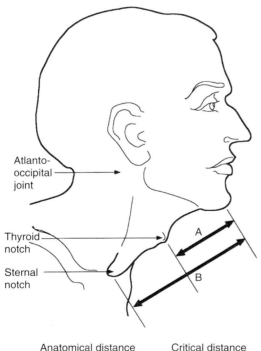

| Anatomical distance | Critical distance |
|---|---|
| A = Thyro-mental distance (Patil distance) | 6.0 cm |
| B = Sterno-mental distance (Savva distance) | 12.5 cm |

**Figure 4**   The Savva and Patil measurements indicating critical distances. The head is fully extended on the neck.

a useful bedside test for predicting preoperative difficulties.

## RADIOLOGICAL INVESTIGATIONS

The original work by White and Kander using X-rays of the head and neck has been repeated, extended and subjected to more detailed analysis [12]. Due mainly to economic factors, these investigations are not easily available and therefore tend not to be used as a routine. However, they are very useful when trying to ascertain what may have caused any difficulty.

When an X-ray is requested to try to predict a difficult airway, the following views are essential. Anteroposterior and lateral views of the neck and thoracic inlet are required. This X-ray will indicate any laryngeal or tracheal deviations or narrowing. It will also show the cervical spines. These pictures are very important and can reveal much information. The lateral X-ray in Fig. 5 shows a classical 'bamboo' spine.

Lateral views of the head and neck are also required. The first of these should be in the neutral position, i.e. with the patient looking straight ahead with the mouth closed. The second should be taken with the head extended as far as possible on the atlas. A comparison between these two films will indicate the degree of extension of the occiput upon the atlas.

The most sophisticated method of examining the atlanto-occipital movement is the use of magnetic resonance imaging (MRI). Two examples are shown (Figs 6 and 7), illustrating the normal movement and other detailed anatomy. Other measurements and comparisons of one distance with another have been made. However, these are usually more in the research rather than the clinical fields [13].

Tracheal abnormalities *per se* are usually difficult to predict but are usually associated clinically with stridor or changes in the voice. Although an anteroposterior chest X-ray continues to be the gold standard world-wide, computerized tomography (CT) scanning (Fig. 8) gives an excellent picture.

## COMBINATION OF TESTS

One of the major problems associated with predicting a difficult airway is that there is a

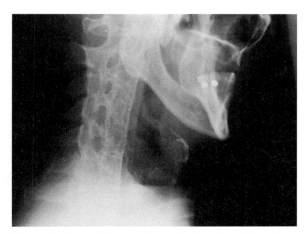

**Figure 5**   Lateral X-ray of a neck showing a 'bamboo spine'.

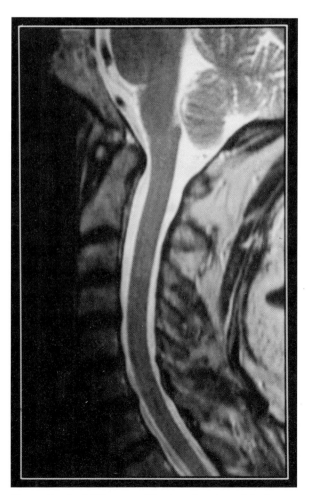

**Figure 6**   An MRI scan of the head and neck in the neutral position.

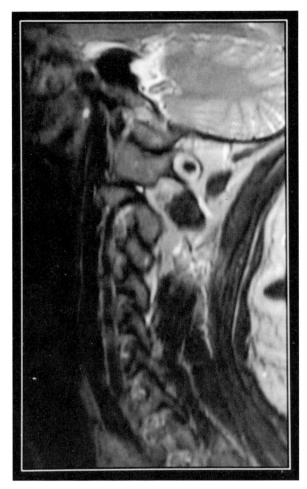

**Figure 7**   An MRI scan of the head and neck with the occiput fully flexed on the atlas.

modified Mallampati assessment in association with a Patil measurement, found that the combination produced a high sensitivity and specificity:

- The sensitivity of such a test calculates the percentage of the difficult airways that are predicted.
- The specificity relates to those producing very low false positives.

The Wilson risk score, for example, used five individual factors and was more successful in producing greater sensitivity and specificity. Latterly, Arne and colleagues have also produced a scoring system based on a multiple factorial analysis [16]. During the investigations they included most of the factors discussed earlier but also included the presence of additional airway pathology, particularly in otorhinolaryngology patients. This investigation produced both a high sensitivity and specificity, resulting in figures consistently greater than 90% for both categories.

## PREGNANCY

Females can have their airway characteristics altered by the physiological changes of pregnancy. In the normal population, the incidence of failed intubation is around 1 in 2303 patients [17]. In pregnant females it has been reported to be around 1 in 300 patients [18]. The main reason for this significant change is that the tissues increase in size as a result of fluid retention. In addition, total body water can increase which will promote capillary engorgement, particularly in the mucosa of the airway passages. Pregnancy-induced hypertension (pre-eclampsia) can also increase the degree of fluid retention and laryngeal oedema has been associated with this condition. It is therefore very wise to consider such patients at greater risk than is normal, despite an apparently normal clinical upper airway examination.

The prediction of a difficult airway therefore follows routine lines. In general, provided five or six simple tests taking no longer than 2–3 min are performed, the majority of cases will be identified. Sadly, despite the application of these tests, a few patients are recorded each year as having produced tremendous difficulty at intubation although they had been otherwise apparently normal.

However, a possible explanation for such an

tremendous variation between observers. These have been subject to many investigations and those of Oates et al. [14] and Tham et al. [15] confirm these variable factors. Consequently, as most tests are subject to individual variation, it means that they are not reproducible from one centre to another.

Such differences also compound the false positives and negatives that result following some of these examinations. It is not surprising, therefore, that the success rate using individual tests is fairly low and, in addition, is also associated with high false positives (e.g. 50% prediction with 5% false positives).

Such results have stimulated other researchers to use combinations of these tests to try to obtain more meaningful results. Frerk [5], using a

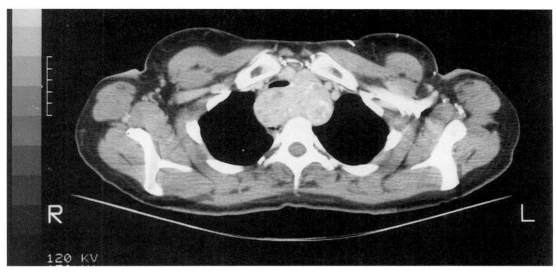

**Figure 8**   A CT scan of a deviated and narrowed trachea.

anomaly may rest with recent investigations using MRI in both children and adults. Under general anaesthesia, it is well known that unless the jaw is supported, the tongue will obstruct the airway. When MRI was used to investigate what happened to the airway in sedated and anaesthetized patients, not only was the tongue a cause of obstruction, but also the anteroposterior diameter of the pharynx was decreased at the soft palate level. Therefore, it may well be wise to accept a concept that airway characteristics are altered by sedation and anaesthesia, and these alterations are usually detrimental to that airway [19, 20].

## RESPONSE TO A PREDICTED DIFFICULTY

In general, if a difficulty is predicted, most anaesthetists would assume that obtaining a good view of the larynx will be more difficult. However, this is not always true. Difficulty with laryngoscopy is usually associated with abnormality of the upper airway. Classifying the degree of difficulty with intubation is based on the classical observations of Cormack and Lehane [21]. However, these classical gradings are, by and large, not relevant when predicting a difficult airway, although they are paramount in describing a difficult laryngoscopy.

What does the anaesthetist in training do when

(s)he predicts a difficult intubation? It would be wise, in the first instance, to summon more experienced assistance. The more experienced anaesthetist will make a decision in regard to management, namely, can the patient be managed another way, for example, under epidural or spinal anaesthesia?

If tracheal intubation is mandatory the choice is usually between accomplishing intubation under sedation and local analgesia or with the patient anaesthetized but breathing spontaneously. Some anaesthetists might also use a short acting depolarizing muscle relaxant *in the anaesthetized spontaneously breathing patient provided they have demonstrated beforehand that the patient's lungs could be ventilated manually*. Such ventilation can be accomplished using the traditional bag and mask technique, or perhaps with a laryngeal mask airway (LMA).

What would a trainee do when faced with an unexpected difficult intubation after general anaesthesia had been induced? Under such circumstances, failed intubation and ventilation drills are introduced with the prime objective of keeping the patient adequately oxygenated until assistance arrives. The management of both predicted and unpredicted difficulties with the airway are described in greater detail in chapter 6.

## PREDICTING A DIFFICULT AIRWAY

Although predicting a difficult intubation is based on the examinations and tests that have been discussed, predicting a difficult airway is not as easy [1]. The factors involved in predicting a difficult intubation are certainly contributory. Others could include, for example:

- difficulty with a man who has a dense beard as the facemask may be difficult to apply;
- tracheal stenosis caused by tumours or strictures;
- anatomical changes after induction of general anaesthesia;
- bronchopleural fistulae;
- asthma.

Each of these conditions is assumed in general to cause potential airway problems and would be managed appropriately.

## KEY POINTS

- Always take a history of previous general anaesthetics and note any correspondence

- Examine
  - Mouth opening
  - Back of mouth – Mallampati
  - Forward movement of the mandible; lower teeth should be able to move beyond upper teeth

- Movement of cervical spine
  - $C_2$–$C_8$ – nodding to and fro
  - Atlanto-occipital joint
  - Delilkan warning sign
  - Usually should move around 90°

- Measurements
  Head fully extended on the neck with the mouth closed
  - Patil distance should be greater than 6.0 cm
  - Savva distance should be greater than 12 cm
  - Wilson risk score: of less than 2 is generally safe but beware of false positives and negatives

- X-rays are of limited value
- Pregnancy
  Difficulties increased due mainly to fluid retention and oedema

- Response to predicted difficulty
  - Seek help
  - Never use muscle relaxants until the airway is fully established

## REFERENCES

1 Benumof J. L. Management of the difficult adult airway with special emphasis on awake tracheal intubation. *Anaesthesiology* 1991; **75:** 1087.
2 Savva D. Prediction of difficult tracheal intubation *British Journal of Anaesthesia* 1994; **70:** 149.
3 Mallampati S. R., Gatt S. P., Gugino L. D. *et al.* A clinical sign to predict difficult tracheal intubation: a prospective study. *Canadian Anaesthetists Society Journal* 1985; **32:** 429.
4 Samsoon G. L. T. and Young J. R. B. Difficult

tracheal intubation: a retrospective study. *Anaesthesia* 1987; **42:** 487.

5 Frerk C. M. Predicting difficult intubation. *Anaesthesia* 1991; **46:** 1005.

6 Wilson M. E. Predicting difficult intubation. *British Journal of Anaesthesia* 1993; **71:** 33.

7 Delilkan A. E. Pre-anaesthetic prediction of difficult intubation – a warning sign. *Malaysian Journal of Surgery* 1979; **5:** 68–72.

8 Calder I., Calder J. and Crockard H. A. Difficult direct laryngoscopy in patients with cervical spine disease *Anaesthesia* 1995; **50:** 756–763.

9 Patil V. U., Stehling L. C. and Zauder H. L. *Fiberoptic Endoscopy in Anesthesia.* Chicago: Year Book Medical Publishers. 1983.

10 Wilson M. E., Speiglhalter D., Robertson J. A. and Lesser P. Predicting difficult intubation. *British Journal of Anaesthesia* 1988; **61:** 211–216.

11 Chou H. C. and Wu T. L. Mandibulohyoid distance in difficult intubation. *British Journal of Anaesthesia* 1993; **71:** 335–339.

12 White A. and Kander P. L. Anatomical factors in difficult direct laryngoscopy. *British Journal of Anaesthesia* 1975; **47:** 468–473.

13 Horton W. A., Fahy L. and Charters P. Disposition of cervical vertebrae, atlanto-axial joint, hyoid and mandible during X-ray laryngoscopy. *British Journal of Anaesthesia* 1989; **63:** 435–438.

14 Oates J. D. L, Oates P. D., Pearsall F. J., Macleod A. D. and Howie J. C. Phonation affects Mallampati class. *Anaesthesia* 1990; **45:** 984.

15 Tham E. J., Gildersleve C. D., Sanders L. D., Mapleson W. W. and Vaughan R. S. Effects of posture, phonation and observer on Mallampati classification. *British Journal of Anaesthesia* 1992; **68:** 32–38.

16 Arne' J., Descoins P., Bresard D., Aries J. and Fusciardi J. A new clinical score to predict difficult intubation. *British Journal of Anaesthesia* 1993; **70:** (Suppl. 1) 1.A1.

17 Cobley M. and Vaughan R. S. Recognition and management of difficult airway problems. *British Journal of Anaesthesia* 1992; **68:** 90–97.

18 Lyons G. Failed Intubation. Six years experience in a teaching maternity unit. *Anaesthesia* 1985; **40:** 759–762.

19 Goudsouzian N. G., Denham W., Cleveland R. and Shorten G. Radiologic localisation of the laryngeal mask airway in children. *Anesthesiology* 1992; **77:** 1085–1089.

20 Shorten G. D., Opie N. H., Grazotti P., Morris I. and Khargure M. Assessment of upper airway in awake, sedated and anaesthetised patients using magnetic resonance imaging. *Anaesthesia and Intensive Care* 1974; **2:** 165.

21 Cormack R. S. and Lehane J. Difficult tracheal intubation in obstetrics. *Anaesthesia* 1984; **39:** 1105–1111.

# 5

# Causes of Difficult Intubation and Intubation Procedures

*Keith R. Murrin*

---

**Introduction**

**Intubation procedure**
  Patient position
  Instruments and technique
  Design of laryngoscope blades
  Muscle relaxation

**Anatomical abnormalities**
  Individual variation
  Disease states

**Musculoskeletal problems**
  Cervical rigidity
  Diffuse idiopathic skeletal hyperostosis
  Polyostotic fibrous dysplasia
  Temporomandibular joint disorders
  Post temporal craniotomy
  Calcification of the stylohyoid ligament
  Pseudoxanthoma elasticum
  Klippel–Feil syndrome

**Inflammatory**
  Bacterial
  Viral
  Non-infective inflammation

**Endocrine**
  Obesity
  Acromegaly
  Thyroid goitre
  Lingual thyroid
  Diabetes mellitus
  Testicular feminization syndrome

**Degenerative diseases**
  Cervical spondylosis
  Pharyngeal pouch
  Laryngocele

**Neoplasm**
  Laryngeal papillomatosis
  Epiglottic or vallecular cysts
  Tumoral calcinosis
  Occipital protuberances

**Trauma**
  Facial injuries
  Sublingual haematoma
  Foreign bodies
  Laryngeal and tracheal trauma

**Key points**

**References**

---

## INTRODUCTION

Difficulty with intubation may not be anticipated preoperatively. However, anticipation of such a possibility can decrease morbidity and mortality, especially in an emergency situation. It is therefore essential to be prepared for impending difficulty at all times. This will enable the operator to prepare and follow a rational plan of action with the correct equipment. Preoperative examination is an important step in the preparation. Intubation difficulty can arise either from inability to visualize the larynx or from obstruction to the passage of the tracheal tube, or from a combination of these.

## INTUBATION PROCEDURE

Difficulty in passing a tracheal tube may be caused by errors in technique, inexperience of the operator, or lack of appropriate equipment.

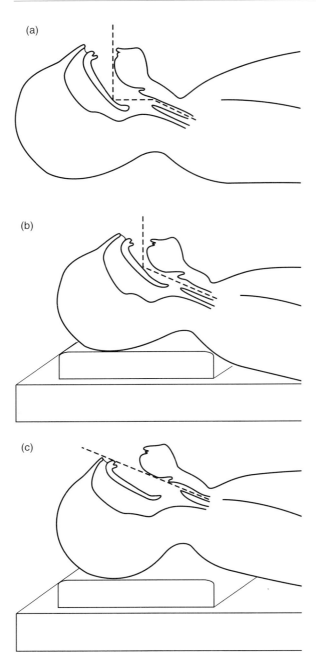

**Figure 1**    (a) Supine position demonstrating the axial planes of mouth, pharynx and trachea. (b) Supine position with flexion of the lower portion of the cervical spine produced by a pillow placed under the occiput, thus producing alignment of the pharynx and trachea.(c) Supine position with flexion of lower portion of the cervical spine and extension of the atlanto-occipital joint. Mouth, pharynx and trachea are in perfect alignment.

## Patient position

Chevalier Jackson stressed the importance of anterior flexion of the lower cervical spine in addition to the more obvious extension of the atlanto-occipital joint [1]. Bannister and Macbeth described the axial alignment of mouth, pharynx and larynx, commonly referred to as 'sniffing the morning air' [2]. The axial planes can be seen in Figs 1a, b and c.

In practice, the lower portion of the cervical spine is maintained in a position of flexion by means of a pillow under the head (Fig. 2). Extension of the atlanto-occipital joint is achieved by traction on the upper teeth or gum with the left index finger, while the middle finger of that hand depresses the mandible, thus opening the mouth. In addition, the middle finger also ensures the lips are not trapped between the teeth and the blade (Fig. 3).

The angle of flexion of the cervical spine, involving the lower cervical vertebrae and the angle of extension at the atlanto-occipital joint, were studied when 10 senior anaesthetists performed laryngoscopy in the course of their normal clinical practice [3]. Measurements of these angles were taken preoperatively and immediately preceding intubation. This study found a common angle of cervical spine flexion of 35° immediately before intubation. Measurement of cervical extension provided a wider scatter of results with a maximum of 20°. The authors, however, suggested an angle of 15° would be an optimal compromise (Fig. 4). The routine preoperative use of the angle finder is proposed by the authors to demonstrate those patients who are unable to achieve the angle of cervical flexion and head extension required for conventional intubation with a rigid blade.

The relative increase in the antero-posterior plane in the head of a child usually makes the use of a pillow unnecessary to achieve flexion of the lower cervical vertebrae.

## Instruments and Technique

The laryngoscope blades in common use are mostly right handed, straight or curved. The tip of the curved laryngoscope blade is inserted into the right corner of the mouth and advanced along the side of the tongue towards the right tonsillar fossa, so that the tongue lies in the recess on the left side of the laryngoscope blade. The tip of the blade is

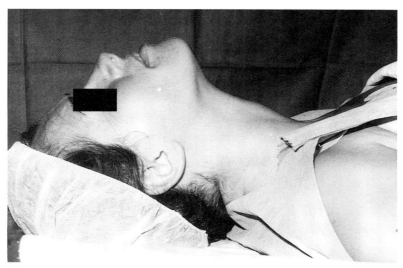

**Figure 2**   Perfect position for intubation. Flexion of the lower portion of the cervical spine produced by a pillow under the head. Axial alignment completed by extension of the altanto-occipital joint (voluntary).

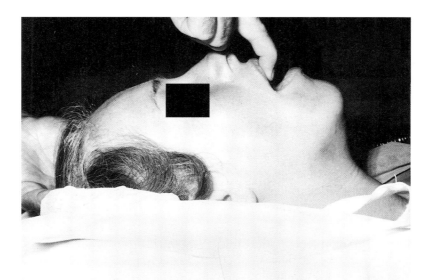

**Figure 3**   Intubation position in the unconscious patient. Note the pillow under the head producing flexion of the lower portion of the cervical spine. Extension of the atlanto-occipital joint is initially produced by caudal pressure from the left hand on the top of the head and upward traction from the index finger of the right hand on the upper teeth or gum.

moved into the mid line when the right tonsillar fossa is visualized. During these manoeuvres, it is important to ensure that the lips and tongue are not trapped between the teeth and the blade (Fig. 5). The blade is then cautiously advanced behind the base of the tongue, elevating it, until the epiglottis is visualized. The tip of the blade is advanced into the vallecula, anterior to the base of the epiglottis, which is lifted forwards to expose the vocal cords (Fig. 6).

Modifications are required when using a straight blade. The straight blade is inserted into the mid line to expose the epiglottis. The tip of the blade is then placed immediately posterior to the epiglottis, directly lifting the structure forwards to expose the underlying glottic aperture (Fig. 7).

(a)

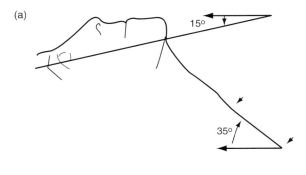

(b)

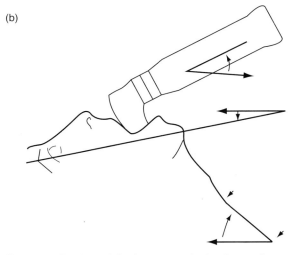

**Figure 4** Flexion of the lower cervical spine and extension of the atlanto-occipital joint during intubation with a conventional rigid laryngoscope.

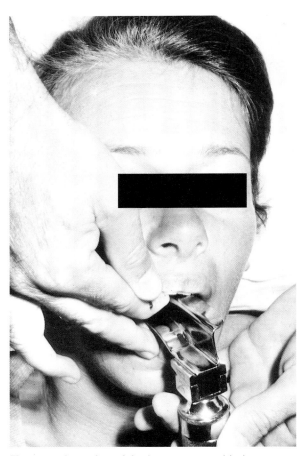

**Figure 5** Insertion of the laryngoscope blade towards the right tonsillar fossa. Maintenance of intubation position with index finger of the right hand depresses the mandible to open the mouth and also clears the lip from the laryngoscope blade and lower dentition or gum.

With both types of laryngoscope blades, traction is applied along the handle, at right angles to the blade, to expose the glottis. This should not be achieved by leverage on the upper teeth or alveolar margins.

These guidelines are intended for a right-handed anaesthetist. Laryngoscope blades are also manufactured for left-handed operators, which should be used with a similar technique on the opposite side.

The tip of the blade may pass inadvertently into the oesophagus, although this is unlikely if the procedure is carried out slowly and methodically. The operator should be alerted by failure to visualize the larynx at the appropriate level and the recognition of oesophageal mucosa. Passage of the tracheal tube without visualizing the larynx may result in oesophageal intubation. Unrecognized, it inevitably leads to hypoxia and eventual death. If there is delay in recognition, subsequent attempts at ventilation may cause gastric distension and regurgitation.

## Design of Laryngoscope Blades

There is no single laryngoscope blade capable of visualizing the larynx in all situations. A unique modification of the conventional Macintosh blade, the McCoy, has a hinge tip, controlled by a lever adjacent to the handle, which enables the operator to elevate the epiglottis, improving the view of the glottic aperture without undue pressure on the teeth or gums [4]. The reader is also

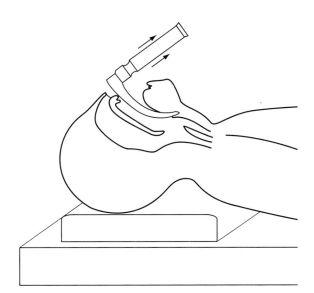

**Figure 6**   Diagram to show final position of the curved laryngoscope blade. N.B. The arrows show the direction of traction of the handle.

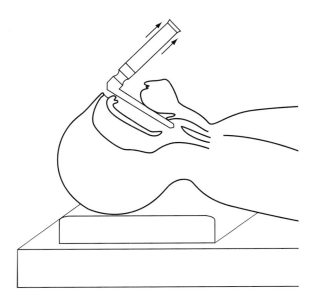

**Figure 7**   Diagram to show the final position of the straight laryngoscope blade. N.B. The arrows show the direction of traction on the handle.

referred to a comprehensive review of blade design by McIntyre [5].

The difficulties commonly confronting the anaesthetist are a protruding sternal region, narrow space between fully parted incisor teeth, reduced infra oral cavity, and the anterior larynx.

These can sometimes be partially or completely overcome using the appropriate shaped blade or laryngoscope. However, familiarity in the use of each variety is essential for a successful outcome.

## Muscle Relaxation

Adequate muscle relaxation should be present before attempting intubation. A common cause of difficulty is to attempt to intubate before a short acting relaxant has worked or after the effect has worn off if the attempt is prolonged. The use of muscle relaxants may be contraindicated with pre-existing respiratory obstruction or obvious anatomical deformities complicating intubation.

Mouth opening may be limited despite adequate muscle relaxation. Occasionally, muscle spasm can be produced by certain drugs such as fentanyl, but it can be antagonized by muscle relaxants [6]. Droperidol may also present a similar picture [7]. Malignant hyperpyrexia is often preceded by abnormal muscle spasm, frequently triggered by the use of suxamethonium or halothane. Myotonia congenita is characterized by abnormal muscle contracture – greatly augmented by suxamethonium.

## ANATOMICAL ABNORMALITIES

### Individual variation

Certain anatomical configurations compatible with a normal existence can give rise to concern during intubation. The most common problem is inability to visualize the larynx which may be encountered in association with the following features:

- short muscular neck (bull neck);
- receding mandible;
- prominent upper incisors;
- 'narrow' mouth with high arch palate;
- limited movement of mandible;
- large breasts.

The X-ray measurements and clinical tests to detect these conditions are discussed in Chapter 4.

### *Maxillary protrusion*

A study of Nigerian patients [8] demonstrated maxillary protrusion in 20% of patients in the surgical population determined by measurement of the distance between the upper incisors and vocal cords. There was a statistically significant correlation between 'upper incisor to vocal cords' and 'tragus of ear to the nasal septum' measurements; thus the latter measurement could be utilized to predict maxillary protrusion. It must be emphasized that malocclusion is usually obvious in these patients and difficulty with laryngoscopy can be anticipated.

### Mandibular coronoid hyperplasia

An infrequent disorder of the mandible is hyperplasia of the coronoid process which, if bilateral, will prevent mouth opening. Bilateral mandibular hyperplasia usually occurs in males. This may not be clinically obvious.

### Abnormal epiglottis

Variations in the size and shape of the epiglottis in adults can give rise to problems during intubation. Hotchkiss et al. [9] report such a case which was investigated using the magnetic resonance imaging (MRI) scan. These authors recommend the MRI scan as a prospective and a retrospective means of assessing a difficult airway. This may be difficult for many reasons.

## Disease States

### Cherubism

In cherubism, there is a painless mandibular enlargement either with or without maxillary involvement [10]. The disease generally regresses during puberty following an earlier period of rapid progression. Thus, adults affected in childhood may only demonstrate mild mandibular enlargement. Occasionally, mandibular surgery is indicated but conservative treatment is generally preferred. The difficulty with visualization of the larynx in these patients is caused by mandibular elongation. It is difficult to displace the soft tissues inside the buccal cavity and pharynx to one side.

### Tracheopathia osteochondroplastica

Tracheopathia osteochondroplastica is a benign dysplasia of the trachea and large bronchi and produces gradual stenosis of the tracheal lumen. Although there are symptoms of airway obstruction, the diagnosis is most commonly made in the autopsy room. However, the more frequent use of bronchoscopy and computerized tomography of the trachea has increased the reporting incidence. Only two cases associated with difficult intubation have been reported in the literature. The second case, reported in 1987 by Smith et al. [11], involved a 64-year-old patient presenting with severe coronary artery stenosis. The chest X-ray demonstrated a stenosing lesion of the trachea. A computerized axial tomography (CAT) scan gives more information than a chest X-ray. The chest X-ray appearances are sometimes mistaken for carcinoma of the trachea because of the irregular narrowing produced by the lesion. Tracheal biopsy is the definitive investigation which should eliminate any doubt about the presence of neoplasm. However, extensive calcification can make the biopsy difficult to obtain.

### Subglottic web

Webs may be congenital or acquired. Congenital webs usually present in infancy or early childhood and the diagnosis is suggested by clinical signs such as stridor, poor cry and feeding problems. A laryngeal web constitutes about 3% of congenital abnormalities of the larynx.

Two patients were reported with unsuspected subglottic webs which caused difficulty with tracheal intubation [12]. One of the cases presented during an awake intubation. Difficult intubation was anticipated in this case. A subsequent fibreoptic nasopharyngoscopy verified movement of the vocal cords and demonstrated the presence of a subglottic laryngeal web. A tracheostomy was performed under local anaesthesia. Interestingly, the patient's earlier notes demonstrated that there had been unsuccessful attempts to intubate the trachea both orally and nasally on previous occasions, but this was attributed to severe temporomandibular joint fixation. Endoscopic visualization is the only method of providing the diagnosis.

Acquired webs or scars may develop as a result of trauma. The most common cause is long-term tracheal intubation for mechanical ventilation. Symptoms at rest rarely occur until at least 75% of the tracheal diameter has been obliterated [13].

### Laryngeal oedema

Laryngeal oedema is most commonly seen with pregnancy, pregnancy-induced hypertension and prolonged labour. This problem may also be related to fluid overload in combination with these conditions.

### Tracheal stenosis

Tracheal stenosis usually results from thyroid, tracheal or mediastinal tumours, previous tracheostomy, prolonged intubation or traumatic lesions. However, tracheal stenosis can be congenital in origin and seen in early childhood presenting as a respiratory difficulty. Sometimes this diagnosis is made in adults, demonstrating that not all cases become clinically significant in childhood.

### Xeroderma pigmentosum

Xeroderma pigmentosum is a rare, autosomal recessive, disease provoked by sunlight. Homozygote carriers of the gene are especially susceptible to ultraviolet light. The sufferer is unable to repair damage in epidermal and connective tissue cells following exposure to the sun. In childhood, the disease may be recognized by dense freckle-like pigmented spots on exposed areas of the skin, most noticeably in the summer months. Death usually occurs before the age of 30 from malignancy originating in the skin.

Atrophy leads to ectropion and microstomia. The use of blind nasal intubation has been described in a patient presenting with an inflamed swollen tongue covered with prominent telangiectasia [14].

### Thalassaemia

A case of difficult intubation associated with thalassaemia has been described [15]. The difficulty with this disorder seems to be related to hypertrophic bone marrow changes which may affect the maxilla, resulting in gross protrusion.

### Mucopolysaccharydosis

This is a group of progressive diseases categorized by excessive storage of the mucopolysaccharides leading to organ dysfunction and anatomical abnormalities. Mucopolysaccharides accumulate in the soft tissue of the oropharynx, the epiglottis, aryepiglottic folds and the tracheal wall. These patients often have a short neck and tracheal rigidity. The problem can be so severe as to warrant the institution of cardiopulmonary bypass before anaesthesia [16]. Hypoxia is poorly tolerated in

these patients since they may well suffer from coronary artery and cardiac valve disease as a result of their condition.

### Morquio syndrome

In contrast to Hurler syndrome, intelligence is normal in this condition. Although most patients with this disease die before the age of 30, many may present for anaesthesia. Jones and Thomas [17] describe a 29-year-old patient with this disorder requiring radical resection of malignant melanoma. Unfortunately the patient died in the immediate postoperative period and the authors outlined the problems that confront the anaesthetist:

- difficulty in intubation because of deformity and redundant pharyngeal mucosa;
- chronic pulmonary disease due to chest deformity and superinfection;
- inadvisability of manipulating the neck because of vertebral abnormalities – there is the possibility of causing atlanto-axial subluxation (degenerate odontoid peg).

## MUSCULOSKELETAL PROBLEMS

### Cervical Rigidity

Reduction in the mobility of the cervical spine occurs with advancing age. The normal range of flexion–extension movements is 90–160° but the movement in any individual will be reduced by 20% by the seventh decade of life [18]. This reduction in mobility could theoretically hinder laryngoscopy, but this does not seem to be a problem in practice. Nichol and Zuck presented an unexpected difficulty with cervical rigidity in a 9-year-old child [19].

### Diffuse Idiopathic Skeletal Hyperostosis

This process of an ossifying diathesis was described as a distinct clinical entity by Crosby and Grahovac [20]. In addition to anterior osteophyte formation, there are calcific ligamentous changes with subsequent ossification. The authors state that this condition may well exist in conjunction with osteoarthritis. In addition to the osteophyte formation there may be rigidity of the spine. Encroachment on the cervical spinal cord can result in neurological problems.

## Polyostotic Fibrous Dysplasia

This is a disorder of a unknown aetiology characterized by an expanding fiberosseous lesion in bone. Fractures may occur in weakened areas including the mandible. The presence of a severe facial deformity can make laryngoscopy difficult. Unfortunately, epidural or spinal blockade is often difficult owing to spinal involvement and vertebral collapse. There may also be accompanying endocrine abnormalities such as acromegaly, hyperparathyroidism, hyperthyroidism and Cushing's syndrome [21].

## Temporomandibular Joint Disorders

Restriction in mouth opening can occur with any of the arthritides. Redick emphasizes that mouth opening is not uncommonly restricted in an otherwise healthy patient [22]. This problem can sometimes be minimized by pushing or pulling the jaw forward before attempting to open the mouth for laryngoscopy or for the insertion of a laryngeal mask [23].

The two movements (gliding and hinge) are made possible by the presence of an articular disc interposed between two synovial compartments. The upper compartment allows gliding movement and the lower compartment functions as a hinge joint. If only the first movement is observed, visualization of the larynx with a rigid laryngoscope may be difficult. The hinge movement allows the mouth to be opened half way and the subsequent gliding movement allows full opening thereafter (Fig. 8). Normal mouth opening in adults is 40 mm (at least two finger breadths) [24].

If temporomandibular disease is unilateral, a jaw thrust with lateral displacement of the mandible towards the affected side will allow reasonably good mouth opening and permit some patients to be intubated with the conventional rigid laryngoscope [25].

## Post Temporal Craniotomy

Surgery involving the temporal fossa can lead to trismus due to a true contracture as opposed to simple muscle spasm. This affects the temporalis muscle either as a result of scar tissue or as a result of an ischaemic process. Ossification can occur in the fibrotic muscle. Patients who have had surgery in the region of the temporal fossa require

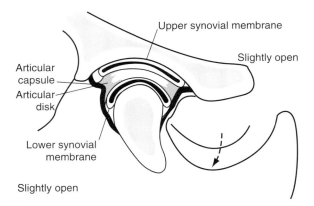

**Figure 8**   Movement of the temporomandibular joint.

meticulous assessment of temporomandibular joint function before anaesthesia [26].

## Calcification of the Stylohyoid Ligament

Calcification of the stylohyoid ligament is an uncommon cause of intubation difficulty [27, 28]. This results from an inability to elevate the soft tissue around the vallecula and hyoid bone. There is shortening and immobility of the stylohyoid ligament and associated muscles.

It has been suggested that patients with calcified ligaments could be identified preoperatively by the presence of a prominent skin crease over the hyoid bone [27]. This crease, however, was absent in the two cases reported by Akinyemi and Elegbe [28]. The common laryngoscopic feature is difficulty in lifting the epiglottis away from the posterior laryngeal wall with a curved laryngoscope.

If this condition is suspected preoperatively, it may be confirmed radiologically. Coincidental findings seen in head and neck X-rays should alert the anaesthetist to the possibility of a difficult intubation.

## Pseudoxanthoma elasticum

Levitt and Collison reported a case of difficult intubation in a patient with this disorder [29]. The difficulty was presumed to be due to calcification and aggregation of elastic fibres in the laryngeal ligaments and cartilage. The problem was overcome with the use of a ventilating bronchoscope.

Calcification and aggregation of elastic tissue is a histochemical characteristic of this condition affecting the skin and mucosa. Clinically, there is difficulty in visualizing the vocal cords because of deformation of the epiglottis and vocal cords.

## Klippel–Feil Syndrome

This involves fusion of a variable number of cervical vertebrae resulting in a short neck with restriction of movement. There may also be abnormalities of the cardiovascular, respiratory, genitourinary and musculoskeletal systems. Burns et al. described the management of a patient suffering from the Klippel–Feil syndrome who presented for Caesarean section [30]. Several important points arose from the case.

- It was considered essential that the airway was secured before the induction of general anaesthesia. This was achieved with a fibreoptic bronchoscope.
- The chosen technique should minimize the known risks of aspiration pneumonitis associated with obstetric anaesthesia.
- Large increases in arterial and intracranial pressure should be avoided.

In patients with pregnancy-induced hypertension (pre-eclampsia), the hypertensive response to tracheal intubation may be severe enough to precipitate pulmonary oedema and intracerebral oedema and haemorrhage.

## INFLAMMATORY

### Bacterial

Difficult intubation can occur in any inflammatory process producing oedema, contracture or abscess formation in the upper respiratory tract. The following conditions have been described.

### *Gangrenous stomatitis*

This is associated with malnutrition, poor oral hygiene and certain illnesses such as measles, scarlet fever, typhoid, syphylis, tuberculosis and leukaemia. The most probable agents are *Borrelia vincenti*, *Fusiformis fusiformis* and *Bacteroides*. Gangrenous stomatitis leads to severe facial deformity from extensive ulceration, circumferential scarring and stenosis of the mouth, and extra-articular anklyosis of the temporomandibular joint. Ventilation through a facemask and a tra-

cheal tube can be extremely difficult. It would seem sensible to have the necessary equipment for transtracheal ventilation at hand whatever method is used in an attempt to intubate the patient. The use of a fibreoptic bronchoscope has been recommended [31] but unfortunately this is not always readily available in underdeveloped countries where the disease is most common.

### *Cicatricial pemphigoid*

Repeated vesicular eruption leads to scarring and thickening of tissues in the upper airway. Increasing involvement of the trachea and larynx can lead to gradual occlusion of the upper airway lumen resulting in stridor and cyanosis. With the cicatricial form of pemphigoid, the most common area of obstruction is at the level of the vocal cords and is often complicated by severe ulceration and deformity of the surrounding mucosa. The use of helium in the inspired gas reduces turbulence and increases the inspiratory flow rate relative to air by 70% [32].

### *Quinsy and retropharyngeal abscess*

Infection in the pharyngeal area can impair visualization of the vocal cords by the formation of oedema, exudate or frank abscess. Inability to open the mouth (trismus) may occur, but this sometimes improves once anaesthesia is established. Heindel [33] emphasizes the dangers of deep neck abscesses in adults. One of the cases presented died from aspiration of the contents of such an abscess during attempts to reintubate the patient.

The hyoid bone limits the spread of infection in the neck. However, it is not uncommon for the infection to spread to adjacent spaces. Localized infections can be drained under general anaesthesia. The anaesthetist may also be called in cases of respiratory obstruction. There is a risk of rupturing the abscess with subsequent aspiration of its contents. Tracheostomy should, therefore, be seriously considered. However, the tracheostomy site may be involved in the infective process.

Awake intubation is the preferred solution if the abscess is located in an area away from the route of intubation. The choice between tracheostomy and fibreoptic intubation can sometimes be made by reference to the CAT or MRI scan. These can demonstrate the position of the abscess. The surgeon must be prepared for an emergency tracheostomy.

## Epiglottitis

This is caused by a rapidly progressive bacterial infection involving supraglottic structures. Distal spread is prevented by the tightly adherent vocal cord mucosa. The causative organism is usually *Haemophilus influenzae* (type B), but occasionally *Staphylococcus aureus*, *Haemolytic streptococcus*, *Neisseria catarrhalis*, *Pneumococcus* or a virus are the causes. It commonly affects children aged from 1 month to 3½ years. For the first 3 months of life passive immunity is usually acquired from the mother; natural immunity is usually acquired after entry into school.

Respiratory arrest can occur quite suddenly in these children. Once the diagnosis has been confirmed the child may need to be intubated. This should always be performed by experienced personnel. Conservative management may be indicated in isolated cases but it is dangerous since results are unpredictable. A review of 749 patients with this disorder revealed a mortality rate of 6.1% with a conservative approach [34]. Increasing awareness has reduced mortality. The incidence of epiglottitis has been reported to be 0.1% of paediatric admissions, 8% presenting with respiratory distress [35]. Most anaesthetists are asked at some time to deal with this disease, especially if they work where the disease is endemic. There are also other causes of epiglottitis, for example inhalation of steam, ingestion of corrosives and diphtheria.

### Epiglottitis is not confined to children

The condition has been described in males between the ages of 29 and 38 [36]. Two of the three patients died from sudden respiratory obstruction. Fatal airway occlusion can occur without preceding stridor. The authors suggest that the patient should sit upright and be given oxygen. The supine position may very well precipitate obstruction. Intubation should be carried out by an experienced anaesthetist. The fibreoptic scope may be of little use due to the difficulty in passing it through swollen oedematous tissues.

The diagnosis is made from the history and can be confirmed with a lateral cervical X-ray, if time permits. Examination of the pharynx should be carried out under anaesthesia. Sudden excitement can precipitate acute complete respiratory obstruction. Tracheal intubation may be carried out following an inhalational induction using a tracheal tube a size smaller than anticipated. Experience has shown that continued intubation (up to 4 days) is preferable to tracheostomy [37–39]. Extubation is usually possible after 48 h.

## Leprosy

This is a rare cause of obstructive granulation tissue in the upper respiratory tract.

## Diphtheria

This membrane-producing disease is now virtually extinct in the Western hemisphere.

# Viral

## Infectious mononucleosis

In the glandular variety, infection is due to the Epstein–Barr virus (EBV), and lymphadenopathy is the predominant feature. Proliferation of tonsillar and adenoidal lymphoid tissue can produce severe pharyngeal obstruction.

## Croup

This is a viral infection which causes oedema below the vocal cords. The majority of cases respond to medical management but a few require intubation with a smaller tracheal tube than calculated.

# Non-infective Inflammation

## Rheumatoid arthritis

Juvenile chronic arthritis and rheumatoid arthritis are clinically and biochemically distinct entities, which occur under and over the age of 16, respectively [40]. However, difficulties in intubation can occur in both cases. Rheumatoid arthritis can be associated with the following:

### Instability of the cervical spine

Approximately 3% of patients with biochemical evidence of rheumatoid arthritis will also have cervical instability. This usually occurs at the atlanto-axial joint but may occur at lower levels. Subluxation of the cervical spine is present in 30% of hospital inpatients with rheumatoid arthritis. Spinal cord compression or transection occasionally occurs, especially with forced flexion.

Preoperatively instability of the cervical spine should be suspected in the following circumstances:

- vestibular symptoms and diplopia due to vertebral artery insufficiency;
- abnormal neurological signs in the limbs;
- inability to maintain extension of the head and neck with loss of the angle between the occiput and cervical spine;
- neck pain radiating into the occiput (neck pain itself is a frequent concomitant of rheumatoid arthritis);
- abnormal protrusion of the axial arch – this can be palpated in the pharynx;
- abnormal radiological appearances:
  - (a) abnormal vertebral movement on flexion;
  - (b) erosion of the odontoid peg;
  - (c) narrowing of the spaces between skull and C1, C1 and C2, with or without the presence of bony erosion;
  - (d) increased distance between the anterior surface of the odontoid peg and the anterior surface of C1. The normal variation in distance is from 2 to 4 mm. Any increase in the distance between the odontoid process and the anterior arch of the atlas on the lateral X-ray of the flexed cervical spine, as compared with the same view in extension, is abnormal.

### Cervical fixation

This commonly affects the lower cervical vertebrae, producing a fixed flexion deformity, which prevents adequate extension of the head. There may be difficulty in introducing the laryngoscopy blade and in seeing the cords. Cervical fixation is often accompanied by temporomandibular joint disease.

### Cricoarytenoid disorders

Glottic stenosis due to diseases affecting the joints can impede the passage of the tracheal tube. A preoperative tracheostomy may be required [41]. It should be suspected if, preoperatively, the rheumatoid patient presents with hoarseness, dyspnoea on exertion, stridor, dysphagia or fullness in the throat. The diagnosis can be confirmed by indirect laryngoscopy which shows decreased cricoarytenoid movement, or bowing of the cords during inspiration.

### Hypoplastic mandible

This may be associated with rheumatoid arthritis. A comprehensive review of anaesthetic problems associated with rheumatoid arthritis is presented

**Table 1** A classification of the difficulties in airway management with rheumatiod arthritis. From D'Arcy *et al.* [42], with kind permission of the authors and Academic Press.

| | Usual clinical characteristics | Quality of airway | Conventional intubation |
|---|---|---|---|
| Group I | Good movement of the neck and jaw | Good | Good |
| Group II | Stiff cervical spine but good jaw movement | Satisfactory | Very difficult |
| Group III | Stiff neck and restricted jaw movements | May obstruct at any time | Impossible |
| Group IV | Stiff neck and jaw with skeletal stunting | Obstructs with sedation | Impossible |

by Jenkins and McGraw [41]. The disorders of the airway which occur with rheumatoid arthritis and their relevance to the anaesthetist have been described by D'Arcy *et al.* [42] (Table 1).

### Ankylosing spondylitis

This inflammatory arthropathy has been reviewed by Sinclair and Mason [43]. Upper airway management can be severely compromised by rigidity of the cervical spine, usually in flexion. This is sometimes accompanied by a tendency to cervical fracture at the C5-C7 level [44], and as a result, the possibility of cord damage. Around 10–40% of these patients have limited mouth opening due to temporomandibular disease [45].

## ENDOCRINE

### Obesity

Shenkman *et al.* [46] recommend that preparation for a difficult intubation should be made in the morbidly obese patient. There may be difficulty in visualizing the vocal cords with the fibreoptic scope due to the presence of pharyngeal folds. There may also be difficulty with ventilation by mask with rapid decrease in oxygen saturation. Obesity is, therefore, 'a persuasive argument' for the insertion of a tracheal tube before the induction of anaesthesia [47]. This is particularly important in obese patients at risk of aspiration. It has been demonstrated that obesity predisposes to the risk of aspiration due to hiatus hernia and increased volume and acidity of the gastric contents [48].

Bond found no correlation between body mass index (kg wt per metre height) and difficulty with laryngoscopy [47]. Meyer confirmed that there is no correlation between body mass index and difficulty of conventional laryngoscopy. He also advocated the use of a rapid sequence induction with the use of a short acting depolarizing muscle relaxant. From his experience with 400 morbidly obese patients, he recommended the use of a Kates–Kessel blade and an introducer in the tracheal tube. He believes that this approach provides optimal intubating conditions in the shortest possible time with the possibility of the early return of spontaneous respiration should any life-threatening problems be encountered. His overall conclusion, however, was that there will be a greater readiness to perform awake intubations in obese patients in the future [49].

The use of a laryngoscope with a handle one half the normal length has been suggested in morbidly obese patients [50]. Alternatively, if obesity produces difficulty in insertion of the laryngoscope blade into the mouth, a 'polio' blade may be used. The practical question that confronts the clinician is what degree of obesity justifies an awake intubation?

## Acromegaly

This disease results from hyperactivity of the pituitary gland. In addition to the other features, it may produce abnormalities in the upper airway. The relevant features are:

- macroglossia;
- thickening of pharyngeal tissues;
- thickening of laryngeal soft tissues and vocal cords;
- recurrent laryngeal nerve palsy;
- decrease in the width of the cricoid arch;
- fixation of the vocal cords;
- prognathism;
- hypertrophy of the aryepiglottic and ventricular folds.

It may be difficult to ventilate an apnoeic acromegalic patient with a mask because of the large nose, hypertrophied nasal cartilages and spreading teeth. Intubation may also be difficult because of

inability to visualize the larynx. The above changes can be so severe as to cause respiratory obstruction and death unrelated to anaesthesia or surgery [51].

## Thyroid Goitre

In the author's experience, visualization of the cords has not been difficult, even in the presence of extremely large goitres. Deviation of the trachea occurs more commonly than compression and may obstruct the subsequent passage of a rigid tracheal tube. A latex armoured tube should be used as it is flexible and will not collapse with compression. A tracheal tube with a smaller diameter than anticipated may be needed.

## Lingual Thyroid

Ectopic thyroid tissue may obscure the larynx. Fogarty described a case which was asymptomatic preoperatively. Ectopic thyroid tissue, however, obscured the view of the larynx [52]. Subsequent ventilation with the mask was also difficult because of the mass at the base of the tongue. The patient was eventually intubated with the aid of a gum elastic bougie.

## Diabetes Mellitus

A correlation has been demonstrated between difficult direct laryngoscopy and severe diabetes [53]. A defective palm print when the hands were covered with black ink and placed on white paper was also demonstrated in these patients. The association between the defective palm print and the difficult laryngoscopy may be explained by tissue glycosylation in both areas.

A difficult intubation occurred as a result of 'stiff joint syndrome' following juvenile onset diabetes [54]. This syndrome is also associated with short stature and joint contractures. In the case described, X-rays of the cervical spine demonstrated extremely limited movement at the atlanto-occipital joint. This was most easily appreciated in flexion and extension views of the cervical spine where it was noticed that the atlanto-ocipital gap remained virtually unchanged during flexion and extension. In healthy patients almost all the extension of the head and neck takes place at the atlanto-occipital joint during intubation.

## Testicular Feminization Syndrome

Difficulties with intubation occurred in two sisters, aged 18 and 21 years, who suffered from the testicular feminization syndrome [55]. The assumed explanation for the difficulty was that the larynx in both girls had retained its prepuberty size and thus would only accept a small tracheal tube.

## DEGENERATIVE DISEASES

### Cervical Spondylosis

Osteoarthritis of the cervical spine may result in anterior osteophyte formation and produce difficulty in visualizing the larynx [56]. The anterior protrusions push the posterior wall of the larynx forwards thus distorting the anatomy. This condition is most likely to be seen in the elderly.

### Pharyngeal Pouch

This well-recognized condition rarely causes difficulty in intubation. It commonly occurs in children. It can also occur in adults, especially trumpet players, glass blowers and rarely as a result of self mutilation [57]. The mouth of the aperture can open and close and mimic the glottis. A tracheal tube can be passed in error into the pouch [58].

### Laryngocele

A laryngocele is an abnormal dilatation of the ventricular saccule of the larynx. The incidence in the United Kingdom is 1 per 2.5 million population per year and it is more common in men than in women. The usual presentation is in the middle age group. Laryngoceles are usually unilateral but can be bilateral. The diagnosis may be made from straight X-rays. An air–fluid interface may be seen on X-ray in a laryngocele. Where doubt exists the lesion may be made more obvious using a Valsava manoeuvre.

Rashid and Warltier recommend the use of the fibreoptic bronchoscope for the management all obstructive lesions of the larynx [59]. The case presented by these authors was an infected laryngocele causing respiratory obstruction preoperatively.

## NEOPLASM

Benign or malignant tumours extending into the airway can obscure the operator's view and obstruct the passage of a tracheal tube.

### Laryngeal Papillomatosis

This is an uncommon, but well-recognized, cause of stridor in childhood which can progress to respiratory failure and death. Most tumours in children are benign; despite certain characteristics of viral infection, electron microscopy has failed to demonstrate characteristic inclusion bodies or viruses. Laryngeal papillomata are seen in the newborn but can occur at any age, and regression may be seen at puberty. Harper et al. described a patient with persistent laryngeal obstruction and respiratory failure who was dependent on hypoxaemia as a stimulant for respiration; relief of hypoxaemia resulted in episodes of apnoea [60]. The history from the parents may suggest the possibility of laryngeal papillomata; huskiness before dyspnoea is the vital clue.

### Epiglottic or Vallecular Cysts

These rarely cause symptoms. They may be observed during laryngoscopy. On some occasions, voice change, stridor, dysphagia, pharyngeal pain or the feeling of something in the throat may cause the patient to be referred for an ENT opinion. They can totally obstruct the view of the glottic opening and occasionally may require aspiration before intubation. Rarely epiglottic cysts may present with rapidly progressive airway obstruction due to secondary infection or bleeding. They are especially dangerous in neonates and infants since the small airway is more significantly obstructed by such a lesion. The most common location for such a cyst is the lingual surface of the epiglottis but they may also occur in the free margin of the vocal cords, the arytenoid and aryepiglottic folds, the pyriform fossa and the ventricle [61]. Ductal cysts occur because of obstruction of the submucosal glands which contain mucus which can be become infected. Saccular cysts are congenital in origin, can contain mucus or air and may become infected. The safest method of intubation is with a fibreoptic scope if these cysts are recognized preoperatively [62]. A gum elastic bougie can facilitate intubation if the condition is discovered unexpectedly. Rapid sequence induction is inadvisable.

## Tumoral Calcinosis

In this rare condition, benign tumours present as soft tissue masses adjacent to large joints. Several factors may contribute to difficult intubation. There may be calcification of the hyoid bone, hyothyroid ligament and cervical intervertebral joints [63]. There may also be forward displacement of the larynx and upper teeth and backward displacement to the tongue. Although only 200 cases have been reported in the world literature, it is important for anaesthetists to be aware of the intubation difficulties associated with this disease.

## Occipital Protuberances

### Occipital lipoma

A case was reported of a large lipoma on the back of the neck, severely limiting extension of the cervical spine [64].

### Decorative hairbands and hairstyle

Decorative hairbands can convert an otherwise normal intubation to one of some difficulty. Removal of the hairband allowing the hair to fall naturally eliminates the cause of the problem. Difficulty due to hairstyle has been described in a Nigerian patient [65]. This problem was solved by placing two pillows under the patient's shoulders, allowing the head to be extended.

## TRAUMA

Trauma to the face and neck can compromise the airway and produce problems with intubation due to haemorrhage, haematoma, oedema and accompanying distortion of the tissues. There may be difficulty in visualizing the larynx and obstruction to the passage of a tracheal tube.

For an exhaustive treatise on this subject, the reader is referred to Chapter 18. Topics relevant to difficult intubation are presented below.

## Facial Injuries

### Mandibular fractures

Fractures of the mandible are frequently bilateral. Problems associated with intubation in patients with mandibular fractures include:

- hypermobility of the tongue, resulting in pharyngeal obstruction;
- distortion of the normal dental configuration which can obstruct the passage of a tracheal tube as well as obscuring the view of the larynx. The author was presented with a patient whose dentures were firmly embedded in the lower posterior pharyngeal wall following facial trauma;
- haemorrhage and oedema involving tissues within the tongue which present a major obstruction to oral intubation;
- trismus prevents adequate opening of the mouth in the conscious patient. Until the patient is anaesthetized it is difficult to be sure which is the cause. Under the effects of general anaesthesia, trismus due to pain rapidly diminishes, allowing normal mouth opening and uncomplicated tracheal intubation. However, trismus due to anatomical deformity will cause difficulty in intubation;
- vomiting or regurgitation of stomach contents may occur. There may be blood clots or food in the stomach;
- cervical injuries may also be present (see Chapter 18).

Definitive surgery for mandibular fractures can sometimes be delayed for 24 h. The risk of gastric aspiration will be much less under these circumstances. Nasal intubation is required for surgical access. If inspection of the mouth and pharynx suggests no obvious difficulty with intubation, then preoxygenation, paralysis with suxamethonium and cricoid pressure is the method of choice. If any doubt exists regarding the ease of intubation, this procedure is best performed in the conscious state. Tracheostomy before surgery is rarely indicated; the fractured mandible is mobile when the patient is unconscious and intubation is rarely a problem for the trained anaesthetist.

### Maxillary fractures (middle third fractures)

Injury to this region may necessitate oral intubation before surgery to secure an airway.

Laryngoscopy and intubation may be impeded by the presence of haemorrhage and anatomical distortion. When the fractures have been surgically corrected, the oral tube can be replaced by a nasal tube for improved surgical access.

## Sublingual Haematoma

Sublingual haematoma has been reported following repeated attempts at intubation with a rigid laryngoscope blade [66]. This increased the difficulties with subsequent attempts in this patient.

## Foreign Bodies

Dentures and items of food have been the commonest causes of obstruction to visualization of the larynx. In one report, there was displacement of a Celestin tube and subsequent difficulty with intubation [67]. The tulip end of the Celestin tube obscured the vocal cords. A Magill forceps was used to squash the end of the Celestin tube. A normal glottic opening was then seen and the trachea was subsequently intubated without difficulty.

## Laryngeal and Tracheal Trauma

Injuries to the trachea, larynx and pharynx can be open or closed (macerated).

### Open Injuries

#### Incisional injuries

Intubation may be difficult for several reasons:

- The tongue and epiglottis may obscure or obstruct the laryngeal opening. This occurs when the incision is above the hyoid bone.
- Haemorrhage into the respiratory tract may obscure vision and also cause airway obstruction. The greatest danger occurs with incisions at tracheal level, when the common carotid or inferior thyroid arteries are lacerated.
- Recurrent laryngeal nerve damage may occur with a low incision.
- If treatment is delayed, infection with cellulitis and oedema may occur.

#### Post surgical

Cervical haematoma most commonly occur following surgery in this area. The risks can be minimized during thyroidectomy by carefully securing

haemastasis at the end of surgery. This same problem may occur following carotid endarterectomy. The degree of internal oropharyngeal oedema seems to be far in excess of the problem anticipated from the external appearance of the patient. The morbidity and the mortality is relatively high in this condition and it has been recommended that the haematoma should be aspirated under local anaesthesia if possible [68]. Unfortunately, local anaesthetic blockade of the superficial cervical plexus is not always possible due to the presence of oedema. The provision of a field block would seem a more reasonable alternative. If general anaesthesia is required, a gaseous induction using helium in the inspired gas has been recommended [69]. The benefit of helium often tends to be forgotten by anaesthetists, but it certainly provides for an easier induction where there is moderate to severe respiratory obstruction.

Patients should be intubated for 8–10 h following re-exploration. One recommendation for a safe time before extubation was when there was an audible leak around a non-inflated cuff after an application of 15 cm of water pressure to a 7 mm tube in adults [69]. It is surprising that this problem only occurs in 3% of patients, as most of these patients are taking platelet-inhibiting therapy before surgery.

### Closed injuries

The most common cause of a closed neck injury is sudden deceleration produced by a car crash. Rupture of the trachea and larynx are often accompanied by surgical emphysema. Symptoms such as pain on swallowing, dyspnoea and haemoptysis may be present. Injury to the larynx and trachea may, however, only become apparent during intubation.

Concomitant cervical spine injuries may prevent the patient being placed in the traditional 'sniffing the morning air' position. Neurological examination and cervical radiology should be carried out to exclude cord damage before attempting intubation.

Muscle relaxants should not be used before intubation in patients with a ruptured trachea or larynx. Inflation will increase surgical emphysema and effective ventilation of the lungs may be impossible. Local anaesthesia may be impracticable because of the injuries. An inhalational induction would therefore seem to be the optimal choice.

Direct trauma to the neck can produce traumatic dislocation of the arytenoid cartilages [70] so that the arytenoid falls anteromedially, causing respiratory obstruction. There may also be relaxation of the corresponding vocal cord. This should not, however, obstruct the subsequent passage of the tracheal tube. Tracheal rupture, as a result of closed injury or laceration, may cause difficulty with intubation. Rapid surgical exploration of the cervical tissues and subsequent manipulation of the tube past the injured segment may overcome this difficulty [71]. Occasionally, with massive cervical injury, the trachea can be intubated directly through the injured area.

### Contusional injuries

In addition, widespread damage to the underlying structures may produce maceration, oedema and damage to the more rigid structures in the throat. The hyoid bone and laryngeal cartilage may be damaged and produce considerable distortion.

### Skiers' neck

In one case, laryngeal deviation was caused by the patient falling on a ski pole. A fracture of the thyroid cartilage was produced and there was narrowing of the larynx. This injury had been forgotten by the patient until he was questioned following a difficult intubation [72].

---

## KEY POINTS

- The ability to perform a successful intubation is crucial in the emergency situation to prevent aspiration of gastric contents.

- Difficulties may not always be anticipated. Unanticipated difficulties usually occur with the physiological variations described at the beginning of the chapter.

- Some medical conditions are associated with difficulty in visualizing the larynx, passing the tracheal tube or a combination of these two factors. Difficulty with intubation may therefore be anticipated with certain clinical syndromes.

- Clinicians are aware of the common causes of difficult intubation. Rare and obscure causes are also presented in this chapter.

- Undue emphasis may have been placed on apparently rare conditions but if the association with difficult intubation is not recognized preoperatively, there may be a catastrophic outcome which is totally avoidable.

- The *conditions* which *commonly* present difficulty with intubation are problems associated with receding mandible, prominent incisors, 'bull' neck, rheumatoid arthritis, neoplasm, pharyngeal abscess and trauma.

- Medi-alert identification bands should be issued to these patients.

## REFERENCES

1 Jackson C. The technique of insertion of intratracheal insufflation tubes. *Surgery, Gynecology and Obstetrics* 1913; **17:** 507.
2 Bannister F. and MacBeth R. G. Direct laryngoscopy and tracheal intubation. *Lancet* 1944; **2:** 651.
3 Horton W. A., Fahy L. and Charters P. Defining a standard intubating position using 'angle finder'. *British Journal of Anaesthesia* 1989; **62:** 6.
4 McCoy E. P. and Mirakhur R. K. The levering laryngoscope. *Anesthesiology* 1993; **48:** 516.
5 McIntyre J. W. R. Laryngoscope design and the difficult adult intubation. *Canadian Journal of*

*Anaesthesiology* 1989; **36**: 94.

6 Askgaard B., Nilson T., Ibler M. *et al.* Muscle tone under fentanyl-nitrous oxide anaesthesia measured with a transducer apparatus in cholecystectomy incisions. *Acta Anaesthesiologica Scandinavica* 1977; **21**: 1.

7 Patton C. M. Rapid induction of acute dyskinesia by droperidol. *Anesthesiology* 1975; **43**: 126.

8 Magbagbeola J. A. O. and Ayeni O. Some aspects of endotracheal anaesthesia in Nigerians. *West African Medical Journal* 1972; **21**: 161.

9 Hotchkiss R. S., Hall J. R., Braun I. F. and Schisler J. Q. An abnormal epiglottis as a cause of difficult intubation – airway assessment using magnetic resonance imaging. *Anesthesiology* 1988; **68**: 140.

10 Maydew R. P. and Berry F. A. Cherubism with difficult laryngoscopy and tracheal intubation. *Anesthesiology* 1985; **62**: 810.

11 Smith D. C., Pillai R. and Gillbe C. E. Tracheopathia osteochondroplastica. A cause of unexpected difficulty in tracheal intubation. *Anaesthesia* 1987; **42**: 536.

12 Capistrano-Baruh E., Wenig B., Steinberg L., Stegnajajic A. and Baruh S. Laryngeal web: a cause of difficult endotracheal intubation. *Anesthesiology* 1982; **57**: 123.

13 Dane T. and King E. G. A prospective study of complications after tracheostomy for assisted ventilation. *Chest* 1975; **67**: 398.

14 Meyer R. J. Awake blind nasal intubation in a patient with xeroderma pigmentosum. *Anaesthesia and Intensive Care* 1982; **10 (1)**: 64.

15 Orr D. Difficult intubation: a hazard in thalassaemia. A case report. *British Journal of Anaesthesia* 1967; **39 (7)**: 585.

16 Nicolson C. S., Black A. E. and Kraras C. M. Management of a difficult airway in a patient with a Hurler–Scheie syndrome during cardiac surgery. *Anesthesia and Analgesia* 1992; **75**: 830.

17 Jones A. E. and Thomas F. C. Morquio syndrome and anaesthesia. *Anesthesiology* 1979; **51**: 261.

18 Kattle F. J. and Mundale M. O. Range of mobility of the cervical spine. *Archives of Physical Medicine* 1959; **40**: 379.

19 Nichol H. C. and Zuck D. Difficult laryngoscopy – 'the anterior' larynx and the atlanto-occipital gap. *British Journal of Anaesthesia* 1983; **55**: 141.

20 Crosby E. T., Grahovac S. Diffuse idiopathic skeletal hyperostosis: an unusual cause of difficult intubation. *Canadian Journal of Anaesthesiology* 1993; **40**: 54.

21 Strauss E. J., Poplak T. M. and Braude B. M. Anaesthetic management of a difficult intubation. *South African Medical Journal* 1985; **68 (6)**: 414

22 Redick L. F. The temporomandibular joint and tracheal intubation. *Anesthesia and Analgesia* 1987; **66**: 675.

23 Tey H. K. Difficult intubation as a result of unsuspected abnormality of the temporomandibular joint [letter]. *Anaesthesia* 1986; **41**: 436.

24 Block C. and Brechner V. L. Unusual problems in airway management (2). The influence of the temporomandibular joint, the mandible, and associated structures on endotracheal intubation. *Anesthesia and Analgesia* 1971; **50**: 114.

25 Patane P. S., Rhagno J. R. and Mahla N. E. Temporomandibular joint disease and difficult tracheal intubation [letter]. *Anesthesia and Analgesia* 1988; **67**: 482.

26 Coonan T. J., Hope C. E., Howes B. J., Holness O. and MacInnis L. Ankylosis of the temporo-mandibular joint after a temporal craniotomy – a cause of difficult intubation. *Canadian Anaesthetists Society Journal* 1985; **32**: 158.

27 Sharwood-Smith G. H. Difficulty in intubation. Calcified stylohyoid ligament. *Anaesthesia* 1976; **31**: 508.

28 Akinyemi O. O. and Elegbe E. O. (1981) Difficult laryngoscopy and tracheal intubation due to calcified stylohyoid ligaments. *Canadian Anaesthetists Society Journal* 1981; **28**: 80.

29 Levitt M. W. and Collison J. M. Difficult endotracheal intubation in a patient with pseudoxanthoma elasticum. *Anaesthesia and Intensive Care* 1982; **10**: 62.

30 Burns A. M., Dorje P., Lawes E. G. and Nielsen M. S. Anaesthetic management of caesarian section in a mother with pre-eclampsia, the Klippel–Feil syndrome and congenital hydrocephalus. *British Journal of Anaesthesia* 1974; **61**: 350.

31 Tassonyi E., Lehmann C., Gunning K., Coquoz E. and Montandon D. Fiberoptically guided intubation in children with gangrenous stomatitis (noma). *Anesthesiology* 1990; **73**: 348.

32 Drenger B., Zidenbaum M., Reifen E. and Leitersdorf E. Severe upper airway obstruction on difficult intubation in cicatricial pemphigoid. *Anaesthesia* 1986; **41**: 1029.

33 Heindel D. J. Deep neck abcesses in adults: management of a difficult airway. *Anesthesia and Analgesia* 1987; **66 (8)**: 774.

34 Cantrell R. W., Ball R. A. and Morioka W. T. Acute epiglottitis. *Transatlantic Pacific Coast Oto-ophthalmol Society Annual Meeting* 1976; **57**: 75.

35 Vetto R. R. Epiglottitis. *Journal of the American Medical Association* 1960; **173**: 990.

36 Warner J. and Finlay W. E. I. Fulminating epiglottitis in adults. Report of three cases and review of the literature. *Anaesthesia* 1985; **40**: 348.

37 Oh T. H. and Motoyama E. K. Comparison of nasotracheal intubation and tracheostomy in the management of acute epiglottitis. *Anesthesiology* 1977; **46**: 214.

38 Tos M. Nasotracheal intubation in acute epiglotti-

tidis. *Archives of Otolaryngology* 1973; **97**: 373.

39 Milko D. A., Marshak G. and Striker T. W. Nasotracheal intubation in the treatment of acute epiglottitis. *Pediatrics* 1974; **53**: 674.

40 Huskisson E. C. and Hart F. D. *Joint Disease: All the Arthropathies* 3rd edn. Bristol: John Wright. 1978.

41 Jenkins J. C. and McGraw W. R. Anaesthetic management of the patient with rheumatoid arthritis. *Canadian Anaesthetists Society Journal* 1969; **16**: 407.

42 D'Arcy E. J., Fell R. H., Ansell B. M. and Arden G. P. Ketamine and juvenile chronic polyarthritis (Still's disease). *Anaesthesia* 1976; **31**: 624.

43 Sinclair J. R. and Mason R. A. Ankylosing spondylitis. The case for awake intubation. *Anaesthesia* 1984; **39**: 3.

44 Murray G. C. and Persellin R. H. Cervical fracture complicating ankylosing spondylitis. *American Journal of Medicine* 1981; **70**: 1033.

45 Resnick D. Temporo-mandibular joint involvement in ankylosing spondylitis. *Radiology* 1974; **112**: 587.

46 Shenkman Z., Shir Y. and Bodsky J. B. Perioperative management of the obese patient. *British Journal of Anaesthesia* 1993; **70**: 349.

47 Bond A. Obesity and difficult intubation. *Anaesthesia and Intensive Care* 1993; **21**: 828.

48 Vaughn R. W., Bauer S. and Wise L. Volume and pH of gastric juice in obese patients. *Anesthesiology* 1975; **43**: 686.

49 Meyer R. J. Obesity and difficult inubation. *Anaesthesia and Intensive Care* 1994; **22**: 314.

50 Datta S. and Briwa J. Modified laryngoscope for endotracheal intubation in obese patients. *Anesthesia and Analgesia* 1981; **60**: 120.

51 Chappel W. F. A case of acromegaly with laryngeal and pharyngeal symptoms. *Journal of Laryngology and Otology* 1896; **10**: 142.

52 Fogarty D. Lingual thyroid and difficult tracheal intubation. *Anaesthesia* 1990; **45**: 251.

53 Reissell E., Orko R., Maunuksela E. L. and Lindgren L. Predictability of difficult laryngoscopy in patients with long-term diabetes mellitus. *Anaesthesia* 1990; **45**: 1024.

54 Salzarulo H. H. and Taylor L. A. Diabetic 'stiff joint syndrome' as a cause of difficult endotracheal intubation. *Anesthesiology* 1986; **64**: 366.

55 Sellers W. F. and Yogendran S. Difficult tracheal intubation. *Anaesthesia* 1987; **42**: 1243.

56 Lee H.-C. and Andree R. A. Cervical spondylosis in difficult intubation. *Anesthesia and Analgesia* 1979; **58**: 434.

57 Hankins W. D. Traumatic hernia of the lateral pharyngeal walls. Trumpet players, glassblowers and self mutilation. *Radiology* 1944; **42**: 499.

58 Bray R. J. Pharyngeal pouch as a cause of difficult intubation. *Anaesthesia* 1977; **32**: 333.

59 Rashid J. and Warltier B. Awake fiberoptic intubation for a rare cause of upper airway obstruction – an infected laryngocoele. *Anaesthesia* 1989; **44**: 837.

60 Harper J. R., Thomas K. and Wirk H. A complicated case of juvenile laryngeal papillomatosis. *Anaesthesia* 1973; **28**: 71.

61 De Santo L. W., Devine K. D. and Weiland L. H. Cysts of the larynx – classification. *Laryngoscope* 1970; **80**: 145.

62 Mason D. G. and Wark K. J. Unexpected difficult intubation. Asymptomatic epiglottic cysts as a cause of upper airway obstruction during anaesthesia. *Anaesthesia* 1987; **42**: 407.

63 Kasuda H., Akazawa S., Shimizu R., Moriguchi H., Masubuchi M. and Miyata M. Difficult endotracheal intubation in a patient with tumoral calcinosis. *Anesthesia and Analgesia* 1992; **74**: 159.

64 Sale J. P. and Skyrme Jones S. An unusual cause of difficult intubation [letter]. *Anaesthesia* 1983; **38**: 1228.

65 Famewo C. E. Difficult intubation due to a patient's hair style [letter]. *Anaesthesia* 1983; **38**: 165.

66 Goldrick K.E. and Donlon J. V. Sublingual haematoma following difficult laryngoscopy. *Anesthesia and Analgesia* 1979; **58**: 343.

67 Brimacombe J. and Swan H. Displacement of a Celestin tube: an unusual cause of difficult intubation. *Anaesthesia and Intensive Care* 1993; **21**: 224.

68 Kunkel J. M., Gomez E. R., Spebar M. J., Delgado R. J., Jarstfer B. S. and Collins G. J. Wound haematomas after carotid endarterectomy *American Journal of Surgery* 1984; **148**: 844.

69 O'Sullivan J. C., Wells D. G. and Wells G. R. Difficult airway management with neck swelling after carotid endarterectomy. *Anaesthesia and Intensive Care* 1986; **14**: 460.

70 Seed R. F. Traumatic injury to the larynx and trachea. *Anaesthesia* 1971; **26**: 55.

71 Sirker D. and Clark M. M. Rupture of the cervical trachea following road traffic accident. *Anaesthesia* 1973; **45**: 909.

72 Bryan A. G. and Jones A. Skier's neck: an unusual cause of difficult intubation [letter]. *Anaesthesia* 1991; **46**: 802.

# 6

# Management of Difficult Intubation

*Peter Latto*

## INTRODUCTION

The delivery of adequate oxygen is of paramount importance to the patient and to the anaesthetist. Under normal circumstances, during general anaesthesia oxygen is delivered from the anaesthetic machine through a breathing system by means of a mask applied to the face, a laryngeal mask airway (LMA) or a tracheal tube. When a facemask is used an oral airway and/or elevation of the jaw may be required to maintain a clear airway.

In an excellent review article Benumof [1] described the *independent* degree of difficulty (ranging from zero to infinity) for *mask ventilation* and for *laryngoscopy and intubation* (Fig. 1). He defines no difficulty with mask ventilation as: 'no external effort and/or internal upper airway device is required to maintain airway patency'. Mask ventilation gets progressively more difficult as one or two person jaw thrusts and oral or nasopharyn-

geal airways are required (see Fig. 1). It is assumed that jaw thrust and an oral airway will always be used together. Infinite difficulty occurs when mask ventilation is impossible when using all these techniques.

No difficulty with intubation occurs when the tube is inserted into the fully visualized larynx with little effort at the first attempt. Things get progressively more difficult when less of the larynx is visible and more force is applied with the laryngoscope. With increasing difficulty the head may be repositioned, there may be more than one attempt at intubation, different laryngoscope blades may be used, pressure may be applied to the front of the neck, and there may be attempts by more than one anaesthetist. An infinitely difficult intubation occurs when there is failure to intubate a paralysed patient when all the above techniques are used.

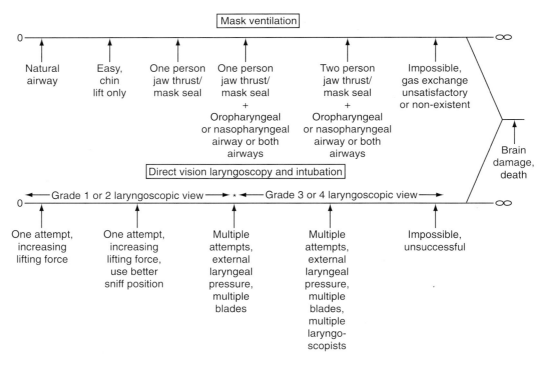

**Figure 1**   Definition of a difficult airway. Airway refers to either mask ventilation or endotracheal tube (ETT) intubation by direct vision laryngoscope. The degree of difficulty can range from zero, which is extremely easy, to infinite, which is impossible. When both mask ventilation and direct vision laryngoscopy are impossible, and no other manoeuvre is successful, brain damage and/or death will ensue. In between these extremes there are several well-defined, commonly encountered degrees of difficulty. The grade of laryngoscopic view refers to Figure 2 and is represented as an approximate continuum above the discrete indices of laryngoscopic difficulty. With permission from Benumof [1].

## DEFINITIONS

Practice guidelines for management of the difficult airway have been drawn up by a task force of the American Society of Anesthesiologists (ASA) [2]. They defined a difficult airway as:

*the clinical situation in which a conventionally trained anesthesiologist experiences difficulty with mask ventilation, difficulty with tracheal intubation or both.*

They stressed the value of descriptions that are quantitative and suggested the following definitions. They acknowledged, however, that other definitions may be preferred by some clinicians.

### 1  Difficult mask ventilation
This occurs when either:

(a)  it is *not* possible for the unassisted anesthesiologist to maintain the $SpO_2$ greater than 90% using 100% oxygen and positive pressure mask ventilation in a patient whose $SpO_2$ was greater than 90% before anaesthetic intervention;

or

(b)  it is *not* possible for the unassisted anesthesiologist to prevent or reverse signs of inadequate ventilation during positive pressure mask ventilation.

### 2  Difficult laryngoscopy
This was defined as a laryngoscopy in which it is *not possible to see any of the vocal cords* when using a conventional laryngoscope.

### 3  Difficult tracheal intubation
This occurs when *more than three* attempts are required for insertion of the tube using conventional laryngoscopic techniques or when it takes *more than 10 min* for tube insertion under the same circumstances.

Other definitions were not excluded. The following points are for consideration:

• Intubation may be succesful in *a much shorter time than 10 min* but the procedure may *still* be considered to be difficult.

• Intubation may be succesfully accomplished *on the first attempt* using a gum elastic bougie but the procedure may *still* be considered to be difficult.

It is clearly valuable to have a quantitative definition that is as widely accepted as possible for purposes of comparison.

A definition more appropriate for the UK anaesthetist might be:

*Any patient in whom it is not possible to intubate when using a laryngoscope and a bougie in an optimum way.*

This would include any patient with a Cormack and Lehane [10] Grade 4 view but should exclude most patients with a grade 3 view of the larynx.

Patients in the category of 'difficulty with mask ventilation' include firstly those with problems of the upper airway and secondly those with thick beards, bronchospasm and marked obesity [3]. Knill defined four practical difficulties with airway management:

• difficulty in maintaining the patency of the upper airway (a term which was preferred to difficulty with mask ventilation);
• difficulty with laryngoscopy;
• difficulty with placement of a tracheal tube;
• difficulty associated with possible contamination of the airway.

He suggested that each of these had different risks and requirements for management. He suggested that it might be appropriate to 'define each type of difficulty clearly and then formulate a simple set of basic management strategies for each that is tailored to its particular risks and management strategies'.

Attempts to include these suggestions in the ASA algorithm had been considered but this had not been possible [4]. The practice guidelines were not intended to be used as rigid rules to be followed, but rather to be a starting point for optimum clinical practice. It was intended that the guidelines should be modified according to local expertise, availability of equipment and preferences [4].

King suggests that problems with mask ventilation and tracheal intubation at induction of anaesthesia have been stressed perhaps at the expense of airway management problems [33]. He included unco-operative patients requiring awake intubation, patients with airway obstruction, irritable airway or cervical spine trauma as having a 'problematic airway' (this term was preferred to the term 'difficult airway').

## INCIDENCE

Difficult intubation can occur unexpectedly in clinical practice. However, some cases of difficulty can be foreseen. It is important, therefore, always to carry out a careful preoperative clinical examination, and also, if possible, to check previous anaesthetic records and if judged necessary to obtain skull, cervical spine and mandibular radiographs. Sia and Edens estimated that 90% of cases of difficult intubation should be anticipated and in only 10% should there be an unexpected problem [6]. In a prospective study of 1200 patients from Cardiff, however, 22 of 43 difficult intubations (51%) were anticipated and 21 (49%) were not [7]. Difficult intubation was anticipated in 84 patients; however, only 22 were actually difficult. It is clear therefore that unexpected cases of difficulty occur commonly in clinical practice and that some cases of anticipated difficulty may be simple to manage. The incidence of very difficult cases requiring awake intubation often with a complex technique is rare, probably about 1–5% of difficult cases. Awake intubation was required in only one of the above 43 patients (2.3%).

An incidence of 2.3% of difficult intubation was reported from a general hospital [8]. The Cardiff Anaesthetic Record System between 1972 and 1977 recorded an incidence of 1%, in which 65% of 109 000 patients had tracheal intubation. However, a smaller unpublished prospective study of intubation problems revealed a 3.6% incidence of difficult intubations in 1200 cases [7]. About half of these intubations were performed by staff in training and the true incidence is probably lower. In another study it was shown that the incidence of difficult intubation was reduced from 3.1% to 1.2% when a consultant attending physician was involved in the management of the case [9].

The number of cases which present a problem with tracheal intubation depends upon the experience of the reporting clinician and the type of patient and surgery involved. Aro and his colleagues found that 85% of difficult intubations could be managed by experienced clinicians with the use of an introducer [8]. In 15% of difficult intubations (0.3% of all intubations) a more complicated approach was necessary.

Some authors classify difficult intubation arbitrarily (including Cardiff data). Others classify according to whether the individual anaesthetist needs to use an intubation aid. Still others categorize according to the type of aid required to intubate successfully. Experienced clinicians may be able to intubate a patient whose cords are not visible. Although they may have no difficulty the record is marked as difficult to warn a trainee who might subsequently intubate the patient. Others who have some difficulty through forgetfulness or pride, omit to mark the form so statistics may not be reliable. A precise definition of difficult intubation is essential before undertaking a prospective evaluation of incidence.

## VIEWS OBTAINED AT LARYNGOSCOPY

Cormack and Lehane [10] defined the different views that can be obtained at laryngoscopy (Fig. 2).

### Implication of the Different Grades on Anaesthetic Management

#### Grade 1
There is general agreement that grade 1 views should present no significant difficulty with intubation.

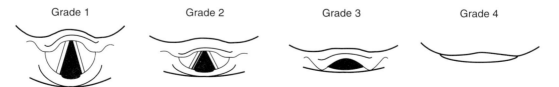

Grade 1     Grade 2     Grade 3     Grade 4

**Figure 2** Grades of laryngoscopic view. Grade 1: most of the glottis is visible and there should be no difficulty in intubation. Grade 2: only the posterior extremity of the glottis is visible. This may give rise to slight difficulty in intubation. Pressure on the front of the neck may improve the exposure of the larynx. Grade 3: no part of the glottis is visible. A bougie is an invaluable aid to intubation in these cases. Grade 4: not even the epiglottis can be seen. An awake intubation should be undertaken in these patients. With permission from Cormack and Lehane [10].

## Grades 2 and 3

It appears that there may be a difference in the clinical management of grade 2 and 3 views in the UK and in the USA. In the USA it appears that multiple attempts, the use of different blades, and the involvement of more than one anaesthetist are often required.

In the UK the use of different blades and multiple attempts may be required less commonly. Wilson [11] in a recent editorial asserted that the use of the gum elastic bougie enables intubation to be accomplished succesfully as long as the epiglottis is visible; that is for grade 2 and 3 views of the larynx. This approach is extremely successful and widely used in the UK.

## Grade 4

This view is very uncommon and *difficulty is often anticipated in advance*. Intubation is best accomplished with the patient awake if a grade 4 view is anticipated. If a grade 4 laryngeal view is encountered unexpectedly under general anaesthesia it is usually not possible to intubate simply using the Macintosh laryngoscope. The safest option when intubation is indicated, and a grade 4 laryngeal view presents under these circumstances, is to maintain oxygenation, wake the patient up, and then perform an awake intubation.

## Other Systems of Classification of Laryngeal Views

Other authors have used a different system of classifying laryngeal views [12, 13]:

**Grade 1** – almost all of cords visible;
**Grade 2** – only half of cords visible;
**Grade 3** – only arytenoids visible;
**Grade 4** – only epiglottis visible;
**Grade 5** – not even epiglottis visible.

The two views of most relevance to anaesthetists are the last in both groups, namely 'only epiglottis visible' and 'not even epiglottis visible.'

Mallampati and his colleagues used yet another system [17]:

**Grade 1** – glottis fully exposed;
**Grade 2** – glottis partly exposed (anterior commissure not seen);
**Grade 3** – glottis could not be exposed (only corniculate cartilages visible);
**Grade 4** – none of glottis or corniculate cartilages could be exposed. (It is assumed that the epiglottis could be seen so this is probably equivalent to a Cormack and Lehane grade 3 view.)

## Prediction of Different Laryngeal Grades and Difficult Intubation

The prediction of difficult intubation is dealt with fully in Chapter 4. It is clear, however, that difficult laryngoscopy (Cormack and Lehane grades 3 and 4) **cannot** always be predicted in advance. In one study only 50% of difficult laryngoscopies were predicted [12]. Therefore clinicians should have an optimum plan for the management of the different grades that might present unexpectedly during general anaesthesia.

## Incidence of Different Laryngeal Grades

Some descriptions include grade 3 and 4 together. It is important to separate them because the clinical management of grade 3 views in our practice is usually straightforward. The clinical management of grade 4 views presents a *much* more formidable challenge.

In a prospective study in 152 patients [14] there was a 75% incidence of grade 1 views of the larynx, an 18% incidence of grade 2 views, a 7% incidence of grade 3 views and no grade 4 views. The best possible view was obtained with backward pressure on the larynx.

### Grade 3 views

It was reported from one publication [15] that an anaesthetist had kept a personal record of 3800 intubations over a 7-year period [16]. The incidence of grade 3 laryngeal views was 1 in 292 (0.34%). The optimum management of such cases presenting unexpectedly is only possible if appropriate training regimens are implemented [15]. This is seen as particularly important in obstetric anaesthesia.

### Grade 4 views

The incidence of grade 4 views when even the epiglottis cannot be seen varies from 0% [14, 15], an estimated 1/200 (0.5%) [10], 3/677 (0.44%) [12] and 0.25, 0.5% and 0.3% in three separate groups [13]. A grade 4 view is therefore a much less common presentation at laryngoscopy than a grade

3 view. Many anaesthetists are incapable of intubating such patients. It is surprising, however, that indirect evidence (our unpublished Cardiff intubation audit) shows that failed intubation appears to be a very rare event. Mallampati [17] had an incidence of his grade 3 views of 19/210 (9%) and of his grade 4 views of 9/210 (4.3%) – a total 13% for grade 3 and 4. This seems very high and would probably have been much less if cricothyroid pressure had been used to improve the view.

## Change in Grade after Backward Pressure on the Cricoid Cartilage

In the Wilson study the incidence of grade 1 and 3 views went from 57.5% to 75.7% and from 9.3% to 5.9%, respectively, with backward pressure on the cricoid cartilage [13]. There was no improvement in the view with cricoid pressure in the one patient with a grade 4 view.

In a prospective series involving a different group of anaesthetists the incidence of grades 1, 3 and 4 were 81.7, 1.3 and 0.3%, respectively [15]. Four cases were reported in whom grade 4 views were converted to grade 3 views when a second anaesthetist took over and used increasing traction on the laryngoscope. A common feature of these cases was that the patients were large and the initial anaesthetists were small with thin wrists. When supervising such cases, the initial anaesthetist should be advised to use additional traction on the laryngoscope handle. It appeared that the different techniques used for laryngoscopy may vary in their effectiveness in securing an optimum view of the cords.

## Difficult Laryngoscopy and Difficult Intubation

It has been stressed that a distinction should be made between difficult laryngoscopy and difficult intubation [15]. Difficult laryngoscopy has been clearly defined as: 'when the cords cannot be seen.'

In order to obtain an optimum view under anaesthesia there are four well known requirements [15]:

- head in the Magill position;
- good muscle relaxation;
- proper use of the laryngoscope;
- backward pressure on the larynx (if necessary).

It appears that many clinicians may not be using an optimum laryngoscopic technique. For beginners there may certainly be difficulty in performing an adequate laryngoscopy. With increasing experience it is usually assumed that the laryngoscopic technique is good but training in the various ancillary intubation techniques may be lacking.

A universally acceptable quantitative definition of difficult intubation is much harder to find. It is clear, however, that in the UK intubation is frequently performed with minimal or no difficulty in patients with grade 3 views of the larynx – even by comparatively inexperienced anaesthetists.

## FAILURE TO INTUBATE AND FAILURE TO VENTILATE

This scenario is every anaesthetist's worst nightmare. It is fortunately extremely uncommon. The mortality from failed intubation, hypoxia during intubation and Mendelson's syndrome was calculated from published figures to range from 6 to 12 per 10 million population [16]. They suggested a minimum figure of 600 deaths per year in the developed world from this cause. Further calculations from Lunn and Mushin's data [18] suggest that these causes could represent 30% of deaths totally attributable to anaesthesia.

Benumof [1] suggested that failed mask ventilation and intubation often used to result in brain damage and death and suggested an incidence (after reviewing the literature) of 0.01–2 cases per 10 000 patients.

## DIFFICULTY WITH MASK VENTILATION

In the Australian Incident Monitoring Study 85 of 2000 reported incidents related to problems with intubation [19]. In 13 of these 85 cases (15%) there was simultaneous difficulty with facemask ventilation. In none of these cases was difficulty in ventilation predicted. These data do not, however, give the incidence of difficulty with facemask ventilation in patients requiring intubation. It is amazing that there does not seem to be any information on this in the literature. The authors of the report commented on the emphasis on intubation in the literature and *the lack of emphasis on the patient who cannot be ventilated or intubated*.

It is clear that in many instances where there is a problem with mask ventilation, the clinical management is saved by the skilful insertion of a tracheal tube.

# FAILED INTUBATION

The incidence of failed intubation has been thoroughly investigated in obstetric anaesthesia. Reported incidences include 1 in 291 cases (0.34%), 1 in 283 cases (0.35%) 1 in 2130 cases (0.05%), and 1 in 800 cases (0.125%) [20–23]. It has been shown that the incidence of failed intubation can be reduced by more than half by improving the training of anaesthetists [23]. *The incidence of failed intubation is approximately eight times higher in obstetric patients than in the general surgical population* [24].

Tunstall has described a failed intubation drill and has stressed that the *prime objective of such drills is to maintain oxygenation and at the same time to prevent aspiration* [25].

The incidence of failed intubation in an Australian series of patients anaesthetized by Rural General Practitioner (GP) anaesthetists was 1 in 200 (0.5%) [26]. It was considered that this high rate occurred because 36% of the GPs attempted intubation in a previously difficult case and preoperative airway assessment was inadequate.

# OUTCOME AFTER FAILED INTUBATION

When commenting on figures for failed intubation it is important to look at the clinical outcome [24]. Lyons reported nine cases of failed intubation in obstetrics with a successful outcome for mother and baby in all the cases [20]. *It seems very unusual for figures on the total number of intubations, the incidence of failed intubation and the outcome in these cases of failed intubation to be provided* [24]. It is clear, however, that there is a significant incidence of mortality and morbidity related to difficulties with intubation in obstetric anaesthesia. King and Adams reported that between 1973 and 1984, 41% of maternal deaths directly attributed to anaesthesia, (data taken from the *Confidential Enquiries into Maternal Deaths in England and Wales*) were caused by intubation difficulties [24]. In one report, 15 of 108 cases (13.8%) of anaesthetic accidents reported to the Medical Protection Society leading to death or serious neurological damage, were caused by intubation problems [27]. In a similar report to the Medical Defence Union 31% of 326 cases of death and cerebral damage relating to errors in anaesthetic technique were associated with intubation problems [28].

# TRAINING FOR MANAGEMENT OF A FAILED INTUBATION

Tunstall stressed that all anaesthetists should be prepared for failed intubation in the parturient [29]. This is also true for failed intubation of other patients presenting with a full stomach. He suggested that there should be a run-through of a failed intubation drill on a mannikin followed by a demonstration of transtracheal ventilation. Tunstall recommends that pressure should be maintained on the cricoid cartilage and the patient placed in the full left lateral and in the head down position. Others leave the patient in the semilateral position and maintain cricoid pressure while the patient is unconscious (this is discussed in greater detail in Chapter 16). It is of critical importance to place obese patients with short necks in an optimum position by elevating the thorax, shoulders and head to bring the anatomical axes into line [30]. This should minimize the chance of failed intubation in such patients.

# CLINICAL MANAGEMENT

## General Considerations

The practical management of a difficult intubation depends on the availability of specialized skills and apparatus, the urgency of the surgery and the type of surgery planned. It is mandatory to ensure that oxygenation is maintained with resumed artificial ventilation at intervals during attempts to pass a tracheal tube. The risk of aspiration of gastric contents should be minimized. When the situation occurs unexpectedly, particularly in obstetric anaesthesia, the patient always has a potentially full stomach and it is important to have a rational and safe plan of action both for failed intubation and failed ventilation. This matter is discussed in detail in Chapter 16.

It is a matter of individual judgement as to how long the clinician should persevere in attempted intubation even if there is adequate oxygenation. A decision will be influenced both by the urgency of the surgery and whether trauma results from the attempts. Desperate and prolonged attempts at intubation resulting in intermittent hypoxia should be avoided. It is essential to avoid trauma and certainly to reduce this to a minimum. Sufficient sets of simple apparatus which might be urgently required should be kept readily available in the theatre suite in a special 'difficult intubation

**Table 1**   Apparatus in Cardiff difficult intubation box.

Clock for timing duration of the procedure
Nasal airways
McCoy laryngoscope
Belscope
Large Macintosh laryngoscope blade
Left-handed Macintosh laryngoscope blade
Straight laryngoscope blade
Polio blade
Plastic tooth bridge
Gum elastic bougie
Stylet
Equipment for retrograde techniques:
    Tuohy needle
    Epidural catheter
    Seldinger wire
Equipment for transtracheal ventilation
    Needle and cannula
Connections from cannula to the anaesthetic machine

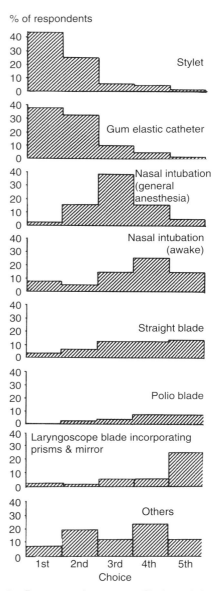

**Figure 3**   Retrospective survey. Choice of simple techniques. From James and Latto [32], with kind permission of the authors.

box' [31], and the contents of the Cardiff box are shown in Table 1. In addition it is essential to have fibreoptic equipment available, together with personnel trained in its use. There have, as yet, been few prospective clinical trials comparing different methods of intubation, and therefore it is not possible to make firm recommendations on the choice of a primary method for any individual patient. Each situation has to be carefully evaluated by the clinician and only then can the exact choice of technique be determined.

## Choice of Technique: Retrospective Survey

A survey of methods chosen by British anaesthetists to facilitate tracheal intubation and expertise with the methods was conducted at a Symposium on Intubation in October 1982 [32] Questionnaires were completed by 163 clinicians. Simple methods were used initially and are shown in order of preference in Fig. 3. One-third of respondents used these methods exclusively and had no experience with any of the complex methods. It is clear that the most popular first and second choices were the gum elastic catheter or bougie and the stylet. The use of simple techniques has changed and the gum elastic bougie has largely displaced other simple techniques in the UK (see page 123). It is also clear that more clinicians are now skilled at fibreoptic intubation and other complex techniques.

## Choice of Technique: Prospective Survey

An unpublished prospective analysis of techniques

used in 43 cases of difficult intubation [7] is shown in Fig. 4, which should be compared with Fig. 3.

## IDENTIFYING THE PRACTICAL PROBLEM

There are many causes of difficult intubation which are discussed in Chapter 5. On a practical level, however, in any particular case of difficulty during induction of a general anaesthetic a

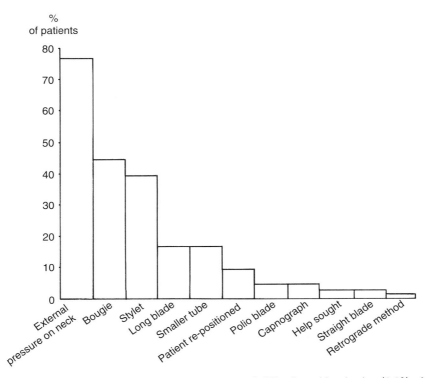

**Figure 4**   Prospective survey. Simple methods used in 43 cases of difficult oral intubation (3.6% of total of 1200 cases). From Eastley *et al.* [7], with kind permission of the authors.

**Table 2**   Some problem orientated solutions to difficult intubation.

| | |
|---|---|
| Inability to open mouth | 1 Inadequate relaxation. Give more relaxant or wait for relaxant already given to become effective<br>2 If trismus is present intubate under local or assess the effect of inhalation anaesthesia in relaxing jaw muscles<br>3 Awake intubation in patients with jaws that are permanently closed |
| Mouth open but difficulty in inserting laryngoscope blade | 1 Detach blade from handle and insert separately<br>2 Use polio blade |
| Laryngoscope deflected by irregular teeth | Use plastic tooth bridge |
| Mouth open but tube deflected by irregular teeth | Use rigid introducer to facilitate positioning the tube |
| Cords partially visible | Initially use either a gum elastic bougie, stylet or other simple technique |
| Epiglottis visible | Use gum elastic bougie |
| Cords not visible | Use gum elastic bougie |
| Epiglottis concealed | Awake intubation is indicated |

specific problem may be identified (Table 2). For cases of both expected and unexpected difficulty clinicians initially use simple familiar techniques and mainly succeed. A plan for difficult intubation is essential.

## Management Algorithms

A number of a algorithms have been described to help in the management of cases of difficult intubation and difficult ventilation. The recommendations of the ASA Task Force on Management of the Difficult Airway [2] are shown in Table 3. An alternative algorithm [1] for difficult airway management is shown in Table 4. Other intubation and airway management algorithms have been described [19]. (See also Chapters 8, 16 and 19.)

Such plans have, however, become increasingly complex and are very difficult to remember in a crisis. Since a number of plans are available it is also necessary to decide which plan is most appropriate for the individual clinician. Algorithms should be of particular value in the management of cases where a difficult airway or difficult intubation are predicted in advance.

**Table 3**  ASA difficult airway algorithm.

1. Assess the likelihood and clinical impact of basic management problems:
   **A** Difficult intubation
   **B** Difficult ventilation
   **C** Difficulty with patient cooperation or consent
2. Consider the relative merits and feasibility of basic management choices:

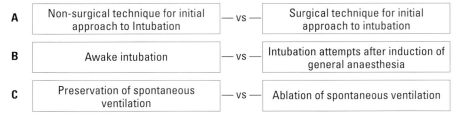

| | | | |
|---|---|---|---|
| **A** | Non-surgical technique for initial approach to Intubation | — vs — | Surgical technique for initial approach to intubation |
| **B** | Awake intubation | — vs — | Intubation attempts after induction of general anaesthesia |
| **C** | Preservation of spontaneous ventilation | — vs — | Ablation of spontaneous ventilation |

3. Develop primary and alternative strategies:

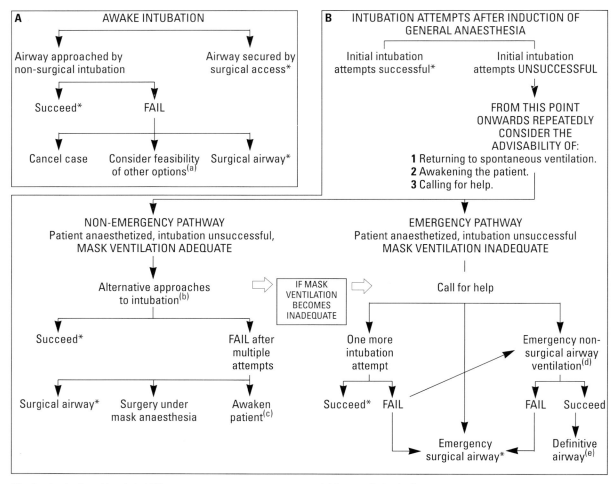

*Confirm intubation with exhaled $CO_2$.
(a) Other options include (but are not limited to): surgery under mask anesthesia, surgery under local anaesthesia infiltration or regional nerve blockade, or intubation attempts after induction of general anesthesia.
(b) Alternative approaches to difficult include (but are not limited to): use of different laryngoscope blades, awake intubation, blind oral or nasal intubation, fibreoptic intubation, intubating stylet or tube changer, light wand, retrograde intubation, and surgical airway access.

(c) See awake intubation.
(d) Options for emergency non-surgical airway ventilation include (but are not limited to): transtracheal jet ventilation, laryngeal mask ventilation, or oesophageal-tracheal combitube ventilation.
(e) Options for establishing a definitive airway include (but are not limited to): returning to awake state with spontaneous ventilation, tracheostomy, or endotracheal intubation.
With permission from Caplan *et al.* [2]

**Table 4**  Difficult airway management algorithm. With permission Benumof [1].

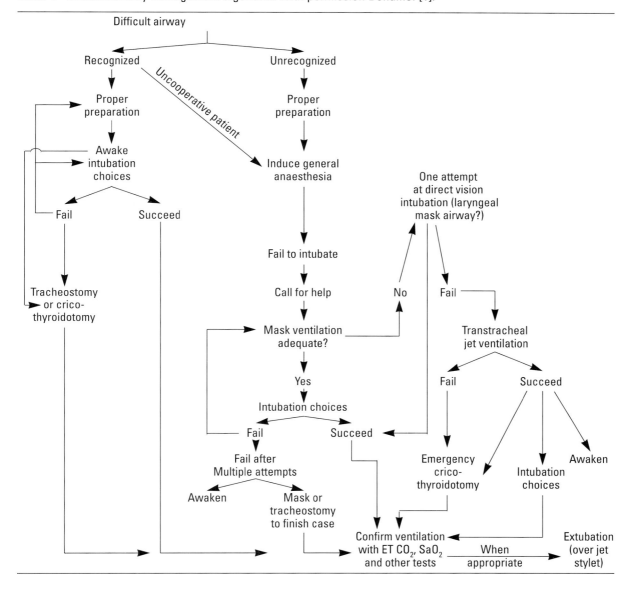

King has recommended that 'the trial-and-error type of cascade algorithm' may be less appropriate than focusing on management of specific problems [33]. He claims that once the specific problem is identified the solution is usually not that difficult – providing that the appropriate equipment is available. Certainly algorithms would appear to be of limited use in the middle of a crisis. There does seem to be some resistance to using the available algorithms and these flow charts do not appear to be commonly displayed in anaesthetic rooms. The detailed study of algorithms is no substitute for the acquisition of expertise with specific complex techniques.

## Application of Specific Techniques in the Algorithm

Only when the anaesthetist has acquired expertise with the various techniques can optimum strategies (as recommended in the various algorithms) be applied. It is important, therefore, that clinicians develop expertise in a wide range of techniques and skills. These should include both simple and complex techniques.

### Simple techniques

- the use of oral and nasal airways;
- optimum laryngoscopy technique;
- the application of cricoid pressure;
- the use of the bougie, the stylet, and the light wand;
- simulated difficult intubation using the bougie;
- blind nasal intubation;
- use of the laryngeal mask airway;
- the administration of local anaesthetic for an awake intubation.

### Complex techniques

- fibreoptic intubation;
- intubation using the laryngeal mask airway;
- retrograde intubation;
- transtracheal needle ventilation;
- use of the Combitube [34].

It is probable that the majority of anaesthetists are lacking in a number of these skills. The reason is simple: the requirement for such skills is infrequent. Furthermore, training in these skills is often woefully lacking. Most anaesthetists 'manage somehow', usually 'getting away with it'. *Lack of the requisite skills introduces an avoidable risk factor and contributes to the morbidity and mortality associated with intubation.*

## Clinical Management in Cases of Anticipated Difficulty

Benumof considers that awake intubation should be performed when problems with airway management are anticipated [1]. Such cases could include patients with upper airway problems, those with obesity, those with with beards and cases of bronchospasm [3]. The degree of anticipated difficulty with airway management may be large. It can therefore be argued that there may be a spectrum of acceptable airway management options. Clearly, at the difficult end of the spectrum, the case for awake intubation is clear and unambiguous.

Cases with minimal airway problems are frequently intubated under general anaesthesia. However, it is clear that difficulties with airway management may *not* be predicted. Indeed, in one study none of the 13 reported cases of ventilation problems were anticipated [19]. There appears to be little emphasis in the literature on predicting such difficulty (in marked contrast to predicting difficult intubation), but anaesthetists are frequently able to identify some of these patients after clinical examination. The anaesthetic management of such patients needs to be modified (see below).

Benumof [1] also suggested that awake intubation is often indicated if a difficult intubation is predicted. This is clearly a much commoner presentation. To quote Benumof: 'First and most most important, the natural airway will be better maintained in most patients when they are awake (No bridges are burned)'. Mason, in a recent editorial [35], stressed the value of teaching awake fibreoptic intubation: 'None of the approaches under general anaesthesia permit the unhurried sequential identification of nasal, pharyngeal and laryngeal structures which is possible in the awake subject and essential when patients with abnormal anatomy or pathology are subsequently encountered'. There are few data available on the frequency of choice of different techniques for awake intubation. Options include fibreoptic, retrograde, blind nasal and spray-as-you-go techniques. Choice is dictated by clinical expertise, apparatus availability and patient requirements.

The disadvantage of awake intubation is that it may be more time-consuming and unpleasant for the patient [1]. If skilfully performed, however, there should be minimal discomfort and the dictates of patient safety should far outweigh the requirement for speed.

The solution then seems quite straightforward. The problem lies in executing the Benumof recommendations. It is clear that in the UK only a very small percentage of the cases where difficult intubation is predicted are in fact intubated awake. There is clearly some risk in attempting intubation under general anaesthesia in these patients. The risks in the UK are minimized by a combination of the following strategies:

- teaching trainee doctors simulated difficult intubation with the bougie and the optimum use of the bougie;
- proper patient preparation in respect of preoperative fasting and the use of antacids, etc.;
- having expert help readily available;
- making sure that all the apparatus that might be required is readily to hand (in particular the bougie);
- monitoring of oxygen saturation and use of the capnograph to confirm tracheal intubation;

- 'prolonged' oxygen administration prior to induction of anaesthesia;
- checking if possible that ventilation is possible before giving a muscle relaxant;
- use of a short acting depolarizing relaxant (and *avoiding* the use of long acting non-depolarizing relaxants);
- if possible, *not* persisting with prolonged and desperate attempts at intubation (see the options available at this stage in the various algorithms). In our experience prolonged attempts at intubation are comparatively rare. This would appear to be somewhat at variance with clinical practice in the USA because the ASA definition of difficult intubation includes: 'attempts lasting more than ten minutes when using a conventional laryngoscope.' This might imply that such prolonged attempts are not that uncommon in US clinical practice;
- teaching management of failed intubation and failed ventilation.

It is likely that the requirement for transtracheal needle ventilation will be minimized if the above precautions are followed. The laryngeal mask is now used commonly in clinical practice and this has been used succesfully in some cases when failed intubation and ventilation have occurred (see Chapter 8).

The risks of proceeding with an intubation under general anaesthesia when difficulties are predicted are very real. These problems however cannot be entirely eliminated by performing awake intubation when difficulty is predicted because many cases of difficult intubation and airway management are not predicted.

The introduction of teaching programmes in fibreoptic intubation, retrograde intubation and needle ventilation should lead to an improvement in clinical practice. Once clinicians can readily use the fibrescope, the instrument will be used more frequently in appropriate cases. The threshold for the use of the instrument will change.

The absence of expertise in awake intubation with the fibrescope means the anaesthetist has two main options. The first is to call for the assistance of a clinician who is capable of an awake intubation. The second is to attempt an intubation under general anaesthesia. This second option can result in patient morbidity and mortality. It is mandatory to reduce such risks to a minimum and to take great care in selecting an acceptable technique for each patient.

## Anticipating ventilation problems

When a case of very difficult intubation is identified preoperatively and there is doubt about the ability to ventilate, a different management plan should be adopted.

Awake intubation under local anaesthesia is the safest approach (Table 5). Under no circumstances should intubation be attempted under general anaesthesia. For a clinician who has not gained expertise with fibreoptic or retrograde techniques, blind nasal intubation may seem appropriate; it is essential to avoid trauma to the airway and bleeding with its potentially fatal results [36]. Retrograde or fibreoptic techniques are usually preferable. Fibreoptic techniques should not be attempted by the inexperienced clinician in these cases. A retrograde technique can be tried in an emergency since it is easy to perform and should not result in major complications. A clinician with no expertise in either fibreoptic or retrograde techniques might wisely decide to recommend a tracheostomy under local anaesthesia to ensure a secure airway. Occasionally

**Table 5** Plan for anticipated very difficult intubation. Incidence not known but it is less than 5% of difficult intubations.

| Attempt awake oral or nasal intubation | | | Avoid oral and nasal intubation | | | |
|---|---|---|---|---|---|---|
| Fibreoptic technique under local anaesthesia | Retrograde technique under local anaesthesia | Awake oral intubation through laryngeal mask airway | Tracheostomy under local anaesthesia | Consider doing operation under local block | Have equipment available for needle ventilation [137] | Consider cardiopulmonary bypass in cases of distal main airway obstruction [187, 188] |

Obtain expert assistance if required. Obtain capnograph to confirm tracheal tube placement.

even this option may not be available in a patient with a fixed flexion neck deformity.

For very short procedures some clinicians may choose to avoid intubation and manage the patient with a facemask breathing spontaneously. It is important to be aware of the potential danger of difficulty in maintaining the airway under these circumstances [37]. The patient with mucopolysaccharide disease has a short neck, a high epiglottis and infiltration of nasopharyngeal tissues. In these patients an oral airway can push the epiglottis back which can then occlude the larynx. However, a nasopharyngeal airway keeps the epiglottis forward and helps to maintain a clear airway should it be lost. Rapid intubation may often not be possible; and there may be fatal consequences. This approach should therefore be used with extreme caution.

Alternatively, it may be possible to perform the operation under local anaesthesia and avoid intubation. There are real risks to this too. If a local block is insufficient or wears off during surgery then it may be necessary to induce general anaesthesia under emergency conditions. If a complication such as a total spinal occurs, it would be difficult to manage since rapid intubation would not be possible.

These cases represent a considerable challenge to even the most experienced anaesthetist and difficulties in management should not be underestimated. It is important to consider and adopt a plan which minimizes risks to the patient.

## CONFIRMATION OF CORRECT PLACEMENT OF TRACHEAL TUBE

In any case of attempted tracheal intubation it is of paramount importance to confirm that the tube is correctly placed in the trachea. On occasions the tube may be placed in error in the oesophagus. The placement of a tube in the oesophagus *must* be recognized immediately so that the tube can be removed and replaced in the trachea. A number of tests have been described to confirm correct placement. Unfortunately, a number of these can produce misleading results. It is generally agreed that the capnograph provides invaluable information in cases where there may be doubt about the position of the tube. *The capnograph should therefore be available in all locations where anaesthesia is undertaken.* This matter is dealt with in detail in Chapter 11.

## Muscle Relaxants

If difficult intubation is suspected it is important to ensure that the airway can be maintained and positive pressure ventilation applied *before* giving a muscle relaxant. Most clinicians avoid the use of a non-depolarizing relaxant under these circumstances and would prefer a smaller dose of a short acting depolarizing relaxant. If failure to intubate or to ventilate occurs then most patients should start breathing spontaneously in 2–3 min.

## SIMPLE TECHNIQUES

One or more of the following techniques may be required in cases of difficult intubation.

### Head Position and Pressure on Front of Neck

A common difficulty is caused by failure to position the patient properly. The optimum position is flexion of the cervical spine and extension of the head at the atlanto-occipital joint [38]. Simple repositioning may enable the anatomy to become visible and intubation to be successfully accomplished. In addition, pressure directed posteriorly on the cricoid or thyroid cartilage on the front of the neck may render the larynx more easily visible. This is particularly helpful when the larynx is anteriorly placed and therefore difficult to see.

### Cricoid Pressure can Result in Difficult Intubation

Cricoid pressure was described by Sellick in 1961 to avoid aspiration during induction [39]. Backward pressure on the front of the cricoid cartilage obstructs the upper oesophagus, which prevents regurgitation and aspiration prior to intubation (Fig. 5). It also prevents gastric distension during positive pressure ventilation with a facemask. In the original description, the head and neck were fully extended and cricoid pressure was applied before induction of anaesthesia. However, in modern clinical practice the patient is often positioned with the neck flexed and head extended to ensure ease of tracheal intubation. Sellick later recommended that firm cricoid pressure, the onset of unconsciousness and the achievement of full muscular relaxation should be achieved simultaneously [40].

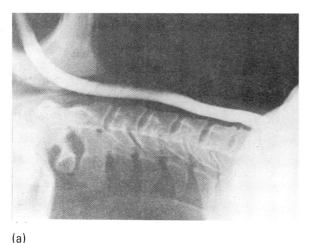

(a)

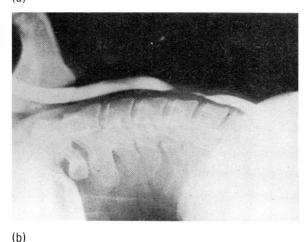

(b)

**Figure 5**   (a) Lateral X-ray of neck showing lumen of upper oesophagus filled by latex tube containing contrast medium.  (b) Obliteration of oesophageal lumen by cricoid pressure at level of C5. From Sellick [39] with kind permission of the editor of the *Lancet*.

With these precautions he believed that the risk of oesophageal rupture from vomiting (not regurgitation) was negligible. The technique was designed to be an alternative to induction in the sitting position.

Anatomical distortion can occasionally result from pressure on the neck rendering intubation more difficult [41, 42]. Crawford described a 'contra cricoid' cuboid support applied to the back of the neck before induction of anaesthesia which minimized this distortion thus reducing the incidence of difficulty caused by the pressure on the front of the neck [42]. The support was 27 cm long, 10 cm wide and 5 cm high.

Posterior displacement of the larynx by back-

ward pressure on the thyroid or cricoid cartilage is frequently used during difficult intubations when the larynx is only partially seen. This enables a better view of the larynx to be obtained in some cases. This can also occasionally distort the anatomy and may require similar 'contra cricoid' pressure to the back of the neck. This may not always be effective in enabling the anaesthetist to visualize the cords.

## Difficult Laryngoscopy Made Easy by Pressure on the Thyroid Cartilage Directed Backwards, Upwards and to the Right (BURP)

The commonest simple aid for managing a difficult intubation is backwards pressure on the cricothyroid cartilage [7]. Some anaesthetists find that the view of the larynx can be improved by leaving the laryngoscope in place and moving the larynx until an optimum view is obtained.

Knill [43] postulated that the best displacement for improving the view would be to push the larynx by applying pressure to the thyroid cartilage (Fig. 6):

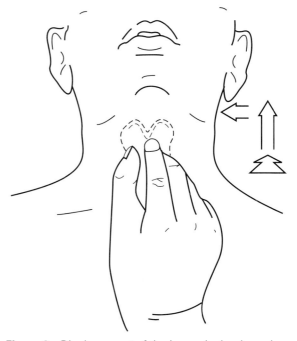

**Figure 6**   Displacement of the larynx by backward, upward and rightward pressure on the thyroid cartilage, or 'BURP'. Arrows indicate the direction of pressure application. With permission from Knill [43].

- posteriorly against the cervical vertebrae;
- as far superiorly as possible;
- laterally to the right.

Pressure was first applied to the thyroid cartilage to push the larynx *back* against the bodies of the cervical vertebrae. The larynx was then displaced as far *upwards* as possible. Lastly pressure was applied to the left side of the thyroid cartilage and the larynx displaced no more than 2 cm to the *right*. Laryngoscopy was then performed and the patient intubated.

Alternatively, laryngoscopy can be performed first. The BURP manoeuvre can then be performed before intubation. This latter sequence is more likely to be used for the unexpected difficult intubation. Two cases were described in which Cormack grade 3 and 4 views were transformed into grade 1 views by this technique.

Three important contributing causes of a difficult intubation were shown to be an anterior larynx, a posteriorly placed tongue and protruding upper teeth [10]. It was postulated that with an anterior larynx or a posteriorly placed tongue, the laryngoscopic line of vision from the incisors to the glottis may be obstructed distally by the base of the tongue. With a prominent premaxilla or elongated incisors, the line of vision is interrupted proximally. The BURP technique, by pushing the larynx upwards and backwards, may improve the view obtained at laryngoscopy The larynx is advanced towards the oropharynx round the base of the tongue. Displacement of the larynx to the right could further improve the view by bringing the larynx towards the mid line [43]. Further work will need to be done before this technique is more widely used in difficult intubations and to establish the clinical circumstances when its use is most appropriate.

## Gum Elastic Bougie or Catheter

A gum elastic bougie was first used as an aid to intubation by Macintosh in 1943 [44] when he found that the tracheal tube could obstruct his view of the cords. The lubricated gum elastic bougie was therefore first threaded through the tube and then gently placed into the trachea. The tube was pushed down into the trachea over the bougie and the bougie removed. The technique was also used when exposure of the larynx was inadequate. The technique is now commonly advo-cated when the cords cannot be seen at laryngoscopy (Figs 7–9). The bougie briefly retains the approximate shape into which it is bent. It is important to keep the bougie in the mid line and to bend the distal end forward after it has been passed through the tracheal tube. The bougie can then be advanced blindly towards the cords and the tube then 'railroaded' over the bougie. It is necessary to check very carefully that the tube has passed into the trachea. In addition to listening to the chest and observing chest movement it is mandatory to listen over the stomach and to measure expired carbon dioxide levels to exclude accidental oesophageal intubation. This technique is our first choice when the cords cannot be seen at intubation and a suitable bougie should therefore be available in every anaesthetic room. The use of the bougie appears to minimize the need to change

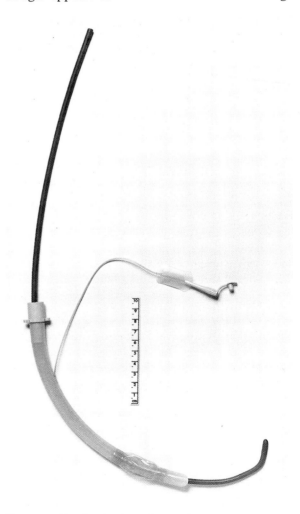

**Figure 7**    Tracheal tube with bougie.

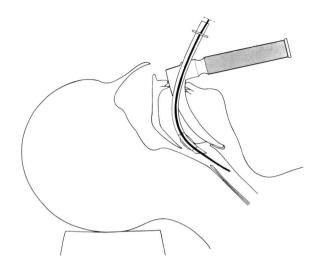

**Figure 8**    Bougie threaded blindly into the trachea.

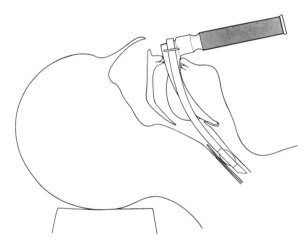

**Figure 9**    Tube railroaded into trachea over bougie and bougie then removed.

laryngoscope blades and the need for more than one clinician to make attempts at first intubation.

*In our clinical practice, the bougie is passed into the trachea on its own. We find this to be technically easier than passing the bougie through the tube as shown in Fig. 8.* This enables an unobscured view of the cords to be maintained. The appropriately curved bougie is passed in the mid line behind the epiglottis in the direction of the cords. The bougie is kept close to the posterior surface of the epiglottis. Once the bougie is in the trachea an assistant threads the tube over the bougie and the tube is then passed in the mid line.

Placement of the bougie into the trachea therefore constitutes the **first** and separate part of the intubation process.

Placement of the tube over the bougie and into the trachea constitutes the **second** and separate part of the intubation process.

It is clear that the bougie is being used with increasing frequency in the UK as an aid to optimum management of difficult intubations. A survey in 1988 showed that 90% of clinicians used this device as a first choice method and only 8% used the stylet [45]. The survey also showed that many clinicians were failing to use the bougie in an optimum manner.

### Optimum use of the gum elastic bougie

#### Clicks and hold up
It has been suggested that blind placement of the bougie in the trachea can be confirmed in three ways [46].

- First, and most important, it is usual to be able to feel a clicking sensation as the tip of the bougie slides over the tracheal cartilages.
- Second, there is a sense of obstruction if the forward passage of the bougie is interrupted as the tip of the bougie hits a small bronchus. It is clearly not necessary to elicit this sign if clicks have already been felt.
- Third, if the patient is not fully paralysed the passage of the bougie may provoke coughing.

These claims were investigated prospectively in 1988 [47]. It was shown that *clicks* were present in 89.7% of cases of tracheal placement of the bougie. The sign was not present if the tip of the bougie went down the centre of the tracheal lumen as the tip did not touch the sides.

**Distal hold up** occurred in all cases of tracheal placement of the bougie. Hold up occurred at 20–40 cm (at a mean distance of 31.9 cm). It was still recommended that clicks should be felt first. Only if these are absent should the bougie be inserted far enough to demonstrate distal hold up.

It is clear that these two signs are most valuable in confirming successful tracheal placement of a bougie when it is not possible to see the the cords. *The authors have recommended that these signs should be taught as part of Cormack's difficult intubation drill* [10].

If the bougie was placed in the oesophagus, both signs were absent in all cases. Under these circumstances, the bougie should be withdrawn and further attempts made to pass it into the trachea provided that arterial desaturation does not occur.

### Tube rotation and use of the laryngoscope

Frequently, staff in training are seen to have difficulty in threading the tracheal tube over the bougie. It is extremely frustrating and potentially very dangerous to be able to insert a bougie successfully into the trachea when intubation is proving difficult, only to fail to pass the tube into the trachea.

Cossham suggested in 1985 that this problem could be minimized by turning the tracheal tube a quarter-turn anticlockwise [48]. This is to prevent the tip of the tube catching on the right vocal cord (Fig. 10). If the tube is rotated a quarter turn clockwise, then the tip can impinge on the arytenoids.

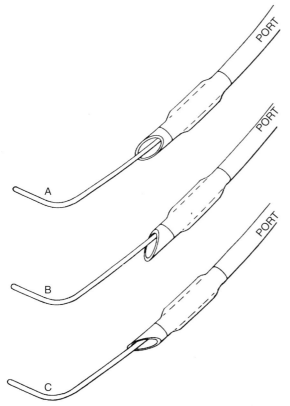

**Figure 10** (A) Tip of tube in a position liable to lodge on the right vocal cord. (B) Clockwise rotation of the tube may lead to the tip becoming lodged behind the arytenoids. (C) One quarter turn anticlockwise of the tube brings it in close contact with the bougie, preventing lodgement. With permission from Cossham [48].

**Table 6** Success at intubation in four groups of patients. Laryngoscope either in or out of the mouth when attempting to pass the tube over the bougie into the trachea. Tube either rotated –90° or not rotated when attempting to pass the tube over the bougie into the trachea. Modified with permission from Dogra *et al.* [49]

| Laryngoscope | Position of tube | Success rate |
| --- | --- | --- |
| No | 0° | 2/25 (8%) |
| No | –90° | 9/25 (36%) |
| Yes | 0° | 12/25 (48%) |
| Yes | –90° | 25/25 (100%) |

These claims were investigated prospectively in 1990 by Dogra and his colleagues [49]. *It was shown that the best results were obtained when the laryngoscope was left in the mouth and the tube was rotated 90° anticlockwise as it passed over the bougie through the cords* (Table 6). It was thought that the improved results with the laryngoscope in the mouth were due to the bougie remaining straight as it passed towards the cords. This eliminates the problems caused by the bougie curving forwards at an acute angle. Similar difficulties can occur when attempting to thread a tracheal tube over a fibrescope.

An alternative approach is to use a tube which has a tapered end [50]. The tip of the Moore tracheal tube is shown in Fig. 11. In a prospective trial this tube was shown to pass more efficiently over the fibrescope than the standard Portex tube. It was also suggested that a 30 cm armoured tube with this tip design should be available for difficult intubations. This type of tube could possibly pass over the gum elastic bougie in the very rare circumstances when there is a hold up at or below the cords with a standard tube. The author has not been aware of any cases of difficulty when an optimum technique was used.

Standard techniques must be used to confirm correct tracheal placement of the tube when it is not possible to see the cords in a bougie-aided intubation.

### Optimum design of the bougie

It is clearly possible to produce a range of different sizes and flexibility of the bougie. The bougie in common use is of 15FG diameter and 60 cm in length. A large bougie might be more difficult to introduce blindly into the trachea. It is probable, however, that a tube would slide more easily into the trachea over a larger bougie. Conversely a

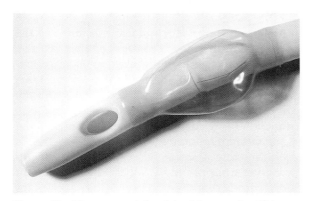

**Figure 11** The tapered tip of the Moore tube. This tube is not yet in commercial production. Photograph reproduced courtesy of Dr A. Pearce.

small bougie might be easier to thread into the trachea, but it is likely that it would be more difficult to thread a tube over a smaller bougie. It is clear that the bougie must bend into a curve and retain that curve for optimum use. Smaller bougies are used in paediatric practice. There have been no prospective trials of different sizes of bougies in adults as the 15FG succeeds in almost every case if used in an optimal way.

Sir Robert Macintosh tried unsuccessfully to obtain a range of sizes from the manufacturer. In 1978 in a private letter to Cormack [23] he wrote:

> I have found the introducer to be of the greatest help, particularly abroad when intubating in difficult (sometimes impossible) circumstances. I can honestly say that armed with an introducer, I have never failed providing I have been able to see the back of an arytenoid.
>
> I have for years tried to persuade different manufacturers (e.g. Portex) to make sets of introducers of say, six different sizes, but to no avail. The answer has always been that there is no demand. To me it is quite clear that young anaesthetists have never been taught the value of an introducer in difficult cases.

### Modification of the bougie
A short length can be cut off either end of the bougie. The hollow tube can then be used for oxygen insufflation [52]. Alternatively, side stream sampling permits capnographic analysis and should confirm tracheal placement of the bougie [53]. Such modifications are not widely

used. It is easy to confirm successful placement of the bougie with other techniques.

In one case of unexpected difficulty, there was failure to intubate using a variety of laryngoscope blades and tubes. A retrograde technique was used and an epidural catheter was passed into the mouth. It was not possible, however, to thread the tube into the trachea over the catheter. Both ends were then cut off a hollow Eschmann Stylet (bougie). The bougie was threaded into the trachea over the epidural catheter and the tube was then passed over the bougie into the trachea [54].

### Case history – failed intubation with improper use of the bougie
A patient presented for a Caesarean section and failed intubation occurred first when using a gum elastic bougie. A second attempt using a smaller tube and a metal introducer also failed [55]. On a third attempt with a bougie, the author was able to pass the bougie successfully into the trachea. However, it was not possible to pass the tube over the bougie. A tracheal tube was passed into the oesophagus, the cuff inflated and the cricoid pressure released. Copious gastric contents were ejected from the tube in the oesophagus. The anaesthetic subsequently proceeded uneventfully with a facemask and the tracheal tube protruding from under the mask. This is clearly one solution to a failed intubation but not one that is likely to be widely used. It is possible that the author would have succeeded with a bougie if the information on the optimum use of the bougie had then been available.

This illustrates the difficulties that occur when the bougie is not used in an optimum manner. *Such incidents are likely to deter users unnecessarily from persevering with this invaluable device.*

### Place of the bougie in current clinical practice
Cormack and his colleagues claim that: 'Over the past decade a consensus view has emerged that the most effective first method of handling a difficult intubation is to use a flexible introducer (gum elastic or soft wire)' [56].

In a recent editorial Wilson wrote: 'The success of this simple tool has quietly but radically altered anaesthetic practice, all that is now required is a view of the epiglottis: even when the cords can not be seen the tip of the gum elastic bougie can be slipped quickly behind the epiglottis, through the cords, and the tracheal tube railroaded over it into position' [11, 14]. He stressed that it was very important for all anaesthetists to be able to deal with the unexpected failure to intubate. He also stressed that if the epiglottis can be seen the gum elastic bougie can be used to facilitate intubation.

Nolan and Wilson [14] showed that the median time taken for intubation using the bougie and simulating an 'epiglottis only' view was only 10 s longer than when intubating in the conventional way with an optimum view of the cords. They recommended that a bougie should be used when a good view of the cords is not obtained immediately.

In a later study, the same authors [57] simulated neck injuries and found that the bougie could be successfully used to intubate all the patients studied. A number of failures occurred when the bougie was not used. They recommended that the bougie should be used as an aid to intubate patients with cervical trauma, particularly if the cords cannot easily be visualized (see Chapter 18).

### The bougie in the patient with crowned front teeth

An important indication for using a fibrescope is to minimize the risk of damage to expensive bridge work or to crowned teeth. Damage to teeth at intubation is a common problem and one that can be particularly distressing to patients. During a conventional intubation, the risk of damaging the teeth can be minimized by not putting any pressure on the top front teeth during the laryngoscopy. This can be helped by avoiding the use of 'undue' force for the laryngoscopy and passing the bougie into the trachea even when the view of the cords is incomplete.

### Use of the gum elastic bougie in the UK and the USA – why is there a different frequency of use?

In 1984, the bougie and the stylet were used with equal frequency in anaesthetic practice in the UK [7]. It is clear that the bougie has now gained a central role in the management of difficult intubation in the UK [45]. This has been a natural process of evolution as clinicians come to appreciate the advantages of the bougie over the stylet.

A letter written by four British anaesthetists working in the USA in 1988 indicated that the device was not readily available in North America [58]. There is no reason to suppose that this situation has changed appreciably. It was claimed that the disadvantage of a rigid introducer inside the tube is that it is often impossible to pass the tube and introducer off the anterior wall of the larynx

and into the trachea. The flexibility of the bougie overcomes this problem and avoids trauma to the laryngotracheal region. This device is particularly indicated when a difficult intubation occurs unexpectedly. It has been suggested that in the USA the common use of fibreoptic techniques and the introduction of training programmes for fibreoptic intubation for residents could have minimized the use of and requirement for other devices [14]. It is significant that a recent description of a difficult intubating trolley in the USA listed four different fibrescopes but no bougie [59]. There is perhaps some reason for cautious optimism as there has been an excellent recent review of the bougie in the American literature [60]. There has been only one study comparing the bougie with the stylet [5]. The study compared the bougie and the stylet when used for simulated difficult intubation. Surprisingly the stylet (in contrast to the bougie) had not previously been evaluated when used for simulated difficult intubation. *These authors clearly demonstrated that the bougie was more effective in facilitating intubation than the stylet. The clinical implications are obvious. The bougie should be used in preference to the stylet.*

In conclusion, it seems that anaesthetists in the UK need to gain more experience and expertise with fibrescopes. By contrast, our colleagues in the USA and elsewhere would assuredly benefit from the widespread introduction of the bougie into their clinical practice.

## Simulated Difficult Intubation and the Gum Elastic Bougie

The trainee faced with a difficult intubation with no view of the cords may panic and not have a clear idea of the correct way to solve the problem. This technique can be taught as part of a difficult intubation training programme [10, 61]. The larynx is first visualized and the laryngoscope blade then lowered so that the epiglottis drops back and conceals the cords. This simulated difficulty can then be managed using Macintosh's method [44]. An Oxford tube (a tube with a right angled bend) was preferred for training in simulated difficulty. Most clinicians however use a curved tube and find this quite satisfactory.

Management of such a situation can be practised under controlled circumstances. This should boost confidence and decrease the incidence both of protracted and failed intubation. It was suggested that this programme should be taught in addition to the Tunstall failed intubation drill [62].

Following the classic pioneering work of Cormack and Lehane in 1984 [10], there have been two major changes in clinical practice.

First, the simulated difficult intubation drill has been introduced as a routine part of the training programmes of all forward thinking anaesthetic departments. It should be taught to *all* trainees as soon as they are confident in dealing with routine intubations. It should also be practised intermittently by senior anaesthetists in order to maintain their expertise. This drill undoubtedly has been responsible for saving lives. In Cormack's obstetric unit, the incidence of failed intubation was only 1 in 800 following the adoption of this simple training procedure [23]. A widely quoted figure for failed intubation in obstetrics is 1 in 300 cases. It was believed that the improvement was due to frequent use of the training drill. Cormack suggested that in any case of a maternal death due to a failed intubation, there would almost certainly be questions asked in court regarding the training programmes of the junior staff. Those responsible for training could be put in a difficult position if such programmes were found to be unsatisfactory.

Secondly, it is clear that, in the UK at least, the bougie has come to be used as a *first step* in the management of the patient presenting with an unexpectedly difficult laryngoscopy or intubation under general anaesthesia.

## Simulated Difficult Intubation with a Bougie through the Laryngeal Mask Airway

A number of methods of intubation through the laryngeal mask airway are described in Chapter 8. The bougie can be passed blindly through the mask into the trachea. In one report the bougie was successfully used in this way in two very difficult patients [63]. The laryngeal mask airway was then removed and a tube threaded over the bougie into the trachea.

These authors suggested that such a technique should be practised as a routine on all patients with laryngeal masks *in situ* to develop confidence in the technique before using it 'in anger' on a patient with intubation problems.

## Intubation through the Laryngeal Mask Airway Using the Bougie

In one prospective study, there was an 84% (21 out of 25) success rate for blind insertion of a bougie through the laryngeal mask and into the trachea [64] and in another, a 90% success rate for blind insertion of a tracheal tube through the mask [65]. If a fibreoptic scope is available the results should be even more successful because the distance between the grille of the mask and the cords is only 3–4 cm. The fibreoptic technique is greatly facilitated because the cords are usually easily seen as soon as the tip of the scope comes through the grille of the laryngeal mask airway.

In another case report of a patient known to be difficult to intubate a laryngeal mask was inserted under local anaesthesia [66]. A gum elastic bougie was then inserted blindly through the laryngeal mask into the trachea. The authors noted that the patient coughed when the bougie entered the trachea. They curved the tip of the bougie up and slightly forwards to facilitate easy passage through the fenestrations of the mask. They marked the bougie to indicate when approximately 4 cms of the bougie had passed through the end of the mask. The bougie should also be marked along its long axis to indicate the orientation of the angulated tip.

Attempted placement of a Cook airway exchanger through the laryngeal mask yielded a success rate of only 30% [67]. These poor results were thought to be due to the fact that the rigid, straight introducer emerges from the posterior aspect of the mask aperture bars and is therefore more likely to pass into the oesophagus. It was noted that the tip of the introducer frequently got caught on the mask aperture bars.

The methods of intubation using the laryngeal mask are discussed in more detail in Chapter 8.

## Introducers

Metal introducers or stylets have been used to facilitate placement of both tracheal catheters [68] and tubes [69–72]. Stylets have been made from a variety of materials including copper wire, coat hangers, knitting needles and brass rods. Unfortunately these are potentially traumatic and usually not sterile. Blunt ended disposable* and non-disposable†‡ introducers are commercially

---

*Spick-stylette Polamedco, Inc, 1625 17th St, Santa Monica, CA 90404, USA.
†Flexiguide Division, Scientific Sales International Inc, PO Box 867, Ravinia Station, Highlands Park, IL 60035, USA.
‡Satinslip intubating stylet-Mallinckrodt.

available and should be safer than the sharp-ended metal in-house variety. Introducers are routinely used with flexible armoured tubes to help in advancing the tube. They are also helpful if a more rigid tube is deflected by irregular teeth. An introducer is most commonly required when visualization of the vocal cords is difficult. Occasionally, the epiglottis can be seen but the cords are completely concealed or only their posterior portions are visible. Sometimes neither the epiglottis nor the cords are visible. Under these circumstances, a lubricated introducer is often bent into a J shape (Figs 12 and 13) and then passed into the tube; both are then directed in the mid line towards the assumed position of the vocal cords. The tip of the rigid introducer is usually kept inside the tracheal tube to minimize the possibility of tracheal trauma. Alternatively the tip of the introducer can protrude past the end of the tube and then be passed blindly into the trachea.

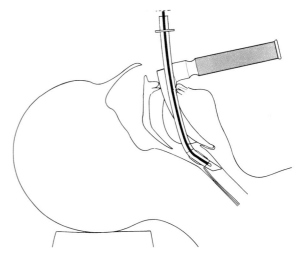

**Figure 13**   Tube with bent stylet used to facilitate intubation.

The tube is then 'railroaded' into position [73]. This technique is potentially traumatic even with a soft, blunt-ended introducer.

A simple adaptation of the stylet was found to be useful in the management of difficult intubations [74]. A well-lubricated silicone coated malleable introducer was used. This was inserted into the tracheal tube so that the tip of the introducer just protruded from the end of the tube. The distal 5 cm of the tube was then bent at an angle of 70–90° (Fig. 14a). The midpoint of the tube was bent at an angle of 70–80° (Fig. 14b). It was claimed that the distal bend gives better access to an anteriorly placed larynx. The bend in the middle enables a clear view of the larynx to be obtained during intubation. This design makes good sense but there are no quantitative data available to confirm its usefulness.

An illuminated flexible stylet has been designed with a 2″ (5 cm) flexible distal end [75]. The stylet is placed inside the tracheal tube and flexion of the distal end is produced by a trigger at the proximal end. A light placed at the tip of the stylet directly illuminates the pharynx and trachea. No data are available on the use of this stylet in cases of difficult intubation and the device is not commercially available. It may have been rendered obsolete by the development of fibreoptic direct vision techniques.

The Salem/Resce intubation guide⋆ (Flexiguide) has a distal tip which can be flexed by oper-

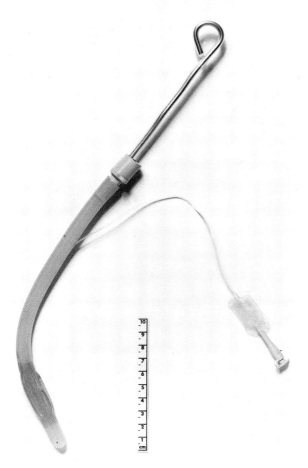

**Figure 12**   Tube with stylet bent into a 'J' shape.

⋆Flexiguide Division, PO Box 867, Ravinia Station, Highland Park, IL 60035, USA.

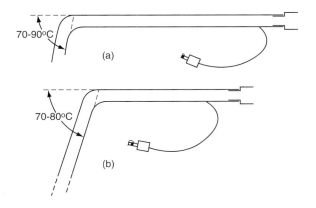

70-90°C

(a)

70-80°C

(b)

**Figure 14** Diagrammatic representation of the distal end (a) and midpoint bends (b) of the tracheal tube. With permission from Smith, Buist and Mansour [74].

ating the control on the proximal handle [76]. It is inserted through the tracheal tube and then guided into the trachea.

A tracheal tube has been designed with a flexible distal end which can be directed towards the larynx.† This tube has a nylon line running under the concave surface from the distal to proximal ends. The proximal end of the nylon line is fixed to a ring loop and when this is pulled the tip of the tube moves anteriorly (Fig. 15). In clinical use the tube is advanced through the nose or mouth and is placed in the pharynx. The tip is advanced towards the cords while traction is exerted on the ring loop to direct the tip of the tube. This device should be particularly useful for nasal intubation and reduce the need to use Magill intubating forceps.

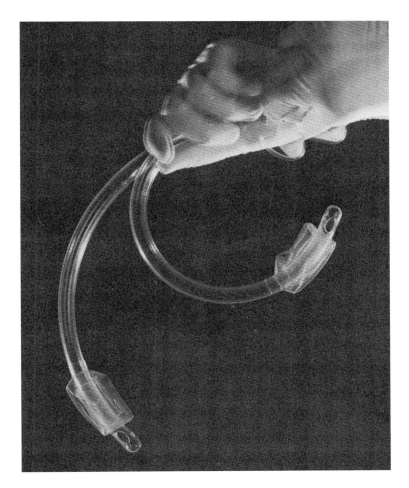

**Figure 15** Double exposure of 'endotrol' tube showing movement caused by pulling on ring loop.

†Endotrol by Mallinckrodt. Obtained from American Hospital Supply (UK) Ltd, Station Road, Didcot, Oxon.

## Use of a Smaller Tracheal Tube

A small diameter tube often facilitates intubation when intubation has been unsuccessful with a tube of an appropriate diameter. In the adult a 7 mm or even a 6 mm internal diameter tube may be chosen. It may then become necessary electively to ventilate the patient because there would be undue resistance to gas flow during spontaneous ventilation. Alternatively, if the smaller tube is unsatisfactory due to difficulty in effecting a seal with the cuff it can be changed using a polythene tube changer [77], stylet [78] or suction catheter [79]. This is not likely to be necessary for short procedures but would be appropriate when longer term ventilation is proposed. A technique employing a small tracheal tube and artificial ventilation is frequently used during operations on the larynx in order to allow good surgical access. Small tubes specially designed for microlaryngeal surgery with internal diameters of 4, 5 and 6 mm with a high volume/low pressure large diameter cuff are commercially available‡ and could also be useful for cases of difficult intubation.

## Laryngoscope Blades and Handles

Many laryngoscope blades have been developed in a search for the impossible – namely the blade that permits easy intubation in all cases. Descriptions of single cases where intubation proved impossible with one blade and success was immediately achieved with another should be taken with a large pinch of salt by the discerning clinician. The design of many laryngoscope blades has been reviewed by McIntyre [80]. He concluded that: 'As there are many individual factors influencing the process of intubation it is not surprising that detailed evaluations of the performance of any particular laryngoscope blade are extremely rare and critical analysis virtually nonexistent'. One study described a theoretical method of analysing laryngoscope blades [81]. It was claimed that such theory was consistent with common clinical opinions and could help in blade design in the future.

It is certainly not necessary to detail all the blades that have been described. If any one blade were better than all the others, it would surely be used exclusively by all clinicians; this is certainly not the case. It is important for clinicians to gain expertise and experience with one blade and not to be misled by the overenthusiastic claims of the inventors of other models. Meaningful comparative evaluations of different blades appear to be very unusual. McIntyre [80] claims, however, that it should be possible for the clinician to select the most appropriate design of blade on the basis of the preoperative examination of the patient. He documented the most appropriate blade for four groups of patients:

- Patients with a protruding sternal region;
- Patients with restricted mouth opening (a narrow space between the incisor teeth);
- Patients with a reduced infra oral cavity;
- Patients with an anterior larynx.

Optimum choice of blade should enable the best possible view of the larynx to be obtained in any particular patient and, at the same time, avoid any trauma. It would appear, however, that we are a long way from this objective in everyday clinical practice.

It has been claimed that: 'In spite of a vast helpful literature, attempted tracheal intubation remains a source of critical incidents, trauma and mortality' [82]. This is true, but improvements in technique and equipment have certainly greatly improved safety and probably decreased the incidence of serious problems in many centres.

The illumination provided by different reusable blades has been evaluated [83]. It was demonstrated that regular sized handles and incandescent bulbs produced better illumination than blades

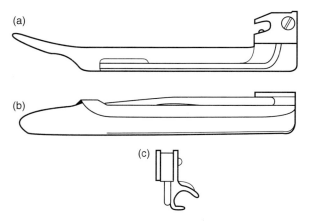

**Figure 16**  The Miller blade. (a) Side view; (b) top view; (c) fitting view. With permission from McIntyre [80].

---

‡MLT endotracheal tube Mallinckrodt. Supplied by American Hospital Supply (UK) Ltd, Station Road, Didcot, Oxon.

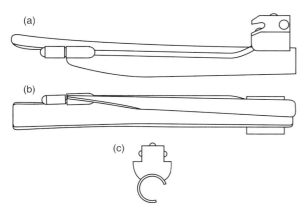

**Figure 17**   The Jackson–Wisconsin blade. (a) Side view; (b) top view; (c) fitting view. With permission from McIntyre [80].

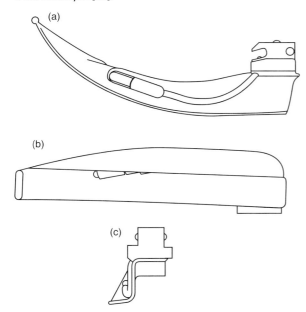

**Figure 18**   The Macintosh blade. (a) Side view; (b) top view; (c) fitting view. With permission from McIntyre [80].

using fibreoptic technology. It was suggested that this was particularly important when dealing with a difficult intubation. The narrow focused light of the fibreoptic blade makes recognition of the glottis more difficult. This may result in the need to move the blade/handle unit in order to demonstrate the glottis.

The blades most commonly used in North America include the Miller, the Jackson –Wisconsin and the Macintosh [80] (Figs 16–18). In North America it is not uncommon to change blades to facilitate the management of a difficult intubation.

In a study in 1973, it was shown that multiple attempts at intubation occurred in 18% of patients and that in 4% of patients intubation was accomplished with a blade other than that originally chosen [84]. With improved clinical expertise it is now likely that change of blade is required much less frequently in the USA.

In the UK it is certainly only rarely necessary to change from the Macintosh blade. The Macintosh blade [85] was described in 1943 and is used almost exclusively in the UK for the intubation of adults (Fig. 19). It has been shown, however, that substantial forces are exerted on the incisor teeth when the Macintosh blade is used [86]. The majority of anaesthetists in this study used the maxillary incisors as a fulcrum of leverage. While it is expected that such force may be applied during a difficult intubation it is surprising that this happened with easy intubations. A blade that provides additional leverage at its tip, such as that described by McCoy [87] should minimize trauma to the incisors.

These results were considered relevant for improving the design of laryngoscope blades in the future.

The standard curved blade described by Macintosh [85] is usually satisfactory for revealing the larynx (Fig. 19). Occasionally, a longer blade of the same design is required for tall patients. The laryngoscope was designed for intubation under

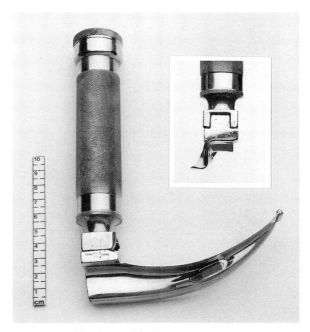

**Figure 19**   Macintosh blade.

spontaneous respiration when the larynx could be exposed at a lighter plane of anaesthesia. The tip of the blade in the vallecula (supplied by the glossopharyngeal nerve) did not touch the dorsal surface of the epiglottis (supplied by the superior laryngeal nerve, a branch of the vagal nerve). The tip of the blade is lifted to expose the cords. Care should be taken to avoid exerting undue pressure on the upper teeth. It is important always to have available at least two working laryngoscopes for any intubation in case the light fails in one.

With a difficult intubation, most clinicians in the UK use an alternative technique rather than another type of laryngoscope blade. Over the years a large number of different designs of the blade have been described. In 1926 Magill described a straight blade laryngoscope, used to pass a catheter with an accompanying expiratory tube into the larynx [88] (Fig. 20). The tip of the blade was placed behind the epiglottis. In 1941, this design was modified and improved by Miller [89]. The Miller blade was shallow with a curve 2 inches (5 cm) back from the tip and had a round, narrow end. This shallow base decreased the risk of damage to the teeth and it was not necessary to open the mouth as widely as with the Magill blade. This type of blade is widely used in North America and is often employed for cases of difficult intubation.

A number of variations in design are available to facilitate intubation. The laryngoscope can be fitted with improved fibreoptic illumination [90, 91]. Most laryngoscopes are designed to allow intubation from the right side of the patient's mouth. A 'left sided entry' laryngoscope blade may be required for patients with deformities of the right side of the face and oropharynx [92]. This is a mirror image of the usual Miller or Macintosh blade and the tube can be introduced from the left side of the mouth. A shorter handle to the laryngoscope may be useful in obese or pregnant patients with large breasts when the usual laryngoscope handle may be impeded [93].

Other options are to detach the blade, pass it into the mouth and then reattach the handle or to use a 'polio' blade (Fig. 21). The handle of a 'polio' laryngoscope is arranged at an angle greater than 90° to the blade to enable easier insertion into the mouth. A ventilation device may be clipped to the standard laryngoscope handle enabling ventilation during intubation [94, 95] (Fig. 22) which would allow a more prolonged attempt at intubation and minimize the risk of hypoxia. A suction channel can also be incorporated in the blade to facilitate immediate suction. Blades with mirrors and prisms are described elsewhere (p.147).

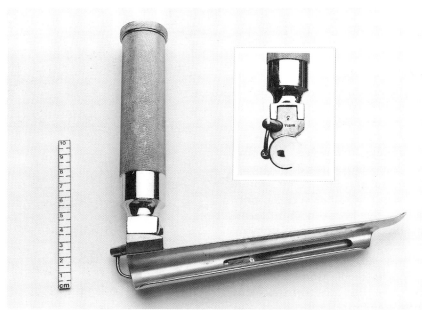

**Figure 20**   Magill blade.

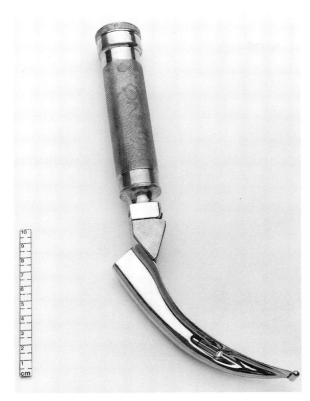

**Figure 21**   Polio blade.

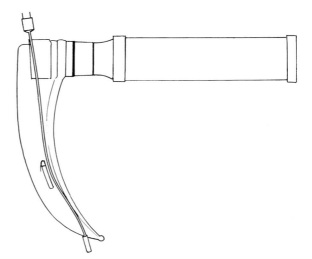

**Figure 22**   The needle attached to the laryngoscope blade, showing the moulding to the shape of the blade. With permission from Galloon [94].

## Other Laryngoscope Blades

### *The Belscope*

The Belscope has a long angulated blade with a 45° bend at the midpoint and a detachable prism (Fig. 23) [96]. There is a marked difference between the shape of the Macintosh blade, and the Belscope. In one report of more than 250 intubations [97] using the Macintosh blade, there were 12 grade 3 views (Cormack and Lehane classification) of the larynx. A good view of the larynx was obtained in all these cases with the Belscope. An introducer was needed in the tube to facilitate intubation in only four of the twelve cases. The prism was not required in any case. It was suggested that this blade should be attached to the normal laryngoscope handle and used in all cases needing intubation in order to gain expertise. In the hands of the author there was an easy learning curve. It was also claimed to minimize damage to the teeth. Due to the angulation of the blade it stays well away from the upper teeth during laryngoscopy and intubation, thus minimizing the risk of dental trauma.

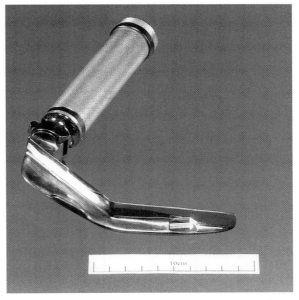

**Figure 23**   The Belscope. Photograph courtesy of Dr M. Ward (Oxford).

### *The Bullard laryngoscope*

The Bullard laryngoscope has an anatomically shaped rigid blade with fibreoptic viewing and light source (Fig. 24). Its use in adults was evaluated in 40 patients in whom intubation difficulty was expected [98]. One disadvantage was that if the intubating forceps are used, the laryngoscope has to be held in the right hand and the forceps in

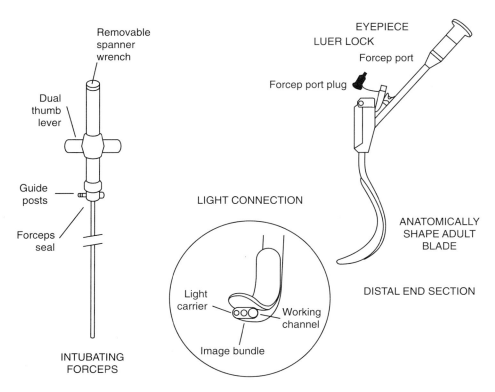

**Figure 24**    Diagram of the Bullard laryngoscope. With permission from Saunders and Giesecke [98].

the left hand. It was also difficult to use in the awake patient.

Laryngeal visualization was attempted in 93 children aged from 1 day to 2 years [99]. Intubation was accomplished using the intubating forceps or a stylet in the tube. The intubation success rate was 97%. As a result of a review of the anaesthetic records and clinical examination, 31% of the patients were expected to present difficulties. Intubation was attempted in 15 paediatric patients and was succesful in 14 (93%). In five of these patients there had been previous failure or great difficulty in intubation. The scope was used successfully in 17 awake infants. Borland and Casselbrant [99] found that it was easy to learn to use this instrument; this contrasted with the difficulties in learning to use fibreoptic devices in this age group.

In another study, a 7FG jet ventilation catheter was passed via the side channel of the Bullard scope into the trachea and used for high frequency jet ventilation [100]. Anaesthesia was maintained with a propofol infusion and vecuronium. This technique enabled pan-endoscopy to be performed in the presence of both normocapnia and cardiovascular stability. It was possible to leave the catheter in

the trachea until the patient was awake. This technique was recommended for the optimum management of patients with laryngeal pathology.

### The Upsher fibreoptic laryngoscope*

This laryngoscope is introduced in the mid line and the curved blade naturally follows the pharyngeal curve towards the larynx (Figs 25 and 26). Most clinicians using this blade will already have considerable experience with the Macintosh blade. It is a sturdy instrument with no moving parts. The scope combines fibreoptic 'round the corner' viewing with the manoeuvrability of the conventional blade. The tip of the blade is advanced until it comes to rest close to the cords under the epiglottis. The tube sits in the semi-enclosed space in the blade and the tip of the tube is initially level with the distal lower border of the blade. The tube is advanced under direct vision through the cords once they are in view. Tubes from 5.5 mm to 9 mm will fit in the scope. It may

---

* Available from Meditron, Unit F2B, Keighley Business Centre, South Street, Keighly BD21 1AG, UK.

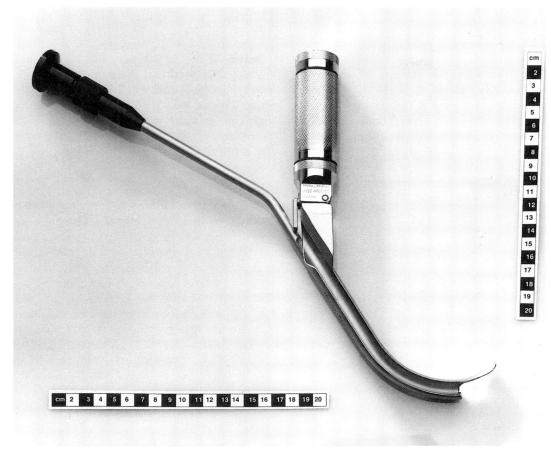

**Figure 25**    The Upsher fibreoptic laryngoscope.

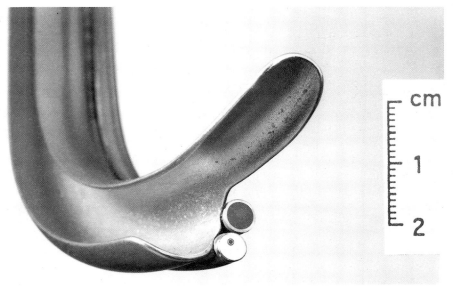

**Figure 26**    The tip of the Upsher fibreoptic laryngoscope with light and viewing channel.

be necessary to lift the handle of the blade to obtain a clear view of the cords. The variable focus eyepiece enables the operator to obtain an uninterrupted view of the procedure. The eyepiece can be attached to a television camera for teaching purposes.

The particular advantage of this device is that it can be succesfully used both when mouth opening is restricted and when neck flexion is contraindicated. It appears to fill an important gap between the conventional Macintosh laryngoscope and the standard fibreoptic laryngoscope. The learning curve is steep and expertise can be acquired rapidly. As with all new devices, it is necessary to practise on a significant number of patients before using it for a difficult intubation.

### The McCoy blade

The McCoy blade is a modified Macintosh blade [87]. There is a hinged distal tip to the blade (Fig. 27). The hinge is approximately 25 mm from the blade tip and is controlled by a lever attached to the proximal end of the blade. This modified blade can be attached to a standard Penlon handle. The tip of the blade is passed into the vallecula. The thumb is then used to depress the lever which elevates the tip of the blade. It was claimed that forward movement of the tip could improve the view of the cords and convert a Cormack and Lehane grade 2 or 3 into a grade 1 or 2. External pressure on the larynx may not be required. It was also suggested that there might be a reduced sympathoadrenal response to intubation with this blade. This is because less force is required to obtain an optimum view of the larynx.

### The combination intubating device

This is a complex device that combines a rigid blade and a flexible fibrescope [101]. The blade is curved and tubular. The tip of the blade is designed to fit in the vallecula. Once the larynx is visualized, a suction catheter is passed through the tube and into the trachea. The tracheal tube is then advanced over the catheter into the trachea. The fibrescope channel is incorporated in the blade. When the bivalve element of the blade is detached, the device can be used for nasal intubation. No forceps or stylet were needed for intubations. The device was used succesfully on 300 adult patients. The authors recommend further evaluation by other investigators. This device would appear to have some features in common with the Upsherscope.

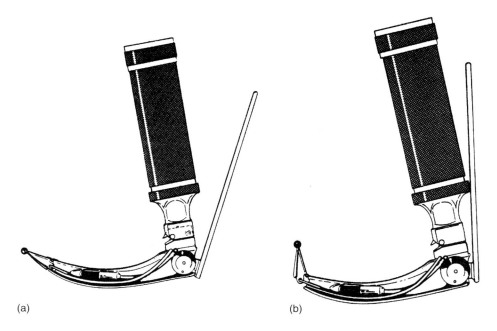

(a)                                    (b)

**Figure 27**   The McCoy laryngoscope. Drawing of the levering laryngoscope blade fitted to a handle showing the blade in a normal position (a) and with the tip elevated (b). With permission from McCoy and Mirakhur [87].

### Other blades

A wide flat blade with a double curve and no flange (Fig. 28) was described by Choi in 1990 [102]. It was claimed that this design combined the advantageous features of both the Macintosh and the Miller blades. Elimination of the vertical flange present in the Macintosh blade should help to minimize damage to the teeth at intubation.

A blade was designed by Bainton in 1987 with a 7 cm tube (Fig. 29) in its distal portion [103]. This was designed for easy visualization of the larynx where the pharyngeal space is restricted by inflam-

mation, tumour or foreign bodies. This bulky, straight bladed device may not work well in patients with an anteriorly placed larynx. It was successfully tested in dogs and in 12 patients with pharyngeal oedema.

## Comparison of Different Laryngoscope Blades

There are surprisingly very few reports comparing intubation statistics from controlled trials of different blades.

### The Belscope and the Macintosh blades and cervical movement

The Belscope and the Macintosh blades are used in different ways. It is essential therefore to practise extensively with the Belscope before using it on a case in whom intubation difficulty is predicted.

A recent study with experienced anaesthetists showed that there was no difference in cervical movement during intubation when using the Belscope (prism attached) or the Macintosh blade [104]. However, intubation took longer with the Belscope and was unsuccessful in two patients despite adequate visualization of the cords.

It was recommended that anaesthetists use the blade with which they are most familiar in patients in whom difficulty in intubation is anticipated. It is probable that the anaesthetists involved in this

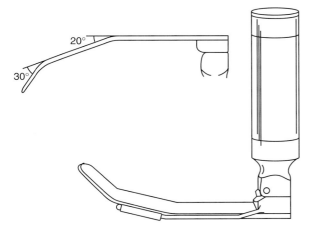

**Figure 28 (a)**   The double-angle blade. Note the incremental curvatures (20° and 30°). With permission from Choi [102].

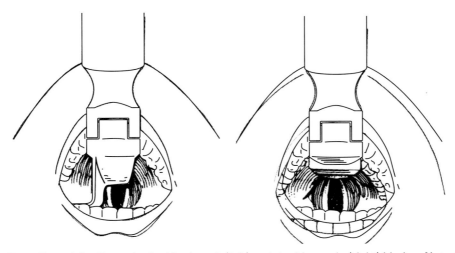

**Figure 28 (b)**   The effect of the flange in the Macintosh (left) and double-angle (right) blades. Note the area of improved vision and more room with the non-flanged double-angle blade. This should also reduce the risk of damaging teeth. With permission from Choi [102].

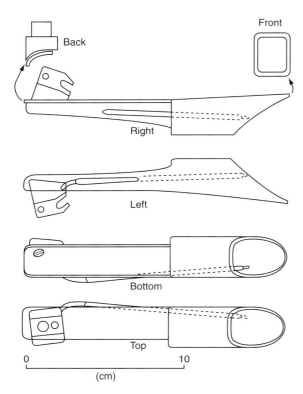

**Fig 29**    Scale drawing of the tubular blade. With permission from Bainton [103].

study were more familiar with the Macintosh blade than with the Belscope.

### Comparison of the Belscope and the Macintosh blades on a mannikin – ease of use by students

In another study, medical students had a higher incidence of failed intubations when using the Belscope on a mannikin than when using a Macintosh blade [105]. There was a 20% failure rate with the Belscope and a 5% failure rate with the Macintosh laryngoscope. The majority of failures occurred in the first five intubation attempts. Intubation was slightly quicker when the Macintosh blade was used but both laryngoscopes resulted in intubation in an acceptable time.

### Rapidity of intubation on a mannikin by first-year anaesthesia residents – a comparison of the fibreoptic with the Bullard laryngoscope

It has been suggested that, in adults, the Bullard laryngoscope may be easier to master than the fibreoptic laryngoscope, have a lower incidence of failed intubations and be quicker and less traumatic. Its main disadvantage was that it was more difficult to use in the awake patient [98].

This theory was tested on a mannikin by 20 first-year anaesthesia residents [106]. It was found that the Bullard laryngoscope and the fibreoptic laryngoscope were equally easy to master. However, passage of the tube took longer with the Bullard laryngoscope. The Bullard laryngoscope was used either with a wire passed blindly into the trachea or with a stylet inside the tube. The wire method was found to be more reliable. It was easy to see the cords with this device but not always easy to pass the tube into the trachea. As expected, the results improved with practice.

The disadvantage of the fibreoptic device is the time taken to prepare it for use. They concluded that 'no technique can be learned easily but any can be improved with practice'.

### Prospective comparison of the Belscope and the Macintosh laryngoscopes in 162 women with full dentition

In this study the grade of laryngoscopic view obtained in each patient was assessed with both the Belscope and the Macintosh laryngoscope [107]. The order of laryngoscopic examination was allocated randomly. Analysis of the data gave a $p$ value of less than 0.001 for improvement of the laryngeal view with the Belscope. Contact of the blade with the upper teeth was commoner with the Macintosh blade. The upper lip needed to be retracted more commonly when the Belscope was used. It was concluded that a consistent improvement in the laryngeal view was obtained with the Belscope and that it was a valuable aid to intubation.

### Prospective comparison of four different blades – Miller, Wisconsin, Macintosh and Belscope

In this study the optimum view obtainable with the these blades was compared in 98 patients [108]. The distance between the blade and the upper incisors was measured at the point of optimum visibility. Of the four blades studied, the Belscope produced the best view. Two patients suffered significant dental trauma with the Wisconsin blade. It was suggested that the use of the Belscope may result in a reduced incidence of upper dental trauma at laryngoscopy.

## Conclusion

It is certain that the reader will finish reading this section feeling extremely confused. It is important for the practising clinician to gain experience and confidence with one blade. Only then should other blades be used. A bewildering array of blades is available to the anaesthetist. It will only be possible to make a rational selection when the results are available of well-conducted trials comparing one blade with another.

*On the basis of the evidence presently available, it would seem reasonable to have available the Macintosh blade, the Belscope and the McCoy laryngoscope.*

### Blind Oral Intubation Using the Augustine Guide™*

This device enables intubation to be accomplished blindly and eliminates the need for head and neck manipulation. Thus it could have a particular role

---

* Augustine Medical, Inc, Eden Prairie MN 53344, USA.

in patients with neck injuries.

The guide consists of a curved positioning blade with a guide channel (Fig. 30) [109]. The curved blade slides down the back of the tongue and the end fits into the vallecula. The distal end has two lateral bulbous protrusions and an indentation in the mid line. Lateral movement of the guide can be recognized by the transmitted palpable lateral movement of the hyoid when the end is properly seated in the vallecula. Anterior movement of the tip lifts the epiglottis to expose the vocal cords. The flexible, hollow stylet is then passed blindly into the trachea. The distal end of the stylet curves anteriorly like the end of a gum elastic bougie. This reduces the chance of the stylet entering the oesophagus.

Tracheal entry is confirmed by easy aspiration into a syringe of 30 ml of air from the tracheal lumen as recommended by Wee [110]. The tube is then threaded over the stylet into the trachea. A bite block can be used to facilitate passage of the guide into the mouth but is not needed as a routine. The ability to use the device competently on difficult cases, will of course, only be acquired by practising on routine cases.

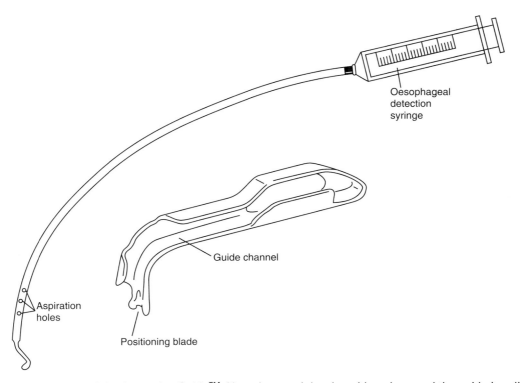

**Fig 30**   The components of the Augustine Guide™. Note the special stylet with syringe and the guide handle with channel. The stylet is inserted into the endotracheal tube, which is then mounted onto the guide channel prior to use. With permission from Carr and Belani [109].

In one study the device was used successfully in six out of seven patients predicted to be difficult to intubate [111]. Difficulty in advancing the guide into the trachea occurred in 22% of attempts. These authors suggested that it might be appropriate to switch to this guide when difficult laryngoscopy occurs unexpectedly. The median time for 31 intubations was 65 s (range 35–90 s).

In one report the success with the device was determined in 50 adult patients in whom the head and neck were kept in the neutral position [112]. Intubation was succesful 96% of the time and was classed as easy in 74% of the patients. Oesophageal intubation was easily recognized whenever it occurred. In a later study the device was used successfully at the first attempt on six patients who were judged as difficult to intubate.

In another report [113] the stylet was used to pass a nasal tube blindly into the trachea in a patient with Treacher–Collins syndrome.

## Nasal Intubation

The term 'blind nasal intubation' was first used by Rowbotham and Magill, who utilized the technique during the First World War [114]. Accidentally, they found that when working with dual insufflation tubes a larger bore tube passed nasally would frequently enter the glottis. The history of nasotracheal intubation has been reviewed by Elder [115], Gold and Buechel [116] and Pederson [117]. By 1937 the most common method of intubation was with a laryngoscope under direct vision. Also widely used were blind nasal intubation, blind oral intubation through a divided airway, and blind oral intubation using the first two fingers of the left hand to palpate the epiglottis or larynx and then sliding the tube posteriorly down behind the epiglottis [118]. However Magill [119] and Lewis [120] still continued routinely to advocate blind nasal intubation rather than direct oral intubation. Anaesthetists of that era were skilled at atraumatic blind nasal intubation but with the advent of muscle relaxants the requirement for the technique largely vanished. In order to maintain the skill, some clinicians practise the technique where nasal intubation is required for elective surgical procedures such as tonsillectomy. Blind nasal intubation has been performed under general [121, 122], or local anaesthesia [116, 123, 124], and even without any form of anaesthesia [125].

Pederson has summarized some of the circum-

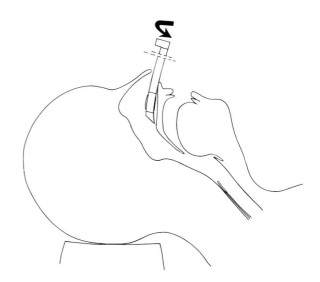

**Figure 31**   Rotation of nasal tube may be required to facilitate passage through the nose (see also Figure 32).

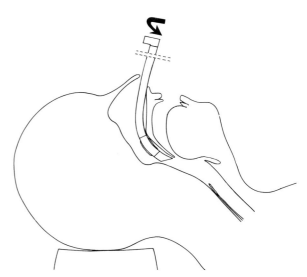

**Figure 32**   Rotation of nasal tube may be required to facilitate passage through the nose.

stances in which awake nasal intubation should be considered [117]:

- decreased airway patency due to inflammation or neoplasm;
- difficult laryngoscopy due to inability to open the mouth, mandibular agenesis, 'bull neck' or buck teeth;
- maxillofacial deformities (after trauma);
- when a mask can not be applied to the face;
- cervical injuries limiting neck movement.

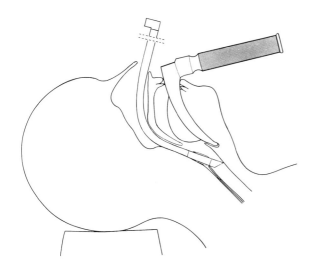

**Figure 33**   Tip of tube stopped at anterior tracheal wall.

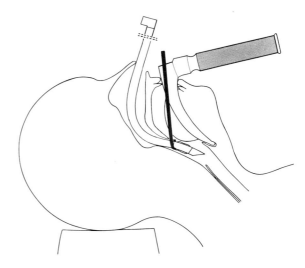

**Figure 35**   Hook used to facilitate passage of nasal tube.

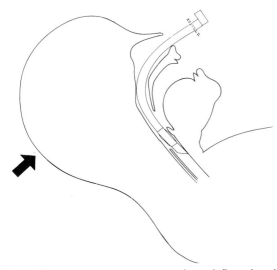

**Figure 34**   Laryngoscope removed, neck flexed and tube then passed into the trachea.

Before performing an awake intubation the anaesthetist should carefully explain the procedure to the patient. The patient is then lightly sedated, and the local anaesthetic administered (see Chapter 7). The patient is positioned with the neck flexed and the head extended at the atlantoaxial joint in the 'sniffing the morning air' position described by Magill [119]. A well-lubricated, curved, nasal tube is gently passed through the most patent nostril into the pharynx. The nasal mucous membranes can be constricted by the use of a phenylephrine spray. The opposite nostril should be occluded with the mouth shut and the chin lifted forwards. The patient is then asked to breathe in deeply and the tube advanced in the mid line while listening for breath sounds. Gold and Buechel successfully intubated 48 out of 50 patients with this method [116]. Confirmation of placement and monitoring of the progress of the tube is facilitated by monitoring carbon dioxide concentrations in the expired air.

Not all nasal intubations are performed so easily. A number of techniques have been described to facilitate the procedure (Table 7). If there is difficulty in passing the tube through the nose a smaller, well lubricated tube should be used and rotated as required (Figs 31 and 32). It is not uncommon to find that the tip of the tube is held up at the anterior tracheal wall and further movement is obstructed. When this happens the situation can usually be resolved by leaving the tube at the laryngeal inlet and flexing the neck when it usually easily passes into the trachea (Figs 33 and 34). The distal end of the tube frequently needs to be manipulated through the cords either with Magill forceps or a hook (Fig. 35). Alternatively a suction catheter can be used to facilitate the passage of the tube into the trachea [133] (Figs 36–38).

Blind nasal intubation may be attempted under general anaesthesia following a failed oral

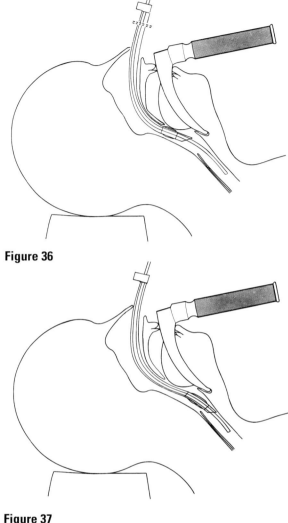

**Figure 36**

**Figure 37**

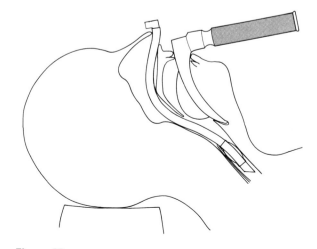

**Figure 38**

intubation. The success rate is increased if the patient hyperventilates. Davies described a technique using nitrous oxide, oxygen, halothane and 7% carbon dioxide [122].

Blind nasal intubation, although a simple procedure, has low reported success rates of 30% [116] and 28% [122] on the first attempt. Davies reported a final success rate of 93%. However, 40% of cases required between four and 12 attempts. It is clear that increased trauma, which may be disastrous, can result from prolonged and rough attempts.

A failure rate of 21% with blind nasal intubation was reported in 61 cases of ankylosis of the jaw [36]. In five cases (8.2%) considerable bleeding occurred and a fatality was reported in a 17-year-old man after hypoxia due to a severe epistaxis. In 60 similar cases the alternative technique of transtracheal ventilation was used without any problems [137].

### The Advanced Trauma Life Support (ATLS) recommendations of the American College of Surgeons

The ATLS recommendations [138] for management of trauma patients with suspected cervical injury have recently been amended. It is now stated that the experience of the clinician dealing with the case is the most important factor in deciding whether to perform oral or nasal intubation. Both blind nasal and oral intubation are accepted for these patients.

Initial advice was to perform blind nasotracheal intubation but this was never widely accepted in the UK. In the USA emergency airway management is often performed by emergency physicians who are not as experienced as anaesthetists in the use of anaesthetic drugs used to facilitate intubation. In the UK intubation of patients with neck injuries is carried out almost exclusively by highly experienced anaesthetists. Most British anaesthetists are not skilled in blind nasal intubation either in anaesthetized or awake patients. Oral intubation with a rapid sequence induction,

**Figures 36–38** Use of suction catheter to facilitate passage of nasal tube through the cords. The suction catheter is passed through the tube into the trachea. The tube is then 'railroaded' over the suction catheter into the trachea and the catheter removed.

**Table 7**   Techniques to facilitate nasotracheal intubation.

| Reference | Used under local anaesthetic (LA) or general anaesthetic (GA) | Technique | Number of patients | Success rate (%) |
|---|---|---|---|---|
| Brodman and Duncalf (1981) [126] | LA or GA | A *soft thin suction catheter* was passed through the nose into the pharynx. The tracheal tube was then passed over the suction catheter. This avoided trauma to nose and pharynx | More than 20 | 100% |
| Mackinnon and Harrison (1979) [127] | Not stated | A *16FG Jacques rubber catheter* was placed on the end of the nasal tube. The Jacques catheter was passed through the nose into the mouth and the tracheal tube was then gently passed through the nose. The catheter was then disconnected from the tube. This was designed to prevent nasal and pharyngeal trauma | Not stated | Not stated |
| Nolan (1969) [128] | GA | A nasotracheal tube can get stuck in the nasopharynx in a patient with a prominent arch of the atlas vertebra. Traction on a *suction catheter* passed through the tube and out of the mouth lifted the tip of the tube into oropharynx. The catheter was then removed and the tube passed into the trachea | 1 | 1(100) |
| Tahir (1970) [129] | LA or GA | Obstruction to the tube in the nasopharynx can occur at the base of the occipital bone, the first cervical vertebra or from lymphoid tissue in children. A *suction catheter* is used as in Nolan's technique | Not stated | Not stated |
| Yamamura et al. (1959) [130] | LA | A children's *laryngoscope bulb* on the end of a vinyl covered line was placed inside and just distal to the end of the nasotracheal tube. The room lights were dimmed. Intubation was then effected by observing the light transilluminating the neck in the midline and then advancing the tube | 30 | 29(96.7) |
| Schneider-man (1966) [131] | LA | A *clear plastic tube* was connected to the proximal end of the tracheal tube. Condensation of moisture on the tube occured during expiration and cleared during inspiration. The tube was advanced into the larynx using this sign | Not stated | Not stated |
| Findlay and Gissen (1961) [132] | LA | A nasotracheal tube was advanced to the pharyngeal inlet where loud breath sounds indicated the tip was near the glottis. A *No. 12 nasogastric* tube was then advanced through the tube into the trachea. The tracheal tube was then advanced over the nasogastric tube into the trachea | 11 | 11(100) |
| Dryden (1976) [133] | Not stated | On occasions the passage of the tube becomes obstructed near the introitus of the larynx despite neck flexion and changes in head position. A *suction catheter* was fed down the tube into the trachea and it was then possible to advance the tube into the trachea | Not stated | Not stated |
| Pedersen (1971) [117] | LA | A silk thread was firmly attached to the proximal end of a *suction catheter* which was then advanced through the nose and down to the laryngeal inlet. At this point, there were maximum breath sounds on auscultation. The patient was asked to breathe in deeply and the catheter advanced into the trachea. Local anaesthetic was then injected down the catheter into the trachea and the nasotracheal tube advanced over the taut silk thread and suction catheter | 20 | 100% |
| Adams et al. (1982) [134] | | Tongue extrusion. When the tongue is extruded it shifts the supralaryngeal structures and provides a more favourable path for intubation | Not stated | Not stated |
| Waters (1963) [135] | GA | See retrograde technique (p. 148)) | | |
| Singh (1966) [136] | GA | See technique using a hook (p. 141) | | |

cricoid pressure and manual in-line stabilization of the neck has been recommended for in-hospital management of trauma patients with suspected spinal injury [139]. The gum elastic bougie may play a critical role in the optimum management of such patients [57].

This matter is discussed in more detail in Chapter 18.

### Nasal intubation in the 1990s

Fibreoptic technology, retrograde techniques, the bougie, the laryngeal mask airway and a number of other techniques are all widely available to today's anaesthetist.

In the past, blind nasal intubation was the main solution and only available option to the problem of difficult intubation. Blind nasal intubation was widely used and most clinicians were highly skilled in this technique before the introduction of muscle relaxants into anaesthetic practice. It would seem that, for obvious reasons, blind nasal intubation is used much less frequently by the present generation of anaesthetists. It is likely therefore that expertise in blind nasal intubation will often be lacking in clinicians of our era. For example, the technique was attempted in seven of 85 patients with intubation problems [19]. All these attempts were unfortunately unsuccessful. It seems that today's anaesthetists do not practise the technique enough on elective cases to be able to intubate the difficult case.

#### Maximizing the success rate of blind nasal intubation

It would appear that spontaneous ventilation and hyperventilation will improve the success rate with blind nasal intubation. In some hospitals all blind nasal intubations are undertaken with the patient awake or with the patient anaesthetized but breathing spontaneously [140]. These authors reported from standard textbooks: 'maintenance of spontaneous ventilation of the lungs is essential to identify the glottic opening' for blind nasal intubation during anaesthesia and 'other requirements for successful blind intubation are hyperpnoea and intubation during expiration'.

### Nasopharyngeal Airways

Nasopharyngeal airways have been used in anaesthetic practice for many years. A binasal pharyn-geal airway (BNPA) was described by Elam and his colleagues in 1969 [141, 142]. It consisted of two soft nasopharyngeal tubes connected to a suitable adaptor (Fig. 39). The BNPA was used both for elective surgery and for resuscitation in patients ranging in age from 2 to 92 years. Gastric dilatation was unlikely to occur with the BNPA because excess pressure could be vented through the mouth. The apparatus, however, should not be used in a patient with a full stomach. It was specifically recommended for patients in whom intubation was impossible or difficult and in the absence of personnel skilled at intubation.

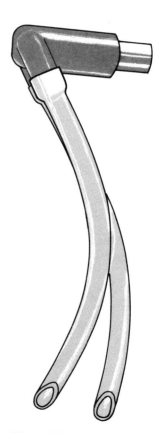

**Figure 39**   Binasal pharyngeal airway assembly. Two Rusch nasopharyngeal tubes are attached to a Puritan rubber adaptor. Redrawn from Elam *et al.* [141], with kind permission of the International Anaesthesia Research Society.

## SPECIALIZED TECHNIQUES

The most important specialized techniques are now described in separate chapters. These include awake intubation (Chapter 7), fibreoptic techniques (Chapter 10), the use of the laryngeal mask airway (Chapter 8) and emergency airway access (Chapter 13).

Specialized techniques may be required if simple measures fail. The choice is determined by the availability of apparatus and the skill and experience of the operator. Although laryngoscope blades with prisms and mirrors are rarely used now they are included in this chapter for the sake of historical completeness.

### Light Wand

In 1957, Macintosh described a lighted stylet as an aid to intubation [143]. The device was claimed to combine the best features of a rigid metal and a gum elastic introducer. The malleable introducer

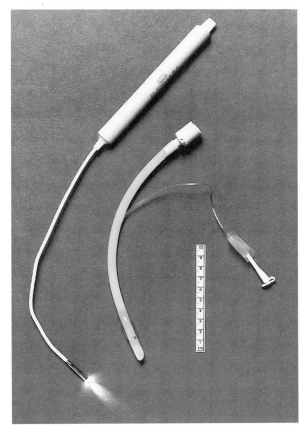

**Figure 40**   The lighted stylet or 'light wand'.

was eighteen inches (45 cm) in length and had a light on the end. Berman in 1959 described a lighted stylet that was claimed to be useful if the laryngoscope light failed [144].

The lighted stylet or light wand† has been used to facilitate intubation both under local and general anaesthesia. The light wand has a battery handle and a copper stylet covered in white plastic. There is a bulb on the distal end of the stylet (Fig. 40). There have been a number of reports of the bulb falling off the end of the 'light wand' [145–147]. In order to overcome this problem, a device has been designed with the bulb and wire enclosed in a clear plastic coating (Tube-Stat, Concept Corporation, Clearwater, FL 33516, USA).

In Ducrow's original description intubation was performed with a red rubber tube [148]. The patient was given oxygen, anaesthetized and then given suxamethonium. The suitably curved, lubricated light wand was inserted into a 10" (25 cm) length of size 22 suction catheter. The light wand was then passed in the midline towards the larynx. The neck was hyperextended and observed for the transilluminating light. When the light was manipulated into the trachea there was a bright patch of illumination in the midline below the cricoid cartilage. The light wand was then removed and a second 10" length of size 18 suction catheter attached to the first piece of suction catheter. The tracheal tube was then threaded over the suction catheter guide into the trachea. The procedure was carried out in a darkened room and used electively on easy cases to gain experience.

Rayburn [149] later modified the method by inserting the light wand directly into a transparent plastic tracheal tube and used the technique under local anaesthesia for difficult intubations. The light wand was inserted just short of the end of the tube and both were bent into a J-shape (Fig. 41). When the tube was in the oesophagus no light was visible; light appeared as it was withdrawn into the pharynx, and was seen as the tip of the tube neared the laryngeal inlet. The tube was then slipped off the end of the light wand into the trachea. Alternatively the light wand could be passed through the tube and manipulated into the trachea prior to threading the tracheal tube into position (Fig. 42). The method was

†Flexi-Lum Surgical Light, Concept Inc, USA. Obtainable in the UK from Henleys Medical Supplies Ltd, London.

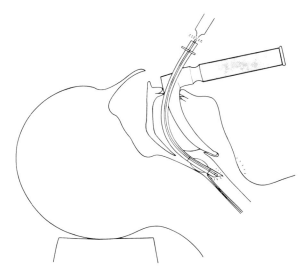

**Figure 41**   The 'light wand' inside a transparent tracheal tube with light transilluminating the tissues of the neck.

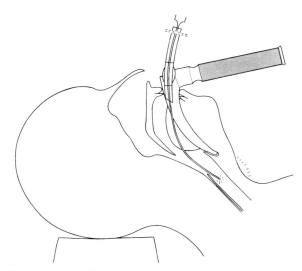

**Figure 42**   The 'light wand' advanced distal to the tracheal tube.

not recommended for children less than 2 years of age but it was successful for cases with a wide variety of causes of difficult intubation.

Despite Rayburn's difficulties in children, a thin fibreoptic bundle and light source have been used to aid intubation in children [150]. The specially designed fine 23.5 cm bundle will just pass through a 4 mm internal diameter tracheal tube and the light shining through the skin of the neck assists location of the larynx.

In 1986, a comparison was made of oral intuba-

tion success rates and times using a technique with a lighted stylet in one group and a Macintosh laryngoscope in the other. The study was performed on anaesthetized, paralysed patients [151]. All 100 patients studied were successfully intubated. In the lighted stylet group 72% were intubated on the first attempt but 28% needed a second or third attempt. Only one patient in the laryngoscope group (2%) was not intubated on the first attempt. There was no significant difference in the time required in the two groups. The time taken to intubate with the lighted stylet improved steadily during the study.

In a second study, a comparison was made of blind oral intubation using the 'light wand' and blind nasal intubation in 23 awake patients in whom difficulty in intubation was predicted [152]. In the 13 patients in the 'light wand' group intubation was accomplished significantly more quickly and with significantly fewer attempts. It was shown that the 'light wand' was suitable for patients with a known difficult airway and this technique was recommended in preference to blind nasal intubation.

A similar study was carried out on 24 adult patients under anaesthesia [153]. Difficulty was anticipated in four patients but not in the other 20. Twenty-two of these patients were successfully intubated using the lighted stylet. An important advantage of the 'light wand' method is that it is unaffected by blood and secretions. This technique was recommended for cases when laryngoscopy produces poor glottic exposure.

In another study intubation using the 'light wand' was attempted on 31 patients [154]. The mean age of the patients was 12.5 years; all patients were known to have abnormal upper airways. Awake intubation was performed in five cases; intubation under general anaesthesia with spontaneous ventilation in 11 cases; and intubation under general anaesthesia with muscle relaxation in 14 patients. Only one failure occurred but there was some difficulty in two patients. The 'light wand' may be used electively or when other techniques have failed. The lighted stylet is also useful for rapid sequence orotracheal intubation. Intubation with the lighted stylet was quicker than intubation with a laryngoscope [155].

It has been claimed that intubation times can be dramatically improved [156] when using the 'light wand' in conjunction with the 'Williams' airway intubator [157]. Williams intubates 90% of his patients using the lighted stylet – an 'indirect visual' intubation technique [157]. The patients are placed with the neck flexed and the head extended and the stylet in the tube is bent to slightly greater than 90°.

Mehta observed the strength of light transmitted through the neck from a lighted stylet in 420 adult patients [158]. The illumination when the tube was in the trachea was graded as excellent in 81% and good in 19% of patients. If the lighted stylet was placed in the oesophagus no transilluminated light was visible in any case. This is therefore recommended as a good test to confirm placement of the tube in the trachea. This test never gives a false result and is rapid, simple and reliable. It does not require elaborate equipment or previous experience.

## Mirrors and Prisms

In 1956, Siker described a curved laryngoscope blade with an attached stainless steel mirror [159]. The laryngoscope was introduced in the usual way and the tube with stylet then directed towards the tip of the laryngoscope until the tip of the tube was seen through the mirror as it approached the vocal cords. It is essential to become accustomed to the inverted appearance of the image (Fig. 43) while manipulating the tube. Expertise should be gained by practising on elective cases. Siker reported successful intubation in three cases in which there had been previous failure with a curved Macintosh or a straight, U shaped cross-sectional Guedel blade.

A modification enables one or two prisms to be applied to a laryngoscope blade [160–162]. Light can be refracted (Fig. 44) through as much as 80° and the view of the larynx is improved. Later versions of the prism were made of plastic and used with a fibreoptic light source. The image is then not inverted and thus the prism technique is easier to use.

## Hooks

A hook, as an aid to nasotracheal intubation, was first described in 1962 [163]. It is particularly helpful in children where the larynx is placed anteriorly. The larynx is visualized with a laryngoscope and the nasal tube passed into the oropharynx. The tube is then advanced over the hook. An assistant advances the tube which is then guided into the larynx with the hook (Fig. 35). The method was claimed to be less traumatic and easier than using Magill forceps. A hook was used in 1965 [164] in an adult patient with a severe fixed flexion neck deformity. An awake blind nasotracheal intubation was attempted. The hook was introduced into the mouth and placed round the distal end of the nasotracheal tube. The tracheal tube was pulled forwards and guided into the trachea using the breath sounds to locate the laryngeal inlet. In 1966, a similar method was used after blind nasal intubation had failed in three patients with ankylosis of the jaw and micrognathia [136]. Specially designed less traumatic hooks are commercially available.

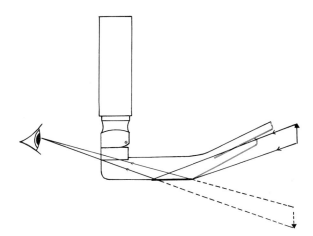

**Figure 43** A mirror attached to the laryngoscope blade gives an inverted image. With permission from Siker [159]

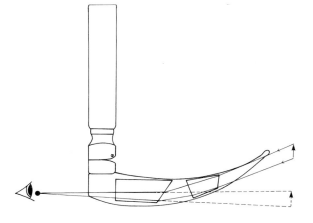

**Figure 44** Prisms attached to the laryngoscope blade give an upright image of the larynx. With permission from Huffman [160–162].

In 1963, Waters [135] used a retrograde method as an aid to intubation. An epidural catheter was passed into the oropharynx through a Tuohy needle inserted through the cricothyroid membrane. A hook was used to deliver the catheter from the mouth. The tracheal tube was then inserted using the catheter as a guide. It may be difficult or impossible to use a hook if jaw opening is restricted.

## Rigid Bronchoscope

Aro and his colleagues [8] used a rigid bronchoscope as an aid to intubation in 12 out of 3402 intubations (0.3%). In a further 68 difficult intubations (2%) an introducer in the tube produced a successful result. The bronchoscope was introduced into the trachea and then a thin atraumatic wire stylet introduced through the bronchoscope. The bronchoscope was then removed and the tube passed over the stylet into the trachea. In their hands the method was simple and safe. In a modification [165] the lubricated bronchoscope is passed inside the tracheal tube, and introduced into the trachea and then the tube slid down over the bronchoscope, which is then removed. These techniques can only be used in patients who are able to open their mouths.

A small adult rigid bronchoscope was used in a patient in whom it was only possible to see the tip of the epiglottis when using a conventional laryngoscope. The cords were easily seen after the bronchoscope had been introduced through the right hand corner of the mouth. A gum elastic bougie was then passed into the trachea. Intubation was carried out by threading the tube over the bougie in the usual manner [166].

A rigid bronchoscope may be required for the management of postintubation tracheal stenosis [167]. If the tracheal lumen was less than 5 mm in diameter Grillo dilated the airway under general anaesthesia with progressively larger paediatric bronchoscopes. This prevented the development of hypercarbia in these spontaneously breathing patients. Positive pressure ventilation was avoided both intra and post-operatively. If the diameter of the tracheal lumen was greater than 6 mm intubation was carried out above the lesion. Cardiopulmonary bypass was not required in any of the 208 patients. Neville in 1969, however, used cardiopulmonary bypass in 35 cases of tracheal disease [168]. He found that the technique was easy to use and did not result in complications.

## Retrograde Methods

Retrograde tracheal intubation was first described in a patient with a pre-existing tracheostomy [169]. The object was to avoid the tracheostomy tube obstructing surgical access during a cervical operation and to ensure an atraumatic and easy tracheal intubation. Following administration of topical analgesia a No. 16 French catheter was introduced through the tracheostomy, directed in a cephalad direction and delivered through the mouth. The catheter was then sutured to the tracheal tube and the catheter pulled from below delivered the tube into the trachea. The catheter was then cut from the tube and the tracheostomy closed for the duration of the operation.

Subsequently a number of retrograde methods have been described employing guides passed percutaneously through the cricothyroid membrane [135, 170–178]. Their main features are shown in Table 8.

Epidural catheters [135, 170–173], central venous catheters [174, 175], a Swan-Ganz wire [176], a Seldinger wire [177, 178] and silk or nylon thread have all been threaded in a retrograde direction through the cricothyroid membrane into the mouth. Techniques have included oral [170] and nasal routes [172] for tracheal intubation. If a patient is unable to open his or her mouth widely the chosen guide such as an epidural catheter should readily enable the patient to spit it out or to be delivered with a hook. A Seldinger wire may be unsuccessful if it cannot be delivered from the mouth and does not pass easily through the nose. Such wires, however, do sometimes pass without difficulty through the nose. A wire usually sits on the posterior pharyngeal wall and cannot be extruded easily by the patient, unlike a non-rigid coiled epidural catheter. No comparison of the use of epidural catheters and flexible wire introducers has been made. It is possible that one particular method may be more successful in an individual patient. Therefore both types of guide should be available.

The technique used by the authors is a modification of that described by Harmer and Vaughan [170] (Figs 45–51). The patient is lightly sedated and has 2 ml of 4% lignocaine injected percutaneously through the cricothyroid membrane. The pharynx is sprayed with 4% lignocaine. The cricoid cartilage is palpated and a small horizontal incision made in the skin above the cartilage after

**Table 8** Retrograde methods of tracheal intubation.

| Reference | LA or GA | Oral nasotracheal | Needle used | Retrograde equipment | Other apparatus | Special instructions | Clinical indication | Number of patients | Success rate |
|---|---|---|---|---|---|---|---|---|---|
| Waters (1963) [135] | Thiopentone and LA in children | Oral | Tuohy with bevel facing cephalad | 1 yard of sterile *vinyl plastic tube* | Hook to remove tube from mouth | Keep catheter taut. Do not use in cases of respiratory obstruction due to laryngeal pathology | Patients with trismus and cases of difficult intubation | Not given | Not given |
| Harmer and Vaughan (1980) [170] | LA | Oral | Tuohy needle | *Epidural catheter* | Large well greased suction catheter | Epidural catheter passed out of mouth. Suction catheter passed over epidural catheter until it reaches the cricothyroid membrane. Large bore armoured ET tube then passed over suction catheter and epidural catheter. Catheters then withdrawn. This avoids trauma of nasal intubation | Difficult intubation | Not stated | Not stated |
| Dhara (1980) [172] | LA | Nasal | Tuohy needle | *Epidural catheter* | 14 FG suction catheter (hook *not* required) | Epidural catheter passed out of mouth. Suction catheter passed through nose and out of mouth. Epidural catheter then threaded through shortened catheter. Suction catheter then removed. (In two patients epidural catheter came straight out of nostril.) Soft red rubber tracheal tube then threaded over epidural catheter | Not stated | 10 (in 6 years) | 10 |
| Bourke and Levesque (1974) [173] | Not stated | Oral and nasal | Large bore needle | *Catheter* | None | Catheter should be threaded through side hole of tracheal tube from outside and in through lumen of tube. This eliminates difficulties in threading tube into the trachea. Distance between cords and cricothyroid membrane is only 1 cm (Fig.52) | Difficult intubation | Not stated | Not stated |
| Powell and Odzil (1967) [174] | LA | Oral and nasal | 17 gauge needle | Bardie intracath. (*central venous catheter*) | Rubber urethral catheter threaded through nose for nasal intubation | Catheter threaded either through lumen of tube or through hole near tip of tube. Keep catheter taut during intubation. Withdraw catheter from above | Ankylosis of the jaw tongue tumours cervical arthritis | 15 | 15 |
| Roberts (1981) [176] | Not stated | Oral or nasal | 16 gauge catheter with stylet | 120 cm teflon coated *Swan–Ganz introducer wire* | Laryngoscope and Magill forceps may be required to deliver the wire from the mouth | Often easy to pass into the nasopharynx and out of the nose | Difficult intubation | Not stated | Not stated |

subcutaneous infiltration with local anaesthetic. A Tuohy needle is inserted into the trachea and its presence confirmed by aspirating air into a syringe filled with sterile water. The syringe is then removed and an epidural catheter inserted into the pharynx. The patient then spits the catheter out of the mouth. The Tuohy needle is removed and a large lubricated suction catheter, which has been kept in a refrigerator to stiffen it, is passed over the epidural catheter into the trachea. Its presence in the trachea should be confirmed with a capnograph. A small soft malleable tracheal tube is then passed over the suction catheter into the trachea and placement also confirmed with a capnograph. If the tube is held up at the laryngeal inlet a gum elastic catheter is passed into the trachea to facilitate its passage. The epidural catheter is then cut off near the skin entry site and the remaining catheter removed from above. The suction catheter should be inserted further into the trachea immediately after removal of the epidural catheter and before attempting to pass the tracheal tube to its final position. This technique can be used in awake patients or under general anaesthesia in patients in whom failed intubation occurs unexpectedly. This technique is reasonably quick and fairly easy even for the tyro.★ In some reports a guide wire or central venous catheter is used alone for retrograde intubations.

This technique was used by physicians trained in emergency medicine in a prehospital mobile emergency unit. The retrograde technique was used in 19 trauma patients under local anaesthesia; in 13 patients after failed intubation with conventional techniques and in six patients as the

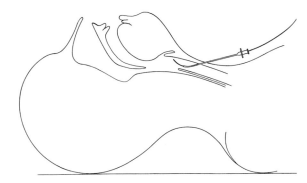

**Figure 46**   Syringe removed and epidural catheter threaded cephalad.

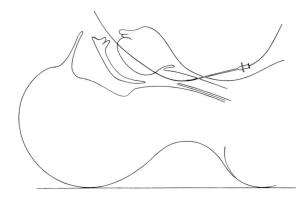

**Figure 47**   Catheter delivered from mouth. Patient may spit it out or passage from the mouth may be facilitated with a hook.

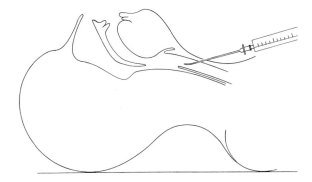

**Figure 45**   Tuohy needle advanced through the cricothyroid membrane into the trachea. On aspiration into the fluid-filled syringe air bubbles demonstrate that the end of the needle is in the trachea.

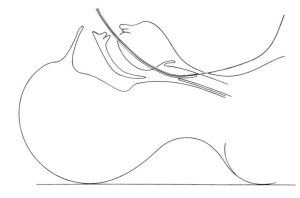

**Figure 48**   Refrigerated suction catheter threaded over epidural catheter and position checked with a capnograph.

★ A video showing this retrograde intubation technique has been prepared by the department of Medical Illustration in Cardiff.

(a)

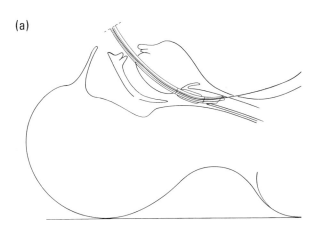

(b)

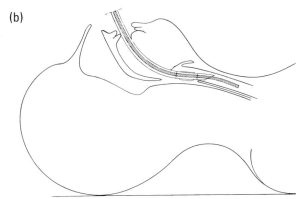

**Figure 49**    (a) Tracheal tube threaded over suction catheter into the trachea. To facilitate passage of the tracheal tube, tension is applied by pulling on both ends of the epidural catheter. The final position of the tube is checked with a capnograph.  (b) The epidural catheter is cut at the neck and pulled from above. The suction catheter is then pushed further into the trachea.

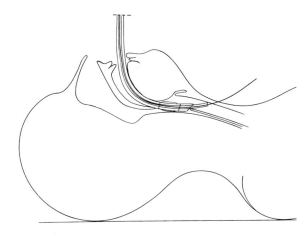

**Figure 50**    The tube may get stuck at the glottis.

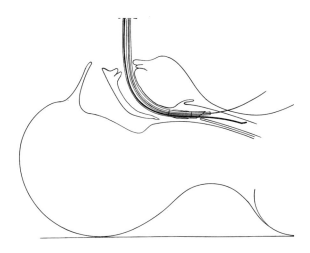

**Figure 51**    Passage of a gum elastic catheter will facilitate passage of the tube.

technique of choice [179]. All cases were intubated successfully in less than 5 min. Intubation was performed apparently without difficulty over either the central venous catheter or the guide wire. Injection of air through the catheter was found to help in location of the catheter tip in the pharynx.

A retrograde technique was used successfully in 25 patients presenting for cardiac operations. These patients had had failed intubations using conventional techniques. In 24 patients the technique was performed under general anaesthesia and in one patient under local anaesthesia [180]. A 60 cm radio-opaque Deseret central venous catheter was used. The tube was passed over the catheter which was held taut as the tube was advanced.

It has been suggested that the J wire is particularly indicated for retrograde intubation [181]. The wire should pass easily through the cords. A rotary movement of the wire enables the tip to be easily seen, grasped, delivered at the back of the pharynx, and pulled out through the mouth. These two reports are unusual. Most clinicians choose to thread the tube over an extra device that is threaded over the wire or catheter. The extra rigidity facilitates successful intubation.

In one report there was failure to intubate over an epidural catheter that had been passed retrogradely. The two ends were then cut off a hollow Eschmann bougie [54]. This bougie was threaded

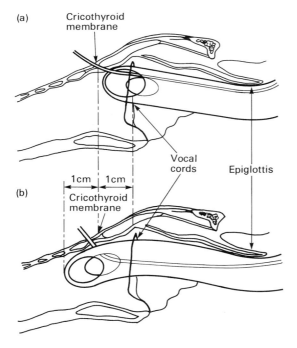

**Figure 52**   Cross-section of larynx and trachea with tracheal tube and catheter guide passing through the cricothyroid membrane. (a) Catheter passes through the end of the tube and 1 cm of the tube passes through the cords. (b) Catheter exits the side hole and 2 cm of the tube passes beyond the cords. After Bourke and Levesque [173], with kind permission of the International Anesthesia Research Society.

over the epidural catheter into the trachea and intubation was successfully accomplished over the bougie. In another report the plastic sheath protector of the guide wire was passed over the wire to facilitate passage of the tube into the trachea [182].

Success rates are high [171, 172, 174] with no reported failures. Bourke and Levesque [173] reported that the tube might not always pass through the cords or could flip out of the trachea as the epidural catheter was withdrawn. They avoided this by passing the epidural catheter through a side hole in the tracheal tube (Fig. 52).

The fibrescope can be used in two distinct ways to facilitate a retrograde intubation.

*Method 1.* Tobias found that even when using a retrograde technique the tube would sometimes not pass through the cords when the catheter guide was removed [183]. It was found that this problem could be helped by passing a fibrescope in conjunction with the retrograde guide (Fig 53). The tube is advanced over the retrograde guide into the trachea. A fibreoptic scope is then advanced through the tube into the trachea before removal of the retrograde guide. The scope acts as a guide for the tube and facilitates the passage of the tube into the trachea. This is similar in principle to the use of a bougie as seen in Fig. 51. The retrograde technique was particularly advocated when multiple attempts at intubation had caused bleeding and there was difficulty in obtaining a clear view with the fibrescope.

*Method 2.* Others have threaded the guide wire through the suction channel of the fibrescope and passed the scope with a tube over it into the

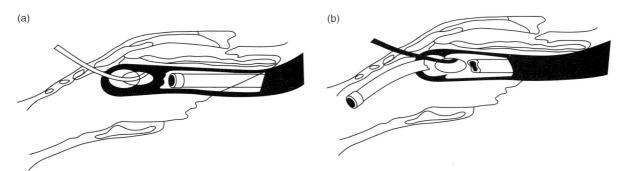

**Figure 53**   Sagittal sections of trachea with endotracheal tube, catheter guide, and tip of flexible laryngoscope. In (a) the endotracheal tube is in place with the catheter guide exiting through the side hole of the endotracheal tube. In (b) the flexible laryngoscope is advanced to act as a stylet before removal of the catheter guide. With permission from Tobais [183].

trachea under direct vision. The wire is used to facilitate localization of the larynx and passage of the scope into the trachea.

In one report there was failure to intubate using a variety of blades, blind nasal intubation and a rigid bronchoscope [184]. A retrograde technique was used to pass a wire into the pharynx. Unfortunately it was not possible to pass the tube into the trachea. The wire was then passed through the suction port of the bronchoscope and the scope and tube were passed into the trachea (retrograde fibreoptic intubation). In another report, a similar technique was used in a patient when intubation failed using conventional techniques [185]. This technique was advocated in patients where difficult intubation is caused by bleeding, cervical deformity or trauma, and in airway obstruction.

Three other cases have been reported where this method was used successfully under local anaesthesia [186]. In these cases the wire was slackened at the cricothyroid membrane when the scope entered the trachea. The scope was then advanced down the trachea towards the carina. The wire was then removed and the tube passed into the trachea over the bronchoscope. This technique could be appropriate for clinicians with limited experience with fibreoptic equipment.

This technique avoids nasal trauma and is appropriate when nasal intubation is contraindicated. It is clear that success is more likely if some kind of additional guide is threaded over the wire or catheter. It is probable that improved results will be obtained if the laryngoscope is left in the mouth when the tube is passed over the retrograde guide. The tube should also be routinely rotated a quarter turn anticlockwise before it passes through the cords [49].

Akinyemi [171] detailed complications occurring with a retrograde method in 12 patients aged from 9 to 25 years with ankylosis of the jaw secondary to cancrum oris. He first attempted blind nasal intubation under general anaesthesia and if four attempts failed used a retrograde technique [135] for nasotracheal intubation. Minor bleeding at the puncture site or from the nose occurred five times, there was difficulty in hooking the catheter through the nose three times and airway problems occurred twice. He concluded that these problems were minor and the technique should be used more frequently.

The technique can be used both in adults and in children [135, 177]. Retrograde techniques are easy to learn and use and do not require complex expensive apparatus. Many hospitals in developed countries cannot afford fibreoptic equipment and hospitals in third world countries are even less likely to have this equipment available. In contrast, the equipment for a retrograde technique should be readily available. It is not ethical to practise on elective cases and in consequence few clinicians have either seen or tried retrograde techniques. This situation can be remedied by video or tape slide presentations and by practice on training models or cadavers. All trainees should receive formal teaching but only 16.5% of the clinicians in a retrospective survey [32] had tried retrograde intubation techniques.

## ACTION TO BE TAKEN FOLLOWING DIFFICULTY IN INTUBATION OR VENTILATION

There are a wide range of options available to the clinician following a difficult intubation. It is important to pass on a detailed description of any difficulties that have been encountered. Failure to do so could have important medico-legal implications. Clearly, if the difficulty in intubation or ventilation has been minimal, the response is likely to be restrained.

### The Anaesthetic Record

A decision has to be made as to whether the procedure is considered to be difficult – a yes or no answer. The Cardiff anaesthetic chart has a box that can be marked for a difficult intubation; thus the incidence of difficult intubation is recorded. The chart also has a box for the use of a bougie or stylet and a box for a fibreoptic intubation. It would also be helpful to record the view obtained of the larynx according to the Cormack and Lehane classification [10].

### The Case Notes

A full record of the difficulties should also be recorded in the notes if the difficulties were more than trivial.

- The *intubation* can be marked as difficult in the patient's *main notes*.

- It should also be helpful to mark the front of the *case notes* in a prominent way in order to alert the anaesthetist before subsequent anaesthetics.
- The *cause of difficulty* should be recorded if apparent. The Cormack and Lehane classification of the view of the larynx should be recorded.
- A note should be made of the *use of ancillary equipment* (gum elastic bougie, stylet, fibreoptic scope, retrograde equipment or transtracheal ventilation).
- Any difficulties with *ventilation* should be noted together with a record of the lowest value of oxygen saturation that resulted.
- The *cause of the difficulty* with ventilation should be recorded if this is apparent.

### Communication with the Patient

- It is important in appropriate cases to *discuss the problem* sympathetically with the patient. This should be done in such a way that the patient is not unduly alarmed. The patient should be informed if any significant difficulty in intubation or ventilation occurred.
- The patient should be given *a letter* with *full details* of the problems to pass on to the anaesthetist involved in any future operative procedure.
- It is possible that *recommendations will be made that an awake intubation is* is indicated in the future.
- It might be considered appropriate for the patient to carry *a Medicalert* to ensure that doctors are aware of the problem in the future.

### Letter to General Practitioner

In some cases, the anaesthetist might also decide to write to the general practioner with details of the problem. He should certainly inform the practitioner if the patient is advised to have an awake intubation in the future.

### What Happens in Practice?

There is considerable room for improvement in our communication systems. Many clinicians are now able to intubate problem patients with minimal difficulty owing to increased levels of expertise with the bougie, fibreoptic scopes and other devices. When this happens there seems to

be less need to make a fuss and to go through the full set of possible responses.

It seems likely that the details of many difficult intubations are not fully documented. Old notes and anaesthetic charts are not always available in the evening before a planned operation. Problems are then more likely to occur with a subsequent anaesthetic carried out by a relatively inexperienced clinician. This tends to happen on busy lists where less time may be taken in assessing patient and carefully reading all the notes. Pride and pressure of work may inhibit some anaesthetists from documenting the difficult cases.

## CONCLUSION

It is important for every clinician to have a clear plan of action when dealing with a difficult or failed intubation. There is no easy totally risk free solution for every case. The risks to the patient should be reduced to a minimum.

Formal training programmes are essential if trainees are to become competent in both the simple and the more complex techniques. Prospective comparison of different techniques to facilitate difficult intubation would be valuable in reaching rational decisions about choice of technique, although the design of studies is difficult due to the low incidence of difficult intubation. At present clinicians may have a real problem in choosing an appropriate technique from the many described in the literature. Clinicians who have a limited range of expertise may find that, if a simple technique fails, they are unable to intubate the patient. Changes in clinical practice are required to increase patient safety.

# KEY POINTS

- Awake intubation is the cornerstone of safe management of the patient with anticipated difficult intubation or airway control.

- It will never be possible to predict all cases of difficult intubation.

- It is important to have a rational policy for the management of unexpected difficult intubation that occurs under anaesthesia.

- The gum elastic bougie should play a central role in the management of both unexpected and expected difficult intubation under anaesthesia.

- The anaesthetist may have a bewildering choice of both equipment and management options at his disposal.

- Algorithms give the clinician the chance for contemplation of the various options.

- Acquiring expertise in particular techniques, however, will always be the foundation of optimum clinical management.

- The laryngeal mask is likely to play an increasingly important role in the management of difficult intubation in the UK.

- Optimum training programmes will include instruction in:
  Simulated difficult intubation with the bougie
  Optimum use of the gum elastic bougie
  Application of local anaesthesia for an awake intubation
  Fibreoptic intubation
  Intubation through the laryngeal mask
  The use of the McCoy laryngoscope and the Belscope
  Transtracheal ventilation and emergency airway access
  Failed intubation drill
  Failed ventilation drill
  Use of the Combitube.

- There may be medicolegal implications if training programmes fail to include instruction in appropriate airway management techniques.

## REFERENCES

1 Benumof J. L. Management of the difficult adult airway. With special emphasis on awake tracheal intubation. *Anesthesiology* 1991; **75**: 1087.

2 Caplan R. A. *et al.* Practice Guidelines for Management of the Difficult Airway. A report by the American Society of Anesthesiologists Task Force on management of the difficult airway. *Anesthesiology* 1993; **78**: 597.

3 Knill R. L. Defining the difficult airway. *Anesthesiology* 1993; **79**: 413.

4 Caplan R. A. Defining the difficult airway. In reply. *Anesthesiology* 1993; **79**: 414.

5 Gataure P., Vaughan R. S. and Latto I. P. Simulated difficult intubation. Comparison of the gum elastic bougie and the stylet. *Abstract Book of the 11th World Congress of Anaesthesiologists*, Sydney: Australia. 1996; 945.

6 Sia R. L. and Edens E. T. How to avoid problems when using the fibreoptic bronchoscope for difficult intubations. *Anaesthesia* 1981; **36**: 74.

7 Eastley R., Latto I. P., Ng W. S., Vaughan R. S., James W. and Draper M. Prospective survey of incidence causes and management of difficult intubation in 1200 patients (unpublished data) 1984.

8 Aro L., Takki S. and Aromaa U. Technique for difficult intubation. *British Journal of Anaesthesia* 1974; **43**: 1081.

9 Deller A., Schreiber M. N., Gromer J. and Ahnefeld F. W. Difficult intubation: Incidence and predictability: a prospective study of 8284 adult patients (abstract). *Anesthesiology* 1990; **73A**: 1054.

10 Cormack R. S. and Lehane J. Difficult tracheal intubation in obstetrics. *Anaesthesia* 1984; **39**: 1105.

11 Wilson M. E. Predicting difficult intubation. *British Journal of Anaesthesia* 1993; **71**: 333.

12 Oates J. D. L., Macleod A. D., Oates P. D., Pearsall F. J., Howie J. C. and Murray G. D. Comparison of two methods for predicting difficult intubation. *British Journal of Anaesthesia* 1991; **66**: 305.

13 Wilson M. E., Spiegelhalter D., Robertson J. A. and Lesser P. Predicting difficult intubation. *British Journal of Anaesthesia* 1988; **61**: 211.

14 Nolan J. P. and Wilson M. E. An evaluation of the gum elastic bougie. Intubation times and incidence of sore throat. *Anaesthesia* 1992; **47**: 878.

15 Williams K. N., Carli F. and Cormack R. S. Unexpected difficult laryngoscopy: a prospective survey in routine general surgery. *British Journal of Anaesthesia* 1991; **66**: 38.

16 Bellhouse C. P. and Dore C. Criteria for estimating likelihood of difficulty of endotracheal intubation

with the Macintosh Laryngoscope. *Anaesthesia and Intensive Care* 1988; **16:** 329.

17 Mallampati S. R., Gugino L. D., Desai S. P. and Freiberger D. A clinical sign to predict difficult tracheal intubation: a prospective study. *Canadian Journal of Anaesthesiology* 1985; **32:** 429.

18 Lunn J. N. and Mushin W. W. *Mortality Associated with Anaesthesia.* London: Nuffield Provincial Hospitals Trust, Association of Anaesthetists of GB and I. 1982; 50, 70, 84.

19 Williamson J. A., Webb R. K., Szekely S., Gillies E. R. N. and Dreosti A. V. Difficult intubation: an analysis of 2000 incident reports. *Anaesthesia and Intensive Care* 1993; **21:** 602.

20 Lyons G. Failed intubation. *Anaesthesia* 1985; **40:** 759.

21 Samsoon G. L. T. and Young J. R. B. Difficult tracheal intubation: a retrospective study. *Anaesthesia* 1987; **42:** 487.

22 Lyons G. and MacDonald R. Difficult intubation in obstetrics. *Anaesthesia* 1985; **40:** 1016.

23 Cormack R. R., Carli F. and Williams K. N. Unexpected difficult laryngoscopy. *British Journal of Anaesthesia* 1991; **67:** 501.

24 King T. A. and Adams A. P. Failed tracheal intubation. *British Journal of Anaesthesia* 1990; **65:** 400.

25 Tunstall M. E. and Sheikh A. Failed intubation protocol: oxygenation without aspiration. *Clinical Anaesthesia* 1986; **4:** 171.

26 Watts R. M. and Bassham M. Training, skills, and approach to potentially difficult anaesthesia in general practitioner anaesthetists. *Anaesthesia and Intensive Care* 1994; **22:** 706.

27 Green R. A. Medico-legal aspects of anaesthesia. In: Kaufman L. (ed.) *Anaesthesia Review*, vol. 4. Churchill Livingstone, London. 1987; 147.

28 Utting J. E. Pitfalls in anaesthetic practice. *British Journal of Anaesthesia* 1987; **59:** 877.

29 Tunstall M. E. Failed intubation in the parturient. *Canadian Journal of Anaesthesiology* 1989; **36:** 611.

30 Davies J. M., Weeks S. and Crone L. A. Difficult intubation in the parturient. *Canadian Journal of Anaesthesiology* 1989; **36:** 668.

31 Allen C. T. B. Apparatus for emergency intubation in laryngeal obstruction. *Anaesthesia* 1976; **31:** 263.

32 James W. and Latto I. P. *Retrospective Intubation Survey.* Unpublished data presented to Welsh Society of Anaesthetists. 1982.

33 King H. K. 'Difficult airway' or 'problematic airway'. *Anaesthesia and Intensive Care* 1994; **22:** 627.

34 Frass M., Frenzer R., Mayer G., Popovic R. and Leithner C. Mechanical ventilation with the Esophageal Tracheal Combitube (ETC) in the intensive care unit. *Archives of Emergency Medicine* 1987; **4:** 219.

35 Mason R. A. Learning fibreoptic intubation: fun-

damental problems. *Anaesthesia* 1992; **47:** 729.

36 Layman P. R. An alternative to blind nasal intubation. *Anaesthesia* 1983; **38:** 165.

37 Kemthorne P. M. and Brown T. C. K. Anaesthesia and the mucopolysaccharidoses. A survey of techniques and problems. *Anaesthesia and Intensive Care* 1983; **11:** 203.

38 Jackson C. The technique of insertion of intratracheal insufflation tubes. *Surgery, Gynecology and Obstetrics* 1913; **17:** 507.

39 Sellick B. A. Cricoid pressure to control regurgitation of stomach contents during induction of anaesthesia. *Lancet* 1961; **ii,** 404.

40 Sellick B. A. Rupture of the oesophagus following cricoid pressure? *Anaesthesia* 1982; **37:** 213.

41 Rosen M. Deaths in obstetric anaesthesia (editorial). *Anaesthesia* 1981; **36:** 145.

42 Crawford J. S. The 'contra cricoid' cuboid aid to tracheal intubation. *Anaesthesia* 1982; **37:** 345.

43 Knill R. L. Anaesthetic techniques. Difficult laryngoscopy made easy with a 'BURP'. *Canadian Journal of Anaesthesiology* 1993; **40:** 279.

44 Macintosh R. R. An aid to oral intubation. *British Medical Journal* 1949; **1:** 28.

45 Dogra S., Falconer R. and Latto I. P. Increased use of gum-elastic bougie in clinical practice. *Anaesthesia* 1990; **45:** 997.

46 Sellers W. F. S. and Jones G. W. Difficult tracheal intubation. *Anaesthesia* 1986; **41:** 93.

47 Kidd J. F., Dyson A. and Latto I. P. Successful difficult intubation. Use of the gum-elastic bougie. *Anaesthesia* 1988; **43:** 437.

48 Cossham P. S. Difficult intubation. *British Journal of Anaesthesia* 1985; **57:** 239.

49 Dogra S., Falconer R. and Latto I. P. Successful difficult intubation. Tracheal tube placement over a gum-elastic bougie. *Anaesthesia* 1990; **45:** 774.

50 Jones H. E., Pearce A. C. and Moore P. Fibreoptic intubation. Influence of tracheal tube tip design. *Anaesthesia* 1993; **48:** 672.

51 Dogra S., Falconer R. and Latto I. P. Successful Difficult Intubation (a reply). *Anaesthesia* 1991; **46:** 72.

52 Amdt G. A. and Ghani G. A. A modification of an Eschmann endotracheal tube changer for insufflation. *Anesthesiology* 1988; **69:** 282.

53 Artu A. A., Schultz A. A. and Bonneu J. J. Modification of an Eschmann introducer to permit measurement of end tidal carbon dioxide. *Anesthesia and Analgesia* 1989; **69:** 129.

54 Freund P. R., Rooke A. and Schwid H. Retrograde Intubation with a modified Eschmann Stylet. *Anesthesia and Analgesia* 1988; **67:** 596.

55 Boys J. E. Failed intubation in obstetric anaesthesia. *British Journal of Anaesthesia* 1983; **55:** 187.

56 Pilkington S., Carli F., Dakin M. J., Romney M., De Witt K. A., Dore C. J. and Cormack R. S.

Increase in Mallampati score during pregnancy. *British Journal of Anaesthesia* 1996; **74:** 638.

57 Nolan J. P. and Wilson M. E. Orotracheal intubation in patients with potential cervical spine injuries. An indication for the gum elastic bougie. *Anaesthesia* 1993; **48:** 630.

58 McCarroll S. M., Lamont B. J., Buckland M. R. and Yates A. B. The gum-elastic bougie: old but still useful. *Anesthesiology* 1988; **68:** 643.

59 Larson C. P. Difficult Intubation Cart. *Journal of Clinical Anaesthesia* 1990; **2:** 432.

60 Viswanathan S., Campbell C., Wood D. G., Riopelle J. M. and Naraghi M. The Eschmann Tracheal Tube Introducer (Gum Elastic Bougie). *Anesthesiology Review* 1992; **XIX:** 29.

61 Cormack R. S. and Lehane J. Simulating difficult intubation. *British Journal of Anaesthetics* 1983; **55:** 1155p.

62 Tunstall M. E. Failed intubation drill. *Anaesthesia* 1976; **31:** 850.

63 Chadd G. D., Ackers J. W. L. and Bailey P. M. Difficult intubation aided by the laryngeal mask airway. *Anaesthesia* 1989; **44:** 1015.

64 Alison A. and McCrory J. Tracheal tube placement of a gum elastic bougie using the laryngeal mask airway. *Anaesthesia* 1990; **45:** 419.

65 Heath M. L. and Allagain J. Intubation through the laryngeal mask. *Anaesthesia* 1991; **46:** 545.

66 McCrirrick A. and Pracilio J. A. Awake intubation: a new technique. *Anaesthesia* 1991; **46:** 661.

67 Brimacombe J. and Berry A. Placement of a Cook airway exchange catheter via the laryngeal mask airway. *Anaesthesia* 1993; **48:** 351.

68 Rowbotham S. Intratracheal anaesthesia by the nasal route for operations on the mouth and lips. *British Medical Journal* 1920; **2:** 590.

69 Caine C. W. Endotracheal intubation. *Anesthesiology* 1948; **9:** 553.

70 Ballantine R. I. W. and Jackson I. Anaesthesia for neurosurgical operations. *Anaesthesia* 1954; **9:** 4.

71 Cass N. M., James N. R. and Lines V. Difficult direct laryngoscopy complicating intubation for anaesthesia. *British Medical Journal* 1956; **ii,** 488.

72 Bowen R. A. An introducer for difficult intubation. *Anaesthesia* 1967; **22:** 150.

73 Edge W. G. and Whitman J. G. Chondro-calcinosis and difficult intubation in acromegaly. *Anaesthesia* 1981; **36:** 677.

74 Smith M., Buist R. J. and Mansour N. Y. A simple method to facilitate difficult intubation. *Canadian Anaesthetists Society Journal* 1990; **37:** 144.

75 Henderson J. B., Bontrager E. and Morse H. T. An articulated stylet for endotracheal intubation. *Anesthesiology* 1970; **32:** 71.

76 Salem M. R., Mathrubhutham M. and Bennett J. Difficult intubation. *New England Journal of Medicine* 1976; **295:** 879.

77 Millen J. E. and Glauser F. L. A rapid simple technic for changing endotracheal tubes. *Anesthesia and Analgesia* 1978; **57:** 735.

78 Finucane B. T. and Kupshick H. L. A flexible stilette for replacing damaged tracheal tubes. *Canadian Anesthetists Society Journal* 1978; **25:** 153.

79 Williams J. H. A method of changing tracheostomy tubes in small children. *Anaesthesia* 1973; **28:** 343.

80 McIntyre J. W. R. Laryngoscope design and the difficult adult tracheal intitubation *Canadian Anaesthetists Society Journal* 1989; **36:** 94.

81 Marks R. R. D., Hancock R. and Charters P. An analysis of laryngoscope blade shape and design: new criteria for laryngoscope evaluation. *Canadian Anaesthetists Society Journal* 1993; **262:** 40.

82 McIntyre J. W. R. Editorial. Tracheal intubation and laryngoscope design. *Canadian Anaesthetists Society Journal* 1993; **40:** 193.

83 Tousignant G. and Tessler M. J. Light intensity and area of illumination provided by various laryngoscope blades. *Canadian Anaesthetists Society Journal* 1994; **41:** 865.

84 Phillips O. C. and Duerksen R. L. Endotracheal intubation: A new blade for direct laryngoscopy. *Anesthesia and Analgesia* 1973; **52:** 691.

85 Macintosh R. R. A new laryngoscope. *Lancet* 1943; **i:** 205.

86 Bucx M. J. L., Snijders C. J., Van Geel R. T. M *et al.* Forces acting on the maxillary incisor teeth during laryngoscopy using the Macintosh laryngoscope. *Anaesthesia* 1994; **49:** 1064.

87 McCoy E. P. and Mirakhur R. K. The levering laryngoscope. *Anaesthesia* 1993; **48:** 516.

88 Magill I. W. An improved laryngoscope for anaesthetists. *Lancet* 1926; **i:** 500.

89 Miller R. A. A new laryngoscope. *Anesthesiology* 1941; **2:** 317.

90 Lewis J. J. Autoclavable Macintosh laryngoscope with high intensity fibreoptic illumination for routine anaesthesia use. *Anesthesiology* 1975; **43:** 573.

91 Greenblatt G. M. Fiberoptic illuminating laryngoscope with remote light source – further development. *Anesthesia and Analgesia* 1981; **60:** 841.

92 Lagade M. R. Use of the Left-Entry laryngoscope blade in patients with right-sided oro-facial lesions. *Anesthesiology* 1983; **58:** 300.

93 Datta S. and Briwa J. Modified laryngoscope for endotracheal intubation of obese patients. *Anesthesia and Analgesia* 1981; **60:** 120.

94 Galloon S. The Toronto ventilating laryngoscope. *British Journal of Anaesthesia* 1973; **45:** 912.

95 Lee S. T. A ventilating laryngoscope for inhalation anaesthesia and augmented ventilation during laryngoscopic procedures. *British Journal of Anaesthesia* 1972; **44:** 874.

96 Bellhouse C. P. An angulated laryngoscope for routine and difficult tracheal intubation. *Anesthesiology*

1988; **69:** 126.

97  Mayall R. M. The Belscope for management of the difficult airway. *Anesthesiology* 1992; **76:** 1059.

98  Saunders P. R. and Giesecke A. H. Clinical assessment of the adult Bullard laryngoscope blade. *Canadian Journal of Anaesthesia* 1989; **36:** S118.

99  Borland L. M. and Casselbrant M. The Bullard laryngoscope. A new indirect oral laryngoscope (paediatric version). *Anesthesia and Analgesia* 1990; **70:** 105.

100  Mendel P. and Bristow A. Anaesthesia for procedures on the larynx and pharynx. The use of the Bullard laryngoscope in conjunction with high frequency jet ventilation. *Anaesthesia* 1993; **48:** 263.

101  Wu T.-L. and Chou H.-C. A new laryngoscope: The combination intubating device. *Anesthesiology* 1994; **81:** 1085.

102  Choi J. J.-I. A new double-angle blade for direct laryngoscopy. *Anesthesiology* 1990; **72:** 576.

103  Bainton C. R. A new laryngoscope blade to overcome pharyngeal obstruction. *Anesthesiology* 1987; **67:** 767.

104  Gajraj N. M., Chason D. P. and Shearer V. E. Cervical spine movement during orotracheal intubation: comparison of the Belscope and Macintosh blades. *Anaesthesia* 1994; **49:** 772.

105  Hodges U. M., O'Flaherty D. and Adams A. P. Tracheal intubation in a mannikin: comparison of the Belscope with the Macintosh laryngoscope. *British Journal of Anaesthesia* 1993; **71:** 772.

106  Dyson A., Harris J. and Bhatia K. Rapidity and accuracy of tracheal intubation in a mannequin: comparison of the Fibreoptic with the Bullard laryngoscope. *British Journal of Anaesthesia* 1990; **65:** 268.

107  Sultana A., Simmons M. and Gatt S. The 'Belscope' – A new angulated laryngoscope: randomised, prospective, controlled comparison with the Macintosh laryngoscope. *Anaesthesia and Intensive Care* 1993; **22:** 98.

108  Watanabe S., Suga A., Asakura N. *et al.* Determination of the distance between the laryngoscope blade and the upper incisors during direct laryngoscopy: comparisons of a curved, an angulated straight and two straight blades. *Anesthesia and Analgesia* 1994; **79:** 638.

109  Carr R. J. and Belani K. G. Augustine Guide™ clinical assessment. *Anesthesia and Analgesia* 1994; **78:** 983.

110  Wee M. Y. K. The oesophageal detector device. Assessment of a new method to distinguish oesophageal from tracheal intubation. *Anaesthesia* 1988; **43:** 27.

111  Krafft P., Fitzgerald R., Pernerstofer T., Kapral S. and Weinstabl C. A new device for blind oral intubation in routine and difficult airway management.

*European Journal of Anaesthesiology* 1994; **11:** 207.

112  Carr R. J. and Belani K. G. Clinical assessment of the Augustine Guide for endotracheal intubation. *Anesthesia and Analgesia* 1993; **76:** S37.

113  Kovac A. L. Use of the Augustine stylet anticipating difficult tracheal intubation in Treacher–Collins syndrome. *Journal of Clinical Anaesthesia* 1992; **4:** 409.

114  Rowbotham E. S. and Magill I. W. Anaesthetics in the plastic surgery of the face and jaws. *Proceedings of the Royal Society of Medicine* 1921; **14:** 17.

115  Elder C. K. Naso-endotracheal intubation: advantages and technique of 'blind intubation'. *Anesthesiology* 1944; **5:** 392.

116  Gold M. I. and Buechel D. R. A method of blind nasal intubation for the conscious patient. *Anesthesia and Analgesia* 1960; **39:** 257.

117  Pederson B. (1971) Blind nasotracheal intubation: a review and a new guided technique. *Acta Anaesthesiologica Scandinavica* 1971; **15:** 107.

118  Sykes W. S. Oral endotracheal intubation without laryngoscopy: a plea for simplicity. *Anesthesia and Analgesia* 1937; **16:** 133.

119  Magill I. W. Endotracheal anaesthesia. *American Journal of Surgery* 1936; **34:** 450.

120  Lewis I. Anaesthesia in general practice. Endotracheal anaesthesia. *British Medical Journal* 1937; **2:** 630.

121  Chandra P. Blind intubation. *British Journal of Anaesthesia* 1966; **38:** 207.

122  Davies J. A. H. Blind nasal intubation with propanidid. *British Journal of Anaesthesia* 1972; **44:** 528.

123  Wycoff C. C. Aspiration during induction of anesthesia: its prevention. *Anesthesia and Analgesia* 1959; **38:** 5.

124  Thomas J. L. Awake intubation. *Anaesthesia* 1969; **24:** 28.

125  Salem J. E. Intubation of conscious patients with combat wounds of upper respiratory passageway in Vietnam. *Oral Surgery* 1967; **24:** 701.

126  Brodman E. and Duncalf D. Avoiding the trauma of nasotracheal intubation. *Anesthesia and Analgesia* 1981; **60:** 618.

127  Mackinnon A. G. and Harrison M. J. Nasotracheal intubation: an atraumatic technique. *Anaesthesia* 1979; **34:** 910.

128  Nolan R. T. Nasal intubation: an anatomical difficulty with Portex tubes. *Anaesthesia* 1969; **24:** 447.

129  Tahir A. H. A simple manoeuvre to aid the passage of a nasotracheal tube into the oropharynx. *British Journal of Anaesthesia* 1970; **42:** 631.

130  Yamamura H., Yamamoto T. and Kamiyama M. Device for blind nasal intubation. *Anesthesiology* 1959; **20:** 221.

131  Schneiderman B. I. An aid for blind naso-endotracheal intubation. *Anesthesiology* 1966; **27:** 93.

132 Findlay C. W. and Gissen A. J. A guided nasotracheal method for insertion of an endotracheal tube. *Anesthesia and Analgesia* 1961; **40:** 640.

133 Dryden G. E. Use of a suction catheter to assist blind nasal intubation. *Anesthesiology* 1976; **45:** 260.

134 Adams A. L., Cane R. D. and Shapiro B. A. Tongue extension as an aid to blind nasal intubation. *Critical Care Medicine* 1982; **10:** 335.

135 Waters D. J. Guided blind endotracheal intubation. *Anaesthesia* 1963; **18:** 158.

136 Singh A. Blind nasal intubation. A report of the use of a hook in three cases of ankylosis of the jaw. *Anaesthesia* 1966; **21:** 400.

137 Layman P. R. Transtracheal ventilation in oral surgery. *Annals of the Royal College of Surgeons of England* 1983; **65:** 318.

138 The American College of Surgeons Committee on Trauma *Advanced Trauma Life Support program for Physicians: Instructor Manual*. Chicago: American College of Surgeons. 1993.

139 Criswell J. C., Parr M. J. A. and Nolan J. P. Emergency airway management in patients with cervical spine injuries. *Anaesthesia* 1994; **49:** 900.

140 Fox D. J. and Rastrelli A. J. Lighted stylet and endotracheal intubation. A reply. *Anesthesiology* 1987; **66:** 852.

141 Elam J. O., Titel J. H., Feingold A., Weisman H. and Bauer R. Simplified airway management during anaesthesia or resuscitation: a binasal pharyngeal system. *Anesthesia and Analgesia* 1969; **48:** 307.

142 Weisman H., Weis T. W., Elam J. O., Bethune R. M. and Bauer R. Use of double nasopharyngeal airways in anaesthesia. *Anesthesia and Analgesia* 1969; **48:** 356.

143 Macintosh R. R. and Richards H. Illuminated introducer for endotracheal tubes. *Anaesthesia* 1957; **12:** 223.

144 Berman R. A. Lighted stylet. *Anesthesiology* 1959; **20:** 382.

145 Stone D. J., Stirt J. A., Kaplan M. J. and McLean W. A. A complication of lightwand-guided nasotracheal intubation. *Anesthesiology* 1984; **61:** 780.

146 Stewart R. D. and Ellis D. G. Lighted stylet and endotracheal intubation. *Anesthesiology* 1987; **66:** 851.

147 Williams R. T. and Stewart R. D. Transillumination of the trachea with a lighted stylet. *Anesthesia and Analgesia* 1986; **65:** 539.

148 Ducrow M. Throwing light on blind intubation. *Anaesthesia* 1973; **33:** 827.

149 Rayburn R. L. Light wand intubation. *Anaesthesia* 1979; **34:** 667.

150 Foster C. A. An aid to blind nasal intubation in children. *Anaesthesia* 1977; **32:** 1038.

151 Ellis D. G., Jakymec A., Kalplan R. M. *et al.* Guided orotracheal intubation in the operating room using a lighted stylet: A comparison with direct laryngoscopic technique. *Anesthesiology* 1986; **64:** 823.

152 Fox D. J., Castro T. and Rastrelli A. J. Comparison of intubation techniques in the awake patient: the Flexi-Lum Surgical Light (lightwand) *versus* blind nasal approach. *Anesthesiology* 1987; **66:** 69.

153 Robelen G. T. and Shulman M. S. Use of the lighted stylet for difficult intubation in adult patients. *Anesthesiology* 1989; **71:** A439.

154 Holzman R. S., Nargozian C. D. and Florence F. B. Lightwand intubation in children with abnormal upper airways. *Anesthesiology* 1988; **69:** 784.

155 Culling R. D., Mongan P. and Castro T. Lightwand guided rapid sequence orotracheal intubation. *Anesthesiology* 1989; **71:** A994.

156 Williams R. T. Lighted stylet and endotracheal intubation. 2 *Anesthesiology* 1987; **66:** 851.

157 Williams R. T. and Harrison R. E. Prone tracheal intubation simplified using an airway intubator. *Canadian Journal of Anaesthesiology* 1981; **28:** 288.

158 Mehta S. Transtracheal illumination for optimal tracheal tube placement. A clinical study. *Anaesthesia* 1989; **44:** 970.

159 Siker E. S. A mirror laryngoscope. *Anesthesiology* 1956; **17:** 38.

160 Huffman J. P. and Elam J. O. Laryngoscopy. *Anesthesia and Analgesia* 1971; **50:** 64.

161 Huffman J. P. The application of prisms to curved laryngoscopes: a preliminary study. *Journal of the American Association of Nurse Anesthetists* 1968; **36:** 138.

162 Huffman J. P. The development of optical prism instruments to view and study the human larynx. *Journal of the American Association of Nurse Anesthetists* 1970; **38:** 197.

163 Bearman A. J. Device for nasotracheal intubation. *Anesthesiology* 1962; **23:** 130.

164 Munson E. S. and Cullen S. C. Endotracheal intubation in a patient with ankylosing spondylitis of the cervical spine. *Anesthesiology* 1965; **26:** 365.

165 Mirakhur R. K. Technique for difficult intubation. *British Journal of Anaesthesia* 1972; **44:** 632.

166 Hex Venn P. The gum elastic bougie. *Anaesthesia* 1993; **48:** 274.

167 Grillo H. C. Surgical treatment of postintubation injuries. *Journal of Thoracic and Cardiovascular Surgery* 1979; **78:** 860.

168 Neville W. Discussion of Grillo H. C. *Journal of Thoracic and Cardiovascular Surgery* 1969; **57:** 52.

169 Butler F. S. and Cirillo A. A. Retrograde tracheal intubation. *Anesthesia and Analgesia* 1960; **39:** 333.

170 Harmer M. and Vaughan R. S. Guided blind oral intubation. *Anaesthesia* 1980; **35:** 921.

171 Akinyemi O. O. Complications of guided blind endotracheal intubation. *Anaesthesia* 1979; **34:** 590.

172 Dhara S. S. Guided blind endotracheal intubation. *Anaesthesia* 1980; **35:** 81.

173 Bourke D. and Levesque P. R. Modification of retrograde guide for endotracheal intubation. *Anesthesia and Analgesia* 1974; **53:** 1013.

174 Powell W. F. and Ozdil T. A translaryngeal guide for tracheal intubation. *Anesthesia and Analgesia* 1967; **46:** 231.

175 Graham W. P. and Kilgore E. S. Endotracheal intubation in complicated cases. *Hospital Physician* 1975; **3:** 60.

176 Roberts K. W. New use for Swan-Ganz introducer wire. *Anesthesia and Analgesia* 1981; **60:** 67.

177 Borland L. M., Swan D. M. and Leff S. Difficult pediatric intubation: a new approach to the retrograde technique. *Anesthesiology* 1981; **55:** 577.

178 McLean Guided blind oral intubation. *Anaesthesia* 1982; **37:** 605.

179 Barrio P. and Riou B. Retrograde technique for tracheal intubation in trauma patients. *Critical Care Medicine* 1988; **16:** 712.

180 Castheley P. A., Landesman S., Fymann P. N., Ergin M. A., Greipp R. and Wolf G. L. Retrograde intubation in patients undergoing open heart surgery. *Canadian Journal of Anaesthesia* 1985; **32:** 661.

181 Gerenstein R. I. J-wire facilitates translaryngeal

guided intubation. *Anesthesiology* 1992; **76:** 1059.

182 King H-K., Wang L-F., Khan A. K. and Wooten D. J. Translaryngeal guided intubation for difficult intubation. *Critical Care Medicine* 1987; **15:** 869.

183 Tobias R. Increased success with retrograde guide for endotracheal intubation. *Anesthesia and Analgesia* 1983; **62:** 366.

184 Carlson C. A. and Perkins H. M. Solving a difficult intubation. *Anesthesiology* 1986; **64:** 537.

185 Lechman M. J., Donahoo J. S. and Macvaugh H. Endotracheal intubation using percutaneous retrograde guidewire insertion followed by anterograde fibreoptic bronchoscopy. *Critical Care Medicine* 1986; **14:** 589.

186 Gupta B., McDonald J. S., Brooks J. H. J. and Mendenhall J. Oral fibreoptic intubation over a retrograde guidewire. *Anesthesia and Analgesia* 1989; **68,** 517.

187 Wilson R. F., Steiger Z., Jacobs J., Sison O. S. and Holsey C. Temporary partial cardiopulmonary bypass during emergency operative management of near total tracheal obstruction. *Anesthesiology* 1984; **61:** 103.

188 Maharaj R. J., Whitton I. and Blyth D. Emergency extracorporeal oxygenation for an intratracheal foreign body. *Anaesthesia* 1983; **38:** 471.

# Awake Intubation

*Keith R. Murrin*

## INTRODUCTION

General anaesthesia is not essential for tracheal intubation. In certain circumstances, it is best if consciousness is maintained.

## ROLE OF AWAKE INTUBATION

Patients who present with difficult intubation fall into two main categories, expected and unexpected. If the problem is expected, there is a choice of cautiously inducing anaesthesia, while maintaining spontaneous respiration, or sedating the patient for an 'awake intubation'. The success of the intubation procedure then depends on the experience of the operator, the availability of suitable equipment and the presence of skilled assistants.

When the problem is unexpected, this will usually be discovered following the induction of anaesthesia and the administration of either depolarizing or non-depolarizing muscle relaxants.

All of the patients presenting with group 1 and 2 laryngoscopic appearances [1] can be intubated conventionally, albeit with a appropriate external manipulation of the thyroid cartilage [2]. Some patients with group 3 laryngoscopic appearances who cannot be intubated with a gum elastic bougie, and all those in group 4, are those at greatest risk.

If a depolarizing muscle relaxant has been employed and there is a risk of aspiration from a full stomach and hypoxaemia before the resumption of spontaneous respiration, the most appropriate immediate action is to insert a laryngeal mask or ventilate with a facemask while maintaining cricoid pressure in the supine position. It should be stressed that preceding induction of anaesthesia in the emergency situation, there should be at least 4 min of preoxygenation. Provided that an appropriate dose of depolarizing muscle relaxant has been employed and there is a normal metabolism of that drug, hypoxia should not intervene before resumption of normal neuro-muscular activity and respiration. With the return of spontaneous respiration, the patient is placed in the lateral position until return of consciousness. An 'awake intubation' can then be performed.

Data presented from the Australian Incident Monitoring Study [3] demonstrated that 15% of difficult intubations involved simultaneous diffi-culties with ventilation using a facemask. If venti-lation is impossible with a facemask or laryngeal mask, oxygenation can be maintained through the cricothyroid membrane utilizing high pressure jet ventilation or high frequency ventilation.

*Note*: If major difficulty with intubation is an-ticipated in the emergency situation with a risk of aspiration, muscle relaxants should not be given. Where appropriate, local anaesthetic techniques should be considered in preference to general anaesthesia.

If grade 4 laryngoscopic appearances are encountered following the administration of a non-depolarizing muscle relaxant in the elective situation, the choice is either to utilize the various indirect methods of intubation, the fibreoptic scope or, following the return of consciousness, awake intubation.

## INDICATIONS FOR AWAKE INTUBATION

Awake intubations should not be limited to those cases in which application of the technique is mandatory [4]. In experienced hands, awake intu-bation can be practised with little discomfort to the patient and therefore its use should be more widespread, increasing the opportunities for trainees to acquire the necessary skills.

Thomas [5] summarized the indications for awake intubations based on the earlier work of Giuffrida *et al.* [6]. They fall under the following major headings:

### Full Stomach

This would include all emergency procedures, especially intestinal obstruction or gastrointestinal

haemorrhage. With the use of local anaesthetic agents, the pharyngeal and laryngeal reflexes are obtunded but when vomiting or regurgitation occurs the patient can usually respond to the threat to his airway; the head and thorax are voluntarily turned to the side and the pharynx is cleared by coughing, retching or swallowing. However, sometimes patient comfort is sacrificed to avoid subsequent aspiration. Walts [7] and D'Hollander [8] recommended that local anaes-thetic be limited to the supraglottic structures and the sedation be minimal. Kopriva *et al.* [9] demon-strated that topical anaesthesia was slightly safer in this respect than sedation with fentanyl. Libman [10] expressed the extreme view that topical anaesthesia should be limited to the lower lip and the outer half of the tongue, while Thomas [5] advocated sparing of the subglottic regions by omission of the transtracheal injection.

Aspiration did not occur in patients with a full stomach when topical anaesthesia was used dur-ing awake intubation [11].

### Moribundity

The use of general anaesthesia is fraught with hazard in the moribund patient. Intubation can often be performed without general anaesthesia, sedation, muscle relaxation or topical anaesthesia.

Cardiovascular instability is often a problem and the sudden start of intermittent positive pres-sure ventilation can produce devastating results with an abrupt reduction in venous return and arterial carbon dioxide tension. Benefit may accrue from the temporary improvement in oxygen delivery when performing the awake intu-bation [12].

### Difficult Intubation

It is highly desirable to maintain spontaneous respiration in cases of difficult intubation. In a patient who is awake and breathing sponta-neously, it is of little importance if a greater length of time is taken to complete the intubation process. There need be no sense of urgency, since hypoxia is unlikely to occur. Some anaesthetists induce anaesthesia with spontaneous respiration and then attempt to ventilate the patient's lungs. If successful, a short acting depolarizing muscle relaxant is then given to aid intubation. Repeated attempts to intubate the trachea may produce laryngeal oedema with subsequent difficulty with ventilation with the mask.

Awake intubation still appears to be more popular in the USA than in the UK, perhaps because of the litigious atmosphere in the USA. This is considered in the chapter on legal implications (see Chapter 21).

## Respiratory Failure

In patients with low arterial oxygen tension it may be inadvisable to produce sudden muscle relaxation and further hypoxia before intubation.

The reader should refer to the papers by Pedersen [13] and Geffin [14] for a detailed list of the individual medical conditions which fall under the above headings. They include:

- clinical evidence of obstruction in the conscious state;
- lesions of the oropharynx, tongue or larynx including neoplasm, infection and haematoma;
- Anticipated difficulties with the face mask, restricted temporomandibular movement and mouth opening, restricted neck and head movement, marked agenesia of the mandible, bull neck, buck teeth and extensive maxillo facial deformity which can occur after burns and trauma;
- gross obesity and abdominal distension;
- cervical instability.

Suderman *et al.* [15], in a ten-year review of 150 patients with traumatic cervical spine injuries with well-preserved neurological function, demonstrated that there were no differences in neurological outcome whether intubation was performed while the patient was awake or under general anaesthesia. However, it should be noted that the data did not reach statistical significance because of insufficient numbers of patients. The safety of awake intubation with cervical spine injury has been demonstrated by a subsequent study [16].

In addition, in-line traction did not affect neurological outcome. However, when traction is applied, this should not be excessive because if it is associated with fracture-dislocations it can produce an ascending neurological deficit. Traction should be applied incrementally with radiological monitoring and with neurological testing. It has been demonstrated that cervical spinal movement can be reduced during tracheal intubation in normal patients by manual in-line traction exerted by an assistant. This was found to be more effective than a collar in reducing spinal movement [17] (see also Chapter 18).

## ADVANTAGES OF AWAKE INTUBATION

### Maintenance of Airway

Muscle tone is preserved and the tongue does not fall backwards to obstruct the pharynx.

### Reduction of Hypoxic and Hypercarbic Events

The incidence of dramatic life-threatening events may well be diminished but hypoxia and hypercarbia as a result of sedation have been demonstrated by blood gas analysis [18] and by end tidal carbon dioxide monitoring [19] during the conduct of awake intubation. It is therefore recommended that preoxygenation should be performed and that supplementary oxygen is provided whenever possible during awake intubation.

The end tidal carbon dioxide concentrations were much higher when both fentanyl and diazepam were administered in combination compared with administration of fentanyl alone [19].

## DISADVANTAGES OF AWAKE INTUBATION

### Aspiration

The risk of aspiration seems to be more related to the degree of sedation than to the extent of the topical analgesia.

### Discomfort

This is minimized with thorough surface analgesia combined with an appropriate degree of sedation.

## DRUGS USED FOR SEDATION DURING AWAKE INTUBATION

Cossham made a strong plea for the adequate use of intravenous sedation to ensure amnesia during awake intubation [20]. It is desirable that intubation of the conscious subject is performed with the aid of sedation provided that patient safety is not compromised. Agents commonly used for this purpose are drugs belonging to the benzodiazepine group (diazepam, midazolam); those belonging to the butyrophenone (droperidol); short acting narcotics (fentanyl); and the infusion of propofol.

## Diazepam

The intravenous use of diazepam is accompanied by an unacceptable incidence of superficial vein thrombosis. This problem is virtually eliminated by the addition of lipid as solvent to form the preparation of Diazemuls. There is often a variation in response [21] and there may be prolonged action with a second peak effect [22, 23].

## Midazolam

This has a shorter duration of action compared with diazepam [24] and is more suitable for brief procedures such as intubation when this is not followed by general anaesthesia. Water soluble midazolam is virtually devoid of thrombophlebitic problems [25]. The dose range is 2–7 mg intravenously for a 70 kg patient.

## Fentanyl

This opioid drug is commonly used with droperidol to produce neuroleptanalgesia. The cough and gag reflex are depressed and the patient often accepts a tracheal tube and is still capable of obeying a command. The dose range is 50–150 μg intravenously for a 70 kg patient.

## Phenoperidine

Phenoperidine is used where more prolonged analgesia is required following intubation. The dose range is 0.5–1.0 mg for a 70 kg patient.

## Propofol

Suppression of pharyngeal and laryngeal reflex activity by propofol has been demonstrated by several studies [26–28] and the widespread use of this drug for the insertion of the laryngeal mask airway (LMA). It is therefore an ideal choice as sedative for awake intubation.

The rate of infusion is dependent on the age and medical condition of the patient. A suitable infusion rate for awake intubation would be 0.7–2.0 mg kg$^{-1}$h$^{-1}$.

## ANTISIALOGOGUE ADMINISTRATION

It is important to premedicate with an antisialogogue such as atropine (0.3–0.6 mg, i.v. or i.m.) hyoscine (0.3–0.4 mg, i.v. or i.m.) or glycopyrrolate (0.2 mg i.v. or i.m.). The reduction in secretions reduces the desire by the patient to swallow repeatedly and increases the effectiveness of the topical local anaesthetic agent.

## LOCAL ANAESTHETIC TECHNIQUES

### Topical Anaesthesia

During the following discussion on topical anaesthesia, reference will be made to surface-active local anaesthetic agents which will not be specifically named but which include:

- cocaine 4–10% (spray or paste);
- lignocaine 4–10% (spray or viscous gel).

Lignocaine, because of its wider safety margin, is the most commonly used agent for this purpose.

### Surface Anaesthesia of the Nasal Mucosa

If nasotracheal intubation is contemplated, vasoconstriction is mandatory to minimize the risk of haemorrhage and increase the diameter of the nasal passages. This has traditionally been achieved with topical 4% cocaine, which has the additional advantage of producing surface anaesthesia. Fry [29] recommends a maximum dose of 200 mg. Xylometazoline (Otravine) has been shown to be at least as effective as cocaine [30].

Gross *et al.* [31] demonstrated that a mixture of 3% lignocaine with 0.25% phenylephrine was an effective substitute for 4% cocaine when applied to the nasal mucosa to prevent bleeding and to provide analgesia.

### *Method*

The nose is packed with ribbon gauze soaked in the local anaesthetic solution. Excess solution must be removed prior to insertion to avoid systemic toxicity. Alternatively, the nasal mucosa may be sprayed with lignocaine or cocaine before intubation.

## Surface Anaesthesia of the Oropharyngeal–Laryngeal Regions

### Gargle

The simplest method of anaesthetizing the mouth is for the patient to gargle with a 4% lignocaine gel; this is bitter, but it can be flavoured to improve patient acceptance [32].

The posterior aspect of the tongue and the epiglottis can be anaesthetized by placing 5% lignocaine ointment on the back of the patient's tongue. The ointment slowly melts and spreads backwards to anaesthetize the epiglottis [14].

Pledgets soaked in lignocaine can be applied to the oral mucosa. This is followed by cricothyroid lignocaine injection. Sedation produces satisfactory conditions for awake intubation without unpleasant recall [33].

### 'Spray-as-you-go'

Surface anaesthesia may be produced by a 'spray-as-you-go' technique, commencing at the nose or mouth and slowly advancing towards the glottis and infraglottic areas. Despite the advantage of the metered dose with the modern canister sprays (Fig. 1), older models such as the Swerdlow (Fig. 2) spray have the advantage of a long blunt-ended nozzle that enables safe entry into the glottis and trachea. Toxicity can be avoided by first placing a calculated safe dose for each patient in the reservoir chamber (Table 1).

**Table 1** Maximum safe dose of local anaesthetic agents (topical application)

| | |
| --- | --- |
| Lignocaine | 3 mg kg$^{-1}$ |
| Cocaine | 1.5 mg kg$^{-1}$ |

### Lozenges

In the past, anaesthesia of the mouth and upper pharynx could be achieved by the administration of an amethocaine lozenge (60 mg) 30 min before intubation. Unfortunately, these have been withdrawn because of toxicity problems. Sidhu *et al.* [34] stated that benzocaine lozenges are almost without effect.

Mongan and Culling [35] demonstrated that sodium benzonatate (Tesalon Pearls) provided rapid and reliable oropharangeal anaesthesia in preparation for awake intubation. Benzonatate, a long chain polyglycol derivative of procaine, is a potent membrane anaesthetic and is supplied in 100 mg capsules. The common use for this preparation is as a non-opioid antitussive and it has been available for nearly 40 years. However, because it is an ester derivative it may cause allergic reactions.

### Ultrasonic nebulizer

An ultrasonic nebulizer containing 10 ml of 4% plain lignocaine (400 mg) inhaled through a mask for 10 min was effective in 95% of 1000 patients

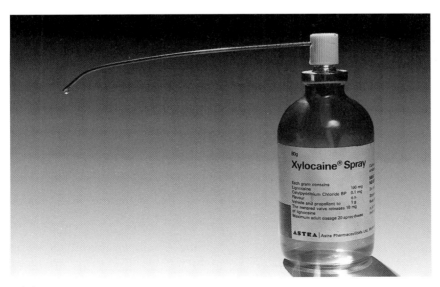

**Figure 1**   Metered-dose spray.

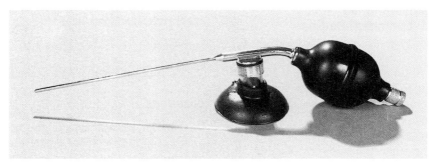

**Figure 2**   Swerdlow spray.

being prepared for bronchoscopy [36]. Serum levels of lignocaine were below the toxic limit of 5 μg ml⁻¹. Nebulized lignocaine has been shown to prevent hypertension and tachycardia during laryngoscopy and tracheal intubation [37]. Bourke *et al.* [38] supported the use of a disposable aerosol nebulizer using a mixture of 4 ml of 4% lignocaine with 1 ml of 1% phenylephrine in combination with diazepam as sedative and a small amount of opiate. A flexible connecting tube between the facemask and the nebulizer allowed the administration to continue with the patient in the sitting or supine position.

### Labat's syringe

The glottis and infraglottic areas can be anaesthetized using Labat's syringe (Fig. 3) or a similar curved applicator. The patient is placed in the sitting position facing the operator. The tongue is extended and held with a gauze swab by the operator or the patient. In the latter situation, the operator is able to utilize an indirect laryngoscope with a warmed mirror for accurate droplet placement. Indirect laryngoscopy is not essential for good results in experienced hands.

The curved applicator of the syringe is introduced over the dorsum of the tongue, which is held extended with a gauze swab, keeping strictly

to the mid line. The patient is requested to take shallow breaths and to avoid coughing. The local anaesthetic solution is then allowed to fall in droplets onto and then through the laryngeal inlet. A slight modification of this technique produced favourable results with the introduction of a Robertshaw double lumen tube in a conscious patient. The absence of a cough reflex during the passage of the tube confirmed surface anaesthesia extended as far distally as the bronchi [39].

Fry [29] recommended additional application to the pyriform fossae with the aid of the indirect laryngeal mirror, thus anaesthetizing the internal branches of the superior laryngeal nerves.

### Cricothyroid puncture

The infraglottic mucosa can be anaesthetised by cricothyroid or transtracheal puncture. The most widely accepted term for this procedure is translaryngeal anaesthesia, although transcricothyroid membrane analgesia would be the least confusing [40]. With the head held in a position of maximum extension, the superior notch of the thyroid cartilage is readily palpable in the midline at the junction of the floor of the mouth and the anterior aspect of the neck. The ring shaped cartilage below the thyroid cartilage is the cricoid cartilage; the gap between these structures which is bridged by the cricothyroid membrane is easily recognized in the majority of patients (Fig. 4). A cross is marked on the skin midway between these structures in the midline thus denoting the point of needle entry.

After sterilization of the skin, a bleb is raised using 1% lignocaine at the designated point of entry. A needle is then introduced at right angles to the skin to penetrate the cricothyroid membrane and enter the lumen of the upper trachea. The use

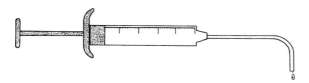

**Figure 3**   Labat's syringe.

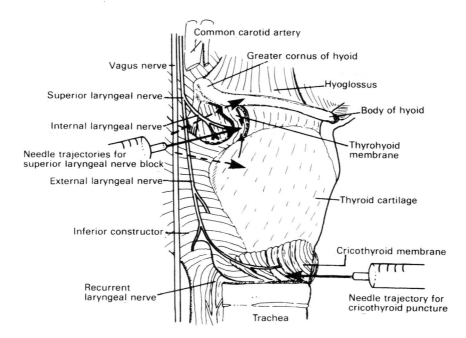

**Figure 4**   Anatomical relationship of hyoid bone, thyroid and cricoid cartilages, showing needle trajectories for cricothyroid puncture and superior laryngeal nerve block. Modified from Zuck [85] with kind permission of the author and the editor of *Anaesthesia*.

of a needle and syringe connected by a short length of flexible tubing, e.g. 21 SWG 'Butterfly' needle, will reduce the possibility of needle breakage or trauma to the larynx. Alternatively, the use of a plastic cannula confers the same benefit.

Following aspiration of air to confirm that the needle tip is in the trachea, 2 ml of local anaesthetic agent are injected. This often produces violent coughing. If performed at the end of inspiration, the local anaesthetic is rapidly coughed in expiration towards the glottic region, thus anaesthetizing the infraglottic mucosa and the lower surface of the vocal cords. If the patient is placed in a reverse Trendelenburg position and a second injection performed on expiration, the anaesthesia will extend to distal regions of the respiratory tract, thus preparing the patient for subsequent bronchoscopy. Violent coughing occurs when the local anaesthetic solution reaches the carina, which also serves to reinforce anaesthesia above the level of injection.

A review of 17 500 cases of cricothyroid puncture reported eight complications [41]:

- four soft tissue infections in the neck;
- two broken needles;
- two cases of severe laryngospasm.

## Regional Blocks

Regional nerve blocks can produce profound analgesia using small quantities of local anaesthetic solution, thus reducing the risk of toxicity from the local anaesthetic agents.

### Maxillary nerve block

This block is reported [42] to produce profound surface analgesia of most of the nasal cavity, thus aiding nasal intubation.

#### Anatomy
Sensory fibres from the second (maxillary) division of the trigeminal nerve pass through the pterygopalatine (sphenopalatine) ganglion to supply the hard and soft palates, septal and lateral walls of the nasal cavity and nasopharynx.

#### Method
A 4 cm needle is angled to 45° at the hub with care being taken to prevent fracture. It is introduced into the greater palatine canal through the greater palatine foramen in the posterolateral aspect of the palate. The needle is then passed into the pterygopalatine (sphenopalatine) fossa as shown in Figs 5–7.

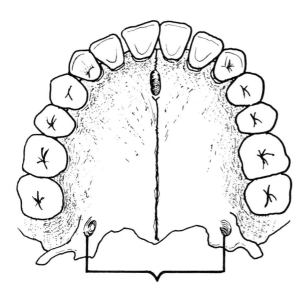

**Figure 5**  Hard palate with the greater palatine foraminae. From Baddour *et al.* [42], with kind permission of the editor of *Anesthesia Progress*.

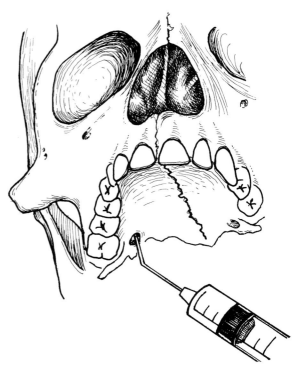

**Figure 6**  Injection into the greater palatine canal. From Baddour *et al.* [42], with kind permission of the editor of *Anesthesia Progress*.

Additional benefit may be gained if a local anaesthetic agent with a vasoconstrictor, or inherent vasoconstrictor properties such as cocaine, is used. The blood supply to the nasal mucosa is reduced by constriction of the sphenopalatine artery as it transverses the pterygopalatine fissure.

### Glossopharyngeal nerve block

Pressure receptors at the root of the tongue that initiate the gag reflex are submucosal and are not blocked with the topical application of local anaesthetic agents [43]. A bilateral block of the glossopharyngeal nerve is required to block these pressure receptors. A bilateral glossopharyngeal nerve block also produces surface anaesthesia of the posterior third of the tongue, tonsillar region, and oropharynx. The gag reflex is also completely suppressed. A major disadvantage is paralysis of the pharyngeal muscles and relaxation of the base of the tongue which may produce sudden respiratory obstruction requiring immediate treatment.

*Note*: A glossopharyngeal nerve block is an additional block in patients who retain an active gag reflex. Therefore, it may follow one of the methods of oral laryngeal topical analgesia or superior laryngeal nerve block. It is important that the superior laryngeal nerve block should always be carried out first to avoid respiratory obstruction.

### Method
After applying surface analgesia to the dorsal aspect of the tongue, it is then depressed and the posterior tonsillar pillar placed under tension. An angled tonsillar needle is inserted behind the posterior tonsillar pillar at its mid point, to a depth of 1 cm (Fig. 8). Following aspiration, 3 ml of local anaesthetic are injected and the procedure repeated on the other side.

### Superior laryngeal nerve block

#### Transmucosal block (Krause's forceps)
The superior laryngeal nerve can be blocked by the oral route along the floor of the pyriform fossa using Krause's forceps.

*Method* Following oropharyngeal anaesthesia the patient is placed in the sitting position facing the operator and asked to stick out the tongue fully. The tongue is held in this position with the aid of a gauze swab. A dental pledget firmly held by Krause's forceps is soaked in local anaesthetic solution. The pledget is then passed into each

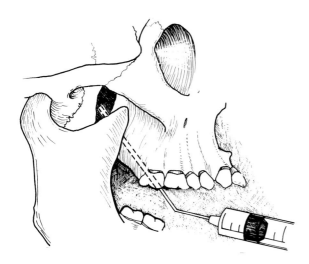

**Figure 7**   Lateral view of the skull showing the path of the needle *into* the pterygopalatine fossa. From Baddour *et al.* [42], with kind permission of the editor of *Anesthesia Progress*.

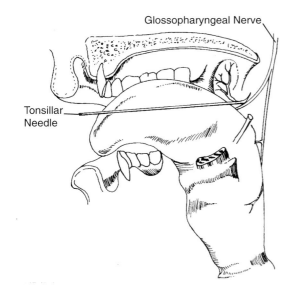

Glossopharyngeal Nerve

Tonsillar Needle

**Figure 8**   Glossopharyngeal nerve block. With permission from De Meester *et al.* [44].

pyriform fossa by following the downward continuation of the tonsillar fossa, close to the lateral pharyngeal wall. The position may be checked by palpating the neck lateral to the superior aspect of the thyroid cartilage. The pledget is held in position for about 1 min to allow the solution to diffuse around the superior laryngeal nerve (Figs 9–11).

## Percutaneous block

***Method*** A cannula should be placed in a vein and intravenous anticonvulsant agents such as diazepam and thiopentone should be immediately available. The cornuae of the hyoid bone and the superior cornuae of the thyroid cartilage are palpated and marked with a skin pencil. This block can be accomplished either by starting from the hyoid landmark or from the thyroid cartilage.

A point is marked on the skin 1 cm medial to the superior cornua of the hyoid bone. A skin weal is raised and a 3 cm, 23 SWG needle is inserted to contact the hyoid bone. The needle is then walked inferiorly off the bone in a caudad direction to pierce the thyrohyoid membrane. In an alternative method, the needle is inserted, after local infiltration, onto the superior cornua of the thyroid cartilage and walked superiorly off the cartilage, piercing the thyrohyoid membrane as in Fig. 4. In both cases an injection of 2 ml of local anaesthetic solution is made following careful aspiration. Aspiration of air indicates that the needle has entered the larynx and must be withdrawn before injection. The block is repeated on the other side. Contact with the nerve is unnecessary. There will be referred pain in the ear if the nerve is hit by the needle [46].

*Warning.* It is important that the thyroid cartilage is not pierced since deposition of local anaesthetic solution can lead to oedema of the vocal cords.

## Systemic Toxicity

Absorption of local anaesthetic agents from the mucous membrane in the upper respiratory tract is extremely rapid, and attention must be paid to safe limits shown in Table 1. Foldes [47] noted objective signs of lignocaine toxicity at venous levels of 5.29 µg ml$^{-1}$. These were tachycardia, moderate hypertension, T-wave flattening and S–T segment depression in the ECG, accompanied by slow activity in the EEG. The most common complication, however, is cerebral excitation which can present as a frank convulsion. This may be preceded by a prodromal period during which the patient describes a perioral tingling sensation and isolated twitching movements. It is important that techniques involving the administration of large doses of local anaesthetic agents should always be performed by skilled personnel in a location with adequate resuscitation facilities.

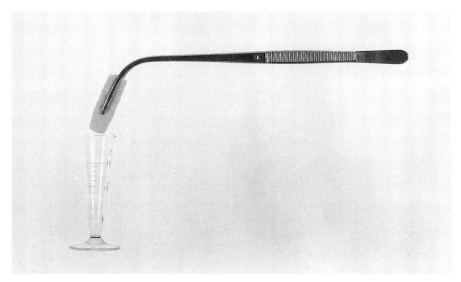

**Figure 9**    Krause's forceps.

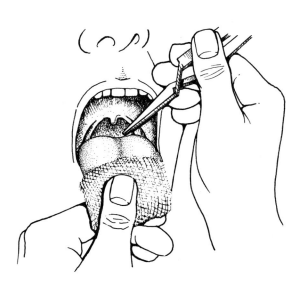

**Figure 10**    Insertion of Krause's forceps. Left hand of operator holding the tongue with a gauze swab. From Macintosh and Ostlere [45], with kind permission of the authors and the publisher, E. S. Livingstone.

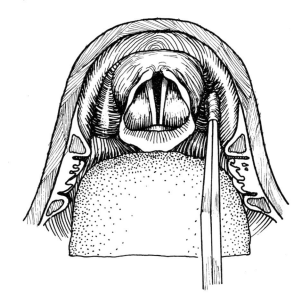

**Figure 11**    Superior view of larynx – final position of Krause's forceps in the pyriform fossa. From Macintosh and Ostlere [45], with kind permission of the authors and the publisher, E. S. Livingstone.

Absorption of local anaesthetic agents from topical anaesthesia prior to intubation has been studied and the following points emerge.

- There is a faster absorption of local anaesthetic agents in children. Differences also exist in children of different age groups [48].
- Peak levels of serum lignocaine [49] occur between 15 and 60 min following topical appli-

cation in adults. This emphasizes the need for careful supervision in the recovery phase.
- Peak levels of active metabolites of lignocaine may occur 3–4 h following administration.
- Measurements of serum lignocaine have been well below the toxic limits despite the administration of amounts which exceeded the manufacturers' recommended values by 25–30%. Indeed, adverse reactions were not observed

even in some patients where levels were greater than those reported to have caused toxicity [49].

- Absorption occurs more rapidly from the alveoli than from other sites in the respiratory tract.
- Selective blocking of the nerves supplying the relevant portions of mucosa subsequently produces much lower blood levels of local anaesthetic agent than topical application [50].

## Cardiovascular Consequences

In adults the pressor response to laryngoscopy and tracheal intubation is attenuated by local anaesthesia and awake intubation, but by no means abolished [51]. Bradycardia, which may be of reflex origin, has been reported in children after laryngeal spraying [52]. This effect may be augmented by concurrent administration of suxamethonium or general anaesthetic agents. Peak levels of lignocaine occur too late to be of value in preventing dysrhythmias during intubation. The pressor response and increase in heart rate are minimized using fibreoptic nasotracheal intubation combined with thorough topical analgesia [53] (see Chapter 2).

## Conclusion

A combination of cricothyroid injection and topical pharyngeal analgesia in the presence of sedation and antisialogogue administration seem the simplest combination of techniques in less experienced hands. The techniques should be carried out only where immediate facilities are available for resuscitation. However, there is a reasonable evidence to suggest that limits set by manufacturers for the use of local anaesthetic agents in this context are unnecessarily low. It would seem that even in children, where absorption is greatest, a dose of 4 mg kg$^{-1}$ of lignocaine is safe [48].

## METHODS OF AWAKE INTUBATION

### Indirect Methods

#### Blind oral intubation

Blind intubation techniques should not be contemplated in patients with lesions of the tongue, pharynx or larynx [14].

A suction catheter can be passed blindly into the trachea to act as a guide for the subsequent passage of a nasotracheal tube. A coude tip may facilitate entry to the trachea in difficult cases [54].

The Augustine Guide™ is a stylet combined with oesophageal detection device. This is a catheter with a moulded tip attached to a large syringe which detects oesophageal placement by the inability to aspirate air into the syringe. A successful intubation has been described with a patient suffering from the Treacher–Collins syndrome [55].

#### Blind nasotracheal intubation

This is associated with a low incidence of success at the first attempt and increased trauma with repeated attempts thereafter. The success rate with blind nasal intubation is much lower than using the fibreoptic scope. A study of 409 elective intubations using a fibreoptic scope demonstrated a success rate of 98.8%, which exceeds the highest rate reported in any series of blind nasotracheal intubations [56].

Blind nasal intubation should be performed gently, preferably with the patient breathing spontaneously. This allows the practitioner to listen to the air-flow associated with respiration or to a whistle attached to the tracheal tube [57].

Stimulation of ventilation can be achieved using either carbon dioxide or doxapram to improve estimation of tip position. Breath sounds disappear when accidental oesophageal placement is performed.

One of the major problems with a nasotracheal intubation is the incidence of nasal bleeding. This renders subsequent fiberoptic visualisation of the larynx extremely difficult. If blind nasotracheal intubation proves unsuccessful, it is advisable to leave the tube in the pharynx as an airway to avoid the possibility of nasal haemorrhage on withdrawal.

Mostert [58] has advised against the abolition of pharyngeal and laryngeal tone when contemplating blind nasal intubation. This is contrary to the practice of some experienced British anaesthetists who even advocate the use of muscle relaxants to facilitate this technique.

Blind nasal intubation can create a false route in the posterior pharyngeal wall. Subsequent withdrawal of the tube can result in brisk haemorrhage [59].

### Laryngeal mask airway (LMA)

It has been demonstrated that the LMA can be inserted in patients ranging from neonates to 9 years of age in the awake state following a spray to the oropharynx with 2% lignocaine solution [60]. After the insertion of the LMA in the conscious state, the patient is anaesthetized with the reassurance of a patent airway. The LMA is then utilized for subsequent passage of a bougie into the trachea [61, 62].

A successful superior laryngeal nerve block greatly reduces the incidence of coughing and laryngospasm with the LMA in anaesthetized patients [63]. This may also be helpful in awake patients.

The LMA can also be used as an introducer for the fibreoptic scope in the awake patient [64]. The tracheal tube is then passed over the fibreoptic scope. The fibreoptic scope and the LMA can then be removed.

### Radiological method

A radio-opaque directable catheter can be used in conjunction with X-ray fluoroscopic control to act as a guide for the tracheal tube [65]. Directable catheters are available in most X-ray departments.

### Light wand

Intubation using a light wand is not recommended in cases of severe obesity, neck oedema or neck tumours, because of the difficulty in illuminating the laryngeal structures [14]. The light wand has been demonstrated to be more efficient than 'blind' nasal intubation [66] and just as efficient as the conventional laryngoscope in routine intubations [67]. It is also suited for use in children [68].

### Retrograde methods

Provided there is access to the cricothyroid membrane, retrograde methods in the conscious or sedated patient, using catheters or wires may provide a simple solution where there is intubation difficulty. Retrograde guidance methods cannot be used in the absence of clearly identifiable landmarks or in the presence of local sepsis [14].

## Direct Methods

### Bougies, stylets and guides

Aids to placement of the tracheal tube are varied. The simplest device is an internal guide which can be wire, aluminium with a teflon coating, or a simple gum elastic bougie. All these have malleable tips and can be bent into any position that aids the subsequent passage of the tracheal tube. A modification of this device is the Salem Resce intubation guide [69], a device that allows the operator to move the tip and thereby the tube anteriorly, posteriorly and sideways by moving a handle guide. A simpler method is merely to use a Magill forceps to grasp the distal end of the tube.

Another method includes a hook which is inserted into a hole at the end of the tube (Murphy's eye). An inadvertent tracheal tear has been described following a difficult intubation using an angulated stylet to guide the tracheal tube through the vocal cords [70].

### Laryngoscope blade

Numerous varieties of laryngoscope blades have been designed but the length of the blade may be more important than the actual design [71]. The use of prisms and the disadvantage of inverted image has been replaced by the incorporation of optical fibres as an additional aid for use with the rigid blade. MacIntyre [72] provides a comprehensive review of laryngoscope blades. However, in the last analysis, none of these blades will cope with every difficult intubation. The long-term solution to difficult intubation is familiarity with, and availability of, the fibreoptic bronchoscope or laryngoscope.

### Laryngeal mirror

A method of intubation of the conscious subject in the sitting position, utilizing the head lamp, laryngeal mirror and the flexible tracheal tube supplied with the fibreoptic bronchoscope has been described [73]. Although this method was utilized for the introduction of the fibreoptic bronchoscope, it could be appropriate for use with patients who are known cases of difficult intubation.

### Fibreoptic intubation

The use of the fibreoptic bronchoscope or laryngoscope as a guide for the subsequent passage of a tracheal tube in cases of difficult intubation are discussed in Chapter 10.

Early pioneering work involving the insertion of the Carlens catheter (double lumen tube) in conscious subjects allowed differential bronchospirometric physiological studies to be performed, thus demonstrating the feasibility of even passing double lumen endobronchial tubes under local anaesthesia. Moreover, bronchoscopy using the rigid scope, was commonly performed under local sedation and anaesthesia before the advent of a ventilating bronchoscope or a fiberoptic scope. Double lumen tubes can be inserted using the fibreoptic bronchoscope as a guide in conscious patients who are known to be difficult to intubate [74].

Although fibreoptic intubation is the method of choice in patients who are difficult to intubate, these facilities are not always available in underdeveloped countries. It is therefore crucial that any anaesthetist working in such areas is versed in the alternative techniques of intubation [75].

It has been demonstrated that patients presenting with difficult airways can be anaesthetized with etomidate, alfentanyl and vecuronium, and ventilated using percutaneous transtracheal high frequency jet ventilation (HFJV) followed by intubation aided by fibreoptic bronchoscopy [76, 77]. This is particularly suitable for patients who are unco-operative, suffering from ischaemic heart disease or impaired pulmonary gas exchange.

Occasionally, it may be advantageous to employ several techniques when confronted with a difficult intubation. A retrograde technique has been reported using a Seldinger wire which was subsequently passed through the suction port of a fibreoptic bronchoscope and guided the scope into the trachea. The tracheal tube was then subsequently railroaded over the scope [78].

## AWAKE INTUBATION IN CHILDREN

Veyckemans *et al.* [79] condemn awake intubation in the neonate and state that it should be only used as a resuscitative measure. They recommend a combination of general and topical anaesthesia. They also emphasize that awake intubation leads to a rise in intracranial pressure in these infants. This finding was subsequently confirmed by Stow [80].

## AWAKE INTUBATION IN PREGNANCY

Sedation, as an adjunct to awake intubation, is not contraindicated in the immediate prepartum patient [81]. If the neonate is depressed, reversal can be achieved with naloxone and flumazenil. It has been demonstrated that the mother can receive adequate sedation for awake intubation and deliver an infant without need of reversal (Apgar Score 8–9) [81].

### Topical Vasoconstrictors in Pregnancy

The use of 3% lignocaine with 0.125% phenylephrine is preferred to cocaine for vasoconstriction before nasotracheal intubation because it is less likely to cause maternal hypertension and impaired uteroplacental blood flow [82]. A study in pregnant ewes suggests that ephedrine is preferable to phenylephrine for vasoconstriction before nasotracheal intubation for the same reason [83].

## KEY POINTS

- The importance of preoperative assessment involving both previous anaesthetic history and relevant clinical examination is stressed [84].

- Emphasis should also be placed on difficult intubation training and in the use of the fibreoptic laryngoscope/bronchoscope.

- A thorough knowledge of the various techniques should also be gained, together with a protocol for failed intubation in both the elective and emergency situations.

- The recommended range of equipment should always be available in all anaesthetic areas accompanied by trained assistance.

- Repeated attempts at intubation may not only reduce the chance of successful intubation, but may also lead to oedema and bleeding, eventually preventing ventilation with a facemask.

# REFERENCES

1 Cormack R. S. and Lehane J. Difficult intubation in obstetrics. *Anaesthesia* 1984; **39:** 1105.

2 Knill R. L. Anaesthetic techniques: difficult laryngoscopy made easy with a 'BURP'. *Canadian Journal of Anaesthesiology* 1993; **40:** 279.

3 Williamson J. A., Webb R. K., Szekely S., Gillies E. R. N. and Dreosti A. V. Difficult intubation: an analysis of 2000 incident reports. *Anaesthesia and Intensive Care* 1993; **21:** 602.

4 Kopman A. F., Wollman S. B., Ross K. and Surks S. N. Awake intubation: a review of 267 cases. *Anesthesia and Analgesia* 1975; **54:** 323.

5 Thomas J. L. Awake intubation. Indications, techniques and a review of 25 patients. *Anaesthesia* 1969; **24:** 28.

6 Giuffridda J. G., Bizzari D. V., Latteri F. S., Berger H. C., Schmookler A. and Flerro F. E. Prevention of major airway complications during anaesthesia by intubation of the conscious patient. *Currrent Research in Anesthesia and Analgesia* 1960; **39:** 201.

7 Walts L. F. Anaesthesia of the larynx in the patient with a full stomach. *Journal of the American Medical Association* 1965; **192:** 705.

8 D'Hollander A. A., Monteny E., Sanders M. and Dubois-Primo J. Intubation under topical supraglottic analgesia in unpremedicated and non fasting patients: amnesic effects of sub hypnotic doses of diazepam and Innovar. *Canadian Anesthetists Society Journal* 1974; **21:** 467.

9 Kopriva C. J., Eltringham R. J. and Siebert M. Q. A comparison of the effects of intravenous Innovar and topical spray on the laryngeal closure reflex. *Anesthesiology* 1974; **40:** 596.

10 Libman R. H. Topical anaesthesia and intubation. *Journal of the American Medical Association* 1976; **236:** 2393.

11 Ovassapian A., Krejcie T., Yelich S. and Dykes M. (1989) Awake fiberoptic intubation in the patient at a high risk of aspiration. *British Journal of Anaesthesia* 1989; **62:** 13.

12 Tomori Z. and Widdicombe J. G. Muscular bronchomotor and cardiovascular reflexes elicited by mechanical stimulation of the respiratory tract. *Journal of Physiology* 1969; **200:** 25.

13 Pedersen B. Blind nasaltracheal intubation. A review and a new guided technique. *Acta Anaesthesiologica Scandinavica* 1971; **15:** 107.

14 Geffin, B. Anaesthesia and the problem upper airway. *International Anesthesiology Clinics* 1990; **28:** 106.

15 Suderman V. S., Crosby E. T. and Lui A. Occasional review: elective oro-tracheal intubation in cervical spine-injured adults. *Canadian Journal of Anaesthesiology* 1991; **38:** 785.

16 Meschino A., Devitt J. H., Koch J. P., Szalai J. P. and Schwartz M. L. The safety of awake tracheal intubation in cervical spine injury. *Canadian Journal of Anaesthesiology* 1992; **39:** 114.

17 Majernick T. G., Houston J. B. and Hughes H. T. Cervical spine movement during orotracheal intubation. *Atlanta Emergency Medicine* 1986; **15:** 417.

18 Redden R. L., Bierry K. A. and Campbell R. L. Arterial oxygen desaturation during awake endotracheal intubation. *Anaesthesia Progress* 1990; **37:** 201.

19 Dohi S., Inomata S., Tanaka M., Ishizawa Y. and Matsumiya M. End tidal carbon dioxide monitoring during awake blind nasotracheal intubation. *Journal of Clinical Anaesthesia* 1990; **2:** 415.

20 Cossham P. S. Difficult Intubation (letter). *Lancet* 1987; **2:** 1034.

21 Dundee J. W. and Haslett W. H. K. The benzodiazepines. A review of their actions and uses relative to anaesthetic practice. *British Journal of Anaesthesia* 1970; **42:** 217.

22 Baird E. A. and Hailey D. M. Delayed recovery from a sedative: correlation of plasma levels of diazepam with clinical effects after oral and intravenous administration. *British Journal of Anaesthesia* 1972; **44:** 803.

23 Kaplan S. A., Jack M. L., Alexander K. and Weinfield R. E. Pharmacokinetic profile of diazepam in man following single intravenous and oral and chronic oral administration. *Journal of Pharmacological Science* 1973; **62:** 1789.

24 Brown C. R., Sanquist F. H., Canup C. A. and Pedley T. A. Clinical electroencephalographic and pharmacokinetic studies of a water-soluble benzodiazepine, midazolam maleate. *Anesthesiology* 1979; **50:** 467.

25 Shou Olesen A. and Huttel M. S. Local reactions to IV diazepam in three different formulations. *British Journal of Anaesthesia* 1980; **52:** 609.

26 McKenzie N. and Grant I. S. Comparison of the new emulsion formulation of propofol with methohexitone and thiopentone for induction of anaesthesia in day cases. *British Journal of Anaesthesia* 1985; **57:** 725.

27 Barker P., Langdon J. A., Wilson I. G. and Smith G. Movements of the vocal cords on induction of anaesthesia with thiopentone or propofol. *British Journal of Anaethesia* 1992; **69:** 23.

28 Wilkins C. J., Cramp P. G. W., Staples J. and Stevens W. C. Comparison of the anesthetic requirement for tolerance of laryngeal mask airway and endotracheal tube. *Anesthesia and Analgesia* 1992; **75:** 794.

29 Fry W. A. (1978) Techniques of topical anaesthesia for bronchoscopy. *Anaesthesia* 1978; **73:** 694.

30 Wight R. G. and Cochrane T. A. A comparison of the effects of two commonly used vasoconstrictors on nasal mucosal blood flow and nasal airflow. *Acta Otolaryngology (Stockholm)* 1990; **109:** 137.

31 Gross J. B., Hartigan M. L. and Schaffer D. W. A

suitable substitute for 4% cocaine before blind naso-tracheal intubation: 3% lidicaine-0.25% phenyl-ephrine nasal spray. *Anesthesia and Analgesia* 1984; **63:** 915.

32 Boulton T. B. Anaesthesia in difficult circumstances; the use of local analgesia. *Anaesthesia* 1967; **22:** 101.

33 Duncan J. A. T. Intubation of the trachea in the conscious patient. *Anaesthesia* 1977; **49:** 619.

34 Sidhu V. S., Whitehead E. M., Ainsworth Q. P., Smith M. and Calder I. A technique of awake fiberoptic intubation: experience in patients with cervical spine disease. *Anaesthesia* 1993; **48:** 910.

35 Mongan P. D. and Culling R. D. Rapid oral intubation for awake intubation. *Journal of Clinical Anaesthesia* 1992; **4:** 101.

36 Palva T., Jokinen K., Saloheimo M. and Karvonen P. Ultrasonic nebuliser in local anaesthesia for bronchoscopy. *Journal of Oto-Rhino-Laryngology* 1975; **37:** 306.

37 Bahman V., Venugopal P. and Con G. P. Effects of aerolised lidocaine on circulatory responses to laryngoscopy and tracheal intubation. *Critical Care Medicine* 1984; **12:** 391.

38 Bourke D. L., Katz J. and Tonneson A. Nebulised anaesthesia for awake endotracheal intubation. *Anesthesiology* 1985; **63:** 690.

39 Kong A. S., O'Meara M. E. and Chung D. C. Awake endobronchial intubation. *Anaesthesia and Intensive Care* 1993; **21:** 261.

40 Allen H. L. Letter: rediscovering the larynx. *Anesthesia and Analgesia* 1983; **62:** 855.

41 Gold M. and Bluechel D. Complications of cricothyroid puncture reviewed. *Anesthesiology* 1959; **20:** 181.

42 Baddour H. M., Hubbard A. M. and Tilson H. B. Maxillary nerve block used prior to awake nasal intubation. *Anaesthesia Progress* 1979; **26:** 43.

43 Cooper M. M. and Watson R. L. An improved regional anesthetic technique for peroral endoscopy *Anesthesiology* 1975; **43:** 372.

44 De Meester T. R., Skinner D. B., Evans R. H. and Benson D. W. Local nerve block anesthesia for peroral endoscopy. *Annals of Thoracic Surgery* 1977; **24:** 278.

45 Macintosh R. R. and Ostlere G. *Local Analgesia. Head and Neck.* Edinburgh: E. S. Livingstone. 1955; p. 10.

46 Gaskill J. and Gillies D. Local Anaesthesia for peroral endoscopy using superior laryngeal nerve block with topical application. *Archives of Otolaryngology* 1966; **84:** 654.

47 Foldes F. F., Malloy R., McNall P. G. and Koukal L. R. Comparison of intravenously given local anaesthetic agents in man. *Journal of the American Medical Association* 1960; **172:** 1493.

48 Eyres L. A., Bishop W., Oppenheim R. C. and Brown T. C. K. Plasma lignocaine concentrations following topical laryngeal application. *Anaesthesia and Intensive Care* 1983; **11:** 23.

49 Jones D. A., McBurney A., Stanley P. J., Tovey C. and Ward J. W. Plasma concentrations of lignocaine and its metabolites during fiberoptic bronchoscopy. *British Journal of Anaesthesia* 1982; **54:** 853.

50 Curran J., Hamilton C. and Taylor T. Topical analgesia before intubation. *Anaesthesia* 1975; **30:** 765.

51 Kautto U.-M. and Heinonen J. Attenuation of circulatory response to laryngoscopy and tracheal intubation; a comparison of two methods of topical anaesthesia. *Acta Anaesthesiologica Scandinavica* 1982; **26:** 599.

52 Mirakhur R. K. Bradycardia with laryngeal spraying in children. *Acta Anaesthesiologica Scandinavica* 1982; **26:** 130.

53 Ovassapian A., Yelich S. J., Dykes M. H. M. and Brunner E. E. Blood pressure and heart rate changes during awake fiberoptic nasotracheal intubation. *Anesthesia and Analgesia* 1983; **62:** 951.

54 Kapp P. J. Endotracheal intubation in patients with fractures of the cervical spine. *Journal of Neurosurgery* 1975; **42:** 731.

55 Kovac A. L. Use of Augustine stylet anticipating difficult tracheal intubation in Treacher–Collins syndrome. *Journal of Clinical Anaesthesia* 1992; **4:** 409.

56 Ovassapian A., Yelich S. J., Dykes M. H. M. and Brunner E. E. Fibro-optic nasotracheal intubation – incidence and causes of failure. *Anesthesia and Analgesia* 1983; **62:** 692.

57 Dyson A., Saunders T. R., Giescheah A. H. and Duncan J. A. T. Intubation of the trachea in the conscious patient. *Anaesthesia* 1977; **49:** 619.

58 Mostert J. W. Contra-indication to awake intubation. *Anaesthesia* 1969; **24:** 495.

59 Edens E. T. and Sia R. L. Flexible fiberoptic endoscopy in difficult situations. *Annals of Otolaryngology* 1981; **90:** 307.

60 Markakis D. A., Sayson S. C. and Schreiner M. S. Insertion of the laryngeal mask airway in awake infants with the Robin syndrome. *Anesthesia and Analgesia* 1992; **75:** 822.

61 Benumof J. L. Use of the laryngeal mask airway to facilitate fibroscope aided tracheal intubation. *Anesthesia and Analgesia* 1991; **74:** 313.

62 Maekawa N., Mikawa K. and Tanaka O. *et al.* The laryngeal mask may be a useful device for fiberoptic airway endoscopy in paediatric anaesthesia. *Anesthesiology* 1991; **75:** 169.

63 Dasey N. and Mansour N. Coughing and laryngospasm with the laryngeal mask. *Anaesthesia* 1989; **44:** 865.

64 Asai T. Fiberoptic intubation through the laryngeal mask in an awake patient with cervical spine injury. *Anesthesia and Analgesia* 1993; **77:** 398.

65 Davidson A. J., Reynolds M. D. and Stewart E. T. Use of a flexible, radio-opaque directable catheter

for difficult tracheal intubations. *Anesthesiology* 1981; **55:** 604.

66 Fox D. S., Castro T. and Rasthelli A. S. Comparison of intubation techniques in the awake patient. The Flexi-lum Surgical Light (Light wand) versus blind nasal approach. *Anesthesiology* 1987; **66:** 69.

67 Ellis D. G., Jakymec A., Kaplan R. H., Stewart R. D., Freeman J. A., Bleyaert A. and Beikebile P. E. Guided orotracheal intubation in the operating room using a lighted stylet: a comparison with direct laryngoscopic technique. *Anaesthesiology* 1986; **64:** 823.

68 Fox D. J. and Matson M. D. Management of the difficult paediatric airway in an austere environment using the light wand. *Journal of Clinical Anaesthesia* 1990; **2:** 123.

69 Salem M. R., Resce T. M. and Ziegler J. Intubation guide. US Patent No 380–2440. 1974.

70 Chortkoff B. S., Perlman B. and Cohen N. H. Delayed pneumothorax following difficult tracheal intubation. *Anesthesiology* 1992; **77:** 1225.

71 Eldor J. and Gozal Y. The length of the blade is more important than its design. *Canadian Journal of Anaesthesiology* 1990; **37:** 268.

72 MacIntyre J. W. Laryngoscope design and the difficult tracheal intubation. *Canadian Journal of Anaesthesiology* 1989; **36:** 94.

73 Richardson R. H. Endotracheal tube bronchoscopy. *Annals of Internal Medicine* 1972; **76:** 512.

74 Pitarn S., Brense A., Cell M. D. and Maler L. E. Awake fiberoptic endobronchial intubation. *Journal of Cardiothoracic Anaesthesia* 1990; **4:** 229.

75 Edwards R. M. Awake, blind nasal intubation (letter). *Anaesthesia and Intensive Care* 1993; **21:** 258.

76 Nakatsuka M. and MacLeod D. A. Hemo-dynamic and respiratory effects of transtracheal high-frequency jet ventilation during difficult intubation. *Journal of Clinical Anesthesia* 1992; **4:** 321.

77 Boucek C. D., Gunnerson H. B. and Tullock W. C. Percutaneous transtracheal high frequency jet ventilation as an aid to fiberoptic intubation. *Anesthesiology* 1987; **67:** 247.

78 Carlson C. A. and Perkins M. H. Solving a difficult intubation (letter). *Anesthesiology* 1986; **64:** 537.

79 Veyckemans F., Matta A., Gribomont B. F. and Kestens-Servaye Pre, per and post operative care of the infant. A safe alternative to awake intubation in neonates. *Acta Anaesthesiologica Belgica* 1985; **3:** 143.

80 Stow P. J., McLeod M. E., Burrows F. A. and Creighton R. E. Anterior fontanelle pressure responses to tracheal intubation in the awake and anaesthetised infant. *British Journal of Anaesthesia* 1988; **60:** 167.

81 Rosenberg D. B. and Gross J. B. Awake, blind nasotracheal intubation for caesarian section in a patient with autoimmune thrombocytopenic perpura and iatrogenic Cushing's syndrome. *Anesthesia and Analgesia* 1993; **77:** 853.

82 Mokriski B. L. K., Malinow A. M. and Gray W. C. Topical nasopharyngeal anaesthesia with vasoconstriction in preeclampsia–eclampsia. *Canadian Journal of Anaesthesiology* 1988; **35:** 641.

83 Ralstan D. H., Shnider S. M. and Delorimeter A. A. Effects of equipotent ephedrine, metara-minolol, mephenteramine and methoxamine on uterine blood flow in the pregnant ewe. *Anaesthesia* 1974; **40:** 354.

84 Benumof J. L. (1991) Management of the difficult adult airway with special emphasis on awake tracheal intubation. *Anesthesiology* 1991; **75:** 1087.

85 Zuck D. A technique for tracheal-bronchial toilet in conscious patient. *Anaesthesia* 1951; **6:** 226.

# 8

# Role of the Laryngeal Mask in Patients with Difficult Tracheal Intubation and Difficult Ventilation

*Takashi Asai and Peter Latto*

## INTRODUCTION

The role of the laryngeal mask airway in the management of difficult airways has been gaining increasing attention. There have been a number of reports of the successful use of the laryngeal mask in patients in whom tracheal intubation or ventilation through a facemask, or both, were difficult.

More than 10% of the published reports of the use of the laryngeal mask refer to this subject. Based on these clinical reports, it has been suggested that the laryngeal mask may be used electively in patients with difficult airways. The laryngeal mask also has a potential role for failed tracheal intubation and failed ventilation through a facemask. The successful insertion of the laryngeal mask facilitates oxygen delivery. It is, however, sometimes difficult to insert the laryngeal mask, and it is not always possible to predict when this difficulty will occur (see Chapter 9).

In this chapter the following topics are discussed.

- the use of the laryngeal mask as the aid to tracheal intubation;
- the techniques of insertion of the laryngeal mask and the subsequent tracheal intubation in fully awake or sedated patients;
- the role of the laryngeal mask in patients with difficult tracheal intubation and ventilation;
- the use of the laryngeal mask in patients with airway problems;
- the possible role of the laryngeal mask outside the operating theatre.

## USE OF THE LARYNGEAL MASK FOR TRACHEAL INTUBATION

The trachea can be intubated by passing a tracheal tube through the laryngeal mask. Since the first description of the technique by Brain [1], several methods of tracheal intubation using the laryngeal mask have been reported [2–7]. These methods have been successfully used in patients with known difficult intubation [5, 6] or in patients in whom tracheal intubation with either a laryngoscope or a fibreoptic bronchoscope, or both, had failed [8, 9].

### Blind Tracheal Intubation through the Laryngeal Mask

A tracheal tube can be passed blindly through the laryngeal mask into the trachea. In one report, the trachea was intubated blindly through the laryngeal mask in 72% of patients at the first attempt and in 96% of patients when time was not limited [10]. Similar results are reported in children [11]. Considerable practice, however, is required to master this blind method (see below).

The reported high success rate of blind tracheal intubation through the laryngeal mask was obtained in patients in whom tracheal intubation was anticipated to be easy [10, 11]. The success rate of correct positioning of the laryngeal mask may be lower in patients in whom tracheal intubation is considered to be difficult. It has been

shown that insertion of the laryngeal mask is more difficult than usual when neck movements are restricted [12]. In addition, blind tracheal intubation through the laryngeal mask is probably more difficult when the laryngeal mask is not correctly positioned. Therefore, in patients in whom tracheal intubation is considered to be difficult, the success rate of blind tracheal intubation through the laryngeal mask is more likely to be lower than in patients with normal airways. It is, however, not known whether the success rate of blind intubation through the laryngeal mask is higher than that of other methods of tracheal intubation (without using the laryngeal mask) in patients in whom tracheal intubation is predicted to be difficult.

The laryngeal mask should not be used in anaesthetized patients who are at risk of pulmonary aspiration of gastric contents. However, it may be used in emergency situations after failed tracheal intubation and ventilation through a facemask. Blind tracheal intubation through the laryngeal mask may not be safe in this situation, because cricoid pressure may be compromised if a tracheal tube is inadvertently pushed into the hypopharynx. This may allow regurgitation of gastric contents into the oropharynx and trachea. A tracheal tube might be passed through the laryngeal mask and be inadvertently inserted into the oesophagus. In this situation, the tracheal tube may drain regurgitated materials, but it is not possible to ventilate either through a tracheal tube or through the laryngeal mask. Therefore, the use of a fibreoptic bronchoscope is recommended when tracheal intubation through the laryngeal mask is attempted in patients at risk of pulmonary aspiration.

### Intubation method

The following procedure should increase the success rate of blind insertion of a tracheal tube (or bougie or lighted bougie) through the laryngeal mask.

- Before insertion of the laryngeal mask, a well-lubricated tracheal tube is inserted into the mask until the tip of the tube just passes through the grille of the mask.
- The tracheal tube is marked (the first mark) at this point where it enters the tube of the laryngeal mask (Fig. 1).
- A second mark is made on the tracheal tube 3 cm above the first mark (Fig. 1). When the

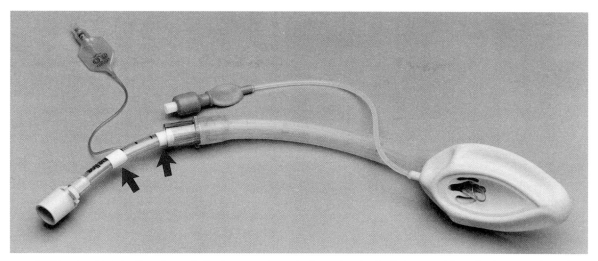

**Figure 1** Tracheal intubation through the laryngeal mask. A tracheal tube is inserted into the laryngeal mask until the tube just passes through the grille of the mask. The tracheal tube is marked at the point where it enters the tube of the laryngeal mask (right arrow). The second mark is made 3 cm proximal to the tracheal tube connector (left arrow). The tip of the tracheal tube would nearly reach to the glottis when the second mark disappears into the tube of the laryngeal mask during insertion of the tracheal tube.

laryngeal mask is inserted in the correct position, the distance between the grille of the mask and the vocal cords is about 3.5 cm in males and 3.0 cm in females [13]. Thus, the second mark on the tracheal tube indicates that the tip of the tracheal tube would almost have reached the vocal cords as the tube is passed through the laryngeal mask.

- The patient's head is extended and the neck flexed as the 'sniffing the morning air' position. The laryngeal mask is inserted, the cuff inflated, and adequacy of ventilation is assessed. If there is either total or a partial obstruction, the mask should be removed and another attempt made. The breathing system can be connected to the tracheal tube and oxygen given throughout the procedure.
- The tracheal tube is inserted into the tube of the laryngeal mask and the tip of the tracheal tube is gently advanced through the grille of the mask. The tip of the tube should curve anteriorly, not laterally. The first mark on the tracheal tube indicates the point where the tip of the tracheal tube just passes the grille of the mask. If resistance is felt at this point, it is likely that the tracheal tube has impacted upon the grille. Resistance will also be felt if the epiglottis lies between the grille and the vocal cords and obstructs the passage of the tube. This will

occur when the first mark, but not the second mark, on the tracheal tube has disappeared into the laryngeal mask.

Resistance of the tube at the grille may be overcome by rotating the tube up to 90° anticlockwise. If resistance is felt after the first, but not the second, mark on the tracheal tube disappears, it is likely that the epiglottis is obstructing the passage. Both the laryngeal mask and the tracheal tube should be removed and the procedure should be either abandoned or another attempt made. When a tracheal tube with a tapered tip (Moore tube) [14] (see Chapter 6) is used, the incidence of impact of the tracheal tube at the grille of the mask should be reduced.

Alternatively, the laryngeal mask can be inserted with a tracheal tube in place. When they are to be inserted together, the tip of the tracheal tube should be positioned just beyond the grille of the mask. This prevents the tracheal tube from impacting upon the grille of the mask during the advance of the tube. It also prevents the tube from passing through the side window of the grille, which may cause lateral deviation of the tube from the laryngeal inlet.

- The tracheal tube is advanced until the second mark disappears into the tube of the laryngeal mask. When resistance is felt at this point, it is likely that the tip of the tracheal tube has now reached the glottis and is pressing on the anterior part of the larynx or tracheal wall. The thyroid cartilage may be pushed anteriorly by the tip of the tracheal tube (see Fig. 33, p. 141, Chapter 10).

If the tube curves laterally, it might impact in the pyriform fossa, and the lateral side of the neck will bulge. This, however, occurs only rarely when the mask is correctly placed. If the side of the neck bulges, the tube should be withdrawn to the first mark and advanced again.

- When resistance is felt and the thyroid cartilage is pushed anteriorly, insertion of the tracheal tube is temporarily stopped, or the tracheal tube is slightly withdrawn. The head is now flexed on the neck as for blind nasotracheal intubation. This flexion of the head disengages the tip of the tracheal tube from the anterior wall of the larynx and aligns the axes of the trachea and the tracheal tube, facilitating insertion of the tube into the trachea.

- If there is no resistance when the tracheal tube is advanced about 5–6 cm beyond the grille of the mask and the thyroid cartilage has not been pushed anteriorly, the tracheal tube may have been inserted into the oesophagus, or alternatively the tube may be in the trachea. Thus, position of the tracheal tube should be examined by auscultation, capnography or an oesophageal detector device. If the tube is not in the trachea, the tube is withdrawn until the first mark comes out of the laryngeal mask and another attempt made to insert the tube into the trachea.

- Correct placement of the tracheal tube in the trachea should be confirmed at the end of the procedure.

## Bougie-aided Tracheal Intubation

A bougie or stylet can be used to aid tracheal intubation through the laryngeal mask [4]. A high success rate may be obtained by using a gum elastic bougie with the tip bent forwards [15]. The shaped bougie is inserted through the laryngeal mask until it passes through the glottis. The entry of the bougie into the trachea can be detected by a typical 'clicking' sensation felt during advancement of the tip of the bougie over the tracheal cartilages and by the inability to advance the bougie further at a point when the tip of the bougie reaches the small bronchi ('hold up') [16].

After insertion of a bougie into the trachea, the laryngeal mask can be removed and a tracheal tube passed over the bougie into the trachea. Alternatively, a small tracheal tube can be passed through the laryngeal mask over the bougie. This technique was used successfully in an awake patient with a past history of a difficult intubation [3]. However, failures have also been reported [17–20].

## Lighted Stylet-aided Tracheal Intubation

A lighted stylet may also be used for tracheal intubation through the laryngeal mask. The transillumination of the tissues of the neck is a reliable sign that the stylet is in the trachea rather than in the oesophagus [21]. The light will disappear as the stylet is advanced behind the sternum.

The lighted stylet should be long enough and flexible enough to pass through the laryngeal mask into the trachea. The Trachlight™ wand (Laerdal Medical Corporation, New York, USA) may be suitable, as it has a long wand (about 35 cm) and the inner rigid stylet can be withdrawn (Fig. 2) [2, 22]. It has been shown that insertion of this lighted stylet through the laryngeal mask into the trachea is easy [22]. The inner metal stylet is partially withdrawn and the Trachlight wand is curved. Transillumination of the tissues enables the user to assess the position of the tip of the stylet during insertion [22]. However, the success rate of tracheal intubation through the laryngeal mask using this stylet is not known.

## Fibrescope-aided Tracheal Intubation

Fibrescope-aided tracheal intubation through the laryngeal mask under direct vision is the most reliable of these methods. The fibrescope can be inserted into the trachea by changing the angle of its tip even if the axes of the tube of the laryngeal mask and the trachea are not aligned [8, 23]. In one study, the trachea was successfully intubated using this technique in 46 of 48 anaesthetized patients known to have difficult airways [6]. By connecting a tracheal tube and the breathing system using a purpose-built swivel connector, oxygen can be delivered while a fibreoptic bronchoscope is passed through the swivel connector, tracheal tube and into the trachea (Fig. 3).

### *Advantages*

There are several advantages of fibrescope-aided tracheal intubation through the laryngeal mask

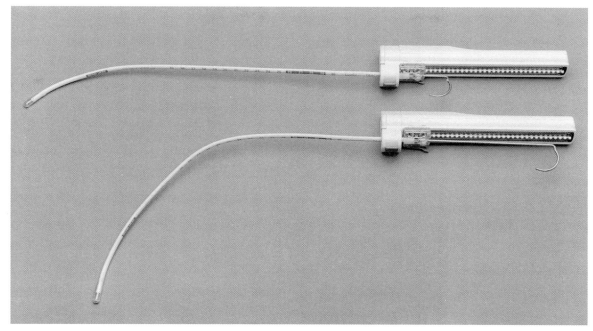

**Figure 2**   Light stylet-aided tracheal intubation. The Trachlight wand™ (Laerdal Medical Corporation) may be suitable for this purpose, as it has a long wand and the inner rigid stylet can be withdrawn (above). The inner metal stylet is partially withdrawn and the wand is curved (below). From Asai and Latto [22] with the permission of the publisher of *British Journal of Anaesthesia*.

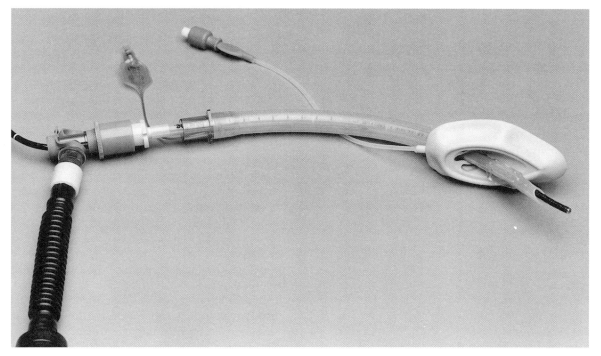

**Figure 3**   Use of a fibreoptic bronchoscope for tracheal intubation through the laryngeal mask. By connecting a tracheal tube and the breathing system using a purpose-built swivel connector, oxygen can be delivered while a fibreoptic bronchoscope is passed through the swivel connector, tracheal tube and into the trachea.

over conventional fibrescope-aided tracheal intubation. Location of the glottis by a fibreoptic bronchoscope without the aid of the laryngeal mask is sometimes difficult, particularly for inexperienced anaesthetists. When the laryngeal mask is in place, the glottis is usually positioned just below the grille of the mask and the distance between these is only a few centimetres (see Fig 2 in Chapter 9) [13]. Location of the glottis with a fibreoptic bronchoscope is therefore easy. For this reason tracheal intubation through the laryngeal mask using a fibreoptic bronchoscope is likely to be easier, particularly for inexperienced anaesthetists, than fibreoptic tracheal intubation without the laryngeal mask. There are, in fact, reports that the glottis was located easily when a fibrescope was inserted through the laryngeal mask in patients with a deviated larynx or with restricted neck movement, where the location of the glottis with the fibrescope alone had been difficult [5, 8].

With the conventional method, it is often difficult to advance a tracheal tube over the bronchoscope as it may impact upon the epiglottis, right arytenoid or hypopharynx [24, 25]. In contrast, tracheal intubation through the laryngeal mask over the fibrescope is usually easy, since obstructions such as the tongue, soft palate and epiglottis are bypassed, and lateral or posterior deviation of the tracheal tube from the glottis is restricted by the laryngeal mask [13, 26]. Tracheal intubation through the laryngeal mask is usually easy even when the larynx is deviated from the mid line once the fibrescope has been inserted into the trachea [8, 23].

## Retrograde Tracheal Intubation

The laryngeal mask has been used for retrograde intubation [27]. The laryngeal mask was inserted under general anaesthesia, and a cannula was then inserted through the cricothyroid membrane in a cephalad direction. A guide wire was passed through the cannula into the larynx and advanced through the vocal cords, the tube of the laryngeal mask and swivel connector. A long Teflon catheter was passed from above over the guide wire into the trachea, and the guide wire removed. A tracheal tube was then passed over the Teflon cannula and advanced through the laryngeal mask into the trachea [27].

The use of the laryngeal mask during these procedures facilitates effective oxygenation. It is,

however, not known whether the technique using the laryngeal mask is easier than conventional retrograde intubation where the laryngeal mask is not used. It has been suggested that the success rate would be increased using a straight guide wire as coiling in the bowl of the laryngeal mask would be less likely to occur [27]. This technique is likely to be difficult and should not be used in preference to anterograde techniques.

## Nasotracheal Intubation

Blind nasotracheal tracheal intubation with the aid of the laryngeal mask in a patient with severe micrognathia has been reported [28] (Fig. 4). After induction of anaesthesia, a laryngeal mask was inserted and a suction catheter was passed through the laryngeal mask into the trachea. Another catheter was passed through the nose and taken out from the mouth. The laryngeal mask was removed and the two ends of the catheters were sutured together. The nasal end of the catheter was gently pulled to remove catheter loop in the oral cavity. A tracheal tube then was passed through a nostril over the catheter into the trachea (Fig. 4). This technique may be indicated in situations where a fibrescope is not available.

## Limitations

There are two major limitations associated with tracheal intubation through the laryngeal mask.

First, a 6.0–6.5 mm ID tracheal tube is the largest size that can be passed through the size 3 or 4 laryngeal mask. A 7.0 mm tracheal tube can be passed through the mask when a size 5 mask is used. It is possible to pass 4.5 mm and 3.5 mm tracheal tubes through the size 2 and 1 masks, respectively. A larger sized tracheal tube, of course, can be used if an introducer has been inserted through the laryngeal mask into the trachea and the mask removed [3, 4, 7, 8]. A modified laryngeal mask with a slit on the side of the tube and the mask has been proposed for the use of a large bore tube [29]. The disadvantage of the modified laryngeal mask is that although the introducer can be easily inserted into the trachea, passage of a tracheal tube over the introducer into the trachea may be difficult [24, 25].

Second, when a standard, uncut 6.0 mm tracheal tube (28–29 cm in length) is passed through the laryngeal mask into the trachea, the

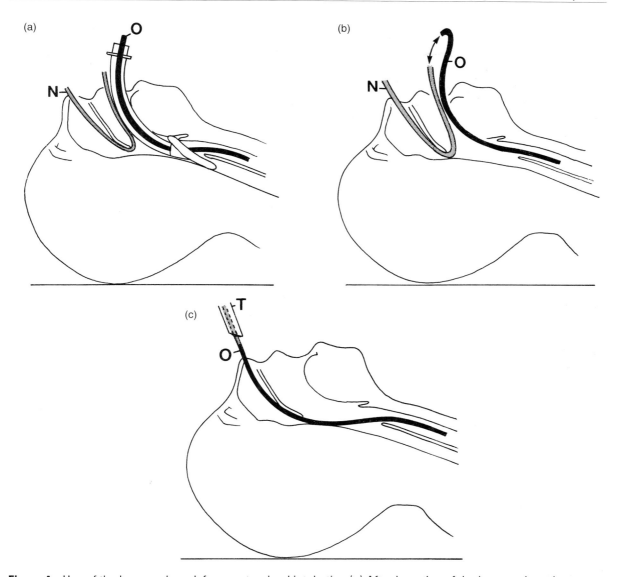

**Figure 4**   Use of the laryngeal mask for nasotracheal intubation.(a) After insertion of the laryngeal mask, a suction catheter (O) is passed through the laryngeal mask into the trachea. Another catheter (N) is passed through the nose and taken into the mouth. (b) The laryngeal mask is removed and the two ends of the catheters are sutured together. (c) The nasal end of the catheter is gently pulled to remove looping of the catheter in the oral cavity. A tracheal tube (T) is then is passed through a nostril over the catheter into the trachea. After Thomson [28] with permission.

cuff of the tracheal tube often lies between the vocal cords [13] (Fig. 5). This may lead to injury to the vocal cords or incomplete protection against pulmonary aspiration. To avoid this problem, the laryngeal mask can be removed after tracheal intubation. However, the tracheal tube may be inadvertently removed during removal of the laryngeal mask. This problem can be minimized by removing the mask while the proximal

end of the tracheal tube is gently being pushed with the tip of another tracheal tube [30]. However, it may be difficult to remove the laryngeal mask with this method as a pilot balloon of a tracheal tube may not be able to pass through the tube of the laryngeal mask. When a bougie is used to push on the tracheal tube, the laryngeal mask can be removed more easily.

A better option is to use a longer tracheal tube,

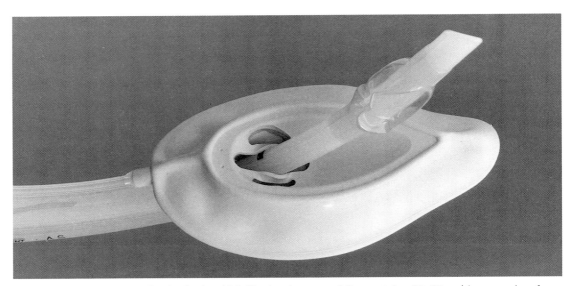

**Figure 5**    When a 6.0 mm tracheal tube (oral Mallinckrodt or nasal Portex tube: 28–29 cm) is passed as far as possible through the laryngeal mask, it projects about 8 cm beyond the grille of the mask. The distance between the grille of the mask and the proximal edge of the cuff of the tracheal tube is 3 cm. When the mask is in place, the distance between the grille of the mask and the vocal cords is often greater than 3 cm and thus, the cuff of the tracheal tube often lies between the vocal cords [13].

such as the 5.0 mm microlaryngeal Portex tube (30.5 cm) or 6.0 mm Mallinckrodt reinforced tube (31 cm). It is thus unnecessary to remove the laryngeal mask. The ST (short)-laryngeal mask has a tube that is 2 cm shorter than conventional length. This allows the tracheal tube to be advanced further through the mask [13]. Only a size 3 ST-laryngeal mask is available in the UK.

## Intubating Laryngeal Mask

The 'intubating' laryngeal mask, a modified device particularly designed for tracheal intubation, is under development by the inventor [31]. A prototype of the intubating laryngeal mask consists of the standard mask, a preshaped metal tube and a handle. The tube of the intubating laryngeal mask is large enough to allow insertion of a 9.0 mm tracheal tube. The mask can be pressed against the hard palate during insertion without insertion of the index finger into the oral cavity, since the tube is made of metal and is rigid. The tube of this prototype is shorter (about 4 cm less) than that of the standard laryngeal mask. Therefore, the cuff of a tracheal tube is less likely to lie between the vocal cords after tracheal intubation through the laryngeal mask. A metal handle is attached to the proximal edge of the tube. The handle is to hold the device and to control the angle of the aperture of the mask.

## INSERTION OF THE LARYNGEAL MASK IN AWAKE OR SEDATED PATIENTS

### Insertion of the Laryngeal Mask in Awake Patients

It is safer to secure the airway when the patient is awake if great difficulty in tracheal intubation or ventilation is predicted. The laryngeal mask can be inserted either when patients are fully awake or when they are sedated. The mask can then be used to facilitate tracheal intubation before induction of anaesthesia (see below). Alternatively, when it is deemed safe, a tracheal tube can be passed through the laryngeal mask either under a deeper level of sedation or after induction of anaesthesia [26]. Several methods of awake tracheal intubation using the laryngeal mask have been reported.

There is one report of insertion of the laryngeal mask in awake infants with the Pierre–Robin syndrome. Ventilation through a facemask was anticipated to be difficult. The laryngeal mask was inserted while the patients were awake and provided a satisfactory airway during induction of anaesthesia [32].

## *Insertion method*

A local anaesthetic, such as 10% lignocaine, is sprayed onto the back of the tongue and oropharynx. Bilateral superior laryngeal nerve block also provides good anaesthesia of the laryngopharynx. The laryngeal mask can then be inserted with minimum discomfort to patients.

Gagging or coughing may, however, occur during insertion of the mask when only topical anaesthesia is applied to the upper airway in the absence of sedation. Small doses of sedatives and an analgesic can be given intravenously to facilitate insertion. When patients are fully awake or lightly sedated, the incidence of gagging may be lower when patients are encouraged to swallow during the insertion. The success rate of insertion and the incidence of complications in awake children are unknown. The laryngeal mask has been used during resuscitation of neonates, and in one study, the laryngeal mask was successfully inserted at the first attempt in all of 20 neonates, without administration of anaesthesia [33].

## Awake Tracheal Intubation through the Laryngeal Mask

The laryngeal mask can be used to aid tracheal intubation in awake patients. This method may be useful, because there is little risk of loss of the airway even if insertion of the mask or tracheal intubation through the laryngeal mask is difficult or impossible.

Awake fibrescope-aided tracheal intubation through the laryngeal mask has been used in patients with a past history of difficult tracheal intubation with a laryngoscope [3] and in those in whom conventional fibrescope-aided tracheal intubation had been difficult or had failed [5, 8].

This method can also be used in patients in whom awake tracheal intubation is indicated, such as in patients with mediastinal masses [8]. This is also useful in patients at high risk of pulmonary aspiration of gastric contents, because airway reflexes will not be lost and pulmonary aspiration is less likely to occur [26].

## ROLE OF THE LARYNGEAL MASK IN PATIENTS WITH DIFFICULT TRACHEAL INTUBATION AND VENTILATION

There have been a number of reports of the successful use of the laryngeal mask in patients in whom difficult tracheal intubation or ventilation through a facemask, or both, were predicted. The reported reasons for difficult tracheal intubation in adults include a previous history of difficult intubation [3, 4, 34], limited mouth opening [4, 35, 36], and restricted neck movements [6, 37]. In neonates and children, Pierre–Robin syndrome [32, 38], Treacher–Collins syndrome [39], Apert syndrome [40] and cleft palate [40] have caused difficulties in tracheal intubation.

The laryngeal mask permitted ventilation in patients in whom tracheal intubation had failed [1, 9, 41–43], and it has also been used when both ventilation through a facemask and tracheal intubation had been difficult [17, 34, 44–46].

These reports of successful use of the laryngeal mask after failed tracheal intubation support a potential role for the laryngeal mask in patients in whom airway management is difficult, but careful consideration is necessary. Principally, the laryngeal mask should not be regarded as a substitute for a tracheal tube, even if the laryngeal mask has successfully enabled ventilation to be accomplished in patients in whom tracheal intubation failed. Tracheal intubation would probably have been preferable to the laryngeal mask in those cases.

There are three occasions when the laryngeal mask may be useful in clinical practice (Tables 1 and 2):

- elective use in patients in whom difficult tracheal intubation or difficulty in ventilation through a facemask, or both, is predicted;
- failed tracheal intubation, but ventilation through a facemask is adequate;
- failed tracheal intubation, failed ventilation through a facemask.

## Elective Use of the Laryngeal Mask

### *Very difficult tracheal intubation is predicted*

Awake tracheal intubation should be performed when great difficulty is predicted. The laryngeal

**Table 1**    Elective use of the laryngeal mask in patients in whom difficult tracheal intubation or ventilation through a facemask, or both, are predicted

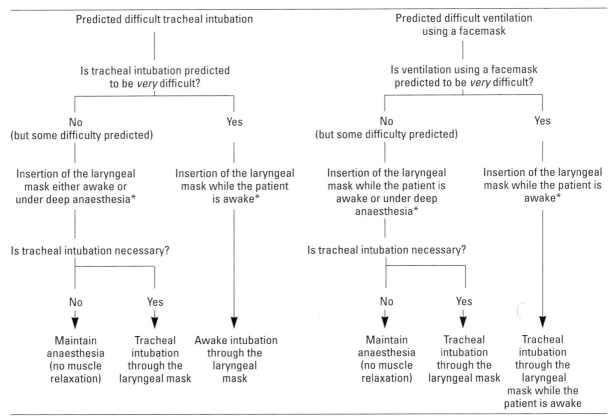

In all cases, where difficulty in tracheal intubation or ventilation is predicted, the use of long acting muscle relaxants should be avoided until the trachea is intubated.

\*    The algorithm only shows the possible use of the laryngeal mask in each situation. There are several alternative methods that are commonly used.

These include:

• Attempts at tracheal intubation under general anaesthesia;

• Awake tracheal intubation with either a laryngoscope or fibreoptic bronchoscope.

mask can be used to facilitate tracheal intubation. In these circumstances, the laryngeal mask should be inserted while the patient is awake. When used in this way, there is little danger to the patient even if insertion of the laryngeal mask fails. If difficulty in insertion of the mask or ventilation occurs, the mask can be promptly removed and the airway remains patent. Once the mask has been successfully inserted, a tracheal tube should be passed through the laryngeal mask while the patient is awake.

### *Some difficulty in tracheal intubation is predicted*

The laryngeal mask may be used to maintain the airway in patients in whom some, but not extreme, difficulty in tracheal intubation is predicted. Once

the laryngeal mask is successfully inserted, maintenance of the airway may be easier than with the facemask [47]. There is, however, a danger of the 'cannot intubate, cannot ventilate' scenario if laryngospasm or bronchospasm occurs while the laryngeal mask is used.

It may be safer to insert the laryngeal mask while the patient remains awake when difficult tracheal intubation is predicted. If it is considered acceptable, the mask might be inserted after induction of anaesthesia. It should be noted, however, that the laryngeal mask does not always provide a patent airway. Insertion of the laryngeal mask may fail in up to 6–8% (up to 33% at the first attempt) of patients who are predicted to be easy to intubate [48, 49], although almost 100%

**Table 2**    Emergency use of the laryngeal mask after failed tracheal intubation or difficulty in ventilation through a facemask, or both

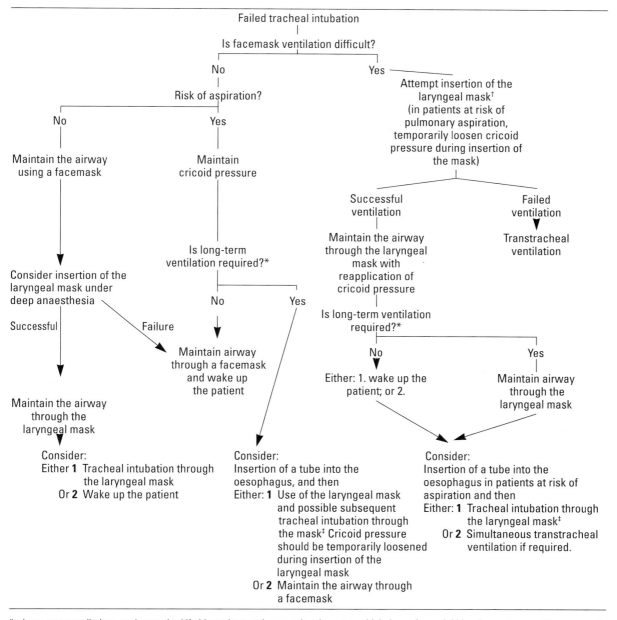

---

\*    Long-term ventilation may be required if either a long acting muscle relaxant or a high dose of an opioid has been given, or if the surgery is very urgent and there is no time to allow the patient to recover consciousness.

†    Attempts at insertion of the laryngeal mask after failed tracheal intubation and after failed ventilation using a facemask would be particularly useful if one is not familiar with other device, such as a transtracheal airway or the Esophageal Tracheal Combitube. The latter are rarely used in the UK.

‡    Attempts at tracheal intubation through the laryngeal mask should ideally be performed by anaesthetists experienced with the technique, and a fibreoptic bronchoscope should be used.

success rate at the first attempt can be achieved by mastering the correct insertion method. The failure rate of insertion of the laryngeal mask is likely to be higher in patients in whom difficult

tracheal intubation is predicted, in particular when neck movement or mouth opening is limited. There are several reports of either failure of insertion or difficulty in ventilation through the laryngeal mask in patients in whom difficult tracheal intubation was predicted [6, 40, 50–52]. In addition, it may not be possible to reinsert the laryngeal mask if it becomes dislodged. Muscle relaxation decreases the pharyngeal integrity [53], which could make insertion more difficult.

It is important to maintain a sufficient depth of anaesthesia to prevent laryngospasm while the laryngeal mask is used. It may be safer not to paralyse these patients. However, in some circumstances a low dose of short acting muscle relaxant may be used to facilitate insertion of the laryngeal mask or to relieve laryngospasm.

Tracheal intubation can be performed with the aid of the laryngeal mask either while the patient is awake or while the patient is deeply anaesthetized. If it is considered safe, a short acting muscle relaxant may be given before tracheal intubation.

### Great difficulty in ventilation through a facemask is predicted

When ventilation through a facemask is predicted to be very difficult or the patient has a history of difficulty in ventilation, the use of regional anaesthesia should be reconsidered. When general anaesthesia is proposed, awake tracheal intubation is the first choice. Insertion of the laryngeal mask and subsequent tracheal intubation through the mask can be performed while the patient is awake.

### Some difficulty in ventilation through a facemask is predicted

When some difficulty in ventilation through a facemask is predicted, the airway might be maintained with the laryngeal mask. The laryngeal mask may be inserted while patient is either awake or anaesthesized, based on the degree of expected difficulty in ventilation through a facemask. If required, tracheal intubation can be performed with the aid of the laryngeal mask.

## Failed Tracheal Intubation, Facemask Ventilation Adequate

There is no need to insert the laryngeal mask in patients in whom tracheal intubation has failed, but ventilation through a facemask is adequate. However, maintenance of a patent airway is probably easier with the laryngeal mask than with a facemask [47]. Thus, the laryngeal mask may be useful in some situations even when ventilation

using a facemask is possible after failed tracheal intubation (see below).

### Patients at low risk of pulmonary aspiration

When the patient is at low risk of pulmonary aspiration and it is considered acceptable to manage the airway without tracheal intubation, the laryngeal mask may be used instead of the facemask. Although there is a risk of causing laryngospasm during insertion, the airway may be easier to maintain with the laryngeal mask than with the facemask. Anaesthesia should be deepened before insertion of the laryngeal mask.

The laryngeal mask might be inserted for the purpose of subsequent tracheal intubation through the mask, but the success rate in this circumstance is not known.

### Patients at increased risk of pulmonary aspiration

#### Long-term ventilation is not required

In patients at increased risk of pulmonary aspiration, insertion of the laryngeal mask should not be attempted when ventilation through a facemask is adequate after rapid sequence induction of anaesthesia and after failed tracheal intubation. Insertion of the laryngeal mask may compromise the situation by causing laryngospasm. This problem is more likely to occur when the depth of anaesthesia and muscle relaxation have become inadequate after a rapid sequence induction of anaesthesia.

Adequate ventilation often cannot be obtained through the laryngeal mask when cricoid pressure is applied before insertion, even when ventilation through the facemask has been effective [12, 23, 54]. In addition, there may be a greater risk of dislodging the laryngeal mask if cricoid pressure is not released during insertion, because the distal part of the mask cannot be positioned correctly in the hypopharynx (Fig. 6). The success rate of tracheal intubation through the laryngeal mask is also low when cricoid pressure is applied before insertion of the mask [10, 23] (see Chapter 9 for detail). Therefore, the mask should not be inserted even for the subsequent tracheal intubation in this group of patients.

The airway should thus be maintained using a facemask and cricoid pressure constantly applied after rapid sequence induction of anaesthesia. Unless surgery is very urgent, the patient should

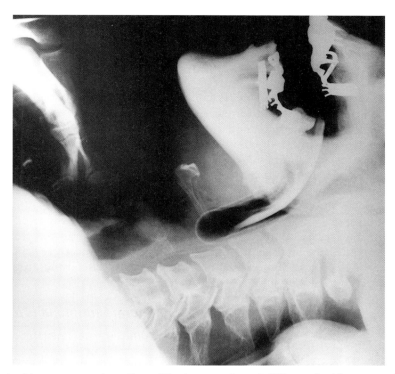

**Figure 6**   Effect of cricoid pressure on insertion of the laryngeal mask. When cricoid pressure is applied before insertion of the laryngeal mask, it prevents correct positioning of the laryngeal mask. When correctly positioned, the tip of the mask should be positioned at the level of the lower edge of cricoid cartilage. The tip of the mask is positioned above the level of both the arytenoid and cricoid cartilages by application of cricoid pressure. X-ray provided by Dr Aoyama and colleagues, University of Occupational and Environmental Health, Japan. (See also Figure 12 in Chapter 9.)

be allowed to recover consciousness and awake tracheal intubation should be attempted.

### Long-term ventilation is required

A long acting muscle relaxant may rarely be given to facilitate tracheal intubation in patients at increased risk of pulmonary aspiration. The anaesthetic management of patients at increased risk of pulmonary aspiration, in whom tracheal intubation has failed, and in whom a long acting muscle relaxation has been given, is a major challenge to anaesthetists. In such a situation, long-term ventilation will be required. Long-term airway management without tracheal intubation may also be required if the surgery is very urgent, and there is no time to allow the patient to recover consciousness.

When a facemask is used for a long duration and, in particular, cricoid pressure is kept applied, maintenance of a patent airway may become more difficult [47]. The effectiveness of cricoid pressure

may also decrease. In addition, gas may be insufflated into the stomach as a result of ineffective cricoid pressure. Furthermore, two people are required for maintenance of a patent airway and for application of cricoid pressure; a third person may therefore be required for other anaesthetic procedures.

Ventilation through the laryngeal mask might be more effective than a facemask in such a situation. Once the laryngeal mask has been successfully inserted, a patent airway can be maintained more easily than when a facemask is used [47]. In addition, one person may be able to apply cricoid pressure and also maintain the airway using the laryngeal mask. Gastric insufflation may be less likely to occur when the laryngeal mask is used than when a facemask is used. Tracheal intubation through the laryngeal mask using a fibreoptic bronchoscope might also be possible. When the laryngeal mask is to be inserted, anaesthesia should be deep enough and cricoid pressure should be temporarily loosened. This, however, increases the chance of regurgitation of gastric contents and subsequent pulmonary aspiration.

A tracheal tube may be intentionally inserted into the oesophagus to drain regurgitated materials before insertion of the laryngeal mask. It is possible to insert the laryngeal mask and to ventilate the lungs through the mask after insertion of a tracheal tube into the oesophagus [55]. However, the position of the laryngeal mask is more likely to be suboptimal if it is placed after a tracheal tube has been inserted into the oesophagus, because the hypopharynx is already occupied by the tracheal tube. Thus, the incidence of dislodgement of the mask is probably greater if the mask is inserted after insertion of a tube into the oesophagus. The position of the mask was not assessed in the above study [55].

A modified laryngeal mask, which enables drainage of regurgitated materials from the oesophagus, is under development by the inventor [56]. The modified laryngeal mask has a second tube, which is attached to the tube of the laryngeal mask, and the orifice of the second tube is in the truncated tip of the mask. Regurgitated material from the oesophagus can be drained through the second tube. By applying negative pressure to the second tube, regurgitated materials from the oesophagus may be less likely to enter the trachea. The effect, however, has not been studied. One of the disadvantages of this modified laryngeal mask is that it is more difficult to insert than the standard mask [56]. It is thus not known whether there is a role for this modified laryngeal mask after failed tracheal intubation in patients at increased risk of pulmonary aspiration.

The decision to use the laryngeal mask in this situation should be made based on the condition of each patient, duration of surgery and the anaesthetist's skill.

## Failed Tracheal Intubation and Failed Facemask Ventilation

The insertion of the laryngeal mask may be tried when both tracheal intubation and ventilation through a facemask have failed. In the UK, equipment for transtracheal ventilation may not be readily available, but the laryngeal mask is widely used. Thus, the use of the laryngeal mask could be the first choice in this situation. The decision to insert the mask should be made at an early stage.

Repeated attempts at insertion of the laryngeal mask should be avoided. If ventilation through the laryngeal mask is inadequate and hypoxia persists, a percutaneous transtracheal airway should be inserted without delay.

In patients at increased risk of pulmonary aspiration, cricoid pressure should be temporarily loosened during insertion of the laryngeal mask to increase the success rate of insertion, although this temporary release may allow regurgitation and pulmonary aspiration [12, 54]. Cricoid pressure should be reapplied after insertion of the mask until the trachea is intubated or until airway reflexes return. Recovery of spontaneous breathing does not guarantee return of airway reflexes [58]. Cricoid pressure applied after insertion of the mask effectively prevents regurgitation of gastric contents [57].

## Long-term ventilation is not required

When the laryngeal mask provides a patent airway and the patient is well oxygenated, the patient should be allowed to recover consciousness unless surgery is very urgent. Awake tracheal intubation, including awake intubation through the laryngeal mask, should then be considered.

## Long-term ventilation is required

When the laryngeal mask has been successfully inserted and adequate ventilation obtained, a decision should be made whether to perform a tracheostomy or continue the anaesthetic and planned surgery while the airway is maintained using the laryngeal mask. Tracheostomy can be performed while the airway is maintained through the laryngeal mask [17, 45, 59].

When a fibrescope is readily available and the relative position of the larynx to the mask can be assessed, fibreoptic tracheal intubation through the laryngeal mask could be tried. It is, however, advisable that this procedure should be performed by anaesthetists who are competent in this method. Once experience has been gained, this method is useful. Each situation will require an assessment of the possible risks, and an appropriate decision made for the individual patient.

## PARTICULAR USE IN PATIENTS WITH AIRWAY ABNORMALITIES

### Restricted mouth opening

It may be difficult to insert either a tracheal tube or the laryngeal mask when the patient's mouth opening is restricted. The laryngeal mask, however, has been successfully inserted to facilitate tracheal intubation in a patient with limited mouth opening [4]. The mask has also been used successfully in a patient with a maxillary tumour with an interdental gap of 6 mm [60]. In the latter report, after induction of anaesthesia, the tip of a fully deflated mask was inserted between the teeth and advanced upwards as far as possible towards the hard palate. The mask was then slid laterally towards the gap behind the molars. The thickest part of the mask (at the level of the aperture bars) was passed through the retromolar gap with some difficulty. The mask was subsequently moved back to the mid line and placed fully into position. The tube of the laryngeal mask was compressed, but not occluded, by the incisors [60].

Although it may be possible to insert the laryngeal mask in patients with restricted mouth opening, great caution is necessary. The use of the laryngeal mask in this situation should be regarded as contraindicated unless the anaesthetist has considerable experience with the device. It would be preferable to insert the mask while the patient is awake in such circumstances.

### Tracheostomy

The laryngeal mask may be useful during surgical or percutaneous tracheostomy. There are several reports of the use of the laryngeal mask during emergency tracheostomy after failed tracheal intubation and ventilation through a facemask [17, 45, 59]. The use of the laryngeal mask in this situation can be justified because it might be the only means of providing oxygenation while the tracheostomy is being performed.

The laryngeal mask may be used during elective tracheostomy in some patients. Caution is necessary if the tracheostomy is being performed because of pathology of the mouth, pharynx or larynx. Caution is also required if the patient is at increased risk of pulmonary aspiration of gastric contents, requires high pulmonary inflation pressures or has tracheomalacia.

The correct insertion of a needle into the lumen of the trachea during percutaneous tracheostomy is easily confirmed using a fibrescope passed through the laryngeal mask [61].

### Tracheal Stenosis

The laryngeal mask has been used in patients with tracheal stenosis [62–64]. Insertion of a tracheal tube increases resistance to ventilation, because it further narrows the diameter of the airway and induces reflex airway constriction [65]. Tracheal intubation may also cause oedema at the stenotic segment. The laryngeal mask does not, in contrast, enter the trachea and thus damage to the airway is unlikely to occur. Airway resistance is lower because the diameter of the tube of the laryngeal mask is much larger than that of the tracheal tube [66]. If the stenosis is in the proximal segment of the trachea, it may be difficult to position a tracheal tube proximal to the stenosis. The laryngeal mask can, however, be used irrespective of the location of the stenosis.

One of the limitations of this technique is that it is not suitable in patients who require high inflation pressures. Anaesthesia can be maintained more safely if the patient is allowed to breathe spontaneously [63]. The laryngeal mask should not be used in patients with tracheomalacia or external compression of the trachea, since it cannot reliably prevent collapse of the trachea [62].

There has been a report of the use of the laryngeal mask during placement of a stent at a stenotic region in the trachea [64]. The upper segment of the trachea became stenotic due to compression by a tumour. After the patient had been anaesthetized and paralyzed, a laryngeal mask was inserted. A catheter containing the stent was passed through the mask into the trachea and a stent was placed at the stenotic region. In this patient, however, there might have been a risk of airway obstruction after induction of anaesthesia. It is thus safer to insert the laryngeal mask and to pass either a catheter or a fibrescope through the laryngeal mask into the trachea, beyond the stenotic region, while the patient is awake. Jet ventilation can be commenced if the airway obstruction occurs after induction of anaesthesia but before placement of a stent.

## EMERGENCY MEDICINE

In emergency situations, airway management is often required. Tracheal intubation is the most reliable method of securing the airway, but it is not easy to master and practice is required to maintain competence [67]. Thus, until a person competent in tracheal intubation arrives, the airway is usually managed by other methods. The facemask and self inflating bag are commonly used, but effective ventilation is sometimes difficult [68, 69]. In some situations, for example when the patient is trapped in crashed car, it may be difficult to intubate the trachea or to apply a facemask.

The Esophageal Obturator Airway has been widely used during cardiopulmonary resuscitation in the USA. Effective ventilation through the Obturator is sometimes difficult, since ventilation may fail owing to difficulty in correct insertion or in securing a proper mask fit [69]. Ventilation is impossible when the Obturator is inadvertently inserted into the trachea. Several serious complications, such as oesophageal, gastric or tracheal rupture, have also been reported (see Chapter 14).

The Esophageal Tracheal Combitube is also recommended during cardiopulmonary resuscitation [70]. It can be inserted blindly, and head and neck movements are not required. Ventilation is possible if the Combitube is inserted into either the oesophagus or the trachea. The device, however, has several disadvantages. It cannot be used in patients with an intact gag reflex, in patients less than 16 years of age or in those less than 1.5 m tall [71]. It is also sometimes difficult to determine whether the tube is in the trachea or oesophagus. Furthermore, if ventilation is performed through the wrong lumen and the patient cannot breathe spontaneously, hypoxia and gastric distension occur. The Pharyngo-Tracheal Lumen Airway [72] shares similar problems [73]. Another disadvantage is that these devices are sometimes not readily available, and the staff are often unfamiliar with them.

The use of the laryngeal mask has been proposed during emergency situations. The device is relatively easy to insert, readily available and more importantly, is not associated with undetected ineffective ventilation owing to oesophageal intubation.

## Cardiopulmonary Resuscitation

The laryngeal mask has been proposed as the initial method of airway control during cardiopulmonary resuscitation, because it is relatively easy to master the technique of insertion, the success rate is high, and airway management is easier than the bag-mask method once the laryngeal mask is successfully inserted.

There have been several studies comparing the effectiveness of ventilation through the laryngeal mask with the combination of facemask, Guedel airway, and self inflating bag when used by unskilled personnel [74–76]. The success rates of insertion of the laryngeal mask and tracheal intubation by medical trainees were 94% and 51%, respectively [67]. Insertion of the laryngeal mask was also quicker (20 s) than tracheal intubation (35 s) [67]. Nurses obtained a significantly higher tidal volume through the laryngeal mask than through the facemask, Guedel airway, and self inflating bag [74]. Adequate ventilation (no increase in end tidal carbon dioxide and arterial oxygen saturation remaining greater than 90% after 2 min of ventilation) was obtained by nurses or medical students in 87% of patients when the laryngeal mask was used, compared with 43% of patients with the facemask. Time of insertion of either the laryngeal mask or the Guedel airway was similar [75].

The success rate of adequate ventilation (tidal volumes exceeding 800 ml within 40 s) achieved by junior doctors, however, was lower with the laryngeal mask than with the facemask. The time to the first successful ventilation was also longer with the laryngeal mask [76].

It appears that although adequate ventilation may not be obtained for the first minute when the laryngeal mask is chosen, once it is in place, ventilation is more effective through the laryngeal mask than the facemask. One of problems is that insertion of the laryngeal mask fails in up to 33% of patients at the first attempt and repeated attempts may prolong hypoxia.

Regurgitation and pulmonary aspiration during cardiopulmonary resuscitation is frequent [77]. There are concerns that use of the laryngeal mask during resuscitation does not prevent regurgitation and pulmonary aspiration. There is also a possibility that the mask may be dislodged during external chest compression.

A multicentre study was performed to study the efficacy of the laryngeal mask during resuscitation at in-hospital arrests until tracheal intubation was performed [78]. In this study, almost all laryngeal masks were inserted by nurses who had attended a training programme. The laryngeal mask was successfully inserted in 160 of 164 patients within two attempts about 3 min from the arrest call. Regurgitation occurred in 34 patients. Twenty of these patients regurgitated before insertion of the laryngeal mask and ten after its removal. Regurgitation was observed in three patients while the laryngeal mask was in place although a self inflating bag had been used in all these patients before insertion of the laryngeal mask. In no case did the laryngeal mask become dislodged during resuscitation.

The laryngeal mask, therefore, may be effectively used as an initial method of airway control until a person competent in tracheal intubation is available. Paramedic ambulance staff in Japan, who are not allowed to perform tracheal intubation, have been allowed to use the laryngeal mask during resuscitation since 1991.

It has also been shown that the laryngeal mask may be useful for resuscitation of neonates [33]. In one study, the laryngeal mask was used during resuscitation of 20 neonates. In all neonates, the laryngeal mask was successfully inserted at the first attempt and provided a clinically patent airway. Positive pressure ventilation was used without any complications directly attributable to its use [33].

Resuscitation while the laryngeal mask is used requires only two people whereas effective bag-mask ventilation with cricoid pressure may need three. Cricoid pressure is effective in preventing regurgitation while the mask is in place [57]. Thus, it is practically possible to introduce cricoid pressure during resuscitation when only two staff are available. However, cricoid pressure may interfere with ventilation [79].

## Difficult Access for Tracheal Intubation or Application of a Facemask

The laryngeal mask has been used in patients in whom access for tracheal intubation or application of a facemask was difficult. A clear airway was obtained in two patients who were trapped in crashed cars, and in whom tracheal intubation or ventilation through a facemask had failed [80]. The laryngeal mask can be inserted by approaching the patient's head from the front and using the 'thumb method' (see Chapter 9).

## Cervical Spine Injury

In patients with cervical spine injuries, it may be possible to insert the laryngeal mask without moving the head and neck [5, 81, 82]. It may, however, be more difficult to insert and insertion of the mask may cause more abrasion of the oropharynx than usual [12].

Once inserted, the use of the laryngeal mask should cause less damage to the unstable spine than the use of a facemask, because the airway can be maintained without moving the head and neck. The laryngeal mask was used in a patient with a cervical spine injury who was hypoxic after failed tracheal intubation [83].

Airway management of patients with cervical spinal injury is discussed elsewhere (see Chapter 18).

## Acute Cerebrovascular Disease

The laryngeal mask has been used in semi-conscious patients with acute cerebrovascular disease, because the pressor effect is less than that of tracheal intubation [84]. There is, however, an increased risk of pulmonary aspiration and rejection of the mask by the patient. In the report, no regurgitation was observed, but one of the six patients rejected the laryngeal mask [84].

## CONCLUSION

The laryngeal mask has been successfully used in patients in whom difficult tracheal intubation or ventilation, or both, were predicted. There have also been reports that the laryngeal mask provided a patent airway after failed tracheal intubation and failed ventilation through a facemask. The laryngeal mask may facilitate tracheal intubation in patients in whom tracheal intubation with a laryngoscope or a fibreoptic bronchoscope, or both, has failed. The laryngeal mask thus has a potential role in the situation of difficult tracheal intubation and difficult ventilation through a facemask. However, the ability of the laryngeal mask should not be overestimated. As with any other piece of equipment, the laryngeal mask may be associated with complications if it is misused. In the future, the laryngeal mask is likely to be used in increasing frequency in management of patients with difficult tracheal intubation or ventilation.

## KEY POINTS

- The laryngeal mask has a potential role in patients in whom tracheal intubation or ventilation through a facemask, or both, are difficult.

- The laryngeal mask may be particularly useful in the 'cannot intubate, cannot ventilate' scenario, as there have been a number of reports that the laryngeal mask provided adequate oxygenation in such a situation where other techniques had failed.

- The laryngeal mask can be used as the aid to tracheal intubation. Several methods have been reported. When a fibreoptic bronchoscope is used, the success rate of tracheal intubation through the laryngeal mask is likely to be the highest.

- It is important to make sure that the depth of anaesthesia is sufficient to minimize the incidence of laryngospasm while using the laryngeal mask.

- The laryngeal mask cannot reliably prevent regurgitation and cricoid pressure often prevents insertion of the mask. Therefore, the use of the laryngeal mask should be avoided in anaesthetized patients at increased risk of pulmonary aspiration unless it is considered to be absolutely necessary.

## REFERENCES

1 Brain A. I. Three cases of difficult intubation overcome by the laryngeal mask airway. *Anaesthesia* 1985; **40**: 353.

2 Asai T. and Morris S. The laryngeal mask airway: its features, effects and role. *Canadian Journal of Anaesthesiology* 1994; **41**: 930.

3 McCrirrick A. and Pracilio J. A. Awake intubation: a new technique. *Anaesthesia* 1991; **46**: 661.

4 Chadd G. D., Ackers J. W. L. and Bailey P. M. Difficult intubation aided by the laryngeal mask airway. *Anaesthesia* 1989; **44**: 1015.

5 Asai T. Fibreoptic intubation through the laryngeal mask in an awake patient with cervical spine injury. *Anesthesia and Analgesia* 1993; **77**: 404.

6 Silk J. M., Hill H. M. and Calder I. Difficult intubation and the laryngeal mask. *European Journal of Anaesthesiology* (Suppl.) 1991; **4**: 47 and 51.

7 Hasham F., Kumar C. M. and Lawler P. G. The use of the laryngeal mask airway to assist fibreoptic orotracheal intubation. *Anaesthesia* 1991; **46**: 891.

8 Asai T. Use of the laryngeal mask for fibrescope-aided tracheal intubation in an awake patient with a deviated larynx. *Acta Anaesthesiologica Scandinavica* 1994; **38**: 615.

9 Loken R. G. and Moir C. L. The laryngeal mask airway as an aid to blind orotracheal intubation. *Canadian Journal of Anaesthesiology* 1992; **39**: 518.

10 Heath M. L. and Allagain J. Intubation through the laryngeal mask. A technique for unexpected difficult intubation. *Anaesthesia* 1991; **46**: 545.

11 White A. P. and Billingham I. M. Laryngeal mask guided tracheal intubation in paediatric anaesthesia. *Paediatric Anaesthesia* 1992; **2**: 265.

12 Asai T., Barclay K., Power I. and Vaughan R. S. Cricoid pressure impedes placement of the laryngeal mask airway. *British Journal of Anaesthesia* 1995; **74**: 521.

13 Asai T., Latto I. P. and Vaughan R. S. The distance between the grille of the laryngeal mask airway and the vocal cords. Is conventional intubation through the laryngeal mask safe? *Anaesthesia* 1993; **48**: 667.

14 Jones H. E., Pearce A. C. and Moore P. Fibreoptic intubation. Influence of tracheal tube tip design. *Anaesthesia* 1993; **48**: 672.

15 Allison A. and McCrory J. Tracheal placement of a gum elastic bougie using the laryngeal mask airways. *Anaesthesia* 1990; **45**: 419.

16 Kidd J. F., Dyson A. and Latto I. P. Successful difficult intubation: use of the gum elastic bougie. *Anaesthesia* 1988; **43**: 437.

17 Denny N. M., Desilva K. D. and Webber P. A. Laryngeal mask airway for emergency tracheostomy in a neonate. *Anaesthesia* 1990; **45**: 895.

18 White A., Sinclair M. and Pillai R. Laryngeal mask airway for coronary artery bypass grafting. *Anaesthesia* 1991; **46**: 234.

19 Smith J. E. and Sherwood N. A. Combined use of laryngeal mask airway and fibreoptic laryngoscope in difficult intubation. *Anaesthesia and Intensive Care* 1991; **19**: 471.

20 Groves J., Edwards N. and Hood G. Difficult intubation following thoracic trauma. *Anaesthesia* 1994; **49**: 698.

21 Mehta S. Transtracheal illumination for optimal tracheal tube placement. *Anaesthesia* 1989; **44**: 970.

22 Asai T. and Latto I. P. Use of the lighted stylet for tracheal intubation via the laryngeal mask airway. *British Journal of Anaesthesia* 1995; **75**: 503.

23 Asai T., Barclay K., Power I. and Vaughan R. S. Cricoid pressure impedes placement of the laryngeal mask airway and subsequent tracheal intubation

through the mask. *British Journal of Anaesthesia* 1994; **72:** 47.

24 Schwartz D., Johnson C. and Roberts J. A maneuver to facilitate flexible fibreoptic intubation. *Anesthesiology* 1989; **71:** 470.

25 Marsh N. J. Easier fibreoptic intubations. *Anesthesiology* 1992; **76:** 860.

26 Asai T. Use of the laryngeal mask for tracheal intubation in patients at increased risk of aspiration of gastric contents. *Anesthesiology* 1992; **77:** 1029.

27 Yurino M. Retrograde and anterograde intubation techniques under general anesthesia through the laryngeal mask airway. *Journal of Anaesthesia* 1994; **8:** 227.

28 Thomson K. D. A blind nasal intubation using a laryngeal mask airway. *Anaesthesia* 1993; **48:** 785.

29 Brimacombe J. Modified Intravent [sic] LMA. *Anaesthesia and Intensive Care* 1991; **19:** 607.

30 Chadd G. D., Walford A. J. and Crane D. L. The 3.5/4.5 modification for fiberscope-guided tracheal intubation using the laryngeal mask airway. *Anesthesia and Analgesia* 1992; **75:** 307.

31 Kapila A., Addy E. V., Verghese C. and Brain A. I. J. Intubating laryngeal mask airway: a preliminary assessment of performance. *British Journal of Anaesthesia* 1995; **75:** 228P.

32 Markakis D. A., Sayson S. C. and Schreiner M. S. Insertion of the laryngeal mask airway in awake infants with the Robin sequence. *Anaesthesia and Analgesia* 1992; **75:** 822.

33 Paterson S. J., Byrne P. J., Molesky M. G., Seal R. F. and Finucane B. T. Neonatal resuscitation using the laryngeal mask airway. *Anesthesiology* 1994; **80:** 1248.

34 Calder I., Ordman A. J., Jackowski A. and Crockard H. A. The Brain laryngeal mask airway. An alternative to emergency tracheal intubation. *Anaesthesia* 1990; **45:** 137.

35 Brain A. I., McGhee T. D., McAteer E. J., Thomas A., Abu-Saad M. A. and Bushman J. A. The laryngeal mask airway. Development and preliminary trials of a new type of airway. *Anaesthesia* 1985; **40:** 356.

36 Thomson K. D., Ordman A. J., Parkhouse N. and Morgan B. D. Use of the Brain laryngeal mask airway in anticipation of difficult tracheal intubation. *British Journal of Plastic Surgery* 1989; **42:** 478.

37 Maltby J. R., Loken R. G. and Watson N. C. The laryngeal mask airway: clinical appraisal in 250 patients. *Canadian Journal of Anaesthesiology* 1990; **37:** 509.

38 Chadd G. D., Crane D. L., Phillips R. M. and Tunell W. P. Extubation and reintubation guided by the laryngeal mask airway in a child with the Pierre–Robin syndrome. *Anesthesiology* 1992; **76:** 640.

39 Ebata T., Nishiki S., Masuda A. and Amaha K. Anaesthesia for Treacher–Collins syndrome using a laryngeal mask airway. *Canadian Journal of Anaesthesiology* 1991; **38:** 1043.

40 Mason D. G. and Bingham R. M. The laryngeal mask airway in children. *Anaesthesia* 1990; **45:** 760.

41 Allen J. G. and Flower E. A. The Brain laryngeal mask. An alternative to difficult intubation. *British Dental Journal* 1990; **168:** 202.

42 Chadwick L. S. and Vohra A. Anaesthesia for emergency Caesarean section using the Brain laryngeal airway. *Anaesthesia* 1989; **44:** 261.

43 de Mello W. F. and Kocan M. The laryngeal mask in failed intubation. *Anaesthesia* 1990; **45:** 689.

44 McClune S., Regan M. and Moore J. Laryngeal mask airway for Caesarean section. *Anaesthesia* 1990; **45:** 227.

45 Lee J. J., Yau K. and Barcroft J. LMA and respiratory arrest after anterior cervical fusion. *Canadian Journal of Anaesthesiology* 1993; **40:** 395.

46 Wheatly R. S. and Stainthorp S. F. Intubation of a one-day-old baby with the Pierre–Robin syndrome via a laryngeal mask. *Anaesthesia* 1994; **49:** 733.

47 Smith I. and White P. F. Use of the laryngeal mask airway as an alternative to a face mask during outpatient arthroscopy. *Anesthesiology* 1992; **77:** 850.

48 McCrirrick A., Ramage D. T., Pracilio J. A. and Hickman J. A. Experience with the laryngeal mask airway in two hundred patients. *Anaesthesia and Intensive Care* 1991; **19:** 256.

49 Ferrut O., Toulouse C., Lançon J. P., Douvier S. and Fayolloe J. L. The laryngeal mask for elective gynecologic surgery. *Anesthesia and Analgesia* 1994; **78:** S110.

50 Collier C. A hazard with the laryngeal mask airway. *Anaesthesia and Intensive Care* 1991; **19:** 301.

51 Christian A. S. Failed obstetric intubation. *Anaesthesia* 1990; **45:** 995.

52 Russell S. H. and Hirsch N. P. Simultaneous use of two laryngoscopes. *Anaesthesia* 1993; **48:** 918.

53 Nandi P. R., Charlesworth C. H., Taylor S. J., Nunn J. F. and Doré C. J. Effect of general anaesthesia on the pharynx. *British Journal of Anaesthesia* 1991; **66:** 157.

54 Ansermino J. M. and Blogg C. E. Cricoid pressure may prevent insertion of the laryngeal mask airway. *British Journal of Anaesthesia* 1992; **66:** 465.

55 Pace N. A., Gajraj N. M., Pennant J. H., Victory R. A., Johnson E. R. and White P. F. Use of the laryngeal mask airway after oesophageal intubation. *British Journal of Anaesthesia* 1994; **73:** 688.

56 Brain A. I. J., Verghese C., Strube P. and Brimacombe J. A new laryngeal mask prototype. Preliminary evaluation of seal pressure and glottis isolation. *Anaesthesia* 1995; **50:** 42.

57 Strang T. I. Does the laryngeal mask airway compromise cricoid pressure? *Anaesthesia* 1992; **47:** 829.

58 Nanji G. M. and Maltby J. R. Vomiting and aspiration pneumonitis with the laryngeal mask airway. *Canadian Journal of Anaesthesiology* 1992; **39:** 69.

59 Dalrymple G. and Lloyd E. Laryngeal mask: a more secure airway than intubation? *Anaesthesia* 1992; **47:** 712.

60 Brain A. I. J.Lecture notes on the laryngeal mask airway and its role in difficult airway management. *First International Symposium on the Difficult Airway*, California, USA. 17–19 September, 1993.

61 Dexter T. J. The laryngeal mask airway: a method to improve visualisation of the trachea and larynx during fibreoptic assisted percutaneous tracheostomy. *Anaesthesia and Intensive Care* 1994; **22:** 35.

62 Asai T., Fujise K. and Uchida M. Use of the laryngeal mask in a child with tracheal stenosis. *Anesthesiology* 1991; **75:** 903.

63 Asai T., Fujise K. and Uchida M. Laryngeal mask and tracheal stenosis. *Anaesthesia* 1993; **48:** 81.

64 Divatia J. V., Sareen R., Upadhye S. M., Sharma K. S. and Shelgaonkar J. R. Anaesthetic management of tracheal surgery using the laryngeal mask airway. *Anaesthesia and Intensive Care* 1994; **22:** 69.

65 Gal T. J. and Suratt P. M. Resistance to breathing in healthy subjects following endotracheal intubation under topical anaesthesia. *Anesthesia and Analgesia* 1980; **59:** 270.

66 Bhatt S. B., Kendall A. P., Lin E. S. and Oh T. E. Resistance and additional inspiratory work imposed by the laryngeal mask airway. A comparison with tracheal tubes. *Anaesthesia* 1992; **47:** 343.

67 Davies P. R., Tighe S. Q., Greenslade G. L. and Evans G. H. Laryngeal mask airway and tracheal tube insertion by unskilled personnel. *Lancet* 1990; **336:** 977.

68 Elling R. and Politis J. An evaluation of emergency medical technicians' ability to use manual ventilation devices. *Annals of Emergency Medicine* 1983; **12:** 765.

69 Bass R. R., Allison E. J. and Hunt R. C. The esophageal obturator airway: a reassessment of use by paramedics. *Annals of Emergency Medicine* 1992; **11:** 358.

70 Frass M., Frenzer R., Zdrahal F., Hoflehner G., Porges P. and Lackner F. The esophageal tracheal combitube: preliminary results with a new airway for CPR. *Annals of Emergency Medicine* 1987; **16:** 768.

71 Bigenzahn W., Pesau B. and Frass M. Emergency ventilation using the Combitube in cases of difficult intubation. *European Archives of Oto-rhino-laryngology* 1991; **248:** 129.

72 Niemann J. T., Rosborough J. P., Myers R. and Scarberry E. N. The Pharyngo-Tracheal Lumen Airway: Preliminary investigation of a new adjunct. *Annals of Emergency Medicine* 1984; **13:** 591.

73 Hunt R. C., Sheets C. A. and Whitley T. W. Pharyngeal tracheal lumen airway training: failure to discriminate between esophageal and endotracheal modes and failure to confirm ventilation. *Annals of Emergency Medicine* 1989; **18:** 947.

74 Martin P. D., Cyna A. M., Hunter W. A., Henry J. and Ramayya G. P. Training nursing staff in airway management for resuscitation. A clinical comparison of the facemask and laryngeal mask. *Anaesthesia* 1993; **48:** 33.

75 Alexander R., Hodgson P., Lomax D. and Bullen C. A comparison of the laryngeal mask airway and Guedel airway, bag and facemask for manual ventilation following formal training. *Anaesthesia* 1993; **48:** 231.

76 Tolley P. M., Watts A. D. and Hickman J. A. Comparison of the use of the laryngeal mask and face mask by inexperienced personnel. *British Journal of Anaesthesia* 1992; **69:** 320.

77 Lawes E. G. and Baskett P. J. F. Pulmonary aspiration during unsuccessful cardiopulmonary resuscitation. *Intensive Care Medicine* 1987; **13:** 379.

78 Results of a multicentre trial. The use of the laryngeal mask by nurses during cardiopulmonary resuscitation. *Anaesthesia* 1994; **49:** 3.

79 Asai T., Barclay K., McBeth C., and Vaughan R. S. Cricoid pressure applied after placement of the laryngeal mask prevents gastric insufflation but inhibits ventilation. *Brisitsh Journal of Anaesthesia* 1996; **76:** 772.

80 Greene M. K., Roden R. and Hinchley G. The laryngeal mask airway. Two cases of prehospital trauma care. *Anaesthesia* 1992; **47:** 688.

81 Brimacombe J. and Berry A. Laryngeal mask airway insertion. A comparison of the standard versus neutral position in normal healthy patients with a view to its use in cervical spine instability. *Anaesthesia* 1993; **48:** 670.

82 Pennant J. H., Pace N. A. and Gajraj N. M. Role of the laryngeal mask airway in the immobile cervical spine. *Journal of Clinical Anaesthesia* 1993; **5:** 226.

83 Pennant J. H., Gajraj N. M. and Pace N. A. Laryngeal mask airway in cervical spine injuries. *Anesthesia and Analgesia* 1992; **75:** 1074.

84 Ito N., Aikawa N., Hori S. *et al.* Laryngeal mask airway in acute cerebrovascular disease. *Lancet* 1992; **339:** 69.

# 9

# Difficulty in Insertion of the Laryngeal Mask

*Takashi Asai*

## INTRODUCTION

The laryngeal mask can be safely inserted blindly without using a laryngoscope and adequate ventilation obtained in the majority of patients [1]. The success rate of insertion is usually greater than 95% even when inserted by inexperienced personnel [2–4]. In up to 8% of cases, however, adequate ventilation through the laryngeal mask may not be obtained; the incidence of failure at the first

attempt is up to 33% [5, 6]. The incidence of failure of insertion of the mask by anaesthetists may
be thus higher than that with tracheal intubation.
Prediction of difficulty in insertion is also not easy.
It is usually not a problem even when insertion of
the mask fails, since the airway is usually managed
either by tracheal intubation or with a facemask.

The laryngeal mask is sometimes not inserted
in the correct position even when adequate
ventilation is obtained [7]. There is, however, no
danger of life-threatening complications, such as
oesophageal intubation. As the mask is inserted
blindly, the exact position is difficult to confirm.
For these reasons, confirmation of the position of
the mask has tended to be ignored. A mask that is
incorrectly inserted, however, is more likely to
become dislodged, obstruct the airway and cause
coughing, laryngospasm or pulmonary aspiration
of gastric contents. Therefore, assessment of the
position of the mask is important to reduce
complications.

The laryngeal mask has been used successfully
to facilitate ventilation in patients in whom ventilation through a facemask, tracheal intubation, or
both, have failed. The use of the laryngeal mask is
incorporated in the failed tracheal intubation algorithm (see Chapters 6 and 8). In this situation, the
small percentage of failure becomes important,
and in patients with difficult airways, the failure
rate may increase. It is, therefore, necessary to recognize in which situations it is likely to be difficult
to insert the mask and to master the technique
that minimizes the incidence of failure.

Some of the causes of failure or misplacement still
remain unclear, although suboptimal method of
insertion is certainly the main cause of failure. In
this chapter, the proper method for placing the mask
and for confirming its correct position will be outlined. Details of misplacement and the reasons
will be covered. The methods of assessment of the
position of the mask and those for minimizing the
incidence of misplacement will be described.
Finally, the effects of cricoid pressure on insertion
of the laryngeal mask and subsequent tracheal intubation through the mask will be discussed.

## ANATOMICAL POSITION

The laryngeal mask is designed to form a seal
around the larynx with the distal part of the mask
conforming to the hypopharynx (Fig. 1) with the

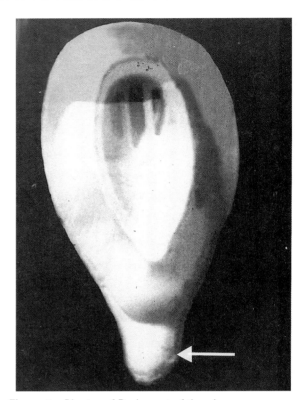

**Figure 1**   Plaster of Paris cast of the pharynx
superimposed on a laryngeal mask, which shows how
the distal part of the mask was designed to occupy
fully the hypopharynx. The tip of the mask rests on the
upper oesophageal sphincter, which is indicated by
an arrow. From Asai and Morris [8] (after Dr Brain)
with permission of the authors and the Canadian
Anaesthetists' Society.

walls of the long axis of the mask facing towards
the pyriform fossae [9]. The hypopharynx, the
laryngeal part of the pharynx, is the pharyngeal
space behind the arytenoid and cricoid cartilages.
Thus, when the mask is inserted correctly, the
distal part of the mask lies posterior to both the
arytenoid and cricoid cartilages and the tip rests
on the upper oesophageal sphincter at the level of
the 5–6th cervical vertebrae (Fig. 2) [6, 10]. The
proximal edge of the mask is positioned below the
base of the tongue, below the level of the tonsils
[11, 12]. The curve of the tube should follow that
of the palate.

The epiglottis is either positioned in the aperture of the mask or compressed by the upper part
of the mask [9]. The aperture of the laryngeal
mask faces directly to the vocal cords, and the

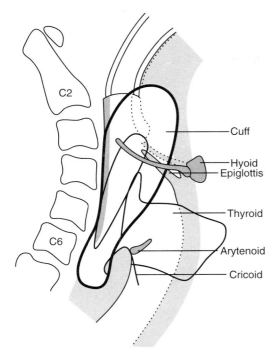

**Figure 2** Correct position of the laryngeal mask. The distal part of the mask occupies the hypopharynx, the space behind both the arytenoid and cricoid cartilages. The tip of the mask rests on the upper oesophageal sphincter at the level of C6. The entire larynx is moved forward and the arytenoid cartilages are rotated in relation to the cricoid cartilage. As a result, the tissues overlying the larynx bulge. From Nandi *et al.* [7], with permission of the authors and Blackwell Scientific Publications.

mean distance between the grille of the laryngeal mask and the vocal cords is 3.1 cm in females and 3.6 cm in males [13]. Thus, when a fibreoptic bronchoscope is passed through the laryngeal mask, the vocal cords are usually easily seen beyond the grille of the mask.

When the cuff is inflated, the thyroid, arytenoid and cricoid cartilages are displaced anteriorly, and the tissues in front of the larynx bulge slightly [1, 7].

## INSERTION

### Standard Insertion Methods

The standard method of insertion recommended by Brain is as follows (details can be obtained from the *Instruction Manual* [11]).

- Before insertion, the cuff should be deflated while the hollow side of the mask is placed on a clean flat surface, with two fingers pressing down on a point just short of the tip (Fig. 3a). The cuff should be deflated fully to impart rigidity to the tip of the cuff. The deflated cuff should be free from wrinkles and its rim should face away from the aperture of the mask (Fig. 3b).
- A lubricant is applied only to the posterior surface of the mask just before insertion. This prevents the cuff tip from rolling over on contact with the palate. Application of lubricant to the anterior surface of the mask should be avoided, as lubricant may block the aperture or be inhaled, causing airway obstruction or coughing.
- The patient's neck is flexed and the head extended ('sniffing the morning air' position) by pushing the occiput from behind with the non-dominant hand. The mouth is opened either by an assistant or with the third finger of the dominant hand.
- The device is held between the thumb and index fingers, as close as possible to the junction of the tube and mask, with the aperture of the mask facing the patient's chin.
- The tip of the cuff is inserted against the inner surface of the patient's upper incisor teeth (Fig. 3c). It is important that at this point the tube should be parallel to the trolley rather than vertical (see *Misplacement*). The mask is then pressed upwards against the hard palate and advanced into the oral cavity, maintaining upward pressure (Fig. 3d).
- The device is advanced using the index finger located at the junction of the tube and the mask. It is essential that the tip of the cuff does not roll over during the advancement of the laryngeal mask.
- A change of direction will be felt as the cuff tip follows the posterior pharyngeal wall downwards. The laryngeal mask is pushed by the index finger as far as possible into the hypopharynx. When the mask is fully advanced, resistance will be felt (Fig. 3e).
- The tube is then held by the non-dominant hand to prevent the mask from moving out of position as the index finger is withdrawn (Fig. 3f).
- With experience, the index finger can advance the mask fully into position. However, if it is

(a)

(b)

(c)

(d)

(e)

(f)

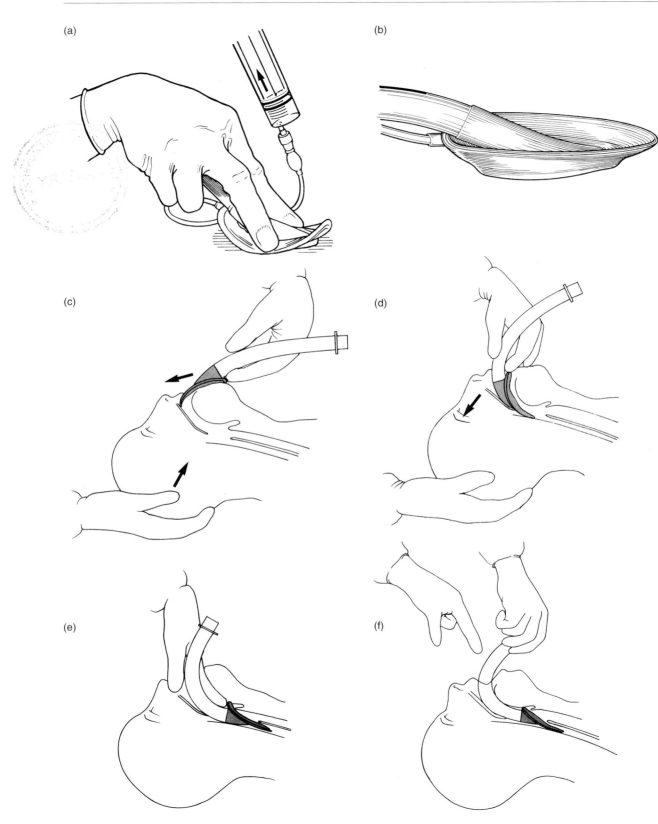

considered that the mask is not fully advanced into the hypopharynx or if the user has small hands, the laryngeal mask may need to be pressed downwards by the non-dominant hand for complete positioning.

- The cuff is inflated with an appropriate volume of air (Table 1). Note that the figures given in Table 1 represent the *maximum* inflation volumes. The tube usually moves out of the mouth slightly (mean distance of 0.7 cm) [13], and the tissues overlying both the thyroid and cricoid cartilage bulge slightly when the cuff is inflated. The tube should not be held or connected to the breathing system during inflation of the cuff. The tip of the mask is likely to be positioned too deeply if the tube is held during inflation (see *Misplacement*).
- The laryngeal mask is connected to the breathing system and adequacy of ventilation is assessed. If it is not possible to ventilate adequately, the mask is removed unless this is considered to be due to closure of the glottis associated with inadequate anaesthesia. After removal, the cuff should again be prepared as described initially and insertion reattempted.

### Insertion of the reinforced laryngeal mask

The technique of insertion of the reinforced laryngeal mask is the same as that for the standard one: the device is held between the thumb and index finger at the junction of the tube and mask and positioned by the index finger.

---

**Figure 3** Standard insertion method. (a) The cuff should be deflated completely while the hollow side of the mask is placed on a clean flat surface, with two fingers pressing down on a point just short of the tip (b) The correct shape of the laryngeal mask for insertion. The deflated cuff should be free from wrinkles and its rim should face away from the aperture of the mask. From Dr Brain [10], with permission. (c) The tip of the cuff is inserted against the inner surface of the patient's upper incisor teeth. Note that the tube should be parallel to the trolley (or floor) rather than vertical. (d) The mask is pressed upwards against the hard palate during insertion. (e) The mask is advanced by the index finger as far as possible into the hypopharynx, until resistance is felt. (f) The tube is held by the non-dominant hand to prevent the mask from moving out of position as the index finger is withdrawn.

**Table 1** Specifications of the laryngeal mask. From Asai and Morris [8], with permission of the authors, the *Canadian Anaesthetists' Society Journal.*

| Size | Patient's weight (kg) | Cuff volume (ml) | Length (cm) (standard/ reinforced) | Internal diameter (mm) (standard/ reinforced) |
|------|------------------------|-------------------|-------------------------------------|-------------------------------------------------|
| 1 | <6.5 | Up to 4 | 8.6/- | 5.3/- |
| 2 | 6.5–20 | Up to 10 | 12.0/13.0 | 7.0/5.1 |
| 2½ | 20–30 | Up to 14 | 13.5/16.5 | 8.4/6.1 |
| 3 | >30 | Up to 20 | 17.5/21.0 | 10.0/7.6 |
| 4 | Adult | Up to 30 | 17.5/21.0 | 10.0/7.6 |
| 5 | Large adult | Up to 40 | 20.0/- | 11.5/- |

## Thumb Insertion Method

The laryngeal mask can be inserted by directing the mask with the thumb instead of the index finger. This method is useful when it is difficult to approach the patient's head from behind, for example when the patient is trapped in a car.

The principle of insertion is the same as the standard method. The mask and the position of the patient's head and neck are prepared as with the standard method. The position of the thumb and index finger differs from that in the standard method. The tip of the thumb, instead of the index finger, is positioned in the space between the tube and the proximal part of the mask (Fig. 4a). The mask is inserted by the thumb while the other fingers are stretched forward over the patient's face during insertion (Figs. 4b–d).

## DIFFICULTY IN INSERTION

### Light Anaesthesia

If anaesthesia is not deep enough, insertion of the mask is more likely to fail. In addition, airway obstruction due to laryngospasm may be misjudged as failure in insertion of the mask.

### Restricted Mouth Opening

When mouth opening is restricted it may be difficult to insert the mask, because the device will not pass between the teeth. Insertion of the index finger, which drives the mask correctly, may also be difficult so that the incidence of misplacement will be increased.

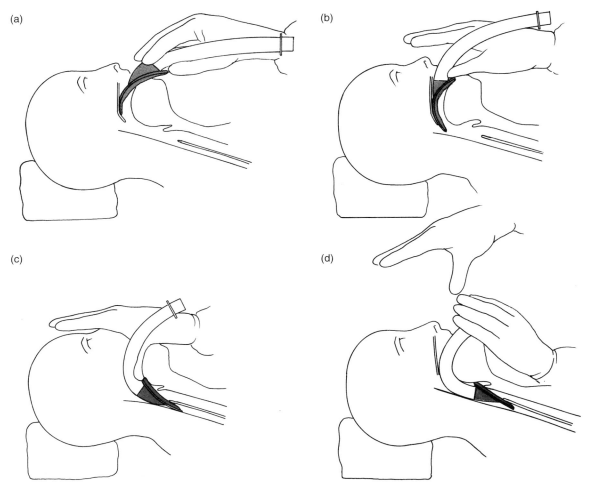

**Figure 4** Thumb insertion method. The laryngeal mask can be inserted by directing the mask with the thumb instead of the index finger. This method is useful when it is difficult to approach the patient's head from behind. (a) The mask is held with the tip of the thumb in the space between the tube and the mask. (b–d) The mask is inserted by the thumb while the other fingers are stretched forward over the patient's face.

## Negotiation of the Posterior Pharyngeal Wall

Difficulty may occur as the tip of the mask passes just behind the tongue, when it changes direction towards the hypopharynx. This difficulty may occur more frequently in children than in adults [14]. Advance of the mask may be difficult when the mask presses the tongue back towards the posterior pharyngeal wall and obstructs the passage. This problem is likely to occur if the mask is advanced vertically to the posterior pharyngeal wall (in this situation, the tube of the laryngeal mask is often vertical, rather than parallel to the trolley) (Fig. 5).

## Restricted Head and Neck Movement

Insertion is best achieved when the neck is flexed and the head extended ('sniffing the morning air' position). Thus, in theory, insertion may be more difficult when the head and neck are either in the neutral position or flexed, because the angle between the oral and pharyngeal axes is acute at the back of the tongue (Fig. 6). It has been confirmed that insertion of the mask may be more difficult if the angle between the oral and pharyngeal axes is less than 90° [15]. It is also not always easy to insert the index finger into the oral cavity to drive the mask fully into position [16]. Although the correct insertion may be more difficult,

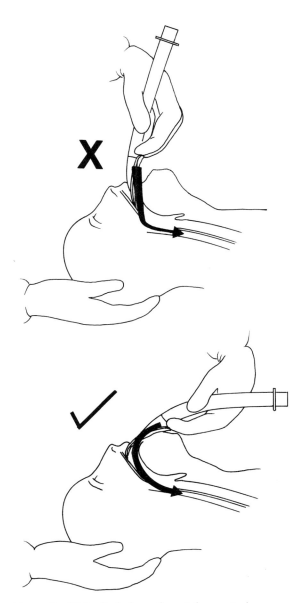

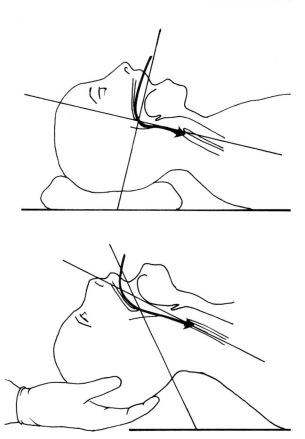

**Figure 6**  Position of the patient's head and neck. If the head and the neck are either in the neutral position or flexed, insertion of the laryngeal mask may be difficult, because the angle between the oral and pharyngeal axes is acute at the back of the tongue (upper). Insertion will be easier when the head is extended on the neck and the lower part of the neck is flexed ('sniffing the morning air' position) (lower). This widens the angle between the oral and pharyngeal axes.

## Pharyngeal Pathology

The tip of the mask may also impact upon an irregularity or swelling in the posterior pharynx, such as tonsillar hypertrophy [11, 12, 14], although the reinforced laryngeal mask can usually be inserted easily [12]. Insertion is also difficult, and may damage tissue, particularly when there is an oropharyngeal tumour. Thus, the use of the laryngeal mask is relatively contraindicated in such situations. There has also been a report of failure of insertion of the laryngeal mask in a patient with an abnormality in the hypopharynx due to large cervical osteophytes [19].

**Figure 5**  Difficulty in insertion at the posterior pharyngeal wall. If the tube is vertical to the trolley, the mask is more likely to impact upon the posterior wall (upper). This problem will be reduced when the tube of the laryngeal mask is held parallel to the trolley (or floor) and inserted by making a smooth curve (lower).

adequate ventilation can often be obtained even when the head and neck are fixed in the neutral position in adults in whom tracheal intubation is considered to be easy [16–18]. The incidence of minor injury to the oropharynx may be greater than usual [16].

## Reinforced Laryngeal Mask

Insertion of the reinforced laryngeal mask requires more skill than insertion of the standard mask. Correct insertion of the reinforced laryngeal mask is even more difficult if the correct method of insertion is not used. With experience, insertion of the reinforced laryngeal mask becomes as easy as the standard device. However, before this experience has been gained, the final correct position might be difficult to achieve, even when the correct method of insertion is used.

## Difficult Tracheal Intubation

Whether it is also difficult to insert the laryngeal mask in patients whose tracheas are difficult to intubate is not clear, although there have been a number of reports of successful insertion of the mask in this group of patients (see Chapter 8). In certain situations, for example when it is difficult to open the mouth, insertion of the mask and tracheal intubation may both be more difficult than usual.

## Cricoid Pressure

When cricoid pressure is applied, it is, in theory, impossible to insert the mask correctly, because the cricoid pressure compresses the hypopharynx in addition to occluding the oesophagus (see below).

## MISPLACEMENT

If anaesthesia is inadequate, airway reflexes occur and the anatomical shapes of the larynx and pharynx are changed, making correct insertion of the distal part of the mask into the hypopharynx more difficult.

## Posterior Deflection ('Downfolding') of the Epiglottis

The tip of the cuff may press the epiglottis downwards during insertion (Figs. 7 and 8). The anteroposterior distance of the pharyngeal space at the level of the tip of the epiglottis is less than 5 mm when the patient is anaesthetized [20]. Thus,

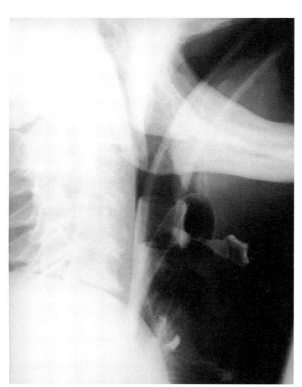 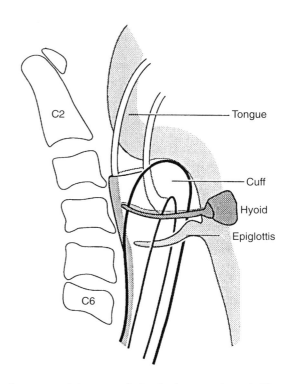

**Figure 7.**  'Downfolding' of the epiglottis. The epiglottis is being pressed downwards by the laryngeal mask. The mask is also advanced too far into the upper oesophagus. From Nandi *et al.* [7], with permission of the authors and Blackwell Scientific Publications.

the epiglottis is likely to be pressed downward when the laryngeal mask is inserted with the tip of the cuff bending towards the aperture of the mask (Fig. 8). The incidence of this misplacement also increases when the mask is inserted with its cuff partially or fully inflated (Fig. 8) [21].

The epiglottis tends to move posteriorly when the patient is paralysed; this is prevented by extension of the head [22]. Thus, when the mask is inserted without extension of the head and flexion of the neck, the epiglottis is more likely to be pressed downward by the mask [16, 17].

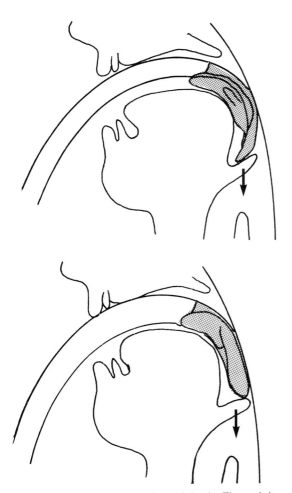

**Figure 8**  'Downfolding' of the epiglottis. The epiglottis is more likely to be pressed downward (arrows) if the laryngeal mask is inserted with the tip of the cuff bending towards the aperture of the mask (upper) or with the cuff partially inflated (lower). After Dr Brain, with permission.

## Migration of the Mask into the Larynx

The tip of the mask may enter the larynx (Fig. 9) or may make contact with the arytenoid cartilages [7]. When the tip of the mask is bent towards the aperture of the mask, the mask is likely to move towards the larynx and impact upon the arytenoid cartilages or glottis. When the tip of the mask is not pressed against the hard palate and posterior pharyngeal wall during insertion, misplacement is also more likely to occur.

## Insufficient Insertion Depth

If the mask is not inserted far enough, the distal part of the mask is positioned above the level of the hypopharynx. Both the glottis and the hypopharynx (oesophageal inlet) may be seen through a fibreoptic bronchoscope, when the bronchoscope is passed through the laryngeal mask. The tip of the mask may press on the arytenoid cartilages, causing an inward displacement of the aryepiglottic folds. The tip of the mask is also likely to enter the larynx. There has been a report of a misplaced mask, where, despite being inserted only in the oropharynx, ventilation was adequate [23].

## Excessive Insertion Depth

The tip of the mask may be advanced too far into the upper oesophagus (Fig. 7). The glottis may be obstructed by the proximal part of the mask. If the laryngeal mask is held or the breathing system is attached during inflation of the cuff, the mask cannot move outwards in the normal way and it remains wedged in the upper oesophageal sphincter.

## Torsion of the Laryngeal Mask

The laryngeal mask may be positioned with the mask twisted around the long axis of the tube. This is more likely to occur when it is rotated during insertion [21] or if it is not correctly fixed in place.

## Folding of the Mask

The mask may fold over on itself if it is inserted with excessive force or if it is not pressed upwards against the hard palate. This is also likely to occur when the cuff is not completely deflated, if the mask is not well lubricated, or if the cuff has

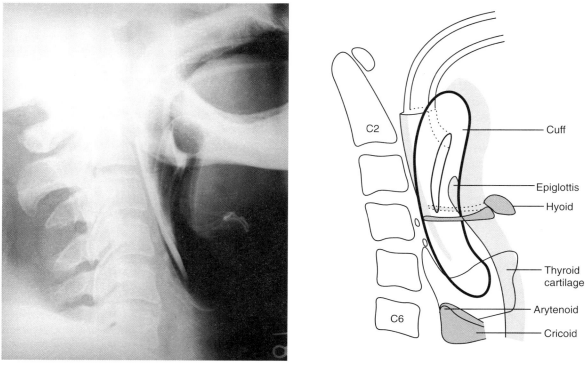

**Figure 9**  Migration of the mask into the larynx. The mask is anterior to the arytenoid cartilages and within the laryngeal inlet. From Nandi *et al.* [7], with permission of the authors and Blackwell Scientific Publications.

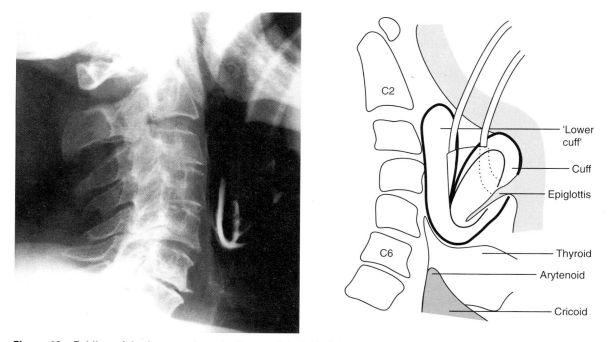

**Figure 10**  Folding of the laryngeal mask. The mask is folded through 180° in the pharynx. From Nandi *et al.* [7], with permission of the authors and Blackwell Scientific Publications.

perished after repeated use. There has been a report in which a mask was inserted easily but was found to be folded through 180° without any apparent airway obstruction (Fig. 10) [7].

## COMPLICATIONS ASSOCIATED WITH MISPLACEMENT

### Airway Obstruction

If the epiglottis obstructs the aperture of the mask, adequate ventilation may not be possible. Tracheal intubation through the laryngeal mask or diagnostic bronchoscopy may also be difficult in this situation. Airway obstruction may occur after insertion of the mask when the tip of the mask is positioned in the larynx. Even when a patent airway is initially obtained, obstruction might occur during anaesthesia, because the mask may obstruct the larynx by expanding due to diffusion of nitrous oxide.

If the mask is not inserted far enough, the tip of the mask may press the arytenoid cartilages anteriorly and displace the arytenoid folds inward, leading to airway obstruction. If an inappropriately small size is used, the mask can be advanced too far into the oesophagus so that the proximal (or cephalad) part of the mask can obstruct the glottis [9].

### Dislodgement

The mask is likely to dislodge when the distal part of the mask does not correctly occupy the hypopharynx, for example when the tip has impacted upon the larynx or when the mask is not inserted far enough.

### Airway Reflexes

When the mask impacts on the larynx, airway reflexes are likely to be induced, leading to laryngospasm, vomiting and possible pulmonary aspiration. If the device is twisted in the oropharynx, the tip of the mask may enter the larynx during anaesthesia and induce airway reflexes or obstruction.

### Damage to the Larynx

Damage to the larynx may, in theory, occur if the tip of the mask enters the larynx and stretches the aryepiglottic folds. This complication is more likely to occur if the device is held during inflation of the cuff and fixed in place, because outward movement of the mask during inflation is prevented.

### Regurgitation and Vomiting

Regurgitation and vomiting are frequently associated with an uncoordinated reflex response. The incidence of regurgitation and vomiting may increase when the upper oesophageal sphincter is overstretched by inflation of the cuff, although it has not been assessed. Again, the cuff is more likely to overstretch the upper oesophageal sphincter if the device is held or connected to the breathing system during inflation of the cuff.

### Insufficient Prevention of Soiling

When the mask is inserted correctly, it can effectively prevent soiling of the larynx from blood in the pharynx. Thus, the laryngeal mask can be used relatively safely during oral surgery [12]. This effect will be lost when the mask is not in the correct position.

### Gastric Insufflation

If the mask does not correctly occupy the hypopharynx and, in particular, if the mask partially obstructs the larynx, gas may be insufflated into the stomach during intermittent positive pressure ventilation. Gastric insufflation may also occur when the glottis is closed due to inadequate depth of anaesthesia. This complication is more likely to occur in small children.

### Difficulty in Tracheal Intubation through the Laryngeal Mask

The trachea can be intubated by passing a tracheal tube through the laryngeal mask into the trachea (see Chapter 8). This may be difficult if the mask is misplaced, for example when the epiglottis is pressed downward by the mask or the tip of the mask has entered the larynx. In this situation, forceful blind tracheal intubation may damage the larynx and pharynx.

## ASSESSMENT OF THE POSITION OF THE MASK

Adequate ventilation through the laryngeal mask is usually assessed by adequate chest expansion with a satisfactory compliance and auscultation. These assessments, however, do not reliably detect misplacement. There are several clinical signs which enable more accurate detection.

### Resistance During Insertion

The mask should be slid into place smoothly. If resistance is felt when the tip of the mask reaches just behind the tongue, the tip may be folded over on itself or impacted upon an irregularity or swelling in the posterior pharynx, such as tonsillar hypertrophy. Resistance will usually be felt when the tip of the mask abuts against the upper oesophageal sphincter. If this resistance is not felt, it is likely that the tip of the mask is folded backward. A 'click' may be felt when the mask passes behind the arytenoid cartilages, immediately before the mask abuts against the upper oesophageal sphincter. This will not be felt if the mask is incorrectly held, for example, by grasping the middle part of the tube.

When the cuff is inflated after insertion of the mask, the tube will move out of the mouth for a mean distance of 0.7 cm [13]. If the tube is seen to be out of the mouth further than usual, the mask is likely to have impacted upon the larynx.

### Bulging of the Neck

When the cuff is inflated, the tissue overlying both the thyroid and cricoid cartilages bulges slightly because the mask pushes the thyroid, arytenoid and cricoid cartilages anteriorly. When no bulge is observed in the neck, the mask may still be in the oropharynx, either because the mask has folded over on itself or because it has not been inserted far enough. When only the tissue over the thyroid cartilage bulges, leaving the tissue over the cricoid cartilage flat, the tip of the mask may have entered the larynx or been inserted only behind the arytenoid cartilages owing to incomplete insertion. The bulge should be symmetrical; if not, the mask may be twisted. This assessment, however, might be difficult in obese patients.

The black line of the tube should be in the mid line, facing cephalad; if not, it is likely that the device is twisting.

### Chest Expansion and Auscultation

Manual ventilation may be difficult if the mask obstructs the airway, even when anaesthesia is deep enough to prevent airway reflexes. Auscultation of breath sounds with a stethoscope placed on the anterolateral part of the neck is useful to detect an inadvertent entry of the mask into the larynx. Stridor may be heard when the tip of the mask partially obstructs the glottis. In this case, the stridor will not be resolved by deepening anaesthesia. Air leakage from between the mask and the pharynx is also detected by auscultation of the neck.

### End Tidal Carbon Dioxide Measurement

Monitoring of end tidal carbon dioxide is useful for assessment of adequacy of ventilation. Observation of the waveforms may be useful in detecting partial obstruction of the airway. Changes in waveforms may also detect lightening of anaesthesia or recovery of muscle tone, since the glottis may be partially closed in these situations.

### Oesophageal Detector Device

The use of the oesophageal detector device to assess the airway patency after insertion of the laryngeal mask has been proposed [24]. The method, however, cannot reliably detect the patency, because the syringe (or bulb) may refill when the mask is not inserted correctly and air leaks into the aperture of the mask from the oral cavity. Conversely, the bulb may fail to refill even when the mask is correctly inserted, but when the vocal cords are closed in response to insertion under inadequate depth of anaesthesia [25].

### Opening the Mouth

When the mask is positioned correctly, the proximal edge of the mask is positioned below the base of the tongue and below the level of the tonsils [11, 12]. Thus, it should be impossible to see the mask upon opening the mouth after insertion. If the mask is seen in the oropharynx, the mask is not inserted far enough.

## CONFIRMATION OF CORRECT POSITION

The correct position can be confirmed by X-ray or magnetic resonance imaging (MRI). The use of a fibreoptic bronchoscope is the most reliable method to detect misplacement of the mask in the clinical setting. Downfolding of the epiglottis at the level of the grille of the mask and torsion of the laryngeal mask are easily detected. If the oesophagus is seen in the aperture of the mask, the mask is not inserted far enough or the mask has folded back on itself.

Fibrescopy, however, cannot always confirm whether the distal part of the mask is correctly inserted into the hypopharynx [26]. It may also be difficult to detect whether the tip of the mask is advanced too far into the oesophageal sphincter. In the past, it was considered that the mask was not in the correct position when part of, or the entire epiglottis was seen through a fibrescope [27, 28]. The epiglottis is, however, sometimes situated in the aperture of the mask even when the mask is in the correct position [26]. Therefore, the presence of the epiglottis in the aperture of the mask is not an indication that the tip of the mask does not lie in the hypopharynx [26].

The mask may be considered to be in the correct position when all of the following criteria are fulfilled, although this cannot detect whether or not the tip of the mask is wedged too far into the upper oesophagus [8]:

- the tissue overlying both the thyroid and cricoid cartilages bulges mildly during inflation of the cuff;
- the glottis is seen through the fibrescope;
- neither the tip of the mask nor the oesophagus is seen in the aperture of the mask; and
- the mask or the tube is not twisted (twist of the tube does not apply to the reinforced laryngeal mask).

## AVOIDANCE OF MISPLACEMENT

### Correct Insertion

The incidence of difficulty in insertion and misplacement can be minimized by using the standard insertion method described by Brain [11]. Anaesthesia should be deep enough to obtund airway reflexes.

Folding of the tip of the cuff is less likely to occur when the posterior surface of the cuff is well lubricated. Insertion may be easier when the neck is flexed and the head extended, because these manoeuvres produce an angle between the oral and the pharyngeal axes of greater than 90° at the back of the tongue (Fig. 6) [29, 30].

When the mask is pressed upward against the hard palate and posterior pharyngeal wall, the tongue will not obstruct passage, and the incidence of posterior deflection of the epiglottis and contact of the cuff with the larynx are also decreased. This can best be achieved with the index finger positioned at the junction of the tube and the mask so that the finger acts as a fulcrum. The tube of the laryngeal mask should be parallel to, rather than at right angles to, the table (Fig. 5). A fully deflated cuff with the tip facing away from the aperture of the mask is less likely to impact on the larynx. The epiglottis tends to move posteriorly when patients are paralysed; this is prevented by extension of the head [22] which should, in theory, reduce the incidence of posterior deflection of the epiglottis by the mask.

### Modified Methods

A number of alternative methods for insertion have been proposed. These include rotation, lateral approach, a partially inflated cuff, jaw thrust, or the use of a laryngoscope [8, 21]. Most of these methods, however, have not been proven to be better than the standard method, and are more likely to result in misplacement [8, 21]. Rotating the laryngeal mask during insertion may be as effective as the standard method, although it may increase the incidence of twisting of the device [21]. Addition of jaw thrusting to the standard method would decrease the incidence of downfolding of the epiglottis, since jaw thrusting widens the anteroposterior distance of the pharyngeal space [31]. These methods can be tried if difficulty is encountered with the standard method.

### Insertion Aids

A few insertion aids have been proposed to reduce the difficulty in advancing the mask over the back of the tongue. A 'skid' spoon has been used to function as an 'artificial hard palate' by covering the soft palate to minimize the resistance in insertion at the posterior pharyngeal wall [32]. A spoon has also been used to pull the tongue forward and downward to facilitate insertion of the mask [33].

Dingley's insertion aid is another device that is intended to facilitate correct insertion of the mask and to reduce the incidence of injury to the oropharynx (Fig. 11) [34]. After insertion of the aid, the laryngeal mask is inserted by the standard method. The incidence of bleeding caused by the insertion of the mask has been shown to be decreased by the use of the insertion aid [34]. Whether or not these aids facilitate correct insertion of the mask, however, is not known.

Difficulty in the final positioning of the reinforced laryngeal mask by the index finger can be decreased by experience. When a tracheal tube is used as a stylet, the final positioning can be achieved by pressing the laryngeal mask [35]. Even when this stylet is used, the laryngeal mask should be held between the thumb and index fingers, as close as possible to the junction of the tube and the mask as usual, and the mask should be inserted as in the standard method except the final positioning [35]. A metal stylet or gum elastic bougie has been suggested for insertion of the reinforced laryngeal mask, but these should not be necessary when the correct insertion technique is used; in fact, the use of the stylet may make the insertion more difficult [35].

## Size of the Mask

A proper size of mask should be used. If too small a size is used, the mask may be inserted too deep into the upper oesophagus and may obstruct the glottis with the proximal part of the mask. The incidence of air leakage may be also higher. Size 4 is generally suitable for both male or female adults of average size (Table 1).

## INCIDENCE

The reported incidence of misplacement of the laryngeal mask varies considerably [8]. This difference may depend on the method of insertion and the experience of the user. The incidence of misplacement can be reduced with experience and by using the correct insertion method [8, 11, 21].

The reported incidence of downfolding of the epiglottis seen on fibrescopy is 0–10% in adults [13, 16, 21, 36], 0–33% in children [14, 27] and 8% in infants [28]. In contrast, when the X-ray or MRI was used, downfolding of the epiglottis was detected in 63% of adults [7] and 74% of children

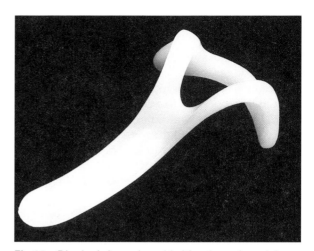

**Fig.11**   Dingley's insertion aid. After insertion of the aid, the laryngeal mask is inserted by the standard method. Photograph provided by Dr J. Dingley, Department of Anaesthetics and Intensive Care Medicine, University of Wales College of Medicine.

[37]. The fact that fibrescopy cannot detect downfolding of the epiglottis that occurred above the level of the grille may explain some of these discrepancies. It is not known how often airway obstruction occurs when the epiglottis is pressed downwards by the mask.

The incidence of suboptimal position diagnosed by fibrescopy was considered to be higher in children than in adults [27, 28]. The epiglottis was seen through the fibrescope within the mask in 49% of children [27], and 56% of infants [28], an incidence higher than in adults [13, 16, 21, 36]. However, the mask may be in the correct position even when the posterior surface of the epiglottis is visible [26].

Brain designed the mask to conform to the hypopharynx and the length of the long axis of the mask aperture to be greater than the distance between the upper border of the thyroid cartilage and the lower border of the cricoid cartilage, that is at the lower border of the hypopharynx. Thus, the mask can be in the correct position even when the epiglottis is enclosed by the mask [26].

If the mask is arbitrarily judged to be correctly inserted when only the glottis or the glottis and the posterior surface of the epiglottis are seen through the fibrescope, the total incidence of misplacement is 20–35% in children and infants as well as in adults [26]. Thus, the difference in the incidence of misplacement between adults and children may not be as great as previously thought.

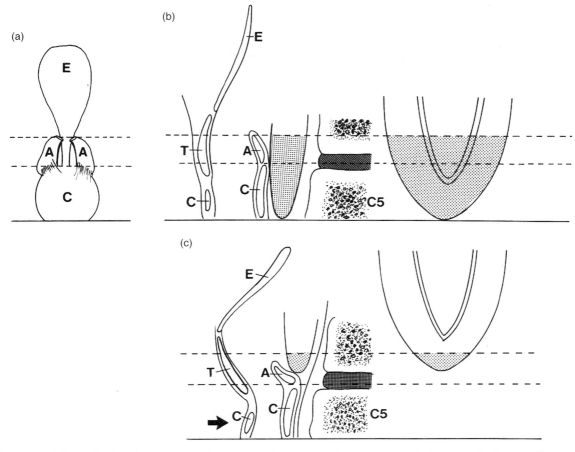

**Figure 12.**   Effect of cricoid pressure on insertion of the laryngeal mask. The dotted area indicates the distal part of the mask that occupies the hypopharynx. (a) Posterior view of the larynx. (b) Correct position of the laryngeal mask. When cricoid pressure is not applied and the mask is correctly positioned, the distal part of the mask fully occupies the hypopharynx, the space behind the arytenoid and cricoid cartilages. (c) Position of the laryngeal mask when cricoid pressure is applied. When cricoid pressure is applied (arrow) before insertion of the laryngeal mask, the mask, in theory, cannot occupy the space behind the cricoid cartilage. The tip of the mask might be wedged in the space behind the arytenoid cartilages. The mask is positioned at least 2 cm more proximal than usual. The arytenoid cartilages can be pushed anteriorly, and thus the mask is more likely to become dislodged. A = arytenoid cartilages, C = cricoid cartilage, E = epiglottis, T = thyroid cartilage, C5 = fifth cervical vertebra (also see Fig. 6 in Chapter 8.) With kind permission of the Editor of the *British Journal of Anaesthesia* [36].

## CRICOID PRESSURE

### Effect of Cricoid Pressure on Insertion of the Laryngeal Mask

#### *Cricoid pressure applied before insertion the laryngeal mask*

Cricoid pressure applied *before* insertion of the laryngeal mask prevents the distal part of the mask from occupying the hypopharynx, because cricoid pressure compresses both the hypopharynx and the oesophageal inlet (Fig. 12, also see Fig. 6 in Chapter 8).

In the past, it was not clear how frequently adequate ventilation was obtained through the laryngeal mask [36, 38–41]. It has been shown that the success rate of both insertion and ventilation through the laryngeal mask is low when cricoid pressure with sufficient force is applied [16]. The success rate of ventilation through the laryngeal mask may be lower when cricoid pressure is applied without support of the neck (single-handed cricoid pressure) compared with cricoid pressure with neck support (bimanual cricoid pressure) [16]. There may also be a greater risk of dislodgement of the mask even if adequate ventilation is obtained, because the distal part of the mask is not positioned correctly.

### Cricoid pressure applied after insertion of the laryngeal mask

Cricoid pressure applied *after* insertion of the laryngeal mask is effective in preventing regurgitation. In one study, cricoid pressure applied after insertion of the laryngeal mask in cadavers effectively prevented regurgitation of dilute barium in the oesophagus at a pressure of 7.8 kPa [42]. Cricoid pressure applied *after* insertion does not usually dislodge the mask [43], but it may decrease adequacy of ventilation through the mask [44].

### Effect of Cricoid Pressure on Tracheal Intubation through the Laryngeal Mask

When cricoid pressure is applied before insertion of the laryngeal mask, the success rate of subsequent tracheal intubation through the laryngeal mask is low. In one study, blind tracheal intubation through the laryngeal mask was successful in 42% of patients at the first attempt when cricoid pressure was applied, and only in 56% even without time limit (the success rates without cricoid pressure in this study were 72% and 96%, respectively) [40]. In another study, the success rate at the first attempt with cricoid pressure was only 15% even when a fibrescope was used for tracheal intubation through the laryngeal mask [36]. Even when cricoid pressure was released after insertion of the mask, tracheal intubation was still difficult, because the larynx was often compressed by a misplaced mask [36].

The effect of application of cricoid pressure *after* insertion of the laryngeal mask on the success rate of tracheal intubation has not been studied formally, but it has been claimed that subsequent tracheal intubation usually does not become difficult [43].

### SUMMARY

The laryngeal mask can be inserted easily and acceptable ventilation obtained in the majority of patients. In addition, there is little danger of life-threatening complications associated with the use of the device. Efforts to reduce any misplacement thus seem to have been largely overlooked. Yet, several complications caused by a misplaced mask have been recognized. In addition, the insertion of the mask is difficult in some situations. The correct insertion is therefore important. The incidence of misplacement can easily be reduced by using the correct method of insertion. All anaesthetists receive formal training in the art of tracheal intubation; the same efforts should be made for the laryngeal mask.

### KEY POINTS

- There are several circumstances where insertion of the laryngeal mask may be difficult.

- The laryngeal mask may not be in the correct position even when adequate ventilation is obtained.

- The incidence of complications is likely to be higher when the laryngeal mask is not placed in the correct position.

- Although it is difficult to confirm the exact position of the mask, there are several useful clinical signs to assess the position.

- Cricoid pressure impedes correct positioning of the laryngeal mask and often obstructs ventilation through the mask.

### REFERENCES

1 Brain A. I. J. The laryngeal mask – a new concept in airway management. *British Journal of Anaesthesia* 1993; **55:** 801.

2 Brodrick P. M., Webster N. R. and Nunn J. F The laryngeal mask airway. A study of 100 patients during spontaneous breathing. *Anaesthesia* 1989; **44:** 238.

3 Davies P. R., Tighe S. Q., Greenslade G. L and Evans G. H. Laryngeal mask airway and tracheal tube insertion by unskilled personnel. *Lancet* 1990; **336:** 977.

4 Maltby J. R., Loken R. G. and Watson N. C. The laryngeal mask airway: clinical appraisal in 250 patients. *Canadian Anaesthetists Society Journal* 1990;

37: 509.

5 Ferrut O., Toulouse C., Lançon J. P., Douvier S. and Fayolle J. L. The laryngeal mask for elective gynecological surgery: a very attractive oral airway dispositive. *Anesthesia and Analgesia* 1994; **78**: S110.

6 Johnston D. F., Wrigley S. R., Robb P. J. and Jones H. E. The laryngeal mask airway in paediatric anaesthesia. *Anaesthesia* 1990; **45**: 924.

7 Nandi P. R., Nunn J. F., Charlesworth C. H., Taylor S. J. Radiological study of the laryngeal mask. *European Journal of Anaesthesiology* 1991; **4** (Suppl.): 33.

8 Asai T. and Morris S. The laryngeal mask airway: its features, effects and role. *Canadian Journal of Anaesthesiology* 1994; **41**: 930.

9 Brain A. I. The development of the laryngeal mask – a brief history of the invention, early clinical studies and experimental work from which the laryngeal mask evolved. *European Journal of Anaesthesiology* 1991; **4** (Suppl.): 5.

10 Brain A. I. Studies on the laryngeal mask: first, learn the art. *Anaesthesia* 1991; **46**: 417.

11 Brain A. I. J. *The Intavent Laryngeal Mask. Instruction Manual* 2nd edn. Intavent: Henley-on-Thames. 1993.

12 Williams P. J. and Bailey P. M. Comparison of the reinforced laryngeal mask airway and tracheal intubation for adenotonsillectomy. *British Journal of Anaesthesia* 1993; **70**: 30–33.

13 Asai T., Latto I. P. and Vaughan R. S. The distance between the grille of the laryngeal mask airway and the vocal cords. Is conventional intubation through the laryngeal mask safe? *Anaesthesia* 1993; **48**: 667.

14 Mason D. G. and Bingham R. M. The laryngeal mask airway in children. *Anaesthesia* 1990; **45**: 760.

15 Ishimura H., Minami K., Sata T., Shigematsu A. and Kadoya T. Impossible insertion of the laryngeal mask airway and orophageal axes. *Anesthesiology* 1995; **83**: 867.

16 Asai T., Barclay K., Power I. and Vaughan R. S. Cricoid pressure impedes placement of the laryngeal mask airway. *British Journal of Anaesthesia* 1995; **74**: 521.

17 Brimacombe J. and Berry A. Laryngeal mask airway insertion. A comparison of the standard versus neutral position in normal healthy patients with a view to its use in cervical spine instability. *Anaesthesia* 1993; **48**: 670.

18 Pennant J. H., Pace N. A. and Gajraj N. M. Role of the laryngeal mask airway in the immobile cervical spine. *Journal of Clinical Anaesthesia* 1993; **5**: 226.

19 Aziz E. S., Thompson A. R. and Baer S. Difficult laryngeal mask insertion in a patient with Forestier's disease. *Anaesthesia* 1995; **50**: 370.

20 Shorten G. D., Opie N. J., Graziotti P., Morris I. and Khangure M. Assessment of upper airway anatomy in awake, sedated and anaesthetised patients using magnetic resonance imaging. *Anaesthesia and*

*Intensive Care* 1994; **22**: 165.

21 Brimacombe J. and Berry A. Insertion of the laryngeal mask airway – a prospective study of four techniques. *Anaesthesia and Intensive Care* 1993; **21**: 89.

22 Boidin M. P. Airway patency in the unconscious patient. *British Journal of Anaesthesia* 1985; **57**: 306.

23 Molloy A. R. Unexpected position of the laryngeal mask airway. *Anaesthesia* 1991; **46**: 592.

24 Ainsworth Q. P. and Calder I. The oesophageal detector device and the laryngeal mask. *Anaesthesia* 1990; **45**: 794.

25 Asai T. The oesophageal detector device is not useful for the laryngeal mask. *Anaesthesia* 1995; **50**: 175.

26 Asai T. Difficulty in assessing the correct position of the laryngeal mask airway. *British Journal of Anaesthesia* 1994; **72**: 366.

27 Rowbottom S. J., Simpson D. L. and Grubb D. The laryngeal mask airway in children. A fibreoptic assessment of positioning. *Anaesthesia* 1991; **46**: 489.

28 Mizushima A., Wardall G. J. and Simpson D. L. The laryngeal mask airway in infants. *Anaesthesia* 1992; **47**: 849.

29 Bannister F. B. and Macbeth R. G. Direct laryngoscopy and tracheal intubation. *Lancet* 1944; **ii**: 651.

30 Brain A. I. J. Laryngeal mask and trauma to uvula. *Anaesthesia* 1959; **44**: 1014–1015.

31 Aoyama K., Takenaka Z., Sata T. and Shigematsu A. The triple airway manoeuvre for insertion of the laryngeal mask airway in paralyzed patients. *Canadian Anaesthetists Society Journal* 1995; **42**: 1010.

32 Harding J. B. A 'skid' for easier insertion of the laryngeal mask airway. *Anaesthesia* 1993; **48**: 80.

33 Rabenstein K. Alternative techniques for laryngeal mask insertion. *Anaesthesia* 1994; **49**: 80.

34 Dingley J. and Whitehead M. J. A comparative study of the incidence of sore throat with the laryngeal mask airway. *Anaesthesia* 1994; **49**: 251.

35 Asai T., Stacey M. and Barclay K. Stylet for reinforced laryngeal mask airway. *Anaesthesia* 1993; **48**: 636.

36 Asai T., Barclay K., Power I. and Vaughan R. S. Cricoid pressure impedes placement of the laryngeal mask airway and subsequent tracheal intubation through the mask. *British Journal of Anaesthesia* 1994; **72**: 47.

37 Goudsouzian N. G., Denman W., Cleveland R. and Shorten G. Radiologic localization of the laryngeal mask airway in children. *Anesthesiology* 1992; **77**: 1085.

38 Brimacombe J. Cricoid pressure and the laryngeal mask airway. *Anaesthesia* 1991; **46**: 986.

39 Brimacombe J., White A. and Berry A. Effect of cricoid pressure on ease of insertion of the laryngeal mask airway. *British Journal of Anaesthesia* 1993; **71**: 800.

40 Heath M. L. and Allagain J. Intubation through the

laryngeal mask. A technique for unexpected difficult intubation. *Anaesthesia* 1991; **46:** 545.

41 Ansermino J. M. and Blogg C. E. Cricoid pressure may prevent insertion of the laryngeal mask airway. *British Journal of Anaesthesia* 1992; **69:** 465.

42 Strang T. I. Does the laryngeal mask airway compromise cricoid pressure? *Anaesthesia* 1992; **47:** 829.

43 Asai T. Use of the laryngeal mask for tracheal intu-bation in patients at increased risk of aspiration of gastric contents. *Anesthesiology* 1992; **77:** 1029.

44 Asai T., Barclay K., McBeth C. and Vaughan R. S. Cricoid pressure applied after placement of the laryngeal mask prevents gastric insufflation, but inhibits ventilation. *British Journal of Anaesthesia* 1996; **76;** 772.

# 10

# Fibreoptic Instruments and Tracheal Intubation in Adults and Children

*Stephen G. Greenhough and Ralph S. Vaughan*

## FIBREOPTIC INTUBATION IN ADULTS

Fibreoptic instruments are being used with increasing frequency in anaesthesia. Their main uses are in airway management, particularly in patients known to be difficult to intubate, in the intensive care unit and in thoracic anaesthesia. Therefore, it seems reasonable that all anaesthetic training programmes should include instruction and practice with these instruments [1]. However, due to the considerable cost per instrument, there may only be one or two per department and, occasionally, there may not be one available. These delicate instruments may be easily damaged entailing either expensive repairs or be rendered useless. It is also possible that cross infection could result without proper cleaning and sterilization of the instrument between cases.

When planning training programmes, it would seem prudent that the following approach be considered:

- Training in the care and cleaning of the instrument.
- Training in the handling of the instrument using dummies and aids

- Training with patients
- Further training to maintain the acquired skills.

An example of a possible training programme is illustrated in Fig. 1. There are many other programmes, the most well-known being that recommended by Dykes and Ovassapian [1]

### The Instrument

#### *Construction* (Fig. 2)

An intubating fibrescope contains bundles of glass or plastic fibres [2]. Each fibre is cladded with a material of low refractive index that prevents light supplied from an external source from leaving the core of the fibre and hence directs this light along the total length of the fibre. This is called total internal reflection. All these fibres are surrounded by a single waterproof covering that allows the instrument to be completely immersed for cleaning and disinfection procedures.

The lengths of fibrescopes vary, but there are certain features common to all instruments. The proximal end has a wide angle lens system that produces a high resolution view of the respiratory tract. There is also a small red arrow that indicates

FIBREOPTIC SCOPE TRAINING SCHEDULE

| Name | DR.  A. N. OTHER | | | | |
|---|---|---|---|---|---|
| 1. Care of scope<br>    (a) General<br>    (b) Cleaning | | | | | |
| 2. Visualization of<br>    Larynx in Dummy | 1 | 2 | 3 | 4 | 5 |
| 3. Intubation in<br>    Dummy | 1 | 2 | 3 | 4 | 5 |
| 4. Visualization of<br>    Larynx in Patients | 1 | 2 | 3 | 4 | 5 |
| 5. Endotracheal<br>    Intubation in<br>    Patients<br>Note: Oral (O) | 1 | 2 | 3 | 4 | 5 |
|     Nasal (N) | 6 | 7 | 8 | 9 | 10 |
|     G.A. (G) | 11 | 12 | 13 | 14 | 15 |
|     Awake/<br>    Sedated (A) | 16 | 17 | 18 | 19 | 20 |

**Figure 1**   An example of a training programme in fibreoptic techniques.

which way the distal tip is pointing initially and can be used thereafter as a reference point with regard to the position of the tip within the respiratory tract. Alongside is the angulation control lever, which is connected to the tip of the fibrescope.

The distance between the control area and the tip of the fibrescope is only moderately flexible. The instrument should not be bent to an angle greater than approximately 45°. Excessive bending can fracture the fibres and can lead to dots appearing at the viewing lens. If too many fibres fracture, the view becomes increasingly indistinct. It also contains a small tube (1.2 mm. diameter) that is attached to the suction port proximally and open to the atmosphere at the tip. This tube is mainly used for suction and injection purposes but, if required, 100% oxygen can be insufflated along this channel. Such a facility can be of considerable advantage in a difficult and prolonged procedure. It is a considerable engineering feat to contain all these components in an instrument with an external diameter as small as 4 mm.

The tip is the most flexible part of the scope and can move between 0° and 120° but all movements are controlled by the angulation lever. The tip contains three main components (Fig. 3), namely:

- the light source;
- the objective lens;
- the orifice for suction, injection of local anaesthetic or other agents, or insufflation.

## Cleaning

The following procedures are recommended for cleaning the instrument after it has been used [3] The fibrescope is washed repeatedly with clear water. The channels are brushed and clean water and air are suctioned through them alternately A leak test is performed to ensure that the outer

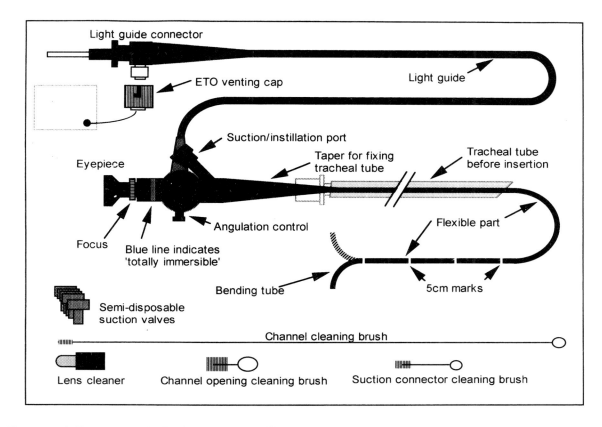

**Figure 2**   A fibreoptic intubating bronchoscope. Kind permission of Dr P. L. Jones

waterproof covering is intact. Finally, the instrument is allowed to dry (see Appendix).

## Disinfection

These processes are repeated with a suitable disinfectant (see Appendix).

## Sterilization

This is a specialized procedure and the reader is recommended to consult the manufacturer's manual [3]. The fibrescope can be soaked in glutaraldehyde for a maximum of 10 h. This is the 'cold' sterilization process. Alternatively, the fibrescope can be sterilized using ethylene oxide gas.

## Storage

The fibrescope should be stored with the tube as straight as possible in a purpose designed cupboard or case.

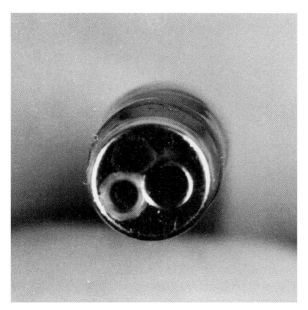

**Figure 3**   The tip of the bronchoscope.

## Training

### *Familiarization with the instrument*

There is no doubt that the initial instruction periods should be spent 'getting to know' the instrument [1, 4–6]. The first lesson is that the total movements are controlled by the proximal end. If the operator's controlling hand rotates to the right, the fibrescope also moves to the right, and vice versa. This is important as the distal end cannot move independently (Figs 4 and 5). Failure to move both hands simultaneously in the same direction as the fibrescope could lead to possible torque damage.

The second lesson is that the operator should know exactly which way the tip is pointing. With the instrument in the normal position, the tip moves forwards and backwards. The only way it can move any other way is if the whole instrument is rotated, e.g. through 90°, to achieve a total sideways movement.

The third lesson is that the fingers of the hand that holds the distal end should always rotate in the same direction as the proximal hand and should not normally release that end. If the distal end is released, the position of the tip could move, particularly in the pharynx, and the operator can lose the 'anatomical bearings'. Furthermore, the first three fingers, which usually hold the distal end, should be used to 'feed' the tube into the airway.

### *Dummies*

It has been shown that practice with dummies enhances the success rates when the trainees start to practise *de novo* with patients [4]. Consequently, the use of dummies is highly desirable. There are several available for this purpose including the Olympus or Ambu Intubation Training Models. Using the instrument with dummies rapidly increases the dexterity of the trainees.

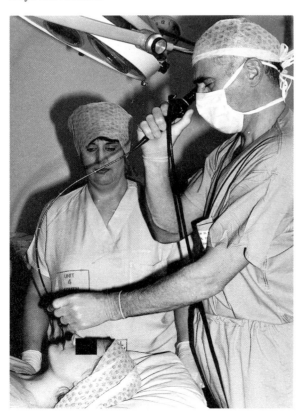

**Figure 4**   This demonstrates how the fibrescope should be held in the anteroposterior position by the operator.

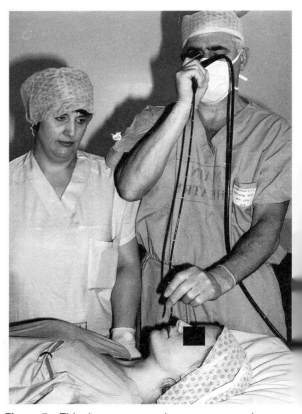

**Figure 5**   This demonstrates the operator moving both hands and body around for an alternative view, e.g. a lateral view.

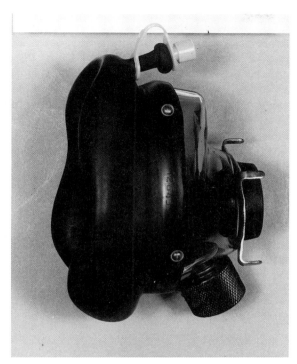

**Figure 6**   Patil Syracuse mask. Note plastic mould and two apertures.

## Intubating aids

Various aids are available for either the nasal or oral approach, and occasionally for both routes.

**Patil Syracuse mask** (Fig. 6)

This modified mask allows the fibrescope to pass either through the nasal passages or the oral cavity and is particularly useful in the early stages of training [7]. More importantly, it allows spontaneous ventilation or enables the anaesthetist to control ventilation if required.

### Aids for the nasal route

These are not used as frequently as the oral varieties. The major problem is possible damage in the nasal passages that can cause much bleeding.

### Aids for the oral route

There are several aids that can be used. For example:

- A special connector can be attached to facemasks, e.g. the Intersurgical Connector (Fig. 7).
- Berman Mark II airway (Fig. 8). This is a modified Guedel airway [8, 9]. When properly placed in the mid line, its distal part is just above the rima glottidis. The Ovassapian [10] and the Williams Airway Intubator [11] are used for the same purpose.
- Laryngeal mask airway (LMA) (Fig. 9). This airway allows excellent facilities for training [12]. It can be used during spontaneous or artificial ventilation while allowing an excellent view of the cords [13]. Recently, the split laryngeal mask has been used successfully as an aid to training in fibreoptic intubation.

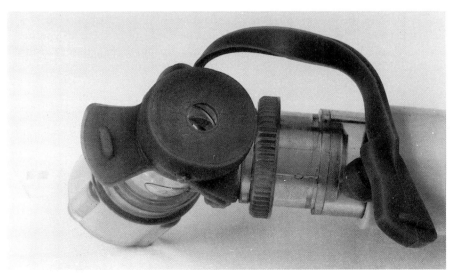

**Figure 7**   An Intersurgical Connector.

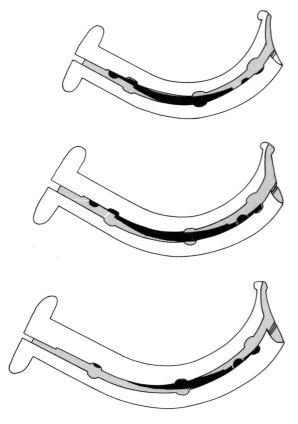

**Figure 8**   Set of Berman Mark II airways. Redrawn from Hogan *et al.* [9], with kind permission of the authors and the editor of *Anaesthesia and Intensive Care.*

## *Fibreoptic intubation*

Training with patients can be accomplished under sedation and local anaesthesia or general anaesthesia. Whichever technique is used, there is a requirement for minimum monitoring that includes an ECG, a blood pressure cuff and a pulse oximeter. Intravenous access is essential before any procedure is undertaken. It must also be remembered that the insertion of a fibrescope into the respiratory tract produces physiological responses. In particular, the cardiovascular responses to fibreoptic intubation are similar to those associated with laryngoscopy [5]. However, these responses can be greater and last longer.

Many different anaesthetic techniques are used for teaching fibreoptic intubation. There is a tendency for the teacher and trainee to concentrate on the task of introducing and advancing the instrument and to rely on auditory alarms. Thus, there is a danger that clinical changes in the patients may be missed. A trained observer is therefore essential during teaching sessions to alert the trainer and trainee to any significant changes [14].

### Sedation and local anaesthesia

It is important when starting to learn to use these instruments to visit a clinic where fibreoptic laryngoscopy and bronchoscopy are performed regularly. In the UK these techniques are usually practised in Otorhinolaryngology (ENT) and Chest Medicine clinics. Sedation usually, but not always, commences with an appropriate premedication [15]. Oral benzodiazapines are commonly used. Atropine should also be given at an appropriate time before endoscopy to decrease upper respiratory tract secretions. Dry conditions allow the more efficient distribution and action of local anaesthetic agents. In addition, atropine prevents reflex bradycardia. Although many patients will have received some form of premedication, they are usually further sedated using appropriate doses of an intravenous benzodiazepine, an anal-

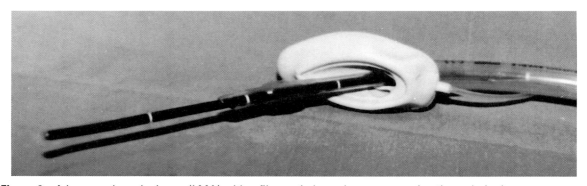

**Figure 9**   A laryngeal mask airway (LMA) with a fibreoptic bronchoscope passing through the lumen.

gesic and occasionally a butyrophenone, e.g. droperidol [5]. Local anaesthesia is introduced either orally, nasally or through the cricothyroid membrane [15]. Additional techniques are described in Chapter 7. Although many physicians use the nasal route, increasing numbers now use the oral route. It is advisable when using this route, to use a 'bite-block'.

Awake intubation is commonly accomplished via the nasal route. Both topical lignocaine and cocaine have been used to produce anaesthesia of the nose. Cocaine also produces local vasoconstriction that can reduce the chances of haemorrhage. Both agents require sufficient time to act. When the oral route is used the tongue and the back of the oral cavity must also be anaesthetized. This is normally performed using topical lignocaine and the 'spray as you go' technique and/or an injection through the cricothyroid membrane [15].

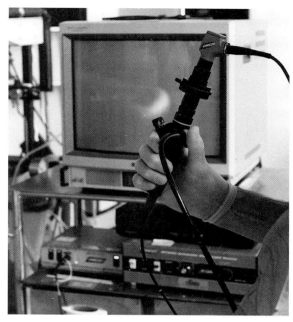

**Figure 11**   A television adaptor for teaching.

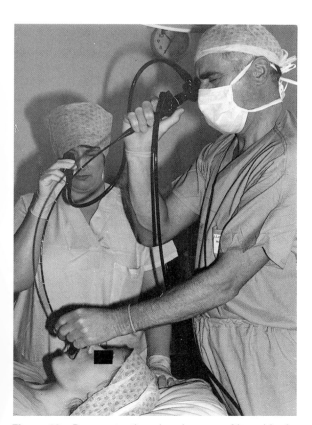

**Figure 10**   Demonstration showing use of 'teaching' viewer.

### General anaesthesia

Several techniques have been described, ranging from a conventional balanced anaesthetic technique to a computerized intravenous propofol infusion regimen [14, 16]. When compared with sedation and local anaesthetic techniques, general anaesthesia has a greater potential for complications. These can include [5]:

- hypoxia;
- hypercarbia;
- dysrhythmias, especially when volatile agents are used;
- awareness.

Some techniques therefore include manual hyperventilation with high concentrations of inspired oxygen and a volatile agent beforehand to try to counteract these complications. The potential for complications makes the need for minimum monitoring and an independent trained observer indispensable.

During these procedures, the trainee will benefit from either a teaching attachment (Fig. 10) or, increasingly, a television camera attached to the fibrescope [17] (Fig. 11). These will help the trainee to become familiar with the anatomical landmarks.

## Intubation Routes

### *Nasal route*

The preoperative visit should include an examination of the nasal passages. The patency of the nasal passages is tested by obstructing one side, then the other, with the patient breathing in and out. Airflow is normally easier through one side than the other. The side with the least resistance to airflow should be used for the passage of the fibrescope and tracheal tube. Either the fibrescope, the tube, or a combination of both, is passed along the floor of the nose. This floor is convex, which usually means in the supine position that the general curve of all instruments should be downwards and backwards with the tip pointing slightly anteriorly. It should be noted that obstructions can be caused by the inferior turbinates or by nasal polyps.

There are various different techniques for nasal intubation:

- Some anaesthetists pass the fibrescope through the nose, into the pharynx, through the vocal cords into the trachea. This technique should enable the operator to detect any unforeseen obstruction such as polyps. However, this technique may have an increased incidence of 'red out' due either to bleeding, or in obese patients, the tip of the fibrescope abutting against folds of endothelium in the pharynx. The tracheal tube is subsequently 'railroaded' over the fibrescope into the trachea.

- Other anaesthetists pass the nasotracheal tube blindly into the pharynx. The fibrescope is then passed through it into the trachea and again the nasotracheal tube is 'railroaded' over the fibrescope. The main disadvantage of this method is that any unforeseen obstruction, such as a nasal polyp, can be dislodged, carried forward, or become impacted in the tube itself. Such trauma can cause much bleeding, increasing the difficulty of the procedure.

With both techniques, it is also advisable to try to increase the 'oropharyngeal space'. This can be achieved by asking the assistant to pull the jaw forward in the same fashion as clearing the airway. Finally, both methods can be complicated by a 'white out'. This is due either to respiratory tract secretions or water condensation covering the objective lens. To prevent this complication, many anaesthetists include an antisialogogue with their premedication, while others insufflate a continuous flow of oxygen down the suction port.

### *Oral route*

The majority of training for fibreoptic intubation has been performed via the nasal route. However, the oral route under general anaesthesia is increasingly used for the same purpose. One of the perceived advantages of this route, particularly in the UK, is that the turnover of patients is greater for any given time. Hence, more training opportunities arise. The main disadvantages are the possible complications of general anaesthesia and muscle paralysis [14]. These include hypoxia, hypercarbia, dysrhythmias and awareness. The other main disadvantage is the pronounced acute angle between the oropharyngeal and the laryngeal–tracheal axes, which can increase technical difficulties. The difficulties can be reduced by using a suitable airway guide and/or displacing the mandible anteriorly to increase the 'pharyngeal space'.

The initial training of fibreoptic oral intubation under general anaesthesia is mainly performed with intubating aids that are specifically designed for teaching and accomplishing orotracheal intubation. The design of the Berman and Ovassapian airways is based on the Guedel airway [8]. The proximal end sits between the teeth and the distal end just above the rima glottidis. The fibreoptic scope can be passed to the end of these airways where the vocal cords usually come into view. The tip of the fibreoptic scope is passed into the trachea and the tracheal tube is passed over the scope into the trachea. The airway is then removed.

Recently, the laryngeal mask airway (LMA) has also proved extremely beneficial in training programmes. It has also been used as an aid to intubation in patients with both normal and abnormal upper airways. After the LMA has been introduced and ventilation shown to be adequate, a fibrescope 'loaded' with a 6.0 mm tracheal tube is introduced into the LMA [13]. The vocal cords are visualized and the fibreoptic scope passed into the trachea. The tracheal tube is passed over the fibrescope into the trachea. The fibrescope is removed and the tracheal tube connected to a breathing system. Artificial ventilation commences and the cuff of the tracheal tube is inflated until an air-tight seal is achieved. Successful

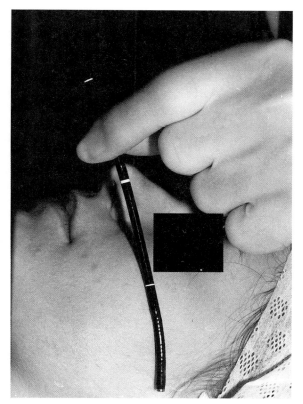

**Figure 12** Measuring the fibrescope against the side of the face from the tragus of the ear to the corner of the mouth. The distance is noted by the left hand.

tracheal intubation is confirmed. However, in approximately 33% of patients, the cuff straddles the vocal cords [18].

There are three ways to prevent possible vocal cord damage under these circumstances, namely:

- use a longer non-standard tracheal tube, e.g. Mallinckrodt nylon reinforced tube or a Portex Microlaryngeal tube;
- use a split LMA that can be removed from the mouth at the same time as the tracheal tube is advanced;
- pass a long gum elastic bougie through the tracheal tube and remove both LMA and tracheal tube. The same tracheal tube can be reintroduced over the bougie into the trachea. Alternatively, a large bore tracheal tube can be introduced.

After all three techniques, confirmation of successful tracheal intubation is essential [19, 20].

There are several techniques used for oral fibreoptic intubation. One example is set out below:

- Measure the distance between the tragus of the ear and the angle of the mouth against the fibrescope (Fig. 12).
- Note that distance by holding the proximal part of the fibrescope between the thumb and first two fingers (Fig. 12).
- Manipulate the tip of the fibrescope approximately 45° in a forward direction (Fig. 13).
- The anaesthetic assistant displaces the jaw slightly downwards and forward (Fig. 14).
- Pass the fibrescope, *in the mid line* to the point where the fingers of the guiding hand touch the lips (Fig. 15).

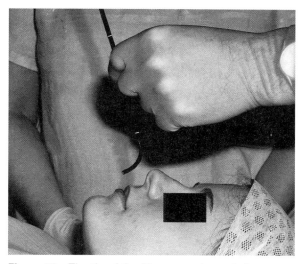

**Figure 13** The tip of the fibrescope is angled anteriorly.

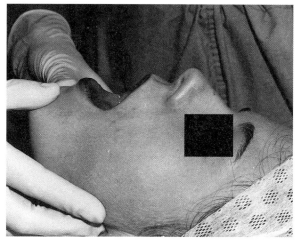

**Figure 14** The assistant displaces the jaw anteriorly.

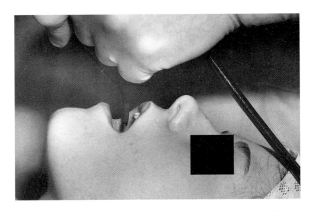

**Figure 15**   The fibrescope is introduced in the mid line until the fingers come to the lips.

- The vocal cords should come into view. The tip of the fibrescope is passed through the cords into the trachea. At this point, the assistant who is holding the jaw may be able to assist by watching for transillumination through the cricothyroid membrane.
- Occasionally, there can be difficulty in the subsequent passage of the tracheal tube. The tip of the tube may impinge against the epiglottis or get stuck in either of the vallecula fossae. To overcome these potential problems, the method recommended by Dogra et al. is of great assistance [21]. In essence, a laryngoscope is inserted into the mouth and the tip of the tube is rotated 90° anticlockwise to pass the obstruction before being returned to the normal position as it passes through the vocal cords into the trachea.

Once the fibreoptic scope has been removed, the tracheal tube is connected to the breathing system. Whatever route is chosen and whichever method is used, it is mandatory that the tube is confirmed to be properly placed in the trachea [19, 20].

There is one additional and convenient method that can also be used to confirm correct placement. As the tip of the fibreoptic scope is withdrawn, both the tip of the tracheal tube and the radio-opaque line contained within its substance can be seen to lie against the tracheal wall.

## Causes and Incidences of Failure

Ovassapian and his colleagues have investigated the incidence and causes of failure with fibreoptic nasal intubations [22]. In a few patients, the scope could not be passed owing to narrowed nasal passages. Of the remainder there were five failures (1.2%) out of 418 attempts. In three, the scope was passed into the trachea but the tube would not pass through the vocal cords.

In 89% of cases visualization of the cords was classified as easy with a mean intubation time of 3 min (Table 1). These intubations were performed by trainees, although the senior more experienced anaesthetists were able to intubate patients in 20–30 s in whom exposure of the cords was easy.

**Table 1**   Ease of laryngeal exposure in 353 intubations. From Ovassapian et al. [22], with kind permission of the International Anaesthesia Research Society.

|  | Easy | Moderately difficult | Difficult |
|---|---|---|---|
| Visualization of vocal cords | 315 (89.2%) | 30 (8.5%) | 8 (2.3%) |
| Mean intubation time (min)* | 3.0 | 6.76 | 16.1 |
| Mean total intubation time (min)† | 16.4 | 19.6 | 28.1 |

*Time from insertion of fibrescope to completion of intubation
†Time from beginning of sedation to completion of intubation

*Easy:* on initial introduction the fibrescope was already aligned for good visualization of the vocal cords so that little or no manipulation of the tip of the scope was needed.

*Moderately difficult:* moderate manipulation of the fibrescope in all directions was necessary to locate the vocal cords.

*Difficult:* extensive manipulation of the fibrescope in all directions, often with changes in position of the operator, was necessary to identify the vocal cords.

Intubation was also easily accomplished in patients in whom there had been previous difficulty. Difficulties occurred when there was distorted airway anatomy, laryngeal pathology, if there was a decreased space between the edge of the epiglottis and the posterior pharyngeal wall and in the presence of bloody secretions. A suction channel is critically important if blood or secretions obscure the view. The causes of difficulty with this method are different from those that occur when using a rigid laryngoscope.

The causes of failure described by Ovassapian and colleagues are illustrated in Table 2 [22]. They include operator inexperience, inadequate local anaesthesia of the airway, distorted anatomy, and the inability to pass a tracheal tube over fibrescope and difficulty in retracting the fibrescope through the tracheal tube [23].

**Table 2**  Causes of failure of fibreoptic intubation. From Ovassapian [23], with kind permission of Raven Press.

- Lack of training and experience
- Presence of secretions and blood
- Inadequate topical anesthesia
- Decreased space between the tip of the epiglottis and the posterior pharyngeal wall
- Large, floppy epiglottis
- Supraglottic cyst or mass
- Inflammation or oedema of the oropharynx
- Severe flexion deformity of the cervical spine
- Distorted airway anatomy
- Inability to advance the endotracheal tube or withdraw the fibrescope

## FIBREOPTIC INTUBATION IN CHILDREN

Children present a special challenge if fibreoptic intubation is required. The causes of difficult intubation in children are usually congenital and may therefore be associated with anaesthetic problems other than the intubation. As the option of awake fibreoptic intubation is not available, the anaesthetist may then be faced with both a difficult general anaesthetic and a difficult intubation. It is clear that there is no place for either the occasional fibreoptic intubator or the occasional paediatric anaesthetist in dealing with these demanding cases.

The following section deals with the use of the fibreoptic laryngoscope in small children. A child for whom a 6.0 mm cuffed endotracheal tube is appropriate can be intubated using any of the described adult techniques.

## Equipment
### Fibreoptic laryngoscopes

The modern fibreoptic laryngoscopes most commonly used for difficult adult intubation have an external diameter of 3.5 mm and a 1 mm diameter suction channel (Fig. 16). These scopes will pass through a tracheal tube as small as 4.5 mm. The suction channel allows local anaesthetic to be sprayed into the larynx and trachea under direct vision and also allows the passage of a flexible guidewire into the trachea. Although at least one manufacturer makes a fibreoptic laryngoscope with an external diameter of 2.0 mm, the author has intubated neonates as small as 1.5 kg using a standard scope and the guidewire technique and

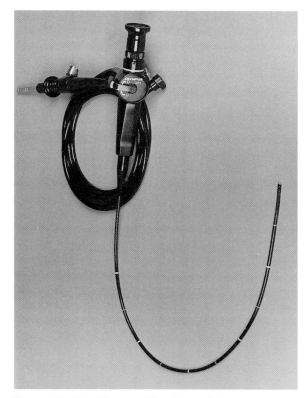

**Figure 16**   The Olympus LF 1 fibreoptic laryngoscope.

feels that the increased versatility and durability of a 3.5 mm fibreoptic laryngoscope makes it a better purchase, even in a paediatric environment.

### Airway maintenance

In general, as inhalational anaesthesia is deepened, the muscle tone in the oropharynx decreases and the airway becomes progressively more difficult to maintain. In the most severe case this loss of muscle tone may well precede the obtunding of laryngeal reflexes. Maintaining the airway in these circumstances may well be more difficult than performing the intubation. Several airways are readily available to help provide airway control.

### Airways

#### Nasopharyngeal
These represent the best solution. The Robertazzi nasopharyngeal airway (Fig. 17), manufactured by Rusch, is made in sizes 20–36FG, allowing for a gradual increase in size as anaesthesia deepens. As the pharyngeal muscle tone decreases a small airway is inserted nasally. If it is of appropriate

length, it will not cause laryngospasm. The size of airway can be increased stepwise as anaesthesia deepens, allowing an adequate depth of anaesthesia to be achieved in even the most difficult patient. The Robertazzi airway is made of soft latex and causes very little nasal trauma.

### Guedel

This is of limited use in the difficult patient because its insertion may be required before the laryngeal reflexes are sufficiently obtunded, the resulting laryngospasm making an already difficult situation impossible. In the more straightforward cases it allows easy airway maintenance with no risk of epistaxis.

### Laryngeal mask airway

This has the same disadvantage as the Guedel airway, in that the patient has to be deeply anaesthetized before the mask airway is inserted. Once in place, it will often provide a very good airway in a difficult patient, and has been advocated as a secure airway, allowing the guided placement of the fibreoptic laryngoscope [24].

## General Anaesthesia

The option of awake intubation with local anaesthesia is not available for most difficult paediatric intubations, with the possible exception of neonates. Most of the intubations will have to be conducted under general anaesthesia. The difficulties of airway maintenance have been discussed and demand an inhalation induction in order to maintain spontaneous respiration. Children under 25 kg should receive atropine 10 μg kg$^1$ before induction of anaesthesia to prevent the bradycardia associated with deep halothane anaesthesia.

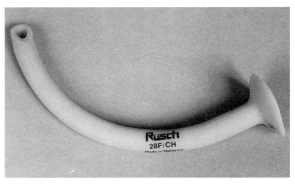

**Figure 17**   The Robertazzi nasopharyngeal airway.

Halothane is the volatile agent of choice administered in oxygen with or without nitrous oxide. Halothane allows a smooth induction of anaesthesia, with minimal respiratory side effects, and allows an adequate depth of anaesthesia for instrumentation and intubation. Local anaesthesia can be used to spray the larynx and upper trachea to reduce further the incidence of laryngospasm during fibreoptic intubation and a dose of 3 mg kg$^1$ of lignocaine may be used. This local anaesthetic solution may be injected down the suction channel of the scope under direct vision.

## Technique of Fibreoptic Intubation

The conventional technique of railroading a tracheal tube over the fibreoptic laryngoscope provides a simple, safe method of intubation for adults and older children. It has some disadvantages for smaller children. If a guidewire is passed through the suction channel of the fibreoptic laryngoscope into the trachea and the guidewire is used to railroad the tracheal tube, then many of these disadvantages are overcome. The guidewire technique allows tubes of any size to be used with a standard laryngoscope and allows multiple tube changes after one instrumentation attempt. This is very significant in children with complex problems as the systemic effects of these disorders may make the prediction of tracheal tube size very difficult.

The guidewire technique may be used following an unaided fibreoptic laryngoscopy [25–27] or, as recently described by Hasan and Black [24], after passing the fibrescope through a laryngeal mask airway. A detailed description of the author's favoured method is as follows:

- Establish deep halothane anaesthesia. The anaesthesia needs to be deep enough to allow tracheal intubation without coughing or breath holding.
- Visualize the larynx using the fibreoptic laryngoscope (Fig. 18a) and spray the larynx and upper trachea with 3 mg kg$^{-1}$ of 1% or 2% lignocaine. Spraying the local anaesthetic is made much easier if an 18 g epidural catheter is inserted down the suction channel and the local anaesthetic injected down the epidural catheter.
- Insert a long cardiac catheter guidewire (145 cm long, 0.035" (0.089 cm) diameter) flexible end first, down the suction channel of the fibre-

optic laryngoscope so that it is just visible in the field of the scope.

- Visualize and approach the larynx and *without* placing the laryngoscope through the vocal cords advance the guidewire into the trachea (Fig. 18b).
- Remove the laryngoscope leaving the guidewire in the trachea (Fig. 18c) Care is required here to avoid inadvertent removal of the guidewire. At this stage anaesthesia can be deepened using a facemask if required.
- Advance an appropriate size, well-lubricated, Mallinckrodt silicone reinforced tracheal tube over the guidewire to the larynx and into the trachea (Fig. 18d). Any difficulty advancing the tube through the larynx can be overcome by rotating the tube at the same time as gently advancing it. Most other tracheal tubes do not allow reliable railroading and cannot be recommended.
- The guidewire can now be passed through a Jackson–Rees T piece and out through the tail of the bag, and the T piece connected to the tracheal tube. The position of the tube can now be confirmed and the degree of leak assessed.
- If the tracheal tube size is satisfactory the tube can be fixed and the guidewire removed (Fig. 18e). Alternatively, the tracheal tube can be removed and a different size tube railroaded over the guidewire.

The skills necessary for fibreoptic laryngoscopy and intubation in small children can be learned by any anaesthetist who is either already familiar with adult fibreoptic laryngoscopy or is prepared to learn conventional fibreoptic laryngoscopy on older children. It should be borne in mind, however, that many of these patients present anaesthetic difficulties requiring skills other than just fibreoptic intubation. Many of the cases are better dealt with by two anaesthetists, one to anaesthetize and monitor the child, the other to perform the intubation.

## THE INTENSIVE CARE UNIT

The fibreoptic bronchoscope can be used in the intensive care unit (ICU) for three purposes, namely:

- It can be used to confirm the position of the tip of the tracheal tube in a similar fashion to the

(a)

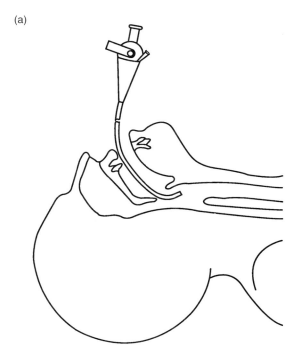

(b)

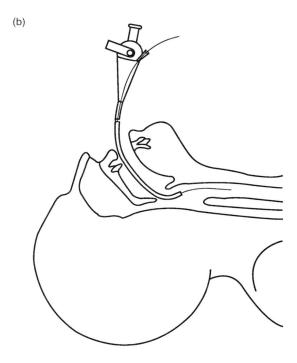

**Figure 18**   The guidewire technique.
(a) Visualize the cords with the laryngoscope.
(b) Pass the guidewire through the cords into the trachea.

(c)

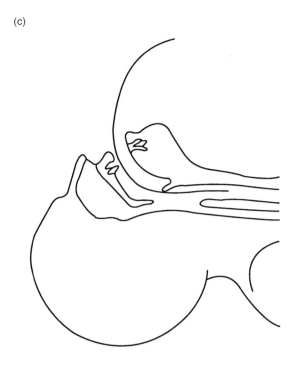

(d)

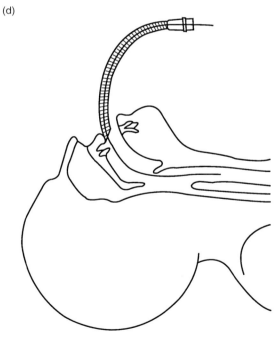

(e)

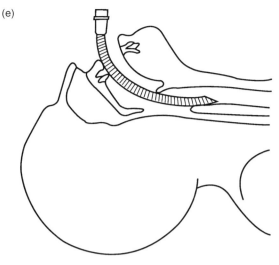

(e) The tube in place and the guidewire removed.

technique described for confirmation of correct placement [23], although using a slightly modified technique. The tip of the fibrescope is positioned just above the carina and the main bronchi identified. The position of the fibrescope at the proximal end of the tracheal tube is noted and marked. The fibrescope is withdrawn and the operator stops when the tip of the fibrescope is alongside the tip of the tracheal tube. The position on the fibrescope at the proximal end of the tracheal tube is again marked. The scope is completely withdrawn and the distance between the two marks measured. This is approximately equal to the distance between the carina and the tip of the tracheal tube. These measurements can be checked daily (or at any time) and recorded on the observation charts. This manoeuvre may lead to a reduction in patient exposure to radiation from repeated chest X-rays. Furthermore, additional oxygen can be insufflated down the suction port during these measurements.

- The fibrescope may be used to obtain secretions from the respiratory tract for bacteriological examination and occasionally, brushings for histological examination.
- The fibrescope can be used to locate and remove plugs of mucus that may have caused lobar or lung collapse. However, as the suction port has such a small diameter, it may not be possible to remove some of these plugs. Under these circumstances, rigid bronchoscopy is usually recommended.

**Figure 18**
(c) Remove the laryngoscope, leaving the guidewire in place.
(d) Railroad the tracheal tube over the guidewire into the trachea.

If a fibrescope is used for any of these purposes, it is essential that it is properly cleaned and sterilized before further use. Failure to do so can lead to cross infection.

## THORACIC ANAESTHESIA

The fibreoptic bronchoscope is used increasingly in thoracic anaesthesia to confirm the position of specialized single and double endobronchial tubes. This aspect is dealt with in Chapter 17.

---

## KEY POINTS

- The anaesthetist must be familiar with the procedures for cleaning, disinfection and sterilization of the instrument.

- Training should proceed along set guidelines. The first step should be for the anaesthetists to familiarize themselves with the instrument, practise on dummies and use intubation aids.

- Sedation and local analgesia techniques must be learned and practised in adults.

- General anaesthesia can be used but there are dangers with prolonged physiological responses, possible hypoxia, hypercarbia and awareness.

- In children, general anaesthesia is used. Specialized personnel and equipment are mandatory.

- The fibreoptic equipment can be used in intensive care and for thoracic anaesthesia.

---

## REFERENCES

1 Dykes M. H. M. and Ovassapian A. Teaching and learning fiberoptic tracheal intubation. In: *Fiberoptic Airway Endoscopy in Anesthesia and Critical Care*. New York: Raven Press, 1990; 163–8.

2 Sloan T. B. and Ovassapian A. The principles of flexible fiberoptic endoscopes. In: *Fiberoptic Airway Endoscopy in Anesthesia and Critical Care*. New York: Raven Press, 1990; 1–14.

3 Olympus Optical Company Co Ltd., San-Ei Building 22-2 Nishi Shinjuku 1-chrome. *Official Operating Manual*. Shinjuku-ku, Tokyo, Japan (USA, UK and Europe).

4 Ovassapian A., Yelich S. T., Dykes M. H. M. and Golman M. E. Learning fiberoptic intubation: Use of simulators v traditional teaching. *British Journal of Anaesthesia* 1988; **61**: 217.

5 Vaughan R. S. Training in fibreoptic laryngoscopy. *British Journal of Anaesthesia* 1991; **66**: 538.

6 Mason R. A. Learning fibreoptic intubation: fundamental problems. *Anaesthesia* 1992; **47**: 729.

7 Patil V., Stehling L. C., Zander H. L. and Koch J. P. Mechanical aids for fiberoptic endoscopy. *Anesthesiology* 1982; **57**: 69.

8 Guedel A. E. A non traumatic pharyngeal airway. *Journal of the American Medical Association* 1933; **100**: 1862.

9 Hogan K., Harper M. H. and Pollard B. J. The use of a pharyngeal guide to aid intubation with the fibreoptic laryngoscope *Anaesthesia and Intensive Care* 1984; **12**: 18.

10 Ovassapian A. and Dykes M. H. M. The role of fiberoptic endoscopy in airway management. *Seminars of Anesthesia* 1987; **6**: 93.

11 William R. T. and Harrison R. E. Prone tracheal intubation simplified using an airway intubator. *Canadian Anaesthetists Society Journal* 1981; **28**: 288.

12 Brain A. I. J. The laryngeal mask – a new concept in airway management. *British Journal of Anaesthesia* 1983; **55**: 801.

13 Silk J. M., Hill H. M. and Calder I. Difficult intubation and the laryngeal mask – a new approach to an old problem. *European Journal of Anaesthesiology* (Suppl.) 1991; **4**: 47.

14 Hartley M. E., Morris S. and Vaughan R. S. Teaching fibreoptic intubation: effect of Alfentanil on the haemodynamic response. *Anaesthesia* 1994; **49**: 4.

15 Issac P. A., Barry J. E., Vaughan R. S., Rosen M. and Newcombe R. G. A jet nebuliser for delivery of topical anaesthesia to the respiratory tract. A comparison with cricothyroid puncture and direct spraying for fibreoptic bronchoscopy. *Anaesthesia* 1990; **45**: 49.

16 Schaefer H. G. and Marsch S. C. V. Comparison of orthodox with fiberoptic orotracheal intubation

under total I. V. anaesthesia. *British Journal of Anaesthesia* 1991; **66:** 60.

17 Smith J. E., Mackenzie A. A. and Scott Knight V. C. E. Comparison of two methods. A fibrescope guided tracheal intubation. *British Journal of Anaesthesia* 1991; **66:** 546.

18 Asai T., Latto I. P. and Vaughan R. S. The distance between the grille of the laryngeal mask and the vocal cords. *Anaesthesia* 1993; **48:** 667.

19 Clyburn P. and Rosen M. Accidental oesophageal intubation. *British Journal of Anaesthesia* 1994; **73:** 55.

20 Anderson K. A. and Hald A. Assessing the position of the tracheal tube. The reliability of different methods. *Anaesthesia* 1989; **44:** 984.

21 Dogra S. S., Falconer R. F. and Latto I. P. Tracheal tube placement over a gum elastic bougie. *Anaesthesia* 1990; **45:** 774.

22 Ovassapian A., Yelich S. J., Dykes M. H. M. and Brunner E. E. Fibreoptic nasotracheal intubation – incidence and causes of failure. *Anesthesia and Analgesia* 1983; 692.

23 Ovassapian A. Fiberoptic tracheal intubation. In: *Fiberoptic Airway Endoscopy in Anaesthesia and Critical Care*, New York: Raven Press. 1990; 57–79.

24 Hasan M. A. and Black A. E. A new technique for fibreoptic intubation in children. *Anaesthesia* 1994; **49:** 1031.

25 Stiles C. M. A flexible fibreoptic bronchoscope for endotracheal intubation in infants. *Anesthesia and Analgesia* 1974; **53:** 1017.

26 Howardy-Hansen P. and Berthelsen P. Fibreoptic bronchoscopic nasotracheal intubation of a neonate with Pierre Robin syndrome. *Anaesthesia* 1988; **43:** 121.

27 Scheller J. G. and Schulman S. R. Fibreoptic bronchoscopic guidance for intubating a neonate with Pierre Robin syndrome. *Journal of Clinical Anaesthesia* 1991; **3:** 45.

# APPENDIX

## Cleaning

1 Wipe the tube with soft moist gauze.
2 Place the distal end in clean water and suction for approximately 10 s alternating with air. Turn off the suction device and disconnect suction line.
3 Remove the suction valve and place in a cleaning solution.
4 Perform leak test procedure.
5 Immerse the entire instrument into the cleaning solution and wash all external surfaces. Remove the instrument, place in clean water and rinse.
6 Insert the purpose made cleaning brushes through all channels to brush the entire suction line.
7 Wash and rinse the suction valve.
8 Reconnect the suction line and suction sterile water and air alternately several times. Continue to aspirate air for approximately 30 s until all the moisture has been expelled and the channel is dry.
9 Dry all external surfaces of the instrument.

## Disinfection

1 Immerse the fibrescope in a disinfectant solution and pump the disinfectant solution through channels using a syringe.
2 Allow the instrument to remain in the disinfectant solution for the recommended period of time.
3 Remove the instrument from the disinfectant solution and suction clean water until the channel is thoroughly rinsed.
4 Thoroughly rinse the outside of the fibrescope. Remove the fibrescope from water and place on a clean, dry surface.
5 Suction air until all the moisture has been expelled and the channel is dry.
6 Wipe the outside surface of the instrument until it is dry.

# 11

# The Detection of Accidental Oesophageal Intubation

*Paul A. Clyburn*

## INTRODUCTION

A fit young woman undergoing diagnostic laparoscopy is anaesthetized by an experienced anaesthetist. Routine preoxygenation is carried out for 3 min and intubation is apparently straightforward. The anaesthetist satisfies himself that the tube is in the trachea by auscultation of both axillae and is further reassured by a normal 'feel' to hand ventilation. Surgery commences but 10 min after induction, the anaesthetist is puzzled by a progressive arterial desaturation. He systematically checks the breathing system, and faced with obvious clinical cyanosis discards the breathing system for a self inflating bag. Bradycardia is followed by ventricular fibrillation and cardiopulmonary resuscitation is commenced. Finally the anaesthetist checks the tracheal tube by direct laryngoscopy and finds the tube in the oesophagus. The tube is resited in the trachea and resuscitation is successful but subsequent recovery reveals irreversible brain damage.

This mythical case scenario is typical of the many cases described in the scientific literature and in medical legal claims. It highlights some of the problems and misconceptions associated with accidental oesophageal intubation. The accidental placement of a tracheal tube in the oesophagus is not uncommon and is, in itself, harmless; but a delay or failure to detect the misplacement and establish the airway will result in harm to the patient.

Undetected oesophageal intubation has been recognized as a problem for more than 40 years [1]. It is a major cause of litigation in the UK [2, 3] and the USA [4], accounting for around 7% of claims involving anaesthetic practice, and frequently results in brain damage or the patient's death. It is a major cause of maternal death [5], and accounts for around 2% of reported critical incidents [6], many of which are associated with a poor outcome [7].

## WHY DOES OESOPHAGEAL INTUBATION GO UNDETECTED?

The incidence of unrecognized oesophageal intubation is not greatly influenced by the experience of the operator – an experienced anaesthetist is as likely to fail to detect oesophageal placement as a trainee [6, 8]. Also, undetected oesophageal intubation occurs as commonly during apparently straightforward intubation as during difficult intubation [6].

During straightforward intubation the tube is seen to pass through the larynx, which should be adequate confirmation of correct placement. However, observation error can occur or the tube may be misplaced during fixation while no longer under direct observation. Moreover, the routine nature of the situation can lead to reduced vigilance. Oesophageal intubation has then occurred under circumstances in which the anaesthetist is convinced of correct placement, particularly when unreliable clinical signs reinforce the belief that all is well. The development of hypoxaemia is delayed, especially when the patient has been preoxygenated [9], and occurs at a time when the causes are legion, preventing prompt diagnosis of cause and effective action.

In contrast, when intubation is difficult, the anaesthetist is alerted to the possibility of oesophageal placement. However, if clinical signs contrive to mislead, (s)he will be reluctant to remove a tube which was difficult to place and will look elsewhere for causes of the resultant hypoxia.

During cardiopulmonary resuscitation there is a particular danger of undetected oesophageal intubation because of the varied experience of personnel and the difficulty of the environment. In all situations the anaesthetist must remain aware of the possibility of oesophageal intubation and not place too great a reliance upon clinical signs.

In addition to misplacement of the tracheal tube, displacement of a correctly placed tube can occur at any time whilst the patient has a tracheal tube in place and is a significant cause of misadventure [8, 10]. Radiological studies reveal that positioning and movement of the patient's head can move the tip of the tracheal tube as much as 5 cm up and down the trachea [11], which can result in extubation and subsequent intubation of the oesophagus. The possibility of this event should be considered every time the patient's head is moved and the correct position of the tube should be reconfirmed. Displacement of the tracheal tube is a particular hazard in the intensive care unit where patients remain intubated for prolonged periods and tube fixation may be inadequate.

## METHODS OF DETECTING CORRECT TRACHEAL TUBE PLACEMENT

Rapid and reliable detection of tracheal tube misplacement and displacement is fundamental to safe management of the compromised airway. As yet there is no ideal method of detection but the features of an ideal monitor are outlined in Table 1. The methods currently available can be divided into clinical and technical tests.

**Table 1** Features of an ideal test for detecting oesophageal intubation.

- Totally reliable without false negative results (failing to detect oesophageal intubation when it occurs).
- No incidence of false positive results (indicating oesophageal intubation when tube is in the trachea).
- Simple and rapid to perform.
- Safe to patient and operator.
- Easy to interpret by inexperienced personnel.
- Capable of continuous monitoring with alarm parameters to detect displacement whilst patient is intubated.
- Portable and easily used outside specialist areas such as during community resuscitation.
- Inexpensive.

## Clinical Tests

There are a number of clinical signs which are used by clinicians to confirm that the tracheal tube is in the trachea, some of which are more useful than others (see Table 2). In addition there are signs which, when present, suggest misplacement of the tracheal tube in the oesophagus.

### Signs which help confirm the tube is in the trachea

The observation of the tracheal tube passing through the larynx should be totally reliable in confirming correct placement. However, as the case scenario above illustrates, human observation error prevents its total reliability and a fixed conviction that misplacement is impossible after direct observation may hinder subsequent diagnosis and corrective action being taken. Furthermore, it is not always possible to visualize the larynx and be sure of correct placement. When a misplacement is suspected, repeat laryngoscopy is usually simple to perform and may provide the diagnosis. If the larynx cannot be visualized, pressing the tube backwards against the soft palate displaces the larynx posteriorly and may bring it into view [12].

Symmetrical outward expansion of the chest wall in response to positive pressure ventilation is thought by many to be a reliable sign of tracheal tube placement. The sign is unreliable because chest expansion may be difficult to assess in obese patients, in the presence of large breasts, or when the patient has a rigid chest wall or lung disease. Furthermore, cadaver studies [13] supported by anecdotal case reports [13–16] have demonstrated chest wall movement mimicking lung ventilation

**Table 2**   Fallibility of common clinical signs.

| Clinical sign | Problem |
| --- | --- |
| Visualization of tube passing through the cords | Observation error<br>Distraction |
| Chest auscultation | Between-patient variability<br>Oesophageal ventilation can produce wall vibration |
| Observation of chest movement | Misleading in obese or in patients with poor chest compliance<br>Oesophageal and gastric distension may expand chest |
| Reservoir bag compliance and refill | Between-patient variation<br>Normal refill of bag from oesophageal gas (especially when fresh gas continues to flow into circuit) |
| Palpation of tracheal tube movement within trachea | Differentiation of tracheal and oesophageal movement difficult |
| Lack of cyanosis | Late indication, especially when patient is preoxygenated<br>Cyanosis is a non-specific sign |
| Presence of water vapour condensing in breathing system | Oesophageal gas may contain water vapour, though absence of vapour suggests oesophageal misplacement |

during oesophageal ventilation. Intermittent distension of the oesophagus with a closed cardio-oesophageal sphincter can lift the mediastinum and expand the chest wall [13]; distension of the stomach by gas leaking through the sphincter may give the appearance of diaphragmatic descent and expansion of the lower chest.

Another popular misconception is that auscultation of breath sounds when properly performed is reliable. However, numerous case reports [13–19], and even studies using blinded observers [20, 21], have demonstrated the unreliability of this sign. The quality of breath sounds varies according to the place of auscultation and the rate and volume of ventilation. Air passing through the oesophagus can produce oesophageal wall vibration which mimics harsh breaths sounds [15] and, without true breath sounds to compare, may be mistaken for lung ventilation. The sensitivity of

this clinical sign can be improved by auscultation over the trachea and the epigastrium to detect the bubbling sound of gastric ventilation, in addition to each lung base and axilla [17, 20, 21].

The characteristic 'feel' of the reservoir bag when ventilating the patient's lungs relies upon the normal compliance of the lung producing refill of the bag during expiration. Lung compliance varies between patients, and moreover, refilling of the bag by insufflated gas from the stomach can also occur [13, 15, 16], especially when fresh gas continues to flow into the breathing system [22]. Even during spontaneous respiration, the expiratory refill of the bag is an unreliable sign [18] as tidal volumes in excess of 50 ml can be produced by a tube in the oesophagus when the patient tries to breath against a closed glottis [23]. High negative intrathoracic pressures generated during obstructed inspiration are transmitted to the compliant oesophagus and gas is sucked in.

Various techniques for palpating the tube to verify tracheal placement have been described. The cuff of the tracheal tube can be felt within the palpable part of the trachea, especially if simultaneously the cuff is deflated and reinflated or the tube moved back and forth [24]. A finger placed on the trachea at the sternal notch or during cricoid pressure may detect vibrations as the tip of the advancing tube passes over the tracheal rings during successful tracheal placement [25]. Alternatively, a gloved hand can be placed in the mouth after intubation and the intra-atytenoid groove identified together with its relationship to the tube [20, 26]. None of these signs can be considered reliable [27].

Sharp compression of the sternum whilst listening over the open end of the tracheal tube for air expelled from the lungs is suggested as a means of differentiating tracheal from oesophageal intubation. This test is unreliable [13] for two reasons: air from the lung can be forced out of the unintubated trachea and be mistaken as coming from an oesophageal tube; and air introduced into the oesophagus and stomach during mask ventilation can be expelled through an oesophageal tube.

## Signs whose presence suggest oesophageal misplacement

The following clinical signs, when present, alert the clinician to the possibility of oesophageal intubation, but their absence should not lead to a complacency that oesophageal intubation could not have occurred.

Oesophageal intubation and ventilation would be expected to be accompanied by progressive gastric distension [28]. This is difficult to detect in obese patients, when gas refluxes back through the lower oesophageal sphincter, or when the stomach is already distended by previous mask ventilation. Overall, this sign is very unreliable [13].

The sound produced by escaping gas during ventilation of an oesophageal placed tube with the cuff deflated is said to be more guttural than that from a tracheal tube. In addition, the more flexible wall of the oesophagus makes it more difficult to achieve an effective seal when the cuff is inflated, though a seal is easily achieved when the cuff of the oesophageal tube is at the level of the cricoid cartilage [13]. These signs are not reliable.

Expired gas from the lung will contain water vapour, which can be seen as condensation in the lumen of clear plastic components of the breathing system. Gas from the oesophagus may also contain water vapour so that the sign is unreliable [20, 27], though the absence of water condensation is highly likely to be due to oesophageal misplacement.

The presence of what appears to be gastric contents in the tube suggests oesophageal intubation [29]. This is unreliable as excessive lung secretions may be mistaken for gastric contents and gastric contamination can occur prior to intubation. The absence of gastric contents should certainly not provide reassurance of tracheal placement.

The presence of cyanosis is a relatively late sign of oesophageal intubation and is non-specific, there being many other causes which may need to be considered. Preoxygenation and the possibility that some degree of ventilation through an unobstructed larynx can still occur when the oesophagus and stomach are ventilated [30], means that arterial desaturation is delayed and not associated with the tube misplacement. The very presence of cyanosis demands prompt action to correct its cause if cardiac arrest or cerebral damage are to be avoided. Pulse oximetry alerts the clinician to desaturation at an earlier stage but is no better at elucidating the cause of the desaturation [31].

In summary, clinical signs are useful pointers and frequently alert the physician to the possibility of oesophageal intubation. However, it is important to realize their limitations and that the absence of contrary clinical signs do not rule out tube misplacement.

**Table 3** Effectiveness of technical tests.

| Test | Effectiveness |
|---|---|
| Capnography | Equipment not routinely available outside of specialized anaesthetic areas<br>Technical reasons can produce false positive results<br>Unsuitable for cardiac resuscitation |
| $CO_2$ colorimetry devices | More portable than capnography but still false positives during cardiac resuscitation |
| Negative pressure device | No reported false negative results to date and simple to use<br>6% false positive results |
| Eschmann introducer – palpable tracheal clicks, progress arrested by carina | Reliability unproven |
| Fibreoptic confirmation | Limited availability for routine confirmation<br>Fragile and easily damaged |
| Transtracheal illumination | Requires darkened room and experienced operator<br>Unreliable, especially in obese, bull neck |
| Chest radiography | Time delay<br>Unreliable at differentiating oesophageal from tracheal intubation |

## Technical Tests

The unreliability of clinical signs at detecting oesophageal intubation has led to the evaluation of a variety of technical tests; some simple using readily available equipment, others involving more complex apparatus (see Table 3). The most reliable technical test is the continued detection of carbon dioxide in expired gas. However, this frequently relies on complex equipment which may not be practical in all situations and simpler negative pressure devices are proving reliable and are being increasingly used.

### Carbon dioxide detection

Provided pulmonary perfusion is adequate, alveolar gas contains carbon dioxide in a concentration of around 5%, while gas emanating from the oesophagus and stomach is usually free of carbon

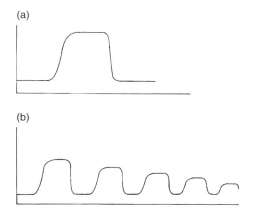

**Figure 1** (a) Normal $CO_2$ waveform from lung ventilation. (b) $CO_2$ waveform diminishing rapidly, suggesting oesophageal ventilation.

dioxide. Capnography, using analysers which display the waveform (Fig. 1a), is a sure way of differentiating oesophageal from tracheal intubation [32–34]. Carbon dioxide can be detected in the stomach or oesophagus [30, 35], either from exhaled alveolar gas forced into the stomach by previous bag ventilation, or from prior ingestion of carbonated drinks[36], but in these situations the carbon dioxide is quickly washed out (Fig. 1b) and should be undetectable within six or so breaths [36, 37]. Capnography is usually available in the operating theatre but is less convenient in other situations where tracheal intubation is performed. Portable, non-quantitative infrared devices such as the Minicap III carbon dioxide detector [38–40] or colorimetric detectors such as the

Fenum detector [41–45] are more convenient though less sensitive alternatives (Fig. 2). It should be remembered that capnography during cardiopulmonary resuscitation is unreliable because of the unpredictable pulmonary carbon dioxide production [46, 47].

### Negative pressure tests (oesophageal detector device) (Fig. 3)

Negative pressure applied to a tube within the oesophagus causes collapse of the soft wall around the tube and aspiration of gas is impossible. In contrast the rigid tracheal rings prevent wall collapse around a tracheal tube and gas is freely aspirated. Aspiration can be performed by attaching a 60 ml syringe [48] or a self inflating rubber or plastic bulb [49] such as an Ellick's evacuator bulb [50] to the tube by means of suitable connections. Free aspiration of gas into the syringe or rapid refill of the bulb confirms tracheal placement. These devices are cheap, simple, and convenient to use, as illustrated by their successful use by paramedics during resuscitation [51]. They have been extensively evaluated under experimental clinical conditions and have proved to be reliable at detecting oesophageal placement (no reported false negatives) [2, 20, 48, 52–54] but produce false positive tests in approximately 6% of cases [53], suggesting oesophageal intubation when the tube is really in the trachea. False positive tests can occur after endobronchial intubation [55], when the tracheal tube bevel abuts against the tracheal wall [56] (the inclusion of a Murphy's eye or the rotation of the tube through 90° before

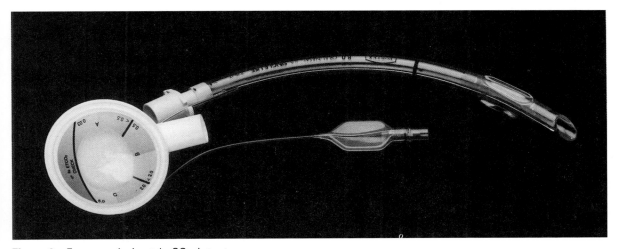

**Figure 2** Fenum colorimetric $CO_2$ detector.

(a)

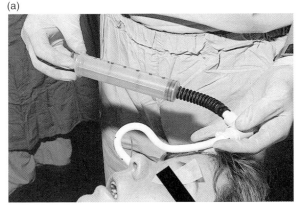

(b)

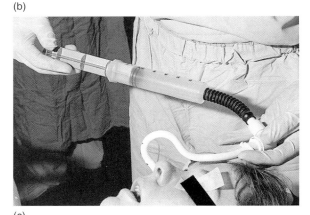

(c)

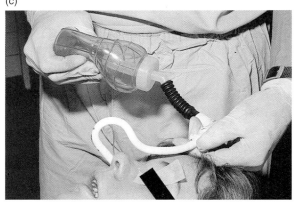

(d)

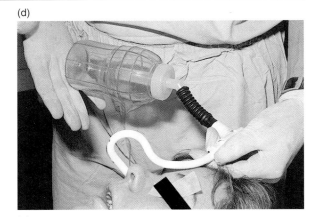

(e)

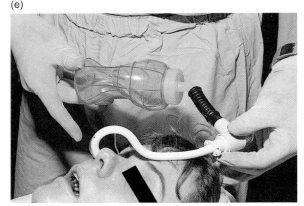

**Figure 3**   Negative pressure oesophageal detector devices. (a) 60 ml syringe before aspiration. (b) Easy aspiration confirming tracheal tube placement. (c) Plastic Ellick's evacuator bulb is squeezed. (d) On release, rapid refill confirms tracheal intubation. (e) Slow or absent refill indicates oesophageal intubation.

repeating the test may overcome this problem), in asthmatics [57], and in cases of upper airway obstruction [58]. The technique is not suitable for small infants [59].

### Fibreoptic confirmation and transtracheal illumination

A fibreoptic laryngoscope or bronchoscope can be used to confirm correct placement of the tracheal tube by visualizing the carina or tracheal rings [60]. The technique is usually only practical when the fibreoptic scope has been used for laryngoscopy or when misplacement is suspected, cannot be confirmed by other means, and the instrument is readily available.

The fibreoptic light wand is a flexible intubating stylet. It has a fibreoptic light emitting from the distal end that will illuminate the end of the tracheal tube [61]. The intensity of transillumination when viewed in a darkened room can differentiate between oesophageal and tracheal intubation. The interpretation requires experience and may be difficult in the presence of neck swelling and obesity.

### Eschmann introducer and similar devices

A flexible intubating stylet such as the Eschmann introducer passed into the trachea through the tube produces characteristic vibrations felt by the guiding hand [62] as the tip of the introducer rubs against the tracheal rings. Furthermore, resistance is encountered after advancing to about 28–32 cm in an adult, while no such resistance is encountered if the tube is in the oesophagus [29] as the introducer freely enters the stomach. Alternatively, a suitably sized lubricated nasogastric catheter can be threaded down the tracheal tube until resistance is met and then gently withdrawn while suction is applied to the catheter [63]. The absence of an abrupt halt to advancement and resistance to withdrawal (due to the collapse of the non-rigid oesophageal wall) are suggestive of oesophageal intubation.

## Miscellaneous methods

The video stethoscope consists of two small microphones placed on each side of the chest with their output displayed on an oscilloscope in an X–Y format. The patterns observed on the oscilloscope can distinguish tracheal from oesophageal ventilation [64]. The technique appears cumbersome and its reliability has not been evaluated.

Whereas the hand cannot detect the difference in gas flow produced from ventilating the trachea or oesophagus, a sophisticated neural network-based computer can learn the subtle differences in ventilatory flow characteristics of tracheal and oesophageal placed tubes and then apply this knowledge to detect oesophageal intubation [65]. Further development and evaluation of computerized flow analysis is required but could provide the foundation for a successful detection device.

Chest radiography is time-consuming, expensive and involves a delay before the film is processed. A 25° oblique view is more reliable than an anteroposterior projection at identifying tracheal placement [66, 67]. The main value of chest radiography is to verify the position of the distal end of the tube and detect endobronchial intubation.

Ultrasound imaging can be used to confirm tracheal tube position [68] but requires the use of a foam cuff or the substitution of saline for air in the cuff.

## CONCLUSION

The routine nature of tracheal intubation can lead to complacency over the danger of undetected oesophageal intubation. Clinical signs are fallible

and overestimation of their reliability may result in the clinician overlooking oesophageal placement as the cause of progressive hypoxia. Thus clinical signs must be backed up by a reliable technical test in **all** situations (see Table 4). Capnography is the most reliable test and when available should be used at induction to confirm tracheal placement. Indeed, continuous capnography is strongly recommended as one of the minimal monitoring standards during general anaesthesia [69]. When capnography is impractical, unavailable, or when carbon dioxide excretion is uncertain, such as during cardiac resuscitation, the negative pressure oesophageal detector device is a simple, portable and reliable alternative.

If oesophageal placement is suspected (see Table 5), visual confirmation is usually possible by laryngoscopy aided by backward pressure on the tube which may bring the larynx into better view.

**Table 4** Minimum confirmation of tracheal tube placement.

| Auscultate over trachea, apices, axillae and epigastrium |
| --- |
| **plus either** |
| • Confirm $CO_2$ concentration > 4% for six breaths |
| **or** |
| • Perform negative pressure test |

**Table 5** Suspicion that the tube is in the oesophagus.

| Confirm tracheal placement by: |
| --- |
| **either** |
| • Capnography waveform observed over at least six breaths (unreliable during cardiac arrest) |
| **or** |
| • Direct laryngoscopy visualizing tube passing through the larynx |
| **or** |
| • Fibreoptic confirmation of tracheal rings |
| If none of above available or possible: |
| • Negative pressure test is simple and reliable |

If tracheal placement cannot be reliably confirmed then tube should be removed, oxygenation maintained by mask ventilation and the trachea reintubated.

**When in doubt – take it out**

If doubt remains the tube should be removed – **'when in doubt, take it out'**. When intubation has been difficult, it may be prudent to secure the route for reintubation should suspicions prove to be unfounded, by first passing a flexible introducing stylet through the tube. An improvement in clinical condition by mask ventilation after the tube has been removed suggests oesophageal misplacement as the cause. Alternatively, the tube may be left *in situ* and a laryngeal mask inserted, which will bypass an oesophageal tube and establish the airway [70].

---

## KEY POINTS

- Accidental intubation of the oesophagus is a common event and, in itself, is of little consequence provided it is quickly detected and the tube resited in the trachea.

- Failure to detect oesophageal intubation and the consequent hypoxia is a major cause of anaesthetic morbidity and mortality.

- Undetected oesophageal intubation is as common during straightforward intubation as during difficult intubation. The experience of the operator is no protection.

- Clinical signs are unreliable and should always be backed up by a reliable test.

- The continued presence of $CO_2$ expired gases, as detected by capnography, is the most reliable test of correct tracheal placement, and where practical should be used after every attempted tracheal intubation.

- When capnography is unavailable or impractical, a negative pressure aspiration test is simple and reliable, though occasionally produces false positives resulting in unnecessary removal of a correctly placed tube.

---

## REFERENCES

1 Edwards G., Morton H. J. V., Pask E. A. and Wylie W. D. Deaths associated with anaesthesia. A report on 1000 cases. *Anaesthesia* 1956; **11**: 194.

2 Baraka A., Salem M. R., Brennar A. M., Nimmagadda U. and Heyman H. J. Use of self inflating bulb in detecting esophageal ventilation. *Anesthesiology* 1992; **77**: A294.

3 Utting J. E. Pitfalls in Anaesthetic practice. *British Journal of Anaesthesia* 1987; **59**: 877.

4 Caplan R. A., Posner K. L., Ward R. J. and Cheney F. W. Adverse respiratory events in anesthesiology. A closed claims analysis. *Anesthesiology* 1990; **72**: 828.

5 Abrams M. E. and Metters J. S. *Report on Confidential Enquiries into Maternal Deaths in England and Wales 1985–1987*. London: HMSO. 1991; 73–87.

6 Holland R., Webb R. K. and Runciman W. B. Oesophageal intubation: an analysis of 2000 incident reports. *Anaesthesia and Intensive Care* 1993; **21**: 608.

7 Cooper J. B., Newbower R. S. and Kitz R. J. An analysis of major errors and equipment failures in anaesthesia management: Considerations for prevention and detection. *Anesthesiology* 1984; **60**: 34.

8 Gannon K. Mortality associated with anaesthesia: a case review study. *Anaesthesia* 1991; **46**: 962.

9 Howells T. H. A hazard of pre-oxygenation. *Anaesthesia* 1985; **40**: 86.

10 Keenan R. L. and Boyan C. P. Cardiac arrest due to anaesthesia. A study of incidence and cause. *Journal of the American Medical Association* 1985; **253**: 2373.

11 Conrardy P. A., Goodman L. R., Lainge F. and Singer M. M. Alteration of endotracheal tube position. Flexion and extension of the neck. *Critical Care Medicine* 1976; **4**: 7.

12 Ford R. W. J. Confirming tracheal intubation – a simple manoeuvre. *Canadian Anaesthetists Society Journal* 1983; **30**: 191.

13 Pollard B. J. and Junius F. Accidental intubation of the oesophagus. *Anaesth Intens Care* 1980; **8**: 183.

14 Cundy J. Accidental intubation of oesophagus. *Anaesthesia and Intensive Care* 1981; **9**: 76.

15 Howells T. H. and Riethmuller R. J. Signs of endotracheal intubation. *Anaesthesia* 1980; **35**: 984.

16 Ogden P. N. Endotracheal tube misplacement. *Anaesthesia and Intensive Care* 1983; **11**: 273.

17 Peterson A. W. and Jacker L. M. Death following inadvertent esophageal intubation: a case report. *Anesthesia and Analgesia* 1973; **52**: 398.

18 Stirt J. A. Endotracheal tube misplacement. *Anaesthesia and Intensive Care* 1982; **10**: 274.

19 Tetsu Uejuma. Esophageal intubation. *Anesthesia and Analgesia* 1987; **66**: 481.

20 Andersen K. H. and Hald A. Assessing the position of the tracheal tube. The reliability of different methods. *Anaesthesia* 1989; **44**: 984.

21 Andersen K. H. and Schultz-Lebahn T. Oesophageal intubation can be undetected by auscultation of the chest. *Acta Anaesthesiologica Scandinavica* 1994; **38**: 580.

22 Baraka A., Tabakian H., Idriss A. and Taha S.

Breathing bag refilling. *Anaesthesia* 1989; **44:** 81.

23 Robinson J. S. Respiratory recording from the oesophagus (letter). *British Medical Journal* 1974; **4:** 225.

24 Chander S. C. and Feldman E. Correct placement of endobroncheal tubes. *New York State Journal of Medicine* 1979; **79:** 1843.

25 Roy R. C. Esophageal intubation. *Anesthesia and Analgesia* 1987; **66:** 482.

26 Charters P. and Wilkinson K. Tactile orotracheal tube placement. A bimanual tactile examination of the positioned orotracheal tube to confirm laryngeal placement. *Anaesthesia* 1987; **42:** 801.

27 Gillespie J. H., Knight R. G., Middaugh R. E., Menk E. J. and Baysinger C. L. Efficacy of endotracheal tube cuff palpation and humidity in distinguishing endotracheal from esophageal intubation. *Anesthesiology* 1988; **69 (Suppl. 3A):** A265.

28 Tessler S., Kupfer Y., Lerman A. and Arsura E. L. Massive gastric distention in the intubated patient. A marker for a defective airway. *Archives of Internal Medicine* 1990; **150:** 318.

29 Birmingham P. K., Cheney F. W. and Ward R. J. Esophageal intubation: a review of detection techniques. *Anesthesia and Analgesia* 1986; **65:** 886.

30 Linko K., Paloheimo M. and Tammisto T. Capnography for detection of accidental oesophageal intubation. *Acta Anaesthesiologica Scandinavica* 1983; **27:** 199.

31 Guggenberger H., Lenz G. and Federle R. Early detection of inadvertent oesophageal intubation: pulse oximetry vs. capnography. *Acta Anaesthesiologica Scandinavica* 1989; **33:** 112.

32 Ionescu T. Signs of endotracheal intubation. *Anaesthesia* 1981; **36:** 422.

33 Murray I. P and Modell J. H. Early detection of endotracheal accidents by monitoring carbon dioxide concentrations in respiratory gas. *Anesthesiology* 1983; **59:** 344.

34 Bashein G. and Cheney F. W. Carbon dioxide detection to verify intratracheal placement of a breathing tube. *Anesthesiology* 1984; **61:** 782.

35 Sum Ping S. T. Esophageal intubation. *Anesthesia and Analgesia* 1987; **66:** 483.

36 Zbinden S. and Schupfer G. Detection of oesophageal intubation: the cola complication. *Anaesthesia* 1989; **44:** 81.

37 Sum Ping S. T. Reliability of capnography in identifying esophageal intubation with carbonated beverages or antacids in the stomach. *Anesthesiology* 1991; **73:** 333.

38 Vukmir R. B., Heller M. B. and Stein K. L. Confirmation of endotracheal tube position: a miniaturised infrared qualitative $CO_2$ detector. *Annals of Emergency Medicine* 1990; **19:** 465.

39 McLeod G. A. and Inglis M. D. The MiniCAP III Detector: assessment of a device to distinguish oesophageal from tracheal intubation. *Archives of Emergency Medicine* 1992; **9:** 373.

40 Petrioanu G., Widjaja B. and Bergler W. F. Detection of oesophageal intubation: can the 'cola complication' be potentially lethal? *Anaesthesia* 1992; **47:** 70.

41 O'Callaghan J. P. and Williams R. T Confirmation of tracheal tube intubation using a chemical device. *Canadian Anaesthetists Society Journal* 1988; **33:** S59.

42 O'Flaherty D. and Adams A. P. The end-tidal carbon dioxide detector. Assessment of a new method to distinguish oesophageal from tracheal intubation. *Anaesthesia* 1990; **45:** 653.

43 Strunin L. and Williams R. T. An alternative to the oesophageal detector device. *Anaesthesia* 1989; **44:** 929.

44 Denman W. T., Hayes M., Higgins D. and Wilkinson D. J. The Fenem $CO_2$ detector device. An apparatus to prevent unnoticed oesophageal intubation. *Anaesthesia* 1990; **45:** 465.

45 Goldberg J. S., Rawle P. R., Zehnder J. L. and Sladen R. N. Colorimetric end-tidal carbon dioxide monitoring for tracheal intubation. *Anesthesia and Analgesia* 1990; **70:** 191.

46 Donahue P. J. More about the esophageal detector. *Anesthesia and Analgesia* 1991; **73:** 671.

47 Muir J. D., Randalls P. B., Smith G. B. and Taylor B. L. Disposable carbon dioxide detectors. *Anaesthesia* 1991; **46:** 323.

48 Wee M. Y. The oesophageal detector device. Assessment of a new method to distinguish oesophageal from tracheal intubation. *Anaesthesia* 1988; **43:** 27.

49 Loan P. B. and Orr I. Another modification of the oesophageal detector device. *Anaesthesia* 1992; **47:** 443.

50 Nunn J. F. The oesophageal detector device. *Anaesthesia* 1988; **43:** 804.

51 Donahue P. L. The oesophageal detector device. An assessment of accuracy and ease of use by paramedics. *Anaesthesia* 1994; **49:** 863.

52 O'Leary J. J., Pollard B. J. and Ryan M. J. A method of detecting oesophageal intubation or confirming tracheal intubation. *Anaesthesia and Intensive Care* 1988; **16:** 299.

53 Zaleski L., Abello D. and Gold M. I. The esophageal detector device: does it work? *Anesthesiology* 1993; **79:** 244.

54 Williams K. N. and Nunn J. F. The oesophageal detector device. A prospective trial on 100 patients. *Anaesthesia* 1989; **44:** 412.

55 Wee M. Y. Comments on the oesophageal detector device. *Anaesthesia* 1989; **44:** 930.

56 Calder I., Smith M. and Newton M. The oesophageal detector device. *Anaesthesia* 1989; **44:** 705.

57 Baraka A. The oesophageal detector device in the asthmatic patient. *Anaesthesia* 1993; **48:** 275.

58 Baraka A. The oesophageal detector device. *Anaesthesia* 1991; **46**: 697.

59 Haynes S. R. and Morton N. S. Use of the oesophageal detector device in children under one year of age. *Anaesthesia* 1990; **45**: 1067.

60 Whitehouse A. C. and Klock L. E. Evaluation of endotracheal tube position with the fibreoptic intubation laryngoscope. *Chest* 1975; **68**: 848.

61 Stewart R. D, LaRosee A., Stoy W. A. and Heller M. B. Use of a lighted stylet to confirm correct endotracheal tube placement. *Chest* 1987; **92**: 900.

62 Kidd J. F., Dyson A. and Latto I. P. Successful difficult intubation. Use of the gum elastic bougie. *Anaesthesia* 1988; **43**: 437.

63 Kalpokas M. and Russell W. J. A simple technique for diagnosing oesophageal intubation. *Anaesthesia and Intensive Care* 1989; **17**: 39.

64 Huang K. C., Kraman S. S. and Wright B. D. Video stethoscope – a simple method for assuring continuous bilateral lung ventilation during anesthesia. *Anesthesia and Analgesia* 1983; **62**: 586.

65 Leon M. A., Rasanen J. and Mangar D. Neural network-based detection of esophageal intuabation. *Anesthesia and Analgesia* 1994; **78**: 548.

66 Batra A. K. and Cohn M. A. Uneventful prolonged misdiagnosis of esophageal intubation. *Critical Care Medicine* 1983; **11**: 763.

67 Smith G. M., Reed J. C. and Choplin R. H. Radiographic detection of esophageal malpositioning of endotracheal tubes. *American Journal of Roentgenology* 1990; **154**: 23.

68 Raphael D. T. and Conrad F. U. III. Ultrasound confirmation of endotracheal tube placement. *Journal of Clinical Ultrasound* 1987; **15**: 459.

69 *Recommendations for Standards of Monitoring during Anaesthesia and Recovery*. London: The Association of Anaesthetists of Great Britain and Ireland. 1988.

70 Pace N. A., Gajraj N. M., Pennant J. H., Victory R. A., Johnson E. R. and White P. F Use of the laryngeal mask airway after oesophageal intubation. *British Journal of Anaesthesia* 1994; **73**: 688.

# 12

# Paediatric Intubation

*Nuala M. Dunne*

## ANATOMY OF THE AIRWAY

There are several differences in the anatomy of the upper airway in children that can make intubation more difficult than in adults. The differences are most pronounced in the neonate [1].

### Tongue

The infant tongue is much larger in relation to the oral cavity and predisposes towards airway obstruction. This is more common in children with Down's syndrome.

### Larynx

The infant larynx lies higher in the neck (C3–4) compared with the adult (C4–6). The higher position of the larynx allows swallowing and nasal breathing to occur simultaneously and places the tongue against the soft palate during normal breathing, causing oral airway obstruction. Children are obligate nose breathers until the age of 3–5 months. The infant larynx is at a more acute angle to the base of the tongue and makes intubation more difficult as it lies anterior to the line of vision obtained with laryngoscopy. The larynx gradually descends, most of this occurring in the first year of life, but does not attain the adult position until the fourth year of life.

### Epiglottis

In the infant the epiglottis is narrow, short and U shaped, and lies posteriorly over the larynx at an angle of 45° (Fig. 1).

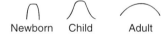

**Figure 1** Changes in the shape of the epiglottis with increasing age. From Brown & Fisk [2] with permission of the publisher, Blackwell Scientific Publications.

### Vocal cords

The vocal cords in infants are angled more forwards and downwards, and predispose to catching the tip of the tracheal tube at the anterior commissure during intubation.

### Cricoid Cartilage

This is the narrowest part of the infant's airway. The tube size selected must therefore be one that passes easily through the cricoid cartilage. The cricoid narrowing and the angulation of the vocal cords have generally disappeared by the age of 10–12 years.

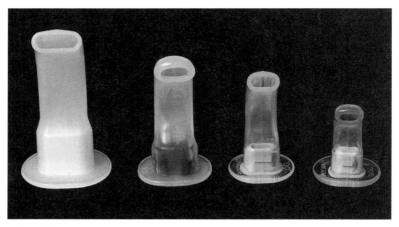

**Figure 2** Paediatric Guedel airways.

**Table 1** The Guedel airway.

| Age | Size | Length (cm) |
|---|---|---|
| Preterm | 00,000 | 3.5, 4.5 |
| Neonate–3 months | 0 | 5.5 |
| 3–12 months | 1 | 6.0 |
| 2–5 yrs | 2 | 7.0 |
| >5yrs | 3 | 8.0 |

### Tonsils

The tonsils and adenoids are small in a neonate but gradually grow to reach a maximum size at 4–7 years and then gradually recede.

### Occiput

The neonate has a relatively large head owing to the advanced development of the brain. This can cause difficulty with intubation as the head may roll around and it may be difficult to visualize the larynx. As the head is large and the distance between cords and carina is short, the tip of the tracheal tube may move up quite considerably with head flexion and down with head extension.

### Trachea

The infant trachea is deviated downwards and posteriorly, whereas in the adult it is straight down. Cricoid pressure therefore has more effect in aiding tracheal intubation in infants.

## PAEDIATRIC EQUIPMENT

### Airways

The Guedel airway is the airway most commonly used in children (Fig. 2). The correct size is one that equals the distance from the mouth to the angle of the mandible (see Table 1).

### Masks

Rendell–Baker masks have the smallest dead space (Fig. 3). The clear plastic Laerdel masks also have a reduced dead space and allow observation of the child's colour (Fig. 4). They are also softer and form a good seal more easily. Laerdel masks

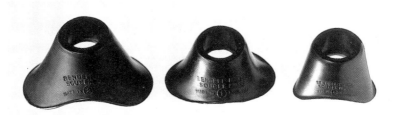

**Figure 3** Rendell–Baker masks.

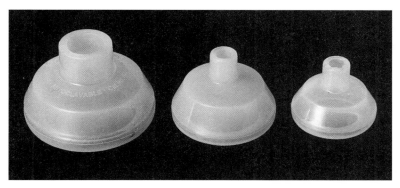

**Figure 4**    Laerdel masks.

are available in three sizes, the middle one being suitable for newborns and infants.

### Laryngoscopes

Owing to the anatomy of the infant's upper airway, a straight-bladed laryngoscope is often more appro-priate and the glottis is viewed by lifting the epiglottis from its posterior surface. Suitable blades include the Anderson–Magill, Robertshaw or Seward (Figs 5 and 6). The Anderson–Magill laryngoscope has a hook on the handle that allows stabilization with the index finger. Older children can usually be intubated in the same way as adults using a standard Macintosh blade. In the USA the Wis-Hipple, Flagg or Miller blades are also commonly used [3]. There are many blades and sizes of handle and it is very much user preference as to choice. Most units have a range of curved and straight-bladed laryngoscopes available.

### Tracheal Tubes

Most tracheal tubes are disposable and made of plastic (Fig. 7). Red rubber tubes are seldom used today. The most commonly used are the Magill type plain tubes, plastic Cole tubes in preterm infants on special care baby units and for resuscitation on maternity units, and preformed plastic RAE tubes. Magill tubes are used both orally and nasally. The Cole tube is quite large, culminating in a shoulder that leads to a small intratracheal section. This is to minimize the risks of endobronchial intubation as the body is too large to pass through the larynx. The RAE tubes are supplied in nasal and oral varieties and have preformed curves. The proximal portion of these tubes is longer than normal and enables the endotracheal connector to be attached further from the airway, providing easier surgical access.

Anaesthetists adopt different methods of selecting tube size. Some use a table like Table 2, while others use the formula 4.0 + age/4 for children older than 1 year. Another method uses the diameter of the patient's little finger.

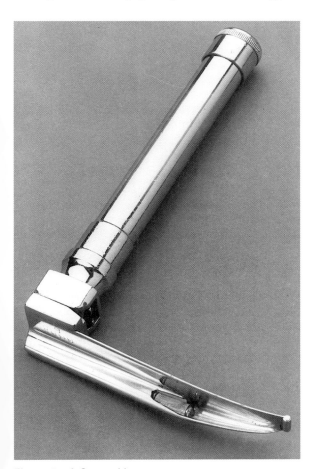

**Figure 5**    A Seward laryngoscope.

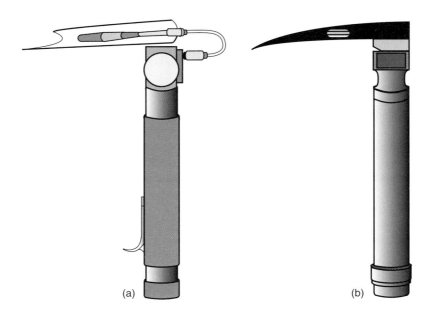

(a)                                    (b)

**Figure 6**   Anderson–Magill (a) and Robertshaw (b) laryngoscopes.

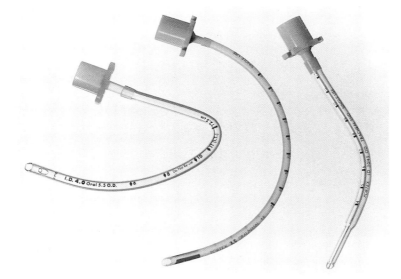

**Figure 7**   Tracheal tubes.

## Bougies

Various sizes of gum elastic bougies are available and are invaluable for aiding intubation. The smallest will pass through a 2.5 mm tracheal tube and can therefore be used in very small neonates.

## Magill Forceps

The paediatric Magill forceps are absolutely invaluable for placing the tip of the tracheal tube through the laryngeal aperture in smaller children.

## Ayre's T Piece

This is the most commonly used breathing circuit for children under 20 kg (Fig. 8). It is suitable for both spontaneous and controlled ventilation. It has no valves which makes the resistance to gas flow as low as possible. The fresh gas flow enters the system as

**Table 2** Tracheal tube size.

| Age | TT size (inner diameter in mm) | Length (cm) Oral | Length (cm) Nasal |
|---|---|---|---|
| Premature | | | |
| < 2 kg | 2.5 | 9 | 11 |
| >2 kg | 3.0 | 10 | 11 |
| Neonate | 3.5 | 10 | 12 |
| 0–6 months | 3.5 | 12 | 14 |
| 6–12 months | 4.0 | 12 | 14 |
| 12–18 months | 4.0–4.5 | 13 | 15 |
| 2 years | 4.5 | 14 | 16 |
| 2–3 years | 4.5–5.0 | 15 | 17 |

TT = tracheal tube.

close to the patient as possible. One arm of the T piece is attached via corrugated tubing to an open-ended distensible bag and the other to the patient.

## Light wand

The light wand can be used when the airway cannot be visualized directly [4]. It has been especially useful in adverse environments for difficult paediatric airway intubation [5]. It consists of a flexible lighted stylet that can be used to transilluminate the airway while the tracheal tube is passed blindly. It is not suitable for use with a tube diameter smaller than 5.5 mm.

## Fibreoptic equipment

The fibreoptic bronchoscope is available in sizes as small as 2.4 mm, which will fit through a size 3 mm tracheal tube. It is important to develop expertise with this equipment and have trained assistance [6].

## INTUBATION AND SPECIAL TECHNIQUES FOR AIRWAY MANAGEMENT

For the less experienced anaesthetist, every paediatric intubation may seem difficult. Even for those more experienced, it is often best to assume that intubation might be difficult until proved otherwise. Adopting this attitude will hopefully lead to rehearsed manoeuvres that can be used if the intubation proves difficult, with all the necessary equipment easily available.

### Inhalational Induction

This is the method of choice with some anaesthetists for all paediatric patients. It is indicated when isolated lesions are obstructing the airway, for example epiglottitis, croup, foreign body aspiration

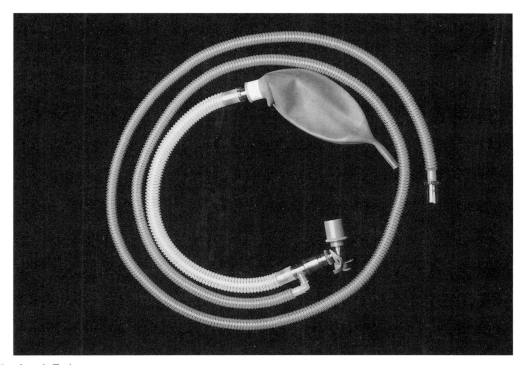

**Figure 8** Ayre's T piece.

and tumours. This used to be the method which was classically taught for dealing with a bleeding tonsil, but has in most centres been superceded by the rapid sequence induction after proper resuscitation.

Anaesthesia is induced using a mask and high gas flows while maintaining spontaneous ventilation. Nitrous oxide is often used to speed up the induction but is contraindicated in severe hypoxia, in the presence of a pneumothorax, subcutaneous emphysema, burns or the acute abdomen. Most anaesthetists use halothane for gaseous induction. Enflurane and isoflurane can be used although the technique is more difficult due to increased airway irritation. Sevoflurane is also being used increasingly for inhalation inductions. Intubation is carried out under deep inhalational anaesthesia or following a muscle relaxant if the ability to hand ventilate the child's lungs has been demonstrated previously.

## Oral Intubation

Older children can usually be intubated in the same way as small adults. It used to be the trend to perform awake intubations in neonates and small infants. This practice has fortunately become less common. It is never easy to intubate a strong, fighting infant, possibly more from mental attitude than sheer physical strength. Research by Anand and other authors has demonstrated the huge stress responses in neonates to inadequate analgesia and anaesthesia [7, 8]. A controlled induction, either gaseous or intravenous, gives much better conditions for intubation.

The glottis is U shaped, floppy and protrudes into the pharynx, obscuring the view of the glottis. Exposure is often best obtained using a straight-bladed laryngoscope in conjunction with a narrow handle (Figs 6 and 9). When intubating infants for the first time, anaesthetists often find great difficulty in sorting out the anatomy. The problem is usually that the laryngoscope has been passed too far and into the oesophagus. If the blade is drawn back slowly the glottis or epiglottis usually comes into view. Some anaesthetists prefer to use a curved blade even in infants. They insert the laryngoscope into the vallecula and employ cricoid pressure to expose the glottis. The author favours the curved blade, finding identification of the anatomy easier and the blade less traumatic. The advantage of passing the curved blade into

the vallecula is in not picking up the epiglottis. This minimizes reflex stimulation and reduces trauma to the glottis. If the epiglottis obstructs the view of the glottis, cricoid pressure is applied to push the larynx backwards. The tube is best passed down on the right side of the mouth and behind the glottis so the view is not obstructed. In neonates and infants, the small Magill forceps are used to place the tip of the tube through the larynx.

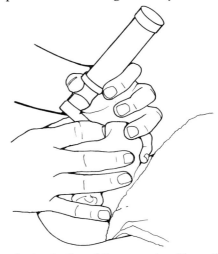

**Figure 9**   Intubation of the neonate with particular attention to the position of anaesthetist's hands and laryngoscope.

The narrowest part of the larynx in children is at the level of the cricoid ring. To help prevent trauma it is important to select an uncuffed tube of a sufficient size to allow a small gas leak at 20 cm $H_2O$ pressure during inflation of the lungs. This is extremely important as the resistance to laminar air flow is proportional to the fourth power of the radius. For example, 1 mm of circumferential oedema in a 4 mm infant airway will reduce the cross-sectional area by 75% and increase the resistance 16 times. The same amount of oedema in an 8 mm adult airway will decrease the cross-sectional area by 44% and increase resistance by only three times.

It is important to have skilled assistance and correct positioning of the patient (Fig. 10). Placing the infant's head in a head ring does not help as it makes laryngoscopy more difficult by increasing the anterior posterior depth of the skull. It is best to place a roll under the shoulders and have the assistant hold the head to prevent side to side movement. This position is also extremely good for ventilating with a face-

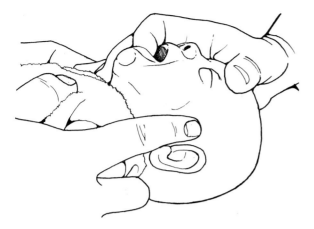

**Figure 10**   The position of the hands of a skilled assistant.

mask. Infants are most frequently intubated with the help of muscle relaxants. Currently, suxamethonium chloride is used less often and non-depolarizing muscle relaxants are used with increasing frequency. Intubation may be necessary under deep inhalational anaesthesia if there is an element of respiratory obstruction.

Mouth opening may be limited despite adequate muscle relaxation. Muscle spasm may be produced by drugs such as fentanyl but can be antagonized by muscle relaxants. Malignant hyperpyrexia is often preceded by abnormal muscle spasm, frequently triggered by using suxamethonium or halothane.

## Awake Intubation

This may be necessary when critical airway lesions are present, such as large tumours, craniofacial defects or after trauma. It used to be the general method for neonates. The child is positioned as for normal intubation with the neck slightly extended, a roll under the shoulders and the head supported against side to side movement. Atropine is usually given intramuscularly or intravenously and the tube introduced following direct laryngoscopy.

## Blind Nasal Intubation

This used to be a popular method of intubation, either in the spontaneously breathing patient or the awake patient if co-operative. It was particularly useful for critical airway lesions and operations in the oropharynx. It is used far less often now with the greater use of fibreoptic equipment.

## Retrograde Intubation

If it is not possible to establish intubation from above, it may be possible to establish an airway from below. This technique initially employed the use of a large bore needle passed through the cricothyroid membrane, an epidural catheter and a retrograde oral tube sequence. Recently it has been performed as a modified Seldinger technique using a 20 gauge needle and a 0.021" (0.053 cm) guide wire. The wire should be placed into the tracheal tube via the Murphy side hole to allow insertion of an extra 1 cm into the larynx before wire withdrawal. This tends to prevent the tracheal tube slipping into the oesophagus.

## INTUBATION AND INTENSIVE CARE

In most children, oral intubation is the option of choice. However, if children are to return to an intensive care unit, for example following cardiac surgery, nasotracheal intubation is often preferred for its increased safety, comfort and ease of nursing.

One of the best methods of intubation is to pass a well-greased tracheal tube of an appropriate size through the left or right nostril. A laryngoscope blade is introduced and the tip of the tube manoeuvred until it lies at the glottic aperture. The length of the tube at the nose is then noted. The tube is subsequently cut with a distance of 3 cm added for a size 3 tube, 4 cm for a size 4 tube, 5 cm for a size 5 tube and so on. This measurement allows 1 cm for strapping the tube after it has been advanced into the trachea. Our preferred method of fixation of the tube is with elastoplast trousers when it has been confirmed to be in the correct position. This is an extremely useful technique as it is very important to get the tube size exactly right for each child, particularly as many are growth retarded or have certain congenital anomalies.

With Down's syndrome, a tube size one half smaller than normal for that age is selected as there tends to be soft tissue hypertrophy. As there is quite a high incidence of postextubation stridor, and hence reintubation in Downs children, a special extubation protocol is used. The children are given 0.5 mg kg$^{-1}$ of dexamethasone 1 h prior to intubation. After extubation, they are immediately allowed to inhale 1 ml of 1:1000 nebulized adrenaline. This is repeated hourly if necessary. It is an extremely successful protocol and children rarely have to be reintubated. The protocol is also employed for children who have been intubated long term (7–21 days).

## DISORDERS OF THE AIRWAY CAUSING DIFFICULTY WITH INTUBATION

### Congenital Anomalies

Many congenital anomalies due to faulty embryological development can produce difficulties with nasal and/or oral intubation.

### Absence of nose

This is an extremely rare condition often associated with a high arched palate. Surgery is required because of feeding difficulties.

### Choanal atresia

Choanal atresia occurs to varying degrees and involves soft tissue or bony obstruction at the posterior border of the hard palate. It may be unilateral or bilateral. It is diagnosed at birth by failure to pass a soft suction catheter into the nasopharynx. Atresia exists if the catheter passes less than a distance of 32 mm. There is a familial tendency that is also often accompanied by congenital heart defects. If it is undiagnosed, feeding can lead to aspiration and secondary pneumonitis. Cyanosis may occur with respiratory obstruction. Corrective surgery for bilateral choanal atresia used to be performed at about 1 year of age but recently primary endonasal puncture in the neonatal period has become more popular. The results have improved with the use of stenting tubes. The infants are best managed with an inhalational induction and oral intubation. As some of these infants will need surgery for congenital heart disease, it is wise to remember not to intubate them nasally following stenting as there may be thinning of the bone with possible disastrous results following the passage of a nasal tube.

### Anterior encephalocoele

This appears as a herniation of cerebral tissue and meninges through a defect in the nasofrontal region of the skull. It is associated with a potentially difficult airway.

### Macroglossia

This describes a tongue that is apparently too large for the oral cavity, due either to a large tongue or a small mouth. Primary macroglossia is a benign condition rarely needing surgical correction. Secondary macroglossia can arise from several causes such as lymphangioma or haemangioma. In the Beckwith–Wiedeman syndrome it is associated with hypoglycaemia, omphalocoele and congenital heart disease. In Down's syndrome the tongue appears large due to a small oral cavity. Macroglossia may cause difficulty with visualization of the vocal cords.

### Maxillofacial cleft

This condition may affect the lip, the palate or both. The incidence of cleft lip and palate is approximately 1 in 700 live births with isolated cleft lip or palate occurring in about one third more. In 1973, Zawistowska et al. classified the abnormalities in 787 patients according to increasing difficulties encountered by the anaesthetist during intubation [9].

The main problem is lack of support for the laryngoscope. Three solutions are suggested:

- The use of a tongue depressor as a support.
- The insertion of the laryngoscope at the extreme right-hand side of the mouth.
- Extension of the head by the assistant to open the mouth and a conventional approach with a curved laryngoscope blade.

Cleft lips are repaired surgically in early infancy and cleft plates delayed until about 1 year of age. Cleft palates are typically associated with Pierre–Robin and Klippel–Feil syndromes [9].

### Cystic hygroma

This is a congenital dysplasia of the lymphatics consisting of multiple, cavernous cysts containing serous, serosanguinous or bloody fluid. They may be unilateral or bilateral and can extend into the mediastinum or axilla. They are usually found in the posterior triangle of the neck (60–70%) or in communication with the axilla (20–30%). The lesions are present at birth and can enlarge rapidly due to bleeding, infection or fluid accumulation. The upper airway may be involved with lesions found in the tongue, lips, floor of mouth, styloid process, larynx, epiglottis and aryepiglottic

**Table 3** Classification of the congenital defects of the maxillofacial cleft. From Zawistowska *et al.* [9].

| Defect | Grade of difficulty |
|---|---|
| Isolated cleft lip | 0 |
| Right-sided cleft of lip and alveolar process<br>Right-sided cleft of lip, alveolar process and palate | 1 |
| Left-sided cleft of the lip and alveolar process<br>Bilateral cleft of lip and alveolar process<br>Left-sided cleft of the lip, alveolar process and palate | 2 |
| Bilateral cleft of lip, alveolar process and palate | 3 |

folds. Airway compromise may necessitate tracheostomy. Incision and drainage tends to lead to chronic fluid loss and reaccumulation may occur in a few days.

## Laryngomalacia

This condition results from flaccid epiglottic and aryepiglottic cartilages that fold in with inspiration. The stridor is usually present from birth and 75% of all cases of congenital stridor are associated with this condition.

## Mandibulofacial dysostosis

These include the Berry, Treacher–Collins and Franceschetti–Zwahlen–Klein syndromes. They result from an embryological disturbance during the formation of the first branchial arch. The resulting deformity produces a hypoplastic and receding mandible, macroglossia, glossoptosis, maxillary protrusion and trismus related to temporomandibular joint abnormalities [10]. There is a high palate and abnormally placed teeth. These children are often difficult to intubate and there is also a problem maintaining an airway even using an artificial airway [11]. The characteristic features are recognizable preoperatively, namely:

- *Ears.* There is deformity of the pinna frequently associated with atresia of the external auditory meatus. Partial or complete deafness may be present.
- *Eyes.* There is an oblique palpebral fissure, notching or a coloboma of the lower eyelid. Meibomian glands are absent and there is no intermarginal strip. The medial two-thirds of the eyelashes are absent. The eyes lie on an oblique axis.
- *Miscellaneous features include*:
  - familial incidence;
  - relationship with hare-lip and cleft palate;
  - long second metatarsal – a constant feature;
  - normal mortality.

## Pierre–Robin syndrome

Micrognathia and glossoptosis in association with cleft palate make up this group of anomalies. It may occur in isolation in about 1 in 30 000 live births or as part of other syndromes. Hemifacial microsomia may also cause problems with airway management [12].

## Klippel–Feil syndrome

This is a congenital musculoskeletal disorder characterized by fusion of the cervical vertebrae, especially synostosis of the atlas and axis. The neck is shortened, immobile and there is often tortocollis. These can be extremely difficult intubations.

## Engelmann's disease (osteopathia hyperostotice scleroticens multiplex infantalis)

A rare disease of the skeleton with limited mouth opening and an immobile neck causing intubation difficulties. Retrograde catheterization techniques have been used to facilitate intubation [13].

## Achondroplasia

This condition is inherited as an autosomal dominant with little clinical variability. It produces a dwarf-like appeareance due to abnormality of cartilage development. Difficulties are due to an angular kyphosis between $C_2$ and $C_3$. Full extension of the head results in the axis of C1–C2 making a forward angle of inclination of 25° with respect to $C_2$–$C_3$. This produces a very anteriorly placed larynx.

## Fetal alcohol syndrome

This occurs in infants of alcoholics. Deformities relevant to the anaesthetist include maxillary and mandibular hypoplasia. Techniques using bougies have been used to intubate these children [14].

## Subglottic cysts

These cysts are present at birth or appear shortly afterwards and are remnants of the thyroglossal duct. They arise from the epiglottic and aryepiglottic folds and may be lined with respiratory or squamous epithelium. Healing of a mucosal lesion after intubation may produce a subglottic cystic lesion, although stenosis is more common. Tracheostomy may be required.

## Kartagener's syndrome

The triad of sinusitis, bronchiectasis and situs inversus is known as Kartagener's syndrome and is probably inherited as an autosomal recessive trait. The syndrome affects 1 in 40 000 of the population. These patients may present for surgical treatment of bronchiectasis. The bronchial anatomy is transposed, the left lung having a short main bronchus and the right lung having a long main bronchus. Selective intubation of the right bronchus presents no difficulty but the use of orthodox equipment in the left main bronchus will obstruct the left upper lobe orifice [15].

## Atrial isomerism

The congenital cardiac defects of right and left atrial isomerism imply right and left sided visceral dominance respectively. In the first, there are two morphological right atria, and in the second, two morphological left atria. Both are associated with functional cardiovascular abnormalities, particularly of venous drainage. In right atrial isomerism there are two trilobar lungs, both with short main bronchi. This is associated with asplenia as the spleen is a left sided structure. In left atrial isomerism there are long main bronchi and polysplenia. Left atrial isomerism presents no problem but right atrial isomerism poses the same problems for intubation as Kartagener's syndrome.

## Craniofacial dysostosis (Crouzon's syndrome)

These patients may present for correction of exophthalmus. Other characteristics are hypertelorism, parrot-beaked nose, high arched palate, nasal obstruction and obliteration of the paranasal sinuses. Brechner (1968) described a patient suffering additionally with the Pickwickian syndrome. A fascinating feature of that case was the presence of a calcified and enlarged anterior longitudinal ligament extending anteriorly down the bodies of the cervical vertebrae and bulging into the pharynx, which produced airway obstruction [16].

## Vascular compression of the trachea

The trachea may be compressed by various vascular ring anomalies (Fig. 11).

These include:

* Double aortic arch, which is the most common. A left and right aortic arch arise from the ascending aorta, encircle the trachea and oesophagus and unite to form a single descending aorta. Symptoms of tracheal compression present in early infancy.
* Anomalous innominate artery. This vessel arises more posteriorly and symptoms of tracheal compression again appear in early infancy.
* Right aortic arch with left ligamentum arteriosus. A vascular ring is formed by the right aortic arch, the left subclavian artery and a left sided ductus or ligamentum arteriosus connecting the left subclavian to the left pulmonary artery.
* Vascular sling. The left pulmonary artery arises from an elongated main pulmonary artery on the right encircling the right main stem bronchus and passing to the left between trachea and oesophagus. Constriction of the right main bronchus, trachea or both may occur.

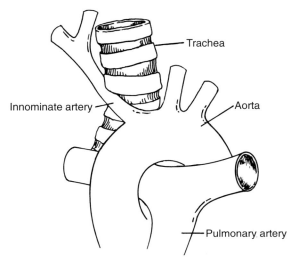

**Figure 11** Compression of the trachea by the innominate artery.

## Mucopolysaccharide disease

Clinical features of this group include:

- skeletal changes;
- coarse facies;
- corneal clouding;
- mental retardation.

### Hurler's syndrome (gargoylism)

This disease may be inherited as an autosomal recessive trait or a sex limited recessive trait affecting males. No physical abnormalities are seen at birth but these develop slowly after 6 months and become apparent in the second year. A grotesque, coarse facial appearance develops. Of great importance to the anaesthetist is the development of a large tongue with a short neck that has limited extension. These children are prone to respiratory failure and may develop initimal thickening of the coronary arteries and valves.

### Hunter's syndrome

This is similar to Hurler's syndrome but the children have a longer lifespan.

### Morquio's syndrome

The degree of facial coarseness is mild to moderate. Sketetal abnormalities are severe. The neck and trunk are short and progressive pectus excavatum develops. Absence or marked hypoplasia of the odontoid peg results in atlantoaxial instability and possible spinal cord compression.

## Acquired Abnormalities

### Infections and immunological disorders

#### Epiglottitis

This is an acute, life-threatening infection of the supraglottic area usually due to *Haemophilia influenzae*. The age of onset is usually 2–8 years. The child should be kept calm and attempts to perform X-rays, physical examination including visualization of the epiglottis should be deferred until a suitably experienced person is available. A surgeon capable of doing a tracheostomy should be available. Induction of anaesthesia with oxygen and halothane should be carried out in the sitting position. Direct laryngoscopy and oral tracheal intubation is performed using a tube one size smaller than normal. This tube is often changed to a nasal one if long-term ventilation is anticipated.

If the oral intubation was difficult such exchange should not be attempted.

#### Laryngotracheal bronchitis (croup)

Children may need intubation or tracheostomy if there is severe respiratory compromise.

#### Subglottic stenosis.

Recurrent croup or stridor may result in subglottic stenosis (Fig. 12). The condition arises most commonly after prolonged intubation, particularly in the neonatal period. This is why it is always important to select a tracheal tube that allows a small leak of gas. The subglottic stenosis may present with respiratory difficulties or be diagnosed at intubation when a tube of the correct size cannot be passed.

#### Peritonsillar abscess

This may be associated with trismus and therefore necessitates a gaseous induction as there is a possibility of a difficult intubation.

#### Ludwig's angina

This condition causes submandibular and sublingual cellulitis. The molar teeth cause the problem and hence it usually occurs in older children. Oedema of the mouth, tongue, neck and deep cervical fascia may make oral intubation impossible.

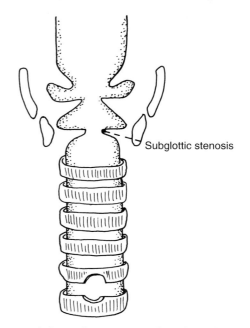

**Figure 12**  Schematic representation of subglottic stenosis.

### Angioneurotic oedema

This is an autosomal dominant disorder of the complement pathway. Deficiency of C1 esterase inhibitor allows unopposed activity of the early complement pathway components. There is episodic swelling of the extremities, face and bowel wall. Any involvement of the larynx is associated with a mortality of 30%.

## Inflammatory

### Juvenile rheumatoid arthritis

This condition is rare below 6 months of age and reaches a peak between the ages of 1 and 3 years. Airway problems are caused by several different factors. Involvement of the temporomandibular joint is common and limits mouth opening. Mandibular hypoplasia may be pronounced and is related to growth impairment exacerbated by steroid therapy. The synovial joints of the larynx may be affected, which can lead to glottic narrowing. Cervical spine involvement occurs in about 50% of cases leading to severe impairment of neck mobility. Preoperative assessment of these children should be very thorough and a difficult intubation anticipated.

## Tumours

### Mediastinal masses

These may include Hodgkin's and non-Hodgkin's lymphoma, teratoma, thymoma, angiomatous tumours, tuberculosis, bronchogenic cysts and oesophageal duplications. Compression and distortion of the trachea may make intubation extremely difficult.

### Papillomatosis

These are multiple tumour growths found in the larynx, pharynx, trachea and occasionally the lung tissue of children. They are benign but often very aggressive and recurrent.

### Haemangiomas

Congenital haemangiomas may occur in the laryngeal and subglottic regions of young infants.

## Trauma

### Laryngeal and tracheal trauma

Open or closed injuries to the larynx and trachea can occur by direct trauma but are unusual in children. Attempts at intubation may cause further damage and intubation is best carried out using a fibreoptic based technique.

### Maxillofacial trauma

Lacerations, bleeding, oedema and fracture of the mandible may make airway management extremely difficult. Blood, vomitus, teeth or bony fragments may occlude the airway. Intubation is best carried out awake or using general anaesthesia with spontaneous ventilation.

## KEY POINTS

- The narrowest part of the infant airway lies at the level of the cricoid cartilage.

- Straight and curved blade laryngoscopes are available and preference lies with the individual anaesthetist.

- Plain, uncuffed tubes are used nasally and orally up to the age of 11 years; cuffed tubes are used for older children.

- Awake intubation of infants and neonates is no longer recommended.

- It is important to have skilled assistance and correct positioning of the patient for easier intubation.

- For children with Down's syndrome select a tube one half size smaller than normal.

- Always make sure the tube is securely strapped in place.

## REFERENCES

1 Ellis H. and Feldman S. *Anatomy for Anaesthetists* Oxford: Blackwell Scientific Publications. 1983.

2 Brown T. C. K. and Fisk G. C. *Anaesthesia for Children* Oxford: Blackwell Scientific Publications. 1979; ch. 1.

3 Ward C. F. Paediatric head and neck syndromes. In Katz R. L. and Stewart D. J. (eds) *Anaesthesia and Uncommon Paediatric Diseases* Philadelphia: W. B. Saunders, 1987; 267.

4 Katz R. L. and Berci G. The optical stylet – a new

intubation technique for adults and children with specific reference to teaching. *Anesthesiology* 1979; **51**: 251.

5 Fox D. J. and Hatson M. D. Management of difficult paediatric airway in an austere environment using the light wand. *Journal of Clinical Anesthesia* 1990; **2**: 123.

6 Woods A. M. Paediatric bronchoscopy, bronchography and laryngoscopy. In: Berry F. A. (ed.) *Anaesthetic Management of Difficult and Routine Paediatric Patients* New York: Churchill Livingstone. 1986.

7 Anand K. J. S. and Hickey P. R. Pain and its affect in the human neonate and fetus. *New England Journal of Medicine* 1987; **317**: 1321–29.

8 Holtby H. M. and Relton J. E. S.Orthopaedic diseases. In: Katz R. L. and Stewart D. J. (eds) *Anaesthesia and Uncommon Paediatric Diseases* Philadelphia: W. B. Saunders. 1987: vol. 1, 372.

9 Zawistowska J., Menzel M. and Wytyczak M. Difficulties and modifications of intubation technique in infants with labial, alveolar and palatal clefts. *Anaesthesia Resuscitation and Intensive Care Therapy* 1973; **1**: 211.

10 Sklar G. S. and King B. D. Endotracheal intubation and Treacher–Collins syndrome. *Anesthesiology* 1976; **44**: 247.

11 Ross E. D. T. Treacher Collins syndrome. An anaesthetic hazard. *Anaesthesia* 1963; **23**: 250.

12 Williams A. J., Williams M. A., Walkwer C. A. *et al.* The Robin anomalad – (Pierre Robin syndrome) – a follow up study. *Archives of Diseases in Childhood* 1981; **56**: 663.

13 Mason J. and Slee I. Anaesthesia and Engelmanns disease. *Anaesthesia* 1968; **21**: 244.

14 Clarren S. K., Smith D. W. The fetal alcohol syndrome. *New England Journal of Medicine* 1978; **298**: 1063.

15 Dunne N. M. and Gillbe C. E. Endobronchial apparatus and its intraoperative management. In: *Baillière's Clinical Anaesthesiology. Thoracic Anaesthesia* London: Baillière Tindall. 1987; 79–98.

16 Brechner V. L. Unusual problems in the management of airways: flexion extension mobility of the cervical vertebrae. *Anesthesia and Analgesia* 1968; **47**: 362.

# 13

# Emergency Airway Access

*Brian Jenkins*

## INTRODUCTION

The maintenance of a clear airway is fundamental to the practice of resuscitation and forms the cornerstone of safe anaesthetic practice. Failure will inevitably lead to cerebral hypoxia and death. This chapter will discuss strategies and devices for maintaining adequate ventilation under adverse conditions. The situation that may threaten the airway are protean; it is important to have a broad knowledge of the techniques involved, as there is as yet no device or technique which is able to handle all situations safely.

## Mortality and Morbidity

In an early audit of perioperative mortality in 1982 [1], Lunn and Mushin stated that four out of the 58 deaths reported were associated with either difficulty with intubation, complete airway obstruction, or severe impairment of ventilation leading to cerebral hypoxia and death. In the Confidential Enquiry into Perioperative Deaths of 1987 [2] it was reported that one in three of the deaths solely attributable to anaesthesia were associated with intubation difficulty.

In a case review study of records from the Medical Protection Society [3], 10 out of 25 deaths associated with anaesthesia were associated with failed intubation, with failures in technique being a significant factor. In a 13 year review of reports to the Medical Defence Union [4], anaesthetic errors in technique were thought to be responsible for 326 cases of brain damage and death. It has been suggested that in a large percentage of these cases there were avoidable factors, some related to lack of adequate training or skills. Although severe difficulties with airway maintenance are rare, they form a large proportion of anaesthetic-related deaths.

## Skills and Techniques

It has been shown radiographically that the main site of airway obstruction during general anaesthesia occurs between the soft palate and the posterior pharyngeal wall [5]. In most cases obstruction can be resolved easily, either by mild traction on the jaw or by means of an oropharyngeal or nasopharyngeal airway. In unconscious or comatose patients in whom airway maintenance may be more difficult, other devices such as the laryngeal mask airway

(LMA) and the tracheal tube may be used. In the vast majority of cases, these artificial aids are adequate to ensure a clear airway, but in a small number of cases they may be inadequate. If such cases are detected preoperatively, most airway management problems may be overcome by elective awake intubation using either a fibreoptic laryngoscope to position the tracheal tube under direct vision or by a retrograde technique involving a transtracheal guide. Some cases may be so difficult to manage because of anatomical abnormalities or other factors that a tracheostomy performed under local anaesthetic may be the safest, and in some instances the only practical alternative.

In a small number of cases, airway maintenance problems may only become apparent when the patient is already unconscious. A muscle relaxant may also have been administered. If, in these cases simple airway aids are insufficient, then a potentially life-threatening situation has already developed. This may deteriorate to the so-called 'cannot intubate, cannot ventilate' scenario.

The main part of this chapter will address emergency airway management of unconscious patients with difficult airways in prehospital, ward and theatre situations.

## THE DIFFICULT AIRWAY

The American Society of Anesthesiologists Task Force on Management of the Difficult Airway gave a definition of the difficult airway for the purposes of their guidelines [6]: 'A difficult airway is defined as the clinical situation in which a conventionally trained anesthesiologist experiences difficulty with mask ventilation, difficulty with tracheal intubation, or both.'

## Failed Intubation

The incidence of failed intubation is low in trained and experienced individuals, but the potential for complications remains high [7, 8]. The incidence is higher in obstetric cases, and has been estimated at 1 in 300 (0.3%) [9], compared with a figure of 0.05–0.35% in the general population undergoing surgical procedures. There are many reasons for intubation failure; major factors are the clinical environment, patient factors, the level of experienced assistance, and the skill and experience of the practitioner.

### Clinical environment

The clinical environment is extremely important as a cause of airway difficulty. Even basic airway management can be compromised by poor working conditions and lack of specialized equipment. In emergency cases, resuscitation may have to be practised in unfavourable conditions simply because of the location of the patient at the time of collapse. Most areas in the hospital environment should have oxygen, suction and basic resuscitation equipment near to hand. These facilities make successful resuscitation more likely, but they will not always be adequate in the most demanding cases of difficult airway management.

### Patient factors

Failed intubation may occur for many reasons. Many emergency patients have airway problems as a result of anatomical variation, acute pathological processes such as trauma, oedema, infection, penetrating injuries or foreign bodies involving the face and cervical spine. Some factors which contribute to difficulty may not be immediately apparent before resuscitation or anaesthetic induction. A detailed history and examination is essential in order to allow adequate preparation. This in turn should make successful management more likely.

### Skill and experience

Many situations of airway difficulty arise through lack of experience and/or poor preparation. Causes include:

- failure to identify anatomical problems during patient assessment;
- failure to check equipment adequately;
- failure to optimally position the patient for intubation;
- the use of induction techniques which are inappropriate to the degree of airway difficulty;
- failure to utilize appropriate equipment (e.g. long-bladed laryngoscope);
- failure to establish adequate anaesthesia before intubation attempts;
- failure to ensure adequate assistance and back-up.

With a more experienced operator and adequate safeguards, a 'difficult airway' may not present any problems. The perceived incidence of difficult airways and of life-threatening complications will thus depend on the experience of the operator and the availability of adequate back-up mechanisms. This is almost certainly a factor in the wide variation in the reported incidence of difficult airways.

Patient harm may occur when there is a failure to apply existing knowledge or to follow basic safety procedures. Examples include:

- failure to utilize appropriate monitoring;
- failure to preoxygenate;
- failure to apply cricoid pressure;
- failure to recognize oesophageal placement of a tracheal tube;
- failure to follow a failed intubation drill;
- when difficulty is experienced, attempting alternative airway management techniques requiring a degree of skill that the operator does not possess.

If a history has been taken, the likelihood of the presence of a full stomach should be estimated. This is vitally important in the risk management of a deteriorating situation. Many techniques of airway management are perfectly justifiable in the absence of food in the stomach, but may be simply too risky in patients with a full stomach except in a 'last ditch' effort to prevent cerebral hypoxia. In these cases, they will usually be seen as a temporary measure until more secure airway protection can be established.

## Unconscious Patient / Difficult Airway

This situation may arise because of:

- failure to recognize intubation difficulty prior to operation, therefore awake intubation was not considered;
- refusal of awake intubation;
- awake intubation felt to be contraindicated;
- patient unconscious, e.g. following trauma, drug overdose or cerebral ischaemia.

Even complete failure of intubation need not necessarily result in disaster as long as oxygenation is possible. However, in a small percentage of cases (0.000 001–0.02%) [10–12] neither intubation nor ventilation are possible by simple means. If immediate and effective management is not rapidly instituted in these patients, cerebral hypoxia and death are inevitable.

Attempting to wake the patient is usually the safest course of action under such circumstances.

Most operations can be delayed for a short time, even in emergency situations. This may allow time to summon senior help, reassess the situation, perform an awake intubation under local anaesthesia, or call a surgeon who is skilled in surgical airway management. However, waking the patient may not always be straightforward. If intubation and ventilation are impossible following induction of general anaesthesia, profound hypoxia may occur before the effects of the administered drugs wear off sufficiently to allow spontaneous respiration.

Some patients may have an increased metabolic rate (obstetric cases, infants), or a degree of respiratory impairment that existed before induction (chronic obstructive airways disease, pneumonia). These conditions decrease the period of total apnoea that is tolerated before cerebral hypoxia ensues. In some septicaemic intensive care patients these two elements of risk may coexist. Malignant hyperpyrexia may present as a case of failed intubation due to profound masseter spasm; in combination with the increased oxygen consumption seen in these cases, a formidable acute airway management problem may ensue.

If spontaneous ventilation via a facemask is adequate, allowing the operation to proceed under controlled circumstances may be a reasonable course of action in emergency situations, e.g. failure to intubate at emergency Caesarean section (see Chapter 16). In this particular situation, other options that may be considered after waking the patient may in themselves present substantial risks. Aspiration of stomach contents may occur when laryngeal reflexes are impaired by local anaesthesia during the preparation for awake intubation. Misplacement of local anaesthetic through an epidural catheter into the spinal space may result in cardiorespiratory collapse in the presence of a difficult or impossible intubation. As in most emergency situations, assessment of the balance of risks should be performed and a risk management strategy formulated to deal with the situation. Because of the difficulty in clearly assessing the situation when under conditions of great stress, airway management algorithms have been devised to guide treatment and help in risk managing difficult and rapidly changing situations. Like most guidelines, they cannot possibly cope with every patient in every situation, but may help standardization of safe management in line with the results of research. Although some algorithms are designed for emergency consultation, ideally the drill should be memorized and practised in simulated emergency situations.

### Repeated attempts at intubation

Airway difficulty in unconscious patients is commonly associated with repeated, increasingly desperate intubation attempts commonly involving increased force and departure from standard practice under conditions of stress. The data from one study strongly suggests that the incidence of complications increases with the number of attempts at intubation [13]. Complications may be minor, major, or life-threatening. These include:

- increased salivation;
- awareness;
- laryngeal/pharyngeal oedema;
- haemorrhage;
- perforated visci;
- stomach distension/regurgitation;
- submucosal passage of the tracheal tube;
- rupture of the trachea [14];
- mediastinal emphysema/surgical emphysema/ pneumothorax.

The reported incidence of minor upper airway complications in this study (e.g. pharyngeal bruises, cut lips) was 5% in patients in whom direct laryngoscopy was easy. In patients who were anticipated to be difficult, the incidence of minor trauma increased to 17%, and in patients who actually proved to be difficult, in whom multiple intubation attempts were made, the incidence of complications was 63% [13]. It is therefore suggested that it is rarely good practice to attempt tracheal intubation repeatedly unless easily correctable factors such as suboptimal positioning of the patient's head and neck were present at the initial attempt. Cases that could be safely managed by admitting defeat and waking the patient may deteriorate to an acutely life-threatening situation if a major complication such as aspiration of stomach contents or upper airway haemorrhage occurs during repeated attempts at intubation. A difficult situation could also be made positively dangerous by the repeated administration of hypnotics, narcotic analgesics and particularly muscle relaxants when the airway is insecure.

## AIDS TO DIFFICULT AIRWAY MANAGEMENT

In order to manage an emergency situation safely, it is better to be an expert in a small number of airway management techniques than to have a small amount of experience in many. Simple intubation aids such as the gum elastic bougie, intubation and light stylets will be used in first-line emergency airway management and are considered in other parts of this book. In this section only a small selection of the many airway management techniques are described. Most of the aids and techniques described will be used when simple management techniques have failed and the airway is in danger. This situation will only occur in a small number of cases of difficult intubation.

Devices and airway management techniques that were initially intended for airway control during cardiopulmonary resuscitation by paramedics are described. Most research with these devices has been performed on elective surgical patients under general anaesthesia. Cases of failed intubation have been successfully managed by such devices and they have a role in the management of certain types of difficult airway. In contrast, the LMA was initially developed for the management of patients undergoing general anaesthesia and has recently been advocated for use by paramedics and other healthcare professionals when the expertise necessary to achieve tracheal intubation is not available. It is likely that there will be further exchanges of techniques and ideas between the fields of prehospital and hospital airway management. It therefore seems appropriate to consider such devices together in one section. The favoured airway management techniques will depend on availability of equipment and the degree of experience gained in their use during elective and non-emergency procedures.

In many studies in which efficiency of ventilation or ease of insertion of an airway are compared, it has been common for similar studies to show conflicting conclusions [15–18]. This seems to suggest that studies of this type have important factors that are difficult to standardize, such as the type and duration of training for each technique. Some techniques may be easy to learn but are inherently less efficient than techniques that require some time and skill to acquire. The easier technique may perform well in comparison with the latter if the learning period is severely limited.

Comparisons between the two techniques should therefore specify the type and duration of training, and the results of such studies may only be valid for a particular set of circumstances.

## Continuous Positive Airway Pressure (CPAP)

The use of a small degree of CPAP via a facemask may be useful (especially in children) to reduce the apposition of the soft tissues of the pharynx and to maintain oxygenation [19]. If intubation has failed and the planned surgical procedure is of short duration, this manoeuvre may be invaluable to enable the operation to be completed. In other cases this may allow an adequate airway to be maintained while the patient is allowed to wake. Continuous positive airway pressure may also be used to preserve 'air space' in an unconscious patient undergoing fibreoptic intubation [20]. The technique is usually only a short-term solution but is simple to perform and may be invaluable in buying time to consider other airway management options.

## Oesophageal Obturator Airway (OOA)

### Introduction

The OOA is a device that was designed for use by unskilled resuscitators to aid airway maintenance in the prehospital situation. The concept was first suggested by Don Michael in 1968 [21]. The device has been in clinical use since 1972, and has been widely used in prehospital cardiopulmonary resuscitation (CPR), especially in the USA [18].

The OOA consists of two basic parts (Fig. 1). The first is a 30 cm plastic oesophageal tube occluded at the distal end. Perforations in this tube are intended to be located in the hypopharynx following correct placement. A large balloon is located at the distal end to create a seal in the oesophagus following successful insertion. This has two main purposes: to prevent gastric distension during ventilation and to prevent aspiration of stomach contents into the lungs. The second part of the device is a facemask with an inflatable cuff designed to make a tight seal with the face, even when used by inexperienced operators. This makes a snap-lock connection with the oesophageal tube, and the device is inserted in one piece following assembly.

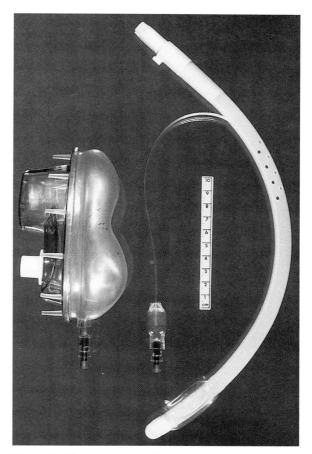

**Figure 1**    The oesophageal obturator airway.

### Insertion

To insert the device, the tip of the tube is first lubricated with a water-soluble gel. The jaw is lifted forward with one hand (Fig. 2a) while the oesophageal tube is slowly and gently introduced into the posterior pharynx with the other (Fig. 2b). The tube is inserted blindly, without a laryngoscope or other aid (Fig. 2c). In the vast majority of cases, the tube should pass easily into the oesophagus. When correctly positioned, the oesophageal balloon should lie below the tracheal bifurcation; the balloon is then inflated. With the mask held firmly over the mouth and nose, the resuscitator expires air down the tube which escapes via the perforations in the tube wall, increasing pressure in the hypopharynx. Because the oesophagus is occluded by the oesophageal balloon and the facemask is held firmly over the mouth and nose, air passes through the patient's glottis to ventilate the lungs. In some cases where

(a)

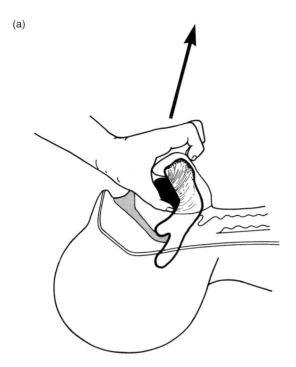

**Figure 2 (a)**   Insertion of the OOA. The thumb is inserted into the mouth and the chin lifted upwards.

(b)

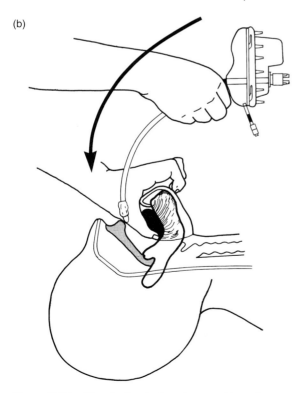

**Figure 2 (b)**   The device is then inserted into the mouth.

(c)

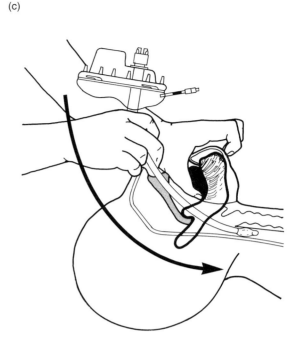

**Figure 2 (c)**   The device is then pushed blindly into the oesophagus. Force should be avoided.

a facial seal is difficult to maintain, two operators may be required to ventilate a patient effectively. A self inflating bag connected to an oxygen supply may be attached to the oesophageal tube in order to ventilate with high concentrations of oxygen.

Following insertion, oesophageal placement and adequate inflation of the balloon should be confirmed by auscultation over both sides of the chest and over the stomach.

Ventilation with the OOA has been compared with facemask/bag ventilation in patients undergoing general anaesthesia by Bryson *et al.* [17]. The results of this study suggested that it was more difficult to obtain a good seal with the mask of the OOA compared with a standard oropharyngeal mask. Lower tidal volumes and less efficient ventilation was noted in the OOA group, particularly in the edentulous. In contrast, Don Michael and colleagues [18] showed a 50% increase in the tidal volumes obtained with an OOA compared with facemask and bag, with tracheal tube ventilation proving marginally more effective than ventilation with the OOA [22]. It is likely that factors such as the degree of skill and the length of training of the operator affect the efficiency of the device, and differences in these factors between the studies may go some way to explaining the contrasting results.

## Oesophageal Gastric Tube Airway

The oesophageal gastric tube airway (OGTA) is a variation on the OOA [23]. It allows the passage of a gastric tube to aspirate gastric secretions and reduce lower oesophageal pressure. Apart from this, it appears to offer few advantages over the OOA, at least in the situation of prehospital CPR airway management [24]. There are relatively few studies involving its use.

## Complications

The incidence of inadvertent tracheal intubation with the OOA is thought to be between 5 and 10% [18]. When recognized, this is not regarded as a major problem and the airway is simply repositioned until the tube is in the oesophagus. The incidence of unrecognized tracheal intubation with this device is unknown; this situation will inevitably result in cerebral hypoxia and death.

The rare, but potentially lethal complication of oesophageal rupture has been well reported. In 1982 Harrison and colleagues surveyed papers published over the previous decade and found a total of 19 reported cases out of an estimated two million insertions [25]. They also pointed out that the incidence of oesophageal rupture in cases in which resuscitation failed is unknown, but the reported incidence is acceptably low in the context of the number of insertions.

## Prehospital resuscitation

The OOA has been extensively used by paramedics in prehospital CPR, especially in the USA. The association of the device with the complication of oesophageal rupture is seen to be a consequence of its extensive use under difficult circumstances rather than a problem which precludes its further use.

It has been suggested that training of paramedics or nurses involved in prehospital resuscitation should not be limited to either tracheal intubation or use of the OOA. The two techniques should be regarded as complementary, with the tracheal tube being used as the airway management technique of choice, and the OOA being used in cases where direct laryngoscopy is not possible [22], or where the skill of tracheal intubation is not available.

Alternative techniques of airway management involving the Combitube and the LMA are likely to be increasingly recommended for use in prehospital CPR as complementary techniques to tracheal intubation. It will only be after they have been used as extensively as the OOA that claims of a reduced incidence of complications associated with their use may be fully justified.

## Laryngeal Mask Airway

### Introduction

The LMA has been used in many situations of airway difficulty, especially in the UK, following increasing acceptance of its use during elective surgical procedures. It has already been demonstrated to be a valuable tool in the management of difficult airways and has been used in many cases of difficult and failed intubation [26–30]. It is being increasingly advocated as a complementary technique to tracheal intubation during CPR (see Chapter 8).

### Difficult and failed intubation

The LMA has been used in several cases of cervical spine immobility, and has been favourably compared with the tracheal tube with regard to the time needed to achieve satisfactory position and the success rate [26]. Other cases of expected severe intubation difficulty have been managed by the LMA, such as contractures due to burns where direct laryngoscopy was thought to be impossible [27].

It has been used in two cases of failed intubation for an emergency caesarean section [28], although its use in this situation as an alternative to waking the patient is certainly controversial [31–33]. However, its use as a tool for managing acute airway obstruction is rapidly becoming established. In many instances it may be a valid alternative to more invasive procedures in preserving the airway in an emergency [29, 30]. However, in cases where pharyngeal anatomy is abnormal such as in laryngeal or buccal neoplasia, or where there is severely limited mouth opening, correct positioning of the LMA may be difficult or impossible. Under these conditions, alternative techniques of airway management such as transtracheal ventilation may be preferable.

The oesophageal detector device [34] has been used to confirm the position of the laryngeal mask [35]. Correct positioning of the laryngeal mask can also be confirmed by passing a fibreoptic laryngoscope through the device and directly visualizing the vocal cords [36].

The LMA can also be used as a means to introduce a tracheal tube in cases of failed or difficult tracheal intubation. A gum elastic bougie [37, 38] or a fibreoptic bronchoscope [39] may be introduced via a LMA to act as a guide for tracheal intubation, or the LMA itself can act as a guide for an uncut, small bore (6.0 mm internal diameter) cuffed tracheal tube [40]. However, maintenance of cricoid pressure has been implicated in a high rate of failure for attempted tracheal intubation through the mask [41], which may limit the use of this technique in emergency situations.

As with any technique which requires a degree of skill, practice in elective patients with normal anatomy is recommended before use in emergency situations.

### Cardiopulmonary resuscitation

The ventilatory efficiency of the LMA has been compared with facemask and bag ventilation when used by inexperienced medical personnel following a short period of training; however, there have been conflicting results. One study suggested that the rate of failure of adequate ventilation with the LMA was lower than with bag and mask [15], while another suggested that it was higher [16].

In a comparison between LMA and tracheal tube placement by paramedics following similar periods of training, a higher incidence of correct placement and adequate ventilation was demonstrated in the LMA group [42]. Two other studies reported a lower incidence of unsatisfactory ventilation in the LMA group compared with a tracheal tube group [43, 44]. A multicentre trial in which the LMA was used by ward nurses following a period of formal training found that satisfactory chest expansion was achieved in 86% of cases [45]. Although regurgitation occurred in 14%, evidence of pulmonary aspiration was present in one case out of 164, an incidence that was regarded as low.

There seems to be a growing consensus that the LMA is a valuable aid in primary resuscitation performed by non-medical personnel. It is seen primarily as a means of securing a patent airway during CPR until tracheal intubation can be performed. Studies have suggested that the amount of training required for its satisfactory use is less than for tracheal intubation. Whether ventilation

via the LMA is more efficient than with a facemask and bag following a similar period of training is at present unclear, but the balance of evidence seems to be shifting in favour of the LMA.

### Complications

The LMA, unlike the tracheal tube and perhaps even the Combitube, does not protect against the risk of regurgitation and aspiration [46–50]. Consequently, considerable debate has ensued concerning the role of the LMA in obstetric anaesthesia for elective Caesarean section [30, 51] and as part of a revised failed intubation drill [52, 53].

The main area of contention seems to be the correct management of failed intubation in a patient at risk from aspiration, when it has been decided that the emergency procedure must be completed. Should LMA placement be attempted, or would it be safer to continue the procedure maintaining the patient's airway by means of a facemask and an artificial airway? There are several arguments against the use of the LMA in this situation. Insertion of the LMA may cause a decrease in lower oesophageal barrier pressure in spontaneously breathing patients, while maintenance of an airway with facemask and oropharyngeal airway may actually result in a rise in barrier pressure [54]. Cricoid pressure is a valuable part of airway management in patients at risk of regurgitation, but maintenance of cricoid pressure has been implicated in a high rate of failure of correct placement of the LMA [41]. To have an airway management tool whose placement requires relaxation of cricoid pressure is a considerable disadvantage, especially in patients at risk of regurgitation. However, some evidence from a study on cadavers suggests that, once the LMA has been correctly placed, it does not further interfere with cricoid pressure [55]. In addition, if ventilation is required at any stage, many regular users of the LMA would contend that prolonged ventilation via the LMA is less likely to result in gastric distension than prolonged ventilation via a facemask (see Chapter 8).

A prototype device combining the LMA with an oesophageal tube has been described recently. It has been suggested that it may help to reduce the incidence of pulmonary aspiration in at-risk cases [56]. However, until more evidence is forthcoming, it has been suggested that the LMA should not be the first choice for maintenance of an airway in a patient with failed intubation at risk of regurgitation [55].

The LMA can certainly play a valuable part in the management of the difficult airway in experienced hands [57], but its ease of use should be balanced against the risk of aspiration in at-risk patients.

## The Oesophageal Tracheal Combitube (OTC)

The OTC is a device developed by Michael Frass and colleagues at the University of Vienna (Fig. 3). It was primarily devised for use in prehospital CPR as a ventilation aid for modestly experienced resuscitators. It is intended to be inserted blindly into the oesophagus in a similar manner to the OOA, but was designed to benefit from the wealth of experience obtained with the older device and to hopefully reduce the complication rate associated with its use.

### Difficult and failed intubation

The OTC has been used in many situations of difficult or impossible intubation. A case of neck impalement with a large splinter of wood has been described in which laryngoscopy was impossible

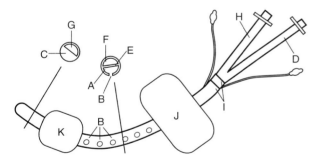

**Figure 3** Lateral and cross-sectional views of the OTC. A = oesophageal lumen; B = perforations of oesophageal lumen (A) between J and K; C = distal closed end of 'oesophageal' lumen (A); D = longer (blue) connector for oesophageal lumen; E = partition wall between lumens A and F; F = 'tracheal' lumen, G = distal open end 'tracheal' lumen (F); H = shorter connector for 'tracheal' lumen (F); I = printed rings on proximal tube (indicate insertion depth – to appose central incisors or alveolar ridges); J = pharyngeal balloon; K = distal balloon (cuff) to seal oesophagus (oesophageal tube position) or trachea (tracheal tube position). Redrawn with permission from Frass, Johnson, Atherton, *et al.* [58].

[59]. Following emergency insertion of the OTC, adequate exchange of gases was possible until an emergency tracheostomy could be performed. It has also been found useful in other cases of acutely threatened airways in which an awake fibreoptic intubation would be difficult even in the most experienced hands. Two cases of acute cervical haematoma from damaged carotid arteries [60] and a case of torrential pharyngeal blood loss in a patient on anticoagulants [61] have been described. All these cases were successfully managed with the OTC. Other situations have occurred in which the OTC has been used after cases of failed intubation [62–65], but its use in these circumstances as an alternative to waking the patient and performing intubation with a local anaesthetic technique has been questioned [66].

### Cardiopulmonary resuscitation

The OTC has been used to maintain an airway during CPR in hospital [67–69]. The airway was regarded as secure and clear throughout CPR manoeuvres, despite the fact that some patients had vomited before intubation. Tracheal suction is not possible through the OTC when in the oesophageal position. Blood gas analysis has demonstrated that the arterial oxygen tension associated with ventilation via the OTC was higher than that observed during tracheal intubation in similar circumstances. This is probably due to a positive end-expiratory pressure (PEEP) effect caused by the increased expiratory resistance associated with the perforations in the 'oesophageal' limb of the OTC [70].

In one study using physicians trained in both techniques, correct placement of the OTC was shown to take less time on average than tracheal intubation [69] despite more time being needed to inflate both the pilot balloons on the OTC; the difference was explained by the fact that successful OTC placement does not require direct laryngoscopy.

The OTC has also been assessed for use during prehospital CPR [71, 72]. Placement of the OTC by paramedics was as successful as tracheal intubation, with 11 out of 14 failed tracheal intubation attempts being successfully managed with the OTC. However, retention of OTC intubating skills after 15 months was generally assessed to be poor [72].

One significant advantage of the OTC compared with the OOA in prehospital CPR is the facility to introduce a gastric tube down the 'tracheal' channel to decompress the stomach when the OTC is in the usual oesophageal position. This may prevent the rise in intragastric and lower oesophageal pressure that is thought to be a significant factor in the aetiology of gastric rupture reported as a complication of the OOA [22].

## The Pharyngo-tracheal Lumen Airway (PTLA)

The PTLA was developed in 1984 as a potential successor to the OOA [73]. It was intended to be used by paramedics and nurses to maintain an airway during prehospital CPR. The device is a double lumen tube, consisting of a long tube with a distal cuff designed to be inflated in the oesophagus, and a shorter tube that protrudes through the larger tube and past a large proximal cuff to ventilate the lungs by pressurizing the hypopharynx (Fig. 4). However, the long tube is also patent at the end, enabling ventilation if it is inadvertently inserted into the trachea. A semirigid spring steel stylet occupies the lumen of the long tube, and needs to be removed if tracheal ventilation via the long tube is required.

The PTLA has been shown to be capable of maintaining effective ventilation and oxygenation

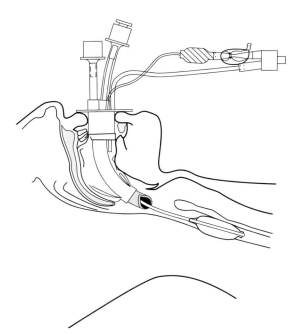

**Figure 4**   Pharyngeo-tracheal lumen airway *in situ*. From Niemann *et al.* [73], with permission.

both in animals and during hospital CPR in six patients as part of a preliminary study [73]. There are few other studies of its clinical use and no reported complications. With the wider experience available with other airway aids such as the OOA, OTC and LMA, it is currently difficult to recommend its use in any situation.

## Retrograde and Fibreoptic Intubation

It is usual to practise these techniques in the awake patient; they require skill and patient co-operation to be consistently successful. Experienced operators may feel confident enough to use the technique in a patient who is asleep, who cannot be intubated but who is easily ventilated. However, in all but the most urgent procedures it is felt that the safest course of action is to wake the patient, postpone the surgical procedure and practise these techniques under more controlled conditions. For many reasons, including the time taken to perform the procedure and the reduced success rate in unconscious patients, they cannot be recommended in a patient who is asleep and cannot be ventilated easily. Under these circumstances, provided the anterior trachea is palpable, a transtracheal approach would be far more appropriate. Retrograde and fibreoptic intubation are discussed in detail in other chapters.

## TRANSTRACHEAL TECHNIQUES

### Introduction

A small number of cases of difficult intubation are also difficult to ventilate. In such cases a transtracheal approach will be favoured by many. It has the advantage that if the equipment required is readily to hand, the procedure can be performed very rapidly. Usually, a small intravenous cannula will be introduced transtracheally, first of all to oxygenate the patient and to buy time to perform a more substantive procedure such as a tracheostomy.

### Detailed Anatomy of the Cricothyroid Membrane

The cricothyroid membrane is a trapezoidal area of approximately 3 cm$^2$. It is located between the inferior border of the thyroid cartilage and the superior border of the cricoid cartilage. With full neck extension, the distance between the upper border and the lower averages 7 mm, and the distance between the left and right edges averages 30 mm. The membrane is located 9–10 mm below the free edge of the true vocal cords, and thus overlies the subglottic region of the larynx [74].

Skin, subcutaneous tissue and fascial layers overlie the cricothyroid membrane. The cricothyroid artery passes transversely across the upper third, although puncture is unlikely to cause significant bleeding due to its small calibre [75]. Major vascular structures such as the thyroid gland and anterior jugular vein are usually well below the cricothyroid membrane, and so haemorrhage from these structures generally only occurs after failure to identify the membrane itself. Ease of identification and absence of vascular structures makes this part of the trachea a favourite site for emergency airway access.

## Emergency Cricothyrotomy
### Transtracheal oxygenation

Once access to the trachea is obtained, what then? As early as 1956, Jacoby demonstrated that adequate oxygenation could be maintained by insufflating 4 l of oxygen per minute directly into the trachea for periods of 30 min [76]. However, under these circumstances, carbon dioxide will not be removed effectively and the plasma level rises rapidly. In the case of complete glottic obstruction, another intratracheal cannula should also be inserted to allow escape of gases and to prevent dangerous increases in intratracheal pressure.

In emergency situations, it is unlikely that there will be ideal conditions for this method of oxygenation. Desaturation is likely to have already occurred, and blood and other secretions are commonly present in the lungs as a result of repeated intubation attempts. Progressive small airway collapse will occur in the absence of ventilation. Under these conditions, the best outcome that could be expected would be the prevention of any further desaturation and to buy time until another technique can be employed or spontaneous respiration resumes. However, the assumption that spontaneous respiration will resume before irreversible cerebral hypoxia ensues may be false. In most circumstances, other methods of improving oxygen delivery such as those described below should be attempted.

### Transtracheal jet ventilation (TTJV)
#### Introduction
There is general agreement that TTJV used in association with a large bore intravenous cannula inserted via the cricothyroid membrane is an effective and efficient technique both to maintain oxygenation and to remove carbon dioxide. Because of its efficacy, it has been suggested that dedicated jet ventilation apparatus be available in all locations where general anaesthesia is practised [10]. It is much quicker to perform than other transtracheal techniques such as tracheostomy and retrograde intubation, which gives it a clear advantage in the 'cannot intubate, cannot ventilate' scenario. It is, however, associated with some potentially lethal complications that will be discussed later. If the patient has been anaesthetized, an intravenous technique of maintaining general anaesthesia will need to be started if the operation is allowed to proceed.

#### Insertion
The patient should be positioned to achieve maximum neck extension. The cricoid and thyroid cartilages are identified and the skin overlying the cricothyroid membrane is fixed by exerting pressure with a finger on each side of the membrane. A 14 gauge intravenous needle and cannula is inserted through the cricothyroid membrane into the trachea and directed towards the carina (Fig. 5). Correct intratracheal position is confirmed by sudden loss of resistance when entering the trachea followed by free aspiration of air through a syringe attached to the needle. This may be most reliably identified when the aspirating syringe contains some water or saline solution. The needle is then removed while the cannula is held at the skin. The high pressure oxygen source is then attached, following fixation of the cannula by taping or suturing to the skin. Immobility of the cannula is vitally important to avoid complications such as subcutaneous and mediastinal emphysema and to maintain patient safety.

#### High pressure oxygen source
A 14 SWG cannula is usually the largest readily available, but even this size will not be large enough to allow spontaneous respiration if used as the sole airway in the case of complete glottic obstruction [77]. With the use of larger cannulae, spontaneous respiration may be possible [78]. However, to ventilate effectively via a small cannula, a means of

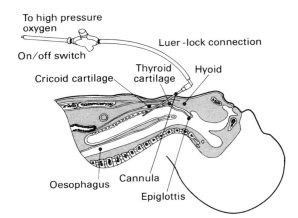

**Figure 5**  Diagram to illustrate positioning of upper airway in relation to larynx and cannula. With kind permission of Layman [115] and the editor of *Annals of the Royal College of Surgeons of England.*

connection to a high pressure oxygen source must be devised. Also, there should be some device to control the intermittent interruption of gas flow, and expiration must be allowed to take place via the glottis. Suitable systems should be capable of maintaining reasonable plasma carbon dioxide tensions while maintaining oxygenation.

The types of acceptable transtracheal jet ventilation systems available have been exhaustively reviewed by Benumof [10]. Systems may use regulated or unregulated oxygen via cylinders, or regulated oxygen directly from the wall outlet, a cylinder reducing valve or via an anaesthetic machine. In systems operating directly from an oxygen supply it is usual to use a jet injector device with a manual control.

The anaesthetic machine oxygen flush mechanism has been shown to be capable of generating a high intermittent pressure that is capable of maintaining adequate ventilation in animals; it has been advocated from many sources [79, 80]. Ventilation is achieved simply by activating the oxygen flush valve to pressurize the lungs and then releasing it to allow sufficient time for expiration to occur. If this method is to be used, then the pressure at which the machine overpressure valve activates should be considered; some apparatus may be incapable of generating sufficient pressure [81]. It is suggested that available machines should be evaluated before deciding on intermittent oxygen flush as a viable means of supplying emergency jet ventilation. An alternative method would be to use a self inflating bag capable of generating a high

pressure [82, 83]. If upper airway obstruction is complete, such a system may have advantages over jet ventilation by reducing the incidence of high peak pressures. Ventilation would certainly be less efficient, but the risk of barotrauma may be reduced.

Ideally, all fittings used to connect to a high pressure source should be designed for this purpose [10]. However, most hospitals that do not use the technique for elective cases are unlikely to have a purpose-built system. Many have assembled connections from readily available equipment, and use the oxygen flush mechanism to achieve adequate ventilation in an emergency situation. In particular, connection of an intravenous cannula hub to an oxygen delivery system in a way capable of achieving adequate ventilation is a problem that has produced a variety of solutions in the anaesthetic literature [79, 80, 82, 84–92]. Probably the most commonly described

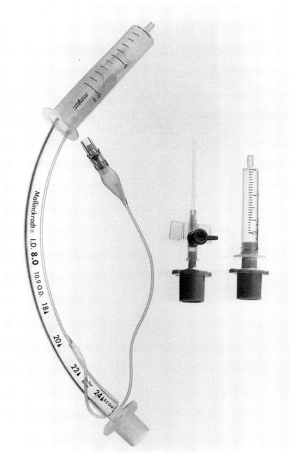

**Figure 6**  Methods for connecting intravenous cannulae to standard airway connectors.

method is to use a 3 ml syringe and a 7–8 mm tracheal tube connector to form a fitting between the female end of the intratracheal catheter and the 15/22 mm standard male connector of an anaesthetic system [82, 84] (Fig. 6). A 5 mm syringe body may be modified to fit a catheter mount connection [85]. It is also possible to connect a 3 mm tracheal tube fitting directly to an intravenous cannula fitting [85]. Yet another way to achieve a connection is by using a 8–9 size tracheal tube inflated inside a 10 ml syringe barrel. Inflation of the pilot balloon forms a seal which enables the i.v. cannula to be connected directly to an anaesthetic system and a high inflating pressure to be applied [90]. Even small bore plastic tubing used in capnography has been suggested for connecting to a high pressure source to produce effective oxygenation [83].

A simpler and probably more effective alternative system has been described using low compliance, high pressure oxygen tubing connected to

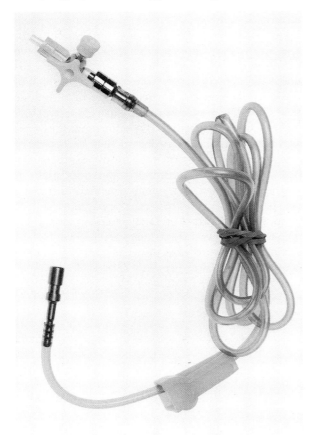

**Figure 7**   A simple system for delivering transtracheal ventilation.

the gas outlet of the anaesthetic machine by means of metallic Luer lock and 15 mm tracheal tube connectors [79] (Fig. 7). Such a system has been shown to be capable of effective ventilation in dogs [80]. This type of direct connection is to be preferred if the oxygen flush mechanism is to be used; most other connections made via an anaesthetic delivery system are unlikely to be capable of providing optimal ventilation because of their high compliance when high pressure oxygen is used. In emergency situations, however, the use of such systems may be the only means of preserving oxygenation.

Whatever delivery system is used, it has been suggested that the preassembled components should be readily available. In an emergency situation a hastily assembled and poorly considered connection system is likely to be dangerous and ineffective.

### Efficacy

Under normal circumstances, gas entering the lungs will be a mixture of 100% oxygen from the jet ventilation system and air entrained by a venturi effect from the upper airway via the patent glottis. Using a 16G cannula, and with a generating pressure of 50 p.s.i. (~345 kPa), the achievable gas flow approximates to 500 ml s$^{-1}$ [93]. This flow rate is sufficient to provide ventilation even in the absence of entrained gases. Entrained gas will add approximately 40% to the total flow rate when the upper airway is patent [93].

Normal blood gas values have been demonstrated during TTJV in animals [80, 83, 94, 95]. In patients, the technique has been associated with adequate carbon dioxide removal and hyperoxia [96–98]. The high arterial oxygen tensions observed could be due to the negligible contribution of entrainment to the total gas flow under normal circumstances [10] or to glottic resistance causing a PEEP effect at the end of expiration. The degree of 'PEEP effect' will depend on the inspiratory/expiratory ratio of the ventilation and the degree of glottic obstruction.

### Complications

Although the technique is highly effective at providing ventilation, it can be associated with potentially lethal complications.

In one of the first reviews of the complications of the technique in 1975, Smith *et al.* described a series of patients in whom the technique was used for acute respiratory distress [86]. The majority of the patients had carcinoma of the tongue or larynx. Out of 28 patients, difficulty with exhalation was experienced in four, two developed subcutaneous emphysema, one mediastinal emphysema, and in one patient a large artery was perforated following an attempt to enter the trachea. The complication rate was higher than in a group of elective patients, but no deaths were seen in either group. Subcutaneous emphysema due to catheter displacement [92] and pneumothorax as a result of barotrauma following use of TTJV [83, 96, 99] have also been reported, but again, no deaths occurred. Minor haemorrhage has been reported in a further series, but does not seem to be a major problem.

The incidence of barotrauma is related to the intratracheal pressure generated. This will depend on the equipment used, anatomical and pathological factors:

- the cross sectional area of the trachea;
- the generating pressure;
- the resistance of the cannula;
- the resistance of the tubes and connectors;
- the compliance/resistance of the lungs and chest wall;
- the inspiratory:expiratory (I:E) ratio;
- the degree of glottic/upper airway obstruction.

In order to reduce the risk of barotrauma, it is important to keep the generated intratracheal peak gas pressures to a minimum. Ideally, the intratracheal pressure should be continuously monitored by means of a second transtracheal cannula.

It cannot be overstressed that the patency of the upper airway is vital for the safety of this technique. If exhalation is prevented, barotrauma and tension pneumothorax are likely. Some early users of this technique suggested the use of subatmospheric pressures in the expiratory phase or a second cannula to act as a 'safety valve' in the event of complete upper airway obstruction [100]. However, if the ability to keep the upper airway clear is in doubt, it will be safer to start to convert to a formal tracheostomy, either by a transcutaneous dilatation technique or by an open surgical method once reasonable oxygenation has been achieved. A supplementary means of clearing the upper airway will be necessary once TTJV has been started. Regular aspiration of blood and other secretions from the oropharynx is mandatory, otherwise they will be entrained into the lung.

## Emergency tracheostomy

The major advantage tracheostomy has over techniques involving small gauge needles is that the internal diameter of the tracheostomy tube will usually allow spontaneous respiration by the patient, albeit against a high resistance when using smaller tubes. It will also allow lower ventilating pressures to be used, which should contribute to the safety of the technique. However, the larger size of the tube to be introduced is likely to cause a proportional increase in trauma caused by placement. Also, because of the size of the tracheostomy tube, more time to perform the procedure safely will generally be needed. It may be possible to have a combined approach, oxygenating the patient via a small transtracheal intravenous cannula while also performing a tracheostomy to ensure a more secure airway.

Percutaneous dilatational tracheostomy (PCDT) techniques may have advantages over the more conventional 'open' technique, especially with regard to reducing the incidence of haematological complications [101–103]. For acute management of the difficult airway, it is difficult to suggest a place for the percutaneous dilatational tracheostomy; it depends on the urgency of airway access needed, the skill of the operator and the particular type of technique employed. The trade-off of safety against speed of surgical access is particularly unfortunate in this situation. Percutaneous dilatational tracheostomy was initially not recommended for use in emergency cases [101], but the more rapid technique of insertion has been suggested as a possible method of surgical access for patients with partial airway obstruction, although this may take up to 10 min to achieve [104]. The most likely niche for this technique will be as a secondary measure of securing the airway when the acute threat has already been resolved.

### Minitracheostomy

Minitracheostomy is a technique which was first described by Matthews and Hopkinson in 1984 as a measure to prevent postoperative sputum retention [105]. The term usually applies to the placement of a size 4.0 mm internal diameter uncuffed tracheostomy through the cricothyroid membrane into the trachea.

*Insertion* The following insertion procedure has been used with the Minitracheostomy II kit (Portex, Oxford) (Fig. 8). The kit consists of a

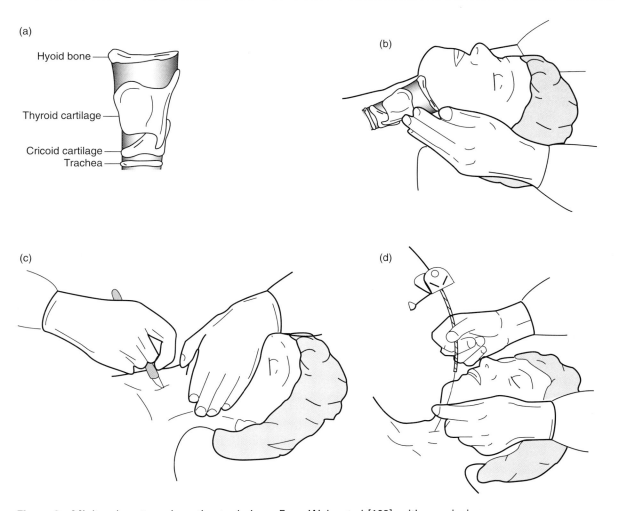

(a)

Hyoid bone

Thyroid cartilage

Cricoid cartilage
Trachea

(b)

(c)

(d)

**Figure 8** Minitracheostomy insertion technique. From Wain *et al.* [109], with permission.

specially designed bevelled blade, an obturator, and the tube itself, which is 4 mm internal diameter and has a flanged 15 mm male connector to enable a direct connection to be made with a standard gas delivery system.

Other kits are available, such as the Melker emergency cricothyrotomy catheter set (Cook Critical Care, Bloomington, Indiana, USA) (Fig. 9) and the Quicktrach (VBM), which differ slightly in insertion methods. Instructions should be read and thoroughly understood before attempting this potentially hazardous procedure.

The minitracheostomy is inserted with the neck in full extension (Fig. 8b). The cricoid and thyroid cartilages are identified, and the positions of the cricothyroid membrane and the overlying skin fixed by pressure of fingers on either side of the membrane. A single vertical incision 3–5 mm in

length is made with the blade supplied (Fig. 8c). Egress of air should be heard as the blade enters the subglottic space. An obturator is then passed through the incision into the trachea, and guided toward the carina. When this is in position, the tube should be gently guided over the obturator into the trachea (Fig. 8d). Correct position is confirmed by bilateral auscultation of the chest and detection of the presence of carbon dioxide in expired gas during gentle manual ventilation.

In severely dyspnoeic patients with a mobile larynx, it may well be difficult to steady the tissues sufficiently to allow insertion of the obturator. This problem can sometimes be solved by transfixing the skin and cricothyroid membrane by means of two needles on either side of the incision [106].

***Acute airway management*** Since its introduction, this technique has become popular for other applications besides prevention of sputum retention. It particular, it has been used as a method of supplying TTJV in the management of acute airway obstruction [107, 108]. Compared with the intravenous cannulae normally used for TTJV, the minitrach has a larger diameter and is purpose-built for intratracheal use, fixation and for direct connection to gas delivery systems. It thus has many advantages over the intravenous cannula for this particular application. However, its larger diameter is associated with a higher incidence of severe haemorrhagic complications. In a series of 60 elective insertions [109], severe haemorrhage necessitating tracheal intubation was reported in two patients, with minor bleeding in five others. It is likely that the incidence of this and other complications would be higher in emergency patients. This must be regarded as a major limitation of the technique, and a significant coagulopathy should be regarded as an absolute contraindication.

The 4 mm internal diameter of the minitrach is probably inadequate to allow spontaneous respiration for more than a short period of time in adults, so that assisted respiration is usually necessary. In a case of complete glottic obstruction, the larger diameter of the minitrach may well allow complete expiration via the cannula without a dangerous rise in intratracheal pressure. However, in these circumstances the airway should still be regarded as precarious, and conversion to a larger tracheostomy is desirable.

Techniques for cricothyrotomy using a Seldinger technique have also been described [110], and kits such as the Minitrach II (Seldinger) and the Melker cricothyrotomy kit (Fig. 9) are now available. It is likely that the incidence of haemorrhagic complications will be reduced compared with the other method of placement, but the time required for successful insertion may increase. The Seldinger technique seems to be becoming the favoured method of cannula insertion through the cricothyroid membrane because of concerns about haemorrhagic complications associated with other methods.

Because of the potential for complications and the skill required for insertion, it is suggested that a large gauge intravenous cannula would be a safer alternative in most emergency situations if a sufficient level of skill has not been developed and maintained by practising this technique in non-emergency cases. Obviously this will only apply if apparatus capable of supplying high pressure oxygen to the intravenous cannula is immediately available. If this is not available and cerebral

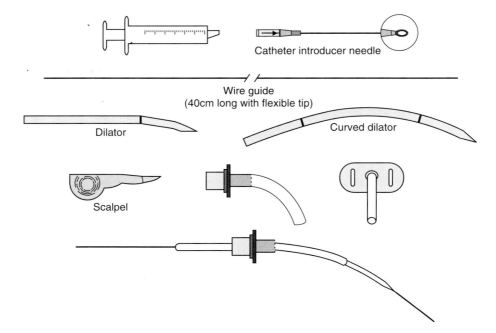

**Figure 9** Melker percutaneous dilatational cricothyrotomy kit. From the manufacturer's literature, Cook Critical Care, Bloomington, Indiana, USA.

hypoxia is imminent, a minitracheostomy technique may well be the best alternative available, although a risky one if sufficient skill and experience have not been obtained.

## EXTUBATION TECHNIQUES

If difficulty with intubation has been experienced, particularly if associated with difficulty with ventilation, then the extubation process may be potentially hazardous. Ideally a means of continuously managing the airway during extubation should be contemplated. General problems associated with extubation are discussed extensively elsewhere in this book (see Chapter 19).

In some cases, especially in patients where reintubation could prove extremely difficult in combination with likely ventilation impairment, e.g. facial haematoma or oedema, elective tracheostomy will usually be the preferred method of postoperative airway management. The stoma would then be maintained until the pathological process which had caused acute respiratory impairment was resolved.

In other situations, particularly where there is no reversible process causing difficulty with intubation, extubation under controlled conditions would seem to be the method of choice. Ideally, this should involve a technique that is able to revert to full airway control at all times during the extubation process. Gum elastic bougies, jet stylets, airway exchange catheters and the fibreoptic bronchoscope [111] have all been suggested for this purpose.

A technique using the jet stylet to aid the extubation of patients suggested by Benumof [111] is outlined here:

- preoxygenate the patient for 5 min;
- aspirate secretions from the pharynx, trachea, nose and nasogastric tube (if present);
- maximally inflate the lungs, then simultaneously deflate the tracheal tube cuff and withdraw the tracheal tube from the larynx over the jet stylet. This sequence should cause a forceful cough after the tube is withdrawn and will help clear the airway of secretions.

If the patient needs to be reintubated using the jet stylet as a guide, the jet stylet may still be kept in an intratracheal position following reintubation by using a catheter mount with a rubber self sealing

diaphragm on the suction port, such as that used during bronchoscopy [112]. This method enables confirmation of correct tracheal tube placement by bilateral chest auscultation and capnography before the jet stylet is withdrawn.

The suction channel of a fibreoptic bronchoscope can also be used to maintain jet ventilation following extubation [111]. The main advantage of this technique is that the trachea is visualized directly, with any intratracheal potential causes for postextubation embarrassment hopefully becoming apparent prior to attempted extubation. A hybrid technique may be used by first performing bronchoscopy on all difficult airway patients before extubation to exclude tracheal abnormalities and provide direct suction, then to introduce a jet stylet catheter to preserve the continuity of airway control in the extubation phase.

## EMERGENCY AIRWAY MANAGEMENT

This section attempts to summarize briefly the current situation with regard to emergency airway management in prehospital and ward situations. An attempt is also made to form a coherent plan of action for the management of the unexpected difficult intubation in these circumstances.

### Prehospital

This will depend on local training initiatives. In many areas of the UK paramedics are trained in tracheal intubation techniques, but training is expensive and time-consuming. Retention of skills has been identified as a problem. The OOA has never been extensively used in the UK, but the LMA seems likely to be used by paramedic services in the future as a complementary technique to tracheal intubation. It is increasingly being suggested as a primary means of airway control when immediate tracheal intubation cannot be achieved for one reason or another. The OTC has the potential to be a valuable tool in prehospital airway management, particularly in patients at risk of aspiration when direct laryngoscopy cannot be achieved. Patients with cervical spine injuries who require immediate airway control would probably be best managed (at least in the prehospital phase) by introducing either the LMA or the OTC with the neck held in neutral position, rather than by risking cervical spine damage during repeated attempts at laryngoscopy.

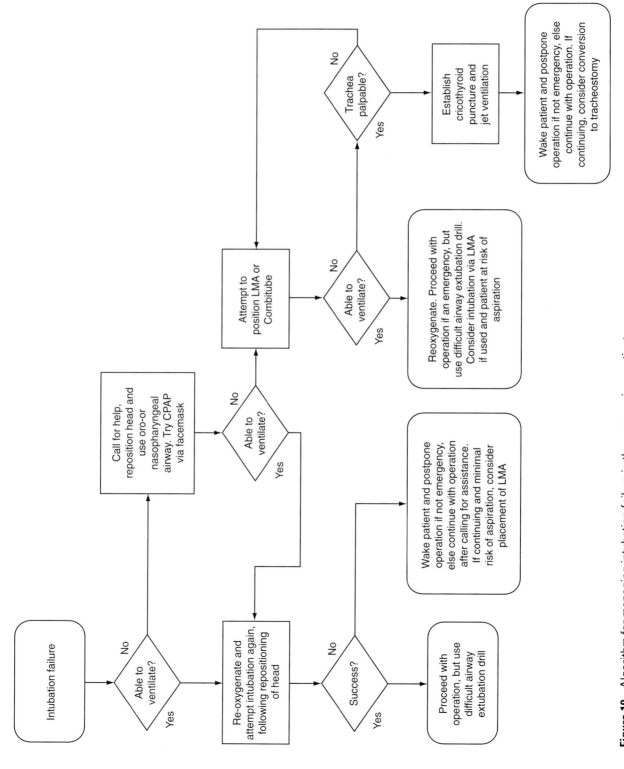

**Figure 10**   Algorithm for managing intubation failure in the unconscious patient.

## Hospital

The results of a recent multicentre study [45] suggest that ventilation via the LMA may be the preferred method of airway maintenance during CPR by nursing staff before tracheal intubation can be achieved. The OTC has also been shown to be very effective in CPR airway management when used by ICU nurses [113]. Both techniques would seem to be an improvement over the poor record of ventilation by facemask and bag in modestly trained staff [114]. Whichever method is employed for primary airway management, there seems to be a consensus that tracheal intubation is still regarded as the airway management of choice during CPR.

## Unexpected Difficult Intubation

### Suggested immediate management

The following notes are intended to act as a guide to the airway management of the unexpected difficult intubation. Obviously, the most important part of management of a difficult intubation is to be aware that a problem exists before attempting tracheal intubation. However, there is as yet no perfect method of detecting a difficult intubation preoperatively. Therefore, preparation of a strategy for the management of cases of unexpected difficult intubation is necessary if disaster is to be avoided (Fig. 10).

In many hospitals the equipment required for difficult airway management is collected in a 'difficult intubation box'. The recent American Society of Anesthesiologists Task Force on Management of the Difficult Airway report [6] made suggestions as to what should be included. This information, and details of the rest of the report, are included elsewhere in this book. Dedicated equipment for TTJV may only be present in a small number of hospitals, but non-commercial systems capable of performing an adequate function should be readily available in most theatre suites. Most simple intubation aids will probably be available, but the skill to use them may not always be present.

Every case is different, and the individual skills of the operator involved will play a large part in which management options are chosen. There are few procedures so urgent that a delay of about 1 h cannot be tolerated. In most situations the safest course of action will be to wake the patient and perform a local anaesthetic procedure. The local anaesthetic procedure should not then be of such a nature as to put the patient at further risk of complications that may then result in resuscitation attempts in a patient with a known difficult airway.

It is assumed that all patients will have been given an adequate dose of induction agent and a short acting muscle relaxant to facilitate intubation. Cricoid pressure should be used in all patients at risk of aspiration. Successful intubation should always be confirmed by capnography and bilateral chest auscultation, particularly when direct laryngoscopy is not possible. Failure to preoxygenate will reduce the time available in which to make decisions, particularly if ventilation is difficult. If possible, *all* patients should be preoxygenated.

Following intubation failure, before any other procedure is contemplated, gentle ventilation should be attempted via facemask and reservoir bag. This may give vital information on the nature of the airway and, if ventilation is difficult, warns the operator before significant desaturation occurs.

### If able to ventilate

- Give 100% oxygen. Call for help. Ventilate gently, taking care not to distend the stomach. Maintain cricoid pressure if there is an aspiration risk.
- Optimize position of head and neck if needed, call for simple intubation aids.
- Attempt intubation again with simple intubation aids. If a second failure is experienced, the options are to:

  - wake the patient (if the operation is not an acute emergency) and convert to a local anaesthetic procedure either immediately or at a later date if the procedure is elective;
  - continue with the procedure if it is an emergency.

If the decision is made to continue with the procedure and the patient is at risk of aspiration, cricoid pressure should be maintained and the lungs ventilated gently until respiration returns. If the patient is considered *not* to be an aspiration risk, placement of a LMA may be considered to aid airway maintenance and to aid blind intubation or fibreoptic aided intubation if required.

### If unable to ventilate

In this situation, the main considerations should be tracheal access and aspiration risk. Patency of the airway should be maintained by any means possible and the patient given 100% oxygen until full control is established.

- Give 100% oxygen, Call for help. Maintain cricoid pressure if the patient is at risk of aspiration. Attempt to maintain airway patency by means of either oropharyngeal or nasopharyngeal airways and/or CPAP via a facemask. If this works, reoxygenate and consider one more attempt at intubation with a tracheal tube and intubation aids or placement of a LMA. If ventilation is difficult, waking the patient and converting to a local anaesthetic technique will usually be the safest option.
- If this fails, attempt to position a LMA or OTC OOA depending on the availability of apparatus and the skill of the operator using it. Consider giving a small amount of suxamethonium if laryngospasm is thought to be a factor. Consider bronchospasm as a reaction to anaesthetic agents. Cricoid pressure may need to be relaxed in order to position the LMA or OTC correctly. If this strategy works, consider waking the patient and converting to a local anaesthetic technique if not a dire emergency. If the procedure has to continue, consider using the LMA to facilitate blind intubation if there is an aspiration risk.
- If previous attempts to secure an airway have failed, cricothyroid puncture and jet ventilation should be attempted if appropriate equipment is available. If this works, consider waking the patient and converting to a local anaesthetic technique if not a dire emergency. If the procedure has to continue, consider converting to a formal tracheostomy, a percutaneous tracheostomy, or cricothyroidotomy with a Minitrach.
- In a number of cases the trachea may be impalpable due to anatomical or pathological processes. If cricothyroid puncture cannot be safely performed and the patient cannot be ventilated using the above techniques, there are not many safe options left. If the operator is a skilled bronchoscopist, conventional or jet ventilation via a rigid bronchoscope or tracheal intubation over a fibreoptic bronchoscope may be considered. If an experienced surgeon is present, an emergency tracheostomy may be attempted. Repeated attempts at placement of a LMA or OTC or OOA may be the strategies most likely to succeed if bronchoscopic skill is inadequate and the skills for open tracheostomy are not available.

Following all cases of difficult intubation, a strategy should be formulated to manage extubation (see previous section).

## SUMMARY

Emergency management of the difficult airway has changed considerably over the last decade, largely because of the development of new devices such as the LMA and the OTC, and of intubation aids such as the fibreoptic laryngoscope. Increased experience and confidence with these new devices will inevitably lead to techniques originally envisaged as 'last ditch' measures becoming part of the guidelines for management of difficult cases. However, with all new techniques comes the responsibility for adequately training medical and paramedical personnel. Poorly understood invasive measures are surely a recipe for disaster, and are likely to lead to justified litigation. Unsuspected difficult airways may cause major problems at any time, and all junior doctors should be trained in basic airway management techniques. Due to the nature of the problem, the management of difficult airways cannot always be left to the most experienced operators. If emergency guidelines for airway management are followed, specialized experience will probably only be necessary during the initial management of a very small number of cases.

## KEY POINTS

- Errors of technique in managing difficult airways are responsible for a large proportion of the deaths associated with anaesthesia.

- The incidence of difficult airways depends on the environment in which resuscitation is practised, patient factors and the skill of the operator.

- Complete failure of intubation need not result in danger to the patient provided oxygenation is maintained by appropriate airway management techniques.

- Repeated attempts at intubation may result in increased complication rates, and in some circumstances may endanger life. In most instances it is far safer to wake the patient and to consider continuing the procedure using a local anaesthetic technique.

- Devices and techniques developed specifically for the management of patients during prehospital rescuscitation may be useful in the management of difficult airways in hospital and vice versa.

- The results of comparisons of efficiency between different airway management devices depend critically on the duration and type of training provided for each device.

- Transtracheal ventilation by means of a small diameter cannula is a valuable technique for maintaining oxygenation during management of a difficult airway in the unconscious patient. However, it is currently rarely used except as a last ditch measure, and consequently few practitioners have experience in using this technique under emergency conditions. Elective placement under local anaesthesia may be considered in known difficult cases.

- Emergency transtracheal oxygenation may be achieved by means of equipment consisting of simple preassembled components pressurized by the oxygen flush mechanism of an anaesthetic machine. However, dedicated purpose-built equipment is usually required for efficient ventilation.

- The safety of emergency transtracheal techniques is critically dependent on a readily palpable cricothyroid membrane. Anatomical variations or pathological processes that result in inability to access the trachea severely limit the options available during emergency airway management. Palpation of the trachea and the cricothyroid membrane should be an invariable routine during the assessment of a difficult airway.

## REFERENCES

1 Lunn J. N. and Mushin W. W. *Mortality Associated with Anaesthesia*. London: The Nuffield Provincial Hospitals Trust. 1982.
2 Buck N., Devlin H. B. and Lunn J. N. *The Report of a Confidential Enquiry into Perioperative Deaths*. London: The Nuffield Provincial Hospitals Trust, 1987.
3 Gannon K. Mortality associated with anaesthesia: a case review study. *Anaesthesia* 1991; **46:** 962.
4 Utting J. E. Pitfalls in anaesthetic practice. *British Journal of Anaesthesia* 1987; **59:** 877.
5 Nandi P. R., Charlesworth C. H., Taylor S. J., Nunn J. F. and Dore C. J. Effect of general anaesthesia on the pharynx. *British Journal of Anaesthesia* 1991; **66:** 157.
6 American Society of Anesthesiologists Practice guidelines for management of the difficult airway: a report by the American Society of Anesthesiologists task force on management of the difficult airway. *Anesthesiology* 1993; **78:** 597.
7 Lyons G. Failed intubation. *Anaesthesia* 1985; **40:** 759.
8 Mallampati S. R., Gatt S. P., Gugino L. D. *et al.* A clinical sign to predict difficult tracheal intubation. *Canadian Journal of Anaesthesiology* 1985; **32:** 429.
9 Cormack R. S. and Lehane J. Difficult tracheal intubation in obstetrics. *Anaesthesia* 1984; **39:** 1105.
10 Benumof J. L. and Scheller M. S. The importance of transtracheal jet ventilation in the management of the difficult airway. *Anesthesiology* 1989; **71:** 769.
11 Bellhouse C. P. and Dore C. Criteria for estimating likelihood of difficulty of endotracheal intubation with a Macintosh laryngoscope. *Anaesthesia and Intensive Care* 1988; **16:** 329.
12 Tunstall M. E. Failed intubation in the parturient (editorial). *Canadian Journal of Anaesthesiology* 1989; **36:** 611.
13 Hirsch I. A., Reagan J. O. and Sullivan N. Complications of direct laryngoscopy: a prospective analysis. *Anesthesiology Review* 1990; **17:** 34.
14 Thompson D. S. and Read R. C. Rupture of the trachea following endotracheal intubation. *Journal of the American Medical Association* 1968; **204:** 995.
15 Tolley P. M., Watts A. D. J. and Hickman J. A. Comparison of the use of the laryngeal mask and face mask by inexperienced personnel. *British Journal of Anaesthesia* 1992; **69:** 320.
16 Alexander R., Hodgson P., Lomax D. and Bullen C. A comparison of the laryngeal mask airway and Guedel airway, bag and facemask for manual ventilation following formal training. *Anaesthesia* 1993; **48:** 231.
17 Bryson T. K. and Benumof J. L. and Ward C. F. The esophageal obturator airway. *Chest* 1978; **74:** 537.

18 Don Michael T. A. and Gordon A. S. The oesophageal obturator airway: a new device in emergency cardiopulmonary resuscitation. *British Medical Journal* 1980; **281:** 1531.

19 Suresh D., Purdy G., Wainwright A. P. and Flynn P. J. Use of continuous positive airway pressure in paediatric dental extraction under general anaesthesia. *British Journal of Anaesthesia* 1991; **66:** 200.

20 Rothfleisch R., Davis L. L., Kuebel D. A. and deBoisblanc B. P. Facilitation of fibreoptic nasotracheal intubation in a morbidly obese patient by simultaneous use of nasal CPAP. *Chest* 1994; **106:** 287.

21 Don Michael T. A., Lambert E. H. and Mehran A. Mouth-to-lung airway for cardiac resuscitation. *Lancet* 1968; **ii:** 1329.

22 Don Michael T. A. The esophageal obturator airway: a critique. *Journal of the American Medical Association* 1981; **246:** 1098.

23 Gordon A. S. An improved esophageal obturator airway. In: Safar P., Elam J. O. (eds) *Advances in Cardiopulmonary Resuscitation.* New York: Springer-Verlag. 1977.

24 Auerbach P. S. and Geehr E. C. Esophageal gastric tube airway in the prehospital setting. *Journal of the American Medical Society* 1983; **250:** 3067.

25 Harrison E. E., Juergen N. H. and Beeman R. W. Esophageal perforation following use of the esophageal obturator airway. *Annals of Emergency Medicine* 1980; **9:** 21.

26 Pennant J. H., Pace N. A. and Gajraj N. M. Role of the laryngeal mask airway in the immobile cervical spine. *Journal of Clinical Anaesthesia* 1993; **5:** 226.

27 Thomson K. D., Ordman A. J., Parkhouse N. and Morgan B. D. G. Use of the Brain laryngeal mask airway in anticipation of difficult intubation. *British Journal of Plastic Surgery* 1989; **42:** 478.

28 Priscu V., Priscu L. and Soroker D. Laryngeal mask for failed intubation in emergency Caesarean section. *Canadian Journal of Anaesthesiology* 1992; **39:** 893.

29 Calder I., Ordman A. J., Jackowski A. and Crockard H. A. The Brain laryngeal mask airway: an alternative to emergency tracheal intubation. *Anaesthesia* 1990; **45:** 137.

30 McClune S. and Moore J. A. Laryngeal mask airway for Caesarean section. *Anaesthesia* 1990; **45:** 1095.

31 Levy D. M. LMA for failed intubation (letter). *Canadian Journal of Anaesthesiology* 1993; **40:** 801.

32 Asai T. and Appadurai I. LMA for failed intubation (letter). *Canadian Journal of Anaesthesiology* 1993; **40:** 802.

33 Brimacombe J. and Berry A. LMA for failed intubation (letter). *Canadian Journal of Anaesthesiology* 1993; **40:** 802.

34 Williams K. N. and Nunn J. F. The oesophageal detector device. A preoperative trial in 100 patients. *Anaesthesia* 1989; **44:** 412.

35 Ainsworth Q. P. and Calder I. The oesophageal detector device and the laryngeal mask. *Anaesthesia* 1990; **45:** 794.

36 Payne J. The use of the fibreoptic laryngoscope to confirm the position of the laryngeal mask. *Anaesthesia* 1989; **44:** 865.

37 Chadd G. D., Ackers J. W. L. and Bailey P. M. Difficult intubation aided by the laryngeal mask airway. *Anaesthesia* 1989; **44:** 1015.

38 Allison A. and McCrory J. Tracheal placement of a gum elastic bougie using the laryngeal mask. *Anaesthesia* 1990; **45:** 419.

39 McCrirrick A. and Pracilio J. A. Awake intubation: a new technique. *Anaesthesia* 1991; **46:** 661.

40 Heath M. L. Intubation through the laryngeal mask: a technique for unexpected difficult intubation. *Anaesthesia* 1991; **46:** 545.

41 Asai T., Barclay K., Power I. and Vaughan R. S. Cricoid pressure impedes placement of the laryngeal mask airway and subsequent tracheal intubation through the mask. *British Journal of Anaesthesia* 1994; **72:** 47.

42 Reinhart D. J. and Simmons G. Comparison of placement of the laryngeal mask airway with endotracheal tube by paramedics and respiratory therapists. *Annals of Emergency Medicine* 1994; **24:** 260.

43 Pennant J. H. Comparison of the endotracheal tube and laryngeal mask in airway management by paramedical personnel. *Anesthesia and Analgesia* 1992; **74:** 531.

44 Davies P. R. F. Laryngeal mask airway and tracheal tube insertion by unskilled personnel. *Lancet* 1990; **ii:** 977.

45 Stone B. J., Leach A. B., Alexander C. A. *et al.* The use of the laryngeal mask airway by nurses during cardiopulmonary resuscitation. *Anaesthesia* 1994; **49:** 3.

46 Cyna A. M. and MacLeod D. M. The laryngeal mask: cautionary tales. *Anaesthesia* 1990; **45:** 167.

47 Griffin R. M. Aspiration pneumonia and the laryngeal mask airway. *Anaesthesia* 1990; **45:** 1039.

48 Nanji G. M. and Maltby J. R. Vomiting and aspiration pneumonitis with the laryngeal mask airway. *Canadian Journal of Anaesthesia* 1992; **39:** 169.

49 Barker P., Murphy P., Langton J. A. and Rowbotham D. J. Regurgitation of gastric contents during general anaesthesia using the laryngeal mask airway. *British Journal of Anaesthesia* 1992; **69:** 314.

50 Lack A. Regurgitation using a laryngeal mask. *Anaesthesia* 1993; **48:** 734.

51 Freeman R. and Baxendale B. Laryngeal mask airway for Caesarean section. *Anaesthesia* 1990; **45:** 1094.

52 Reynolds F. Tracheostomy in obstetric practice:

how about the laryngeal mask airway? *Anaesthesia* 1989; **44**: 870.

53 Ansermino J. M., Blogg C. E. and Carrie L. E. S. Failed tracheal intubation at Caesarean section and the laryngeal mask. *British Journal of Anaesthesia* 1992; **68**: 118.

54 Rabey P. G., Murphy P. J., Langton J. A., Barker B. and Rowbotham D. J. Effect of the laryngeal mask airway on lower oesophageal pressure in patients during general anaesthesia. *British Journal of Anaesthesia* 1992; **69**: 346.

55 Strang T. I. Does the laryngeal mask airway compromise cricoid pressure? *Anaesthesia* 1992; **47**: 829.

56 Akhtar T. M. Oesophageal vent-laryngeal mask to prevent aspiration of gastric contents. *British Journal of Anaesthesia* 1994; **72**: 52.

57 Brain A. I. J. Three cases of difficult intubation overcome by the laryngeal mask airway. *Anaesthesia* 1985; **40**: 353.

58 Frass M., Johnson J. C., Atherton G. L. *et al.* Esophageal Tracheal Combitube (ETC) for emergency resuscitation: anatomical evaluation of ETC placement by radiography. *Resuscitation* 1989; **18**: 95.

59 Eichinger S., Schreiber W., Heint T. *et al.* Airway management in a case of neck impalement: use of the oesophageal tracheal Combitube airway. *British Journal of Anaesthesia* 1992; **68**: 534.

60 Bigenzhan W., Pesau B. and Frass M. Emergency ventilation using the Combitube in cases of difficult intubation. *European Archives of Oto-rhino-laryngology* 1991; **248**: 129.

61 Klauser R., Röggla G., Pidlich J., Leithner C. and Frass M. Massive upper airway bleeding after thrombolytic therapy: successful airway management with the Combitube. *Annals of Emergency Medicine* 1992; **21**: 431.

62 Frass M., Frenzer R., Zahler J., Ilias W. and Leithner C. Ventilation via the esophageal tracheal Combitube in a case of difficult intubation. *Journal of Cardiothoracic Anaesthesia* 1987; **1**: 565.

63 Baraka A. The Combitube oesophageal– tracheal double lumen airway for difficult intubation. *Canadian Journal of Anaesthesiology* 1993; **40**: 1222.

64 Brugger S. Successful intubation with the Combitube of two patients with bull neck. *Acta Medica Austriaca* 1993; **20**: 78.

65 Staudinger T., Tesinsky P., Klappacher G. *et al.* Emergency intubation with the Combitube in two cases of difficult airway management. *European Journal of Anaesthesiology* 1995; **12**: 189.

66 Brimacombe J. The oesophageal tracheal Combitube for difficult intubation. *Canadian Journal of Anaesthesiology* 1994; **41**: 656.

67 Frass M., Frenzer R., Zdrahal F., Hoflehner G.,

Porges P. and Lackner F. The esophageal tracheal Combitube: preliminary results with a new airway for CPR. *Annals of Emergency Medicine* 1987; **16**: 768.

68 Frass M., Frenzer R., Rauscha F., Weber H., Pacher R. and Leithner C. Evaluation of esophageal tracheal Combitube in cardiopulmonary resuscitation. *Critical Care Medicine* 1987; **15**: 609.

69 Frass M., Frenzer R., Rauscha F., Schuster E. and Glogar D. Ventilation with the esophageal tracheal Combitube in cardiopulmonary resuscitation. Promptness and effectiveness. *Chest* 1988; **93**: 781.

70 Frass M., Rödler S., Frenzer R., Ilias W., Leithner C. and Lackner F. Esophageal tracheal Combitube, endotracheal airway, and mask: comparison of ventilatory pressure curves. *Journal of Trauma* 1989; **29**: 1476.

71 Atherton G. L. Ability of paramedics to use the Combitube in prehospital cardiac arrest. *Annals of Emergency Medicine* 1993; **22**: 1263.

72 Staudinger T., Brugger S., Roggla M. *et al.* Comparison of the Combitube with the endotracheal tube in cardiopulmonary resuscitation in the prehospital phase. *Wiener Klinische Wochenschrift* 1994; **106**: 412.

73 Niemann J. T., Rosborough J. P., Myers R. *et al.* The pharyngeo-tracheal lumen airway: preliminary investigation of a new adjunct. *Annals of Emergency Medicine* 1984; **13**: 591.

74 Caparosa R. J. and Zavatsky A. R. Practical aspects of the cricothyroid space. *Laryngoscope* 1957; **67**: 577.

75 Holst M., Halbig I., Persson A. and Schiratzki H. The cricothyroid muscle after cricothyroidotomy. A porcine experimental study. *Acta Otolaryngology (Stockholm)* 1989; **107**: 136.

76 Jacoby J. J., Hamelburg W., Ziegler C. H., Flory F. A. and Jones J. R. Transtracheal resuscitation. *Journal of the American Medical Association* 1956; **162**: 625.

77 Bougas T. P., Cook C. D. Pressure–flow characteristics of needles suggested for transtracheal ventilation. *New England Journal of Medicine* 1960; **262**: 511.

78 Dallen L. T., Wine R. and Benumof J. L. Spontaneous ventilation via transtracheal large-bore intravenous catheters is possible. *Anesthesiology* 1991; **75**: 531.

79 de Lisser E. A. and Muravchick S. Emergency transtracheal ventilation. *Anesthesiology* 1981; **55**: 606.

80 Scuderi P. E., McLeskey H. and Comer P. B. Emergency percutaneous transtracheal ventilation during anaesthesia using readily available equipment. *Anesthesia and Analgesia* 1982; **61**: 867.

81 Meyer P. D. Emergency transtracheal jet ventilation. *Anesthesiology* 1990; **73**: 787.

82 Stinson T. W. A simple connector for transtracheal ventilation. *Anesthesiology* 1977; **47**: 232.

83 Cote C. J., Eavey R. D., Todres D. and Jones D. E. Cricothyroid membrane puncture: oxygenation and ventilation in a dog model using an intravenous catheter. *Critical Care Medicine* 1988; **16**: 615.

84 Patel R. Systems for transtracheal ventilation. *Anesthesiology* 1983; **59**: 165.

85 Hilton P. J. A simple connector for cricothyroid cannulation. *Anaesthesia* 1982; **37**: 221.

86 Smith B. R., Babinski M., Klain M. and Pfaelle H. Percutaneous transtracheal ventilation. *Journal of the American College of Emergency Physicians* 1976; **5**: 765.

87 Dunlap L. B. A modified, simple device for the emergency administration of percutaneous transtracheal ventilation. *Journal of the American College of Emergency Physicians* 1978; **7**: 42.

88 Fisher J. A. A 'last ditch' airway. *Canadian Anaesthetists Society Journal* 1979; **26**: 225.

89 Carlton D. M. and Zide M. F. An easily constructed cricothyroidotomy device for emergency airway management. *Journal of Oral Surgery* 1980; **38**: 623.

90 Gildar J. S. A simple system for transtracheal ventilation. *Anesthesiology* 1983; **58**: 106.

91 Aye L. S. Percutaneous transtracheal ventilation (letter). *Anesthesia and Analgesia* 1983; **62**: 619.

92 Ravussin P. and Freeman J. A new transtracheal catheter for ventilation and resuscitation. *Canadian Anaesthetists Society Journal* 1985; **32**: 60.

93 Spoerel W. E., Narayanan P. S. and Singh N. P. Transtracheal ventilation. *British Journal of Anaesthesia* 1971; **43**: 932.

94 Klain M. and Smith R. B. High frequency percutaneous transtracheal jet ventilation. *Critical Care Medicine* 1977; **5**: 280.

95 Thomas T., Zornow M., Scheller M. S. and Unger R. The efficiency of three different modes of transtracheal ventilation in hypoxic hypercarbic swine. *Canadian Journal of Anaesthesiology* 1988; **35**: 561.

96 Weymuller E. A., Paugh D., Pavlin E. G. and Cummings C. W. Management of difficult airway problems with percutaneous transtracheal ventilation. *Annals Otology Rhinology and Laryngology* 1987; **96**: 34.

97 Jacobs H. B. Transtracheal catheter ventilation: clinical experience in 36 patients. *Chest* 1974; **65**: 36.

98 Monnier P. H., Ravussin P., Savary M. and Freeman J. Percutaneous transtracheal ventilation for laser endoscopic treatment of laryngeal and subglottic lesions. *Clinical Otolaryngology* 1988; **13**: 209.

99 Oliverio R., Ruder C. B., Fermon C. and Curd A. Report on pneumothorax secondary to ball-valve obstruction during jet ventilation. *Anesthesiology* 1979; **51**: 255.

100 Jacobs H. B. Needle-catheter brings oxygen to the trachea. *Journal of the American Medical Association* 1972; **222**: 1231.

101 Clagia P., Firschling R. and Syniec C. Elective percutaneous dilatational trachestomy: a new simple bedside procedure; preliminary report. *Chest* 1985; **87**: 715.

102 Bodenham A., Diament A., Cohen A. and Webster N. Percutaneous dilatational tracheostomy. A bedside procedure on the intensive care unit. *Anaesthesia* 1991; **46**: 570.

103 Hazard P., Jones C. and Benitone J. Comparative clinical trial of standard operative tracheostomy with percutaneous tracheostomy. *Critical Care Medicine* 1991; **19(8)**: 1018.

104 Griggs W. M., Myburgh J. A. and Worthley L. I. G. Urgent airway access – an indication for percutaneous tracheostomy? *Anaesthesia and Intensive Care* 1991; **19**: 586.

105 Matthews H. R. and Hopkinson R. B. Treatment of sputum retention by minitracheostomy. *British Journal of Surgery* 1984; **71**: 147.

106 Baskett P. J. F. Life support techniques. *Resuscitation Handbook*. London: Gower. 1989; 28.

107 Squires S. S. and Frampton M. C. The use of mini-tracheostomy and high-frequency jet ventilation in the management of acute airway obstruction. *Journal of Laryngology and Otology* 1986; **100**: 1199.

108 Matthews H. R., Fischer B. J., Smith B. E., Hopkinson R. B. and DeMeester T. R. Minitracheostomy: a new delivery system for jet ventilation. *Journal of Thoracic and Cardiovascular Surgery* 1986; **92**: 673.

109 Wain J. C., Wilson D. J. and Mathisen D. J. Clinical experience with minitracheostomy. *Annals of Thoracic Surgery* 1990; **49**: 881.

110 Corke C. and Cranswick P. A Seldinger technique for minitracheostomy insertion. *Anaesthesia and Intensive Care* 1988; **16**: 206.

111 Benumof J. L. Management of the difficult adult airway: with special emphasis on awake tracheal intubation. *Anesthesiology* 1991; **75**: 1087.

112 Goskowicz R., Gaughan S., Benumof J. L. and Ozaki G. T. It is not necessary to remove a jet stylet in order to determine tracheal tube location. *Journal of Clinical Anaesthesia* 1992; **7**: 732.

113 Staudinger T., Brugger S., Watschinger B. *et al.* Emergency intubation with the Combi-tube: comparison with the endotracheal airway. *Annals of Emergency Medicine* 1993; **22**: 1573.

114 Lowenstein S. R., Hansbrough J. F., Libby L. S., Hill D., Mountain R. D. and Scroggin C. H. Cardiopulmonary resuscitation by medical and surgical house officers. *Lancet* 1981; **ii**: 679.

115 Layman P. R. Transtracheal ventilation in oral surgery. *Annals of the Royal College of Surgeons of England* 1983; **65**: 318.

# 14

# The Combitube

*Brian Jenkins*

## INTRODUCTION

Tracheal intubation is generally agreed to be the 'gold standard' of airway management during cardiopulmonary resuscitation (CPR). It enables direct connection of ventilation devices to the respiratory tract and maintains a seal that prevents tracheal soiling. However, for resuscitation of patients in a prehospital situation, training paramedical services to the skill level required to be regarded as competent in this technique takes considerable time, effort and money. Even when an investment in training has been made, retention of skills has been shown to be a major problem [1].

### The Oesophageal Obturator Airway

With prehospital CPR in mind, the concept of using a device to obstruct the oesophageal lumen and to ventilate the lungs indirectly by increasing intrapharyngeal pressure was first described by Don Michael in 1968 [2]. The main advantage of such a device is that direct laryngoscopy is not required; training in its use would therefore require less skill and medical input. The oesophageal obturator airway (OOA) was developed from this concept, and has been extensively used [3], especially in the USA. The incidence of major side effects associated with its use is reported to be low [4]. The main disadvantages of the oesophageal obturator airway are perceived to be [5, 6]:

- Inadvertent tracheal placement (in which case ventilation is impossible, and the OOA has to be resited).
- Difficulty in obtaining a good seal with the mask, causing leakage of ventilatory gas and decreased efficiency.

Also, maintenance of an airway seal with this device requires operator skill, and both hands are usually needed to maintain effective ventilation.

### The Pharyngeo-Tracheal Lumen Airway

The pharyngeo-tracheal lumen airway (PTLA) (Fig. 1) [7, 8] is an artificial airway that was designed to overcome the main limitations of the OOA. It is a double lumen tube, which allows ventilation following either oesophageal or tracheal placement, and its insertion is aided by a stylet that occupies one of the luminae. The stylet needs to be removed when the smaller, distal tube is located in the trachea. The upper balloon is inflated by the mouth of the resuscitator.

## THE OESOPHAGEAL TRACHEAL COMBITUBE

Like the PTL, the oesophageal tracheal Combitube (OTC) is an artificial airway that was designed to overcome the limitations of the OOA. The OTC allows for ventilation following either oesophageal or tracheal intubation, but is designed for blind oesophageal placement. It

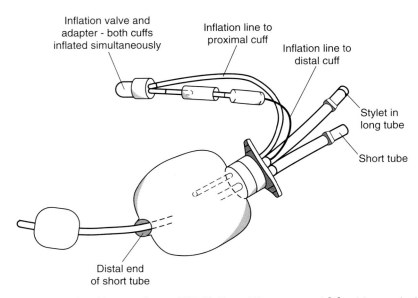

**Figure 1**    The pharyngeo-tracheal lumen airway (PTLA). From Niemann *et al.* [8], with permission.

effectively combines the functions of the OOA and a tracheal tube. Balloons are inflated to form seals in the hypopharynx and the oesophagus. The tube is held in the correct position by the pharyngeal balloon, and after insertion there should be no need to hold or externally fixate the tube to ensure that correct positioning is maintained. Like the OOA, it was designed to be used by personnel untrained in tracheal intubation as an airway management tool during prehospital CPR. Most of the initial research on this airway was performed by Michael Frass and colleagues at the University of Vienna.

The OTC is felt to have distinct advantages over the PTLA [9]. It is rigid enough not to require a stylet, so that when the distal tube is located in the trachea following blind intubation adequate ventilation can be achieved by simple reconnection of the breathing system to the alternative tube. It has a smaller diameter than the PTLA and is perceived to be easier to insert.

## Structure

The OTC (Sheridan Catheter Corporation, Argyle, New York, USA) is a polyvinyl chloride double lumen tube, with luminae that end at approximately the same level, separated by a partition (Fig. 2). One lumen ('oesophageal') is blind at the distal end. It has eight perforations that are intended to be located at the level of the lower

pharynx following correct placement. The proximal part of this lumen ends in a tube with a blue 25 mm connector to connect to a ventilating system. The other lumen ('tracheal') is open at the distal end and unperforated throughout. It also forms a tube at its proximal end with a shorter transparent 25 mm connector. This can also be connected directly to a ventilating bag. The external diameter at the distal end is 13 mm.

The designation of the proximal connectors into oesophageal and tracheal refers to the lumen that should be used to ventilate when the named structure has been intubated. In other words, the oesophageal lumen is used for ventilation of the lungs when the tip of the tube is located in the oesophagus. In this position the tracheal lumen also lies within the oesophagus (Fig. 3), and a gastric tube may be passed through it to aspirate stomach contents if required. If the tube has inadvertently been placed in the trachea, the tracheal lumen may be used for ventilation of the lungs without need for repositioning. In this position the oesophageal lumen has no function.

There are two balloons, one smaller distal and one larger proximal. The distal balloon maintains a seal in either the oesophagus or the trachea, and the proximal balloon fixes the OTC in the hypopharynx. Between the balloons are the perforations in the blind-ending oesophageal lumen.

There are two circumferential marks on the tube approximately 8 cm from the distal end of

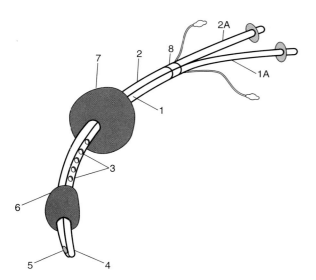

**Figure 2** The oesophageal tracheal Combitube. 1 = 'oesophageal obturator' lumen; 1A = short tube for lumen 1; 2 = 'tracheal' lumen; 2A = short tube for lumen 2; 3 = perforations of lumen 1; 4 = distal blind end of lumen 1; 5 = open end of lumen 2; 6 = distal cuff; 7 = pharyngeal balloon; 8 = printed rings indicating depth of insertion. From Frass *et al.* [23], with permission.

the tube; these are intended to aid correct placement (Fig. 2).

## Insertion of the OTC

Insertion is aided by full muscle relaxation. The patient's head should be held in a neutral position. The operator stands to one side of the patient, using one hand to lift the tongue and mandible forward and the thumb and forefinger of the other hand to guide the OTC gently into the lower pharynx. Insertion continues until the two positioning marks are level with the teeth or with the alveolar ridges in edentulous patients. At this stage the upper balloon is inflated with 100 ml of air (without holding the tube) to seal the upper airway and to fix the OTC in the correct position. The lower balloon is then inflated with 10–15 ml of air to maintain a seal in the oesophagus or the trachea and prevent oesophageal distension due to air leakage around the lower balloon when the tube is placed in the oesophagus. The upper balloon presses against the base of the tongue and apposes the soft palate to the posterior pharyngeal wall, wedging the balloon behind the hard palate and sealing off the laryngopharynx from the orophar-

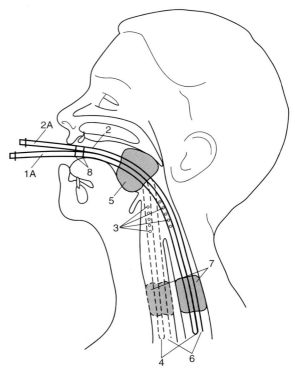

**Figure 3** Cross-section of the oesophageal tracheal Combitube (OTC) in oesophageal (continuous lines) and tracheal (dotted lines) position. 1 = 'oesophageal' lumen; 1A = longer, blue connector leading to lumen 1; 2 = 'tracheal' lumen; 2A = shorter, clear connector leading to lumen 2; 3 = perforations of lumen 1; 4 = distal blocked end of lumen 1; 5 = pharyngeal balloon; 6 = distal open end of lumen 2; 7 = distal cuff (for sealing of either the oesophagus or the trachea); 8 = printed rings indicating depth of insertion. From Frass *et al.* [9], with permission.

ynx and nasopharynx (see Fig. 4). The design of the balloons is such that the volumes of air required for maintenance of a seal and for tube fixation are similar in patients of differing size and body build.

## Tracheal Tube Insertion

If a tracheal tube needs to be inserted while the OTC is in position, the upper balloon should be deflated, and then the lower balloon. When successful tracheal intubation has been achieved, the OTC may be removed. Ventilation via the OTC may be employed between intubation attempts with the tracheal tube.

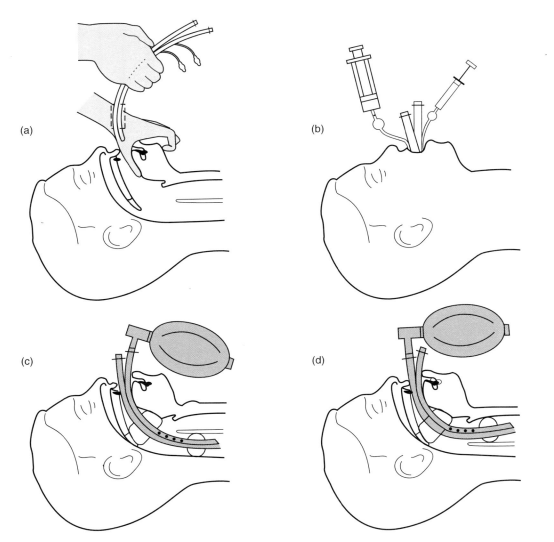

**Figure 4**    (a) Blind insertion of the OTC; (b) inflation of the pharyngeal balloon and then the distal cuff; (c) ventilation in the oesophageal position of the OTC; (d) ventilation in the tracheal position of the OTC. From Frass *et al.* [12], with permission.

## Ventilation

If the described insertion technique has been fol- lowed, it is most likely that the end of the tube will be located in the upper oesophagus. It is therefore usual to attempt ventilation first through the oesophageal lumen. When the distal balloon is located in the oesophagus, ventilation is achieved via the perforations in the wall of the oesophageal limb. The distal cuff occludes the oesophagus and the proximal cuff occludes the upper airway, so that inflating gas pressurizes the laryngopharynx and inflates the lungs via an open glottis (Fig. 3).

Because the upper airway is occluded, expiration must also be achieved via the perforations in the oesophageal limb (Fig. 3). Oesophageal place- ment of the distal balloon is confirmed on hearing bilateral breath sounds over the chest on ausculta- tion when ventilating the oesophageal lumen. Stomach auscultation should also be performed to ensure that gastric distension is not occurring due to insufficient inflation of the distal balloon.

If the end of the tube is located in the trachea and ventilation is attempted via the oesophageal lumen, chest inflation will not occur. The stomach will become distended. In contrast to the OOA, ventilation can still be achieved without repositioning the tube simply by using the tracheal limb of the OTC for ventilation. As described, this lumen has an open distal end and is thus able to function as a tracheal tube. While ventilating using the tracheal limb, correct placement is again confirmed by bilateral chest auscultation and capnography.

Initial trials in animals [10] produced encouraging results, suggesting that the OTC was able to function in the manner for which it was originally designed. The adequacy of ventilation via the OTC was then studied in adult patients undergoing routine surgery under general anaesthesia [11]. A randomized cross-over design was used to compare ventilation via the OTC with tracheal ventilation. Patients were allocated into one of two groups. The first group were ventilated via an tracheal tube for 20 min, followed by removal of the tracheal tube, OTC insertion, and ventilation via the OTC for a further 20 min. In the second group, the order of insertion of tracheal tube and OTC was reversed. After each period of ventilation, arterial blood was sampled for gas analysis and pH measurement. The same ventilation parameters were used throughout the study. In all but one of the 32 patients, placement of the OTC in the oesophagus was achieved at the first attempt. The only patient in whom tracheal placement occurred was excluded from further analysis.

Results showed a significantly higher mean arterial oxygen tension in the patients following ventilation with the OTC compared with ventilation with the tracheal tube. No significant differences in mean arterial carbon dioxide tension or pH were demonstrated between the two groups. An explanation for the observed high oxygen tension in the OTC group is suggested in the next section.

## Ventilation Characteristics

Other studies in which blood gas tensions were examined [12, 13] have shown that a high arterial oxygen tension is a feature of OTC ventilated patients compared with patients ventilated via an tracheal tube. This phenomenon was investigated in a paper by Frass and colleagues [9]. Twelve adult patients classified as American Society of Anesthesiologists (ASA) levels I and II undergoing routine abdominal surgery were studied. Patients with respiratory disorders were excluded. All anaesthetics were administered by the same person using a standard technique that included muscle relaxants. A 16 SWG catheter was introduced into the trachea to measure intratracheal pressure. In randomized order, each patient was ventilated by mask, tracheal tube and OTC for 20 min with each airway. Ventilation parameters were matched between patients. At the end of each period arterial blood samples were taken for gas analysis.

The study group consisted of five males and seven females with ages ranging from 20 to 52 years. Mean arterial oxygen tension in the OTC group was significantly greater than in the tracheal tube group, but not the mask group. Significant differences in mean arterial carbon dioxide tension and pH were seen between all groups, with mask ventilation being associated with the highest carbon dioxide and lowest pH, then OTC, then tracheal tube. Air leakage was highest with mask (29.8 ± 14%), then OTC (15.1 ± 9.6%), then tracheal tube (6.3 ± 9.0%). Expiratory flow time was significantly longer in the OTC than the tracheal tube group. Ventilation with the OTC produced a small endotracheal positive end-expiratory pressure (PEEP) (2.1 ± 1.2 mmHg), which was quantitatively similar to that seen with mask ventilation.

The PEEP effect is thought to be produced by expiratory resistance to gas flow from the perforations in the oesophageal limb of the OTC. This effect would be likely to be more pronounced with increasing frequency of respiration or in any situation in which less time was allowed for expiration. In certain circumstances, this effect may be advantageous in that it simulates physiological PEEP seen in spontaneously breathing patients. Loss of physiological PEEP following tracheal intubation may prove disadvantageous, especially in critically ill patients [14]. It may also be a problem in patients with chronic respiratory disease in whom expiratory resistance is necessary to maintain the patency of small airways during expiration.

## Applications

The OTC can be inserted blindly without head and neck movement, which may be important in some trauma patients. Because the proximal balloon acts as an upper airway obturator, blood, secretions and foreign bodies from the upper airway are prevented from being swallowed or inspired. If the preferred oesophageal positioning is obtained, gastric aspiration may be achieved via the open-ended 'tracheal' lumen following insertion of a stomach tube.

## Cardiopulmonary resuscitation: studies with the OTC

In the report that demonstrated adequacy of ventilation in adult patients undergoing surgery [11], 21 patients who required CPR and were intubated with the OTC were also described. Acceptable blood gas results were achieved in all patients, despite the fact that three patients had vomited prior to introduction of the OTC. These results encouraged further studies into the use of the OTC during CPR.

In the first of these studies [12], effectiveness of ventilation was assessed in 31 patients requiring CPR following cardiac arrest calls, either in intensive care or in a general hospital ward setting. All patients had coronary artery disease; patients with chronic obstructive airways disease or infective lung disease were excluded from further analysis. There were two parts to this study; the first examined the adequacy of ventilation by OTC and a reservoir bag, using an estimated inspired oxygen concentration of 40%. The second part compared the efficiency of ventilation with the OTC and with a tracheal tube (internal diameter 8 mm) in a group of 15 patients. All patients in the second part of the study were mechanically ventilated using the same parameters, but treatment groups were neither randomized nor reversed. Arterial blood gas samples were taken after 20 min of ventilation.

In the bag-ventilated patients, an adequate level of ventilation and oxygenation was demonstrated ($paO_2$ 111.6 mmHg $\pm$ 26.4, $paCO_2$ 36.8 mmHg $\pm$ 7.0, pH 7.4 $\pm$ 0.08). In the mechanically ventilated group, patients ventilated using the OTC were again reported to have significantly higher mean arterial oxygen tensions than those in the tracheal tube group.

Four patients died during resuscitation attempts before blood gas analysis could be performed. In all OTC patients, oesophageal placement was achieved after blind insertion. In postmortem examinations of patients who died within 24 h following CPR, there was neither macro- nor microscopic evidence of pulmonary aspiration.

In another study [13], the promptness and effectiveness of ventilation using the OTC for airway management during CPR was investigated. Patients were randomly allocated to either OTC or tracheal intubation groups. If the allocated airway could not for any reason be used the patients were excluded from further analysis. Patients were also excluded if they had chronic respiratory disease or if the OTC was inadvertently introduced into the trachea. The physicians taking part in the study had been trained in the technique of tracheal intubation and had achieved at least three successful intubations. Induction agents and muscle relaxants were used to facilitate placement of the OTC and tracheal tubes.

Forty-three patients met the criteria of the study. The time required for correct placement was significantly shorter in the OTC group (27.3 $\pm$ 8.4 s) compared with the tracheal intubation group (39.7 $\pm$ 10.0 s), despite the fact that more time was required for balloon inflation with the OTC. The differences in total intubation time were thought to be partially explained by the fact that direct laryngoscopy is unnecessary to position the OTC correctly. Ventilation via the OTC was again demonstrated to produce higher mean arterial oxygen tensions than ventilation via the tracheal tube. Long-term survival was similar in both groups.

The utility of the OTC in the prehospital phase of CPR has also been investigated [15]. Patients were allocated on alternate days to receive either tracheal intubation or OTC placement as the initial means to secure the airway. In addition, OTC placement was attempted if first attempts at tracheal intubation were unsuccessful. Successful placement was achieved in 80 of 86 patients, and 11 out of 14 patients were managed successfully with the OTC following failed attempts at tracheal intubation. In another study [16], paramedics were assessed following training with the OTC for successful placement, recognition of oesophageal placement and retention of skills. In 69% of patients the OTC was successfully placed, with recognition of oesophageal placement in all cases. In addition, 64% of cases of failed tracheal intubation were successfully managed with the OTC. However, 15 months after the training, 9 out of the 11 paramedics studied were deemed to have inadequate retention of skills.

## The OTC in the intensive care unit and long-term ventilation

The OTC has also been used in ICU patients. In a study by Frass et al. [17], six patients were ventilated in the ICU for 2–8 h with the OTC in the oesophageal position following placement during management of CPR on a general ward. The OTC performed satisfactorily under these circumstances.

The effectiveness of OTC intubation by ICU nurses for CPR airway management has been compared with tracheal intubation by ICU physicians [18]. It was concluded that airway management with the OTC when used by ICU nurses was as effective as tracheal intubation performed by intensivists during CPR on the ICU.

The OTC has been used to maintain a clear airway in patients requiring tracheostomy for elective respiratory management in the ICU [19]. In six patients with varying degrees of respiratory incapacity, the OTC performed satisfactorily in maintaining an adequate airway while tracheostomy was performed. Since the OTC is usually placed in the oesophagus, full tracheostomy could be performed without withdrawal, thus avoiding many of the potential complications associated with withdrawal of a tracheal tube during this procedure [20].

## The OTC in failed and difficult tracheal intubation

There have been a few cases described in which airway management with the OTC has proved to be effective in situations where tracheal intubation had proved to be difficult or impossible.

In a case in which patient's neck and pharynx were impaled with a splinter of wood, preventing laryngoscopy, the OTC was used successfully to ventilate the patient's lungs until an emergency tracheostomy could be performed [21].

A case was described in which a patient with severe rheumatoid arthritis was unable to be intubated with a standard tracheal tube, but in whom a secure airway was maintained with the OTC [22]. There were no complications of the technique, and extubation was performed with the patient awake at the end of the general anaesthetic.

A case of unforeseen difficult tracheal intubation in a patient with respiratory insufficiency has been described [23]. The OTC was correctly positioned in 15 seconds, and the patient was able to be adequately ventilated and oxygenated. An open lung biopsy was performed with the OTC in situ.

Other such cases have been described where the OTC was able to manage successfully situations of failed tracheal intubation [24, 25]. The oesophageal detector device [26] was used to confirm correct oesophageal placement of the OTC on one such occasion [24].

The OTC has also been suggested for elective use in cervical spine injuries, poor access to the head in the prehospital setting, potential subluxation of the atlantoaxial joint, and in patients such as opera singers where tracheal intubation is a relative contraindication.

## The OTC in failed intubation and difficult ventilation

Use of the OTC in cases of failed intubation per se remains controversial [27], but in the 'cannot intubate, cannot ventilate' situation there seems to be a growing consensus that it could be a valuable adjunct. The OTC has been used in situations of acute threat to the airway in which the usual fallback measure of waking the patient and proceeding to a local anaesthetic technique was considered unworkable. Two cases of rapidly developing cervical haematomas have been described in which direct laryngoscopy was not possible and the airway was in immediate danger [28]. Another case was described in which there was massive oropharyngeal haemorrhage in a patient on thrombolytic therapy [29]. On each of these occasions the OTC was used to secure the airway until emergency tracheostomy or tracheal intubation could be performed under controlled circumstances.

Two other cases, one of limited mouth opening and the other of profuse vomiting during intubation, were successfully managed with the OTC [30]. Both cases were emergencies in which tracheal intubation had failed and in which mask ventilation was extremely difficult, resulting in acute hypoxia. Following placement of the OTC, adequate oxygenation was achieved in both cases.

A recent report by the American Society of Anesthesiologists task force on difficult airway management [31] concluded that the OTC should be added to the list of suggested items to be included in a portable kit for the management of difficult airways, with particular reference to its potential use in the 'cannot intubate, cannot ventilate' scenario.

## Precautions and Complications

The Combitube is not recommended for patients under the age of 16 or below 150 cm in height. Patients should ideally not have intact gag reflexes. It should not be used as an airway in patients known to have ingested caustic liquids. Aspiration of tracheal secretions is impossible with the OTC in the oesophageal position, which may be a problem in patients with copious tracheal secretions.

Oesophageal [32–34] and gastric [32, 35, 36] rupture have been described as complications associated with use of the OOA during prehospital CPR. It has been postulated that, in some cases, oesophageal rupture may be caused by stomach contraction against an occluded distal oesophagus [4]. It is believed that the incidence of these potentially fatal complications should be lower with the OTC due to its shorter length; it is not long enough to reach the thoracic oesophagus where the majority of these complications occur. Also, with the OTC in the oesophageal position the tracheal limb is open, preventing large pressure rises in the distal oesophagus. As with the OOA, oesophageal stenosis and other pathology involving the oesophagus should be absolute contraindications to its use.

A radiological study of the position of the OTC

following insertion during CPR [37] confirmed that after blind insertion in all ten patients studied, the OTC was placed in the position intended by the design theory. When the proximal balloon was hyperinflated, the anatomical position was generally unchanged. However, difficulties with ventilation through the OTC following incorrect placement have been reported. Two cases were described [38] in which recommended insertion techniques were employed, but in which ventilation could not be achieved via either limb of the OTC. The upper balloon had occluded the glottis, resulting in total inability to ventilate via either limb (Figs 5 and 6). Both situations were satisfactorily resolved by partial withdrawal of the OTC until breath sounds were heard over the chest.

## Summary

The OTC is an interesting device that has performed satisfactorily in a variety of circumstances, and seems to be a worthy successor to the oesophageal obturator airway. There are many published papers demonstrating that patients ventilated with the OTC have higher arterial oxygen tensions than patients ventilated with tracheal tubes at the same inspired oxygen concentration. There are several cases in which it has proved useful in unexpected cases of difficult intubation where direct laryngoscopy was difficult or impossible. There have also been a few cases described in which situations of difficult ventilation have been successfully managed by using the OTC. It

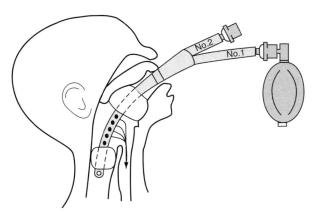

**Figure 5**  Correct position of the Combitube in the oesophagus, allowing passage of gas from the side orifices into the trachea. From Green and Beger [38], with permission.

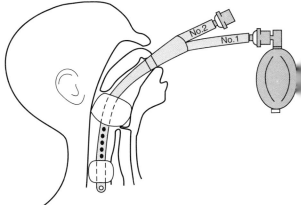

**Figure 6**  Excessive insertion depth of the OTC, causing obstruction of the glottic opening. Ventilation not possible. From Green and Beger [38], with permission.

has been included in the latest ASA guidelines for difficult airway management. It is not yet widely used, so that it is too early to comment on its safety record and potential for complications. However, in theory at least, it should be safer than the oesophageal obturator airway when used under similar circumstances. Its extra lumen enables ventilation to be accomplished even when the tube is placed in the trachea, although no data are yet available to evaluate its function when used in this manner.

## KEY POINTS

- The OTC was initially designed to be used by non-medical personnel during prehospital resuscitation.

- Ventilation may be achieved following either oesophageal or tracheal placement.

- Ventilation with the OTC in the oesophageal position produces higher plasma oxygen tensions than in patients ventilated via tracheal tubes. This is likely to be due to a 'PEEP effect' associated with expiration through small perforations in the oesophageal limb. No data are yet available to assess the ventilation characteristics of the OTC following tracheal placement.

- The OTC has been used during prehospital and hospital CPR. It has been demonstrated to be at least as easy to insert and as effective as a tracheal tube in these situations.

- The OTC has been used to maintain the airway during tracheostomy, and may have significant advantages over the tracheal tube in this circumstance.

- Several cases of failed and difficult intubation have been successfully managed using the OTC, and it may be particularly useful in procedures where the neck cannot or should not be extended and in the 'cannot intubate, cannot ventilate' situation. It has been included in the latest ASA guidelines for difficult airway management.

- The OTC has been used when there has been an acute threat to the airway where direct laryngoscopy has proved to be difficult or impossible. All reported cases were successfully managed.

- Two cases have been reported where ventilation could not be achieved via either the oesophageal or tracheal limb following insertion. They were successfully managed by partial withdrawal of the OTC.

# REFERENCES

1 Shea S. R., MacDonald J. R. and Gruzinski G. Prehospital endotracheal airway or esophageal gastric tube airway: a critical comparison. *Annals of Emergency Medicine* 1985; **14:** 102.

2 Don Michael T. A., Lambert E. H. and Mehran A. Mouth-to-lung airway for cardiac resuscitation. *Lancet* 1968; **ii:** 1329.

3 Don Michael T. A. and Gordon A. S. The oesophageal obturator airway: a new device in emergency cardiopulmonary resuscitation. *British Medical Journal* 1980; **281:** 1531.

4 Don Michael T. A. The esophageal obturator airway: a critique. *Journal of the American Medical Association* 1981; **246:** 1098.

5 Don Michael T. A. Comparison of the esophageal obturator airway and endotracheal intubation in prehospital ventilation. *Chest* 1985; **87:** 814.

6 Auerbach P. and Geehr E. Inadequate oxygenation and ventilation using the EGTA in the prehospital setting. *Journal of the American Medical Association* 1983; **250:** 3067.

7 Hooks P. J., Scarberry E. H. and Bryan-Brown C. W. The pharyngeal tracheal lumen (PTL) airway: a one handed emergency resuscitation tube. *Anesthesia and Analgesia* 1984; **63:** 229.

8 Niemann J. T., Rosborough J. P., Myers R. and Scarberry E. N. The pharyngeo-tracheal lumen airway: preliminary investigation of a new adjunct. *Annals of Emergency Medicine* 1984; **13:** 591.

9 Frass M., Rödler S., Frenzer R., Ilias W., Leithner C. and Lackner F. Esophageal tracheal Combitube, endotracheal airway, and mask: comparison of ventilatory pressure curves. *Journal of Trauma* 1989; **29:** 1476.

10 Frass M., Frenzer R., Ilias W., Lackner F., Hoflehner G. and Losert U. The esophageal tracheal Combitube (ETC): animal experiment results with a new emergency tube. *Anästhesia, Intensivtherapie, Notfallmedzin* 1987; **22:** 142.

11 Frass M., Frenzer R., Zdrahal F., Hoflehner G., Porges P. and Lackner F. The esophageal tracheal Combitube: preliminary results with a new airway for CPR. *Annals of Emergency Medicine* 1987; **16:** 768.

12 Frass M., Frenzer R., Rauscha F., Weber H., Pacher R. and Leithner C. Evaluation of esophageal tracheal Combitube in cardiopulmonary resuscitation. *Critical Care Medicine* 1987; **15:** 609.

13 Frass M., Frenzer R., Rauscha F., Schuster E. and Glogar D. Ventilation with the esophageal tracheal Combitube in cardiopulmonary resuscitation. Promptness and effectiveness. *Chest* 1988; **93:** 781.

14 Mathru M., Venus B., Rao T. L. K. and Matsuda T. Noncardiac pulmonary oedema precipitated by tracheal intubation in patients with inhalation injury. *Critical Care Medicine* 1983; **11:** 804.

15 Staudinger T., Brugger S., Roggla M. *et al.* Comparison of the Combitube with the endotracheal tube in cardiopulmonary resuscitation in the prehospital phase. *Wiener Klinische Wochenschrift* 1994; **106:** 412.

16 Atherton G. Ability of paramedics to use the Combitube in prehospital cardiac arrest. *Annals of Emergency Medicine* 1993; **22:** 1263.

17 Frass M., Frenzer R., Mayer G., Popovic R. and Leithner C. Mechanical ventilation with the esophageal tracheal Combitube (ETC) in the Intensive Care Unit. *Annals of Emergency Medicine* 1987; **4:** 219.

18 Staudinger T., Brugger S., Watschinger B. *et al.* Emergency intubation with the Combitube: comparison with the endotracheal airway. *Annals of Emergency Medicine* 1993; **22:** 1573.

19 Wiltschke C., Kment G., Swoboda H. *et al.* Ventilation with the Combitube during tracheotomy. *Laryngoscope* 1994; **104:** 763.

20 Stock M. C., Woodward C. G., Shapiro B. A., Cane R. D., Lewis V. and Pecaro B. Perioperative complications of elective tracheostomy in critically ill patients. *Critical Care Medicine* 1986; **14:** 861.

21 Eichinger S., Schreiber W., Heint T. *et al.* Airway management in a case of neck impalement: use of the oesophageal tracheal Combitube airway. *British Journal of Anaesthesia* 1992; **68:** 534.

22 Yurino M. Esophageal tracheal Combitube overcomes difficult intubation: flexion deformity of the cervical spine due to rheumatoid arthritis. *Journal of Anaesthesia* 1994; **8:** 233.

23 Frass M., Frenzer R., Zahler J., Ilias W. and Leithner C. Ventilation via the esophageal tracheal Combitube in a case of difficult intubation. *Journal of Cardiothoracic Anaesthesia* 1987; **1:** 565.

24 Baraka A. The Combitube oesophageal– tracheal double lumen airway for difficult intubation. *Canadian Journal of Anaesthesiology* 1993; **40:** 1222.

25 Brugger S. Successful intubation with the Combitube of two patients with bull neck. *Acta Medica Austriaca* 1993; **20:** 78.

26 Williams K. N. and Nunn J. F. The oesophageal detector device. A preoperative trial in 100 patients. *Anaesthesia* 1989; **44:** 412.

27 Brimacombe J. The oesophageal tracheal Combitube for difficult intubation. *Canadian Journal of Anaesthesiology* 1994; **41:** 656.

28 Bigenzhan W., Pesau B. and Frass M. Emergency ventilation using the Combitube in cases of difficult intubation. *European Archives of Oto-rhino-laryngology* 1991; **248:** 129.

29 Klauser R., Röggla G., Pidlich J., Leithner C. and Frass M. Massive upper airway bleeding after thrombolytic therapy: successful airway management with the Combitube. *Annals of Emergency Medicine* 1992; **21:** 431.

30 Staudinger T., Tesinsky P., Klappacher G. *et al.* Emergency intubation with the Combitube in two cases of difficult airway management. *European Journal of Anaesthesiology* 1995; **12:** 189.

31 American Society of Anesthesiologists. Practice guidelines for management of the difficult airway: a report by the American Society of Anesthesiologists task force on management of the difficult airway. *Anesthesiology* 1993; **78:** 597.

32 Johnson K. R., Genovesi M. G. and Lassar K. H. Esophageal obturator airway: use and complications. *Journal of the American Society Emergency Physicians* 1976; **5:** 36.

33 Harrison E. E., Jurger N. H. and Beeman R. N. Esophageal perforation following use of the oesophageal obturator airway. *Annals of Emergency Medicine* 1980; **9:** 21.

34 Strate R. G. and Fischer R. P. Midesophageal perforations by esophageal obturator airways. *Journal of Trauma* 1976; **16:** 503.

35 Crippen D., Olvey S. and Graffis R. Gastric rupture: an esophageal obturator airway complication. *Annals of Emergency Medicine* 1981; **10:** 370.

36 Adler J. and Dykan M. Gastric rupture: an unusual complication of the esophageal obturator airway. *Annals of Emergency Medicine* 1983; **12:** 224.

37 Frass M., Johnson J. C., Atherton G. L. *et al.* Esophageal tracheal Combitube (ETC) for emergency intubation: anatomical evaluation of ETC placement by radiography. *Resuscitation* 1989; **18:** 95.

38 Green K. S. and Beger T. H. Proper use of the Combitube (letter). *Anesthesiology* 1994; **81:** 513.

# 15

# Complications of Tracheal Intubation

*Michael Harmer*

## INTRODUCTION

Tracheal intubation confers many advantages for patient, anaesthetist and surgeon. In most patients, the technique is easily performed and relatively free from serious complications. Nevertheless, both minor and occasionally very serious sequelae occur following laryngoscopy and intubation. Equally important are the undesirable consequences arising from drugs and procedures used for intubation such as the side effects of depolarizing muscle relaxants. Although the incidence of complications is related, as with all procedures, to the experience and expertise of the clinician, it is advisable even in experienced hands to confine tracheal intubation to those instances in which clear cut indications exist.

The undesirable consequences of tracheal intubation can be classified in a number of ways: topographically relating to lesions of lips, teeth or larynx; aetiologically relating to complications such as trauma, reflexes, chemical reactions; but probably the most useful classification for the practising anaesthetist is chronological order with complications being related to laryngoscopy, the act of intubation, the period of intubation, extubation and the post extubation period.

Laryngoscopy and intubation are associated not only with trauma, but also with acute, but transient, physiological disturbances. The possibility of respiratory obstruction and other respiratory accidents and disturbances dominates the period.

Complications while the patient is intubated generally relate to equipment problems or failure.

At extubation, physiological disturbances mirror those found at intubation. Acute respiratory embarrassment may accompany extubation, and this period is again one of great anxiety for the anaesthetist. The details of problems associated with extubation are covered in Chapter 19.

Short-term complications after extubation may be either immediate serious problems related to respiratory exchange or later unpleasant, but less severe, problems such as sore throat and muscle pains. Serious late sequelae result from the progression of pathological changes initiated during intubation and are particularly prevalent following long-term intubation. The complications and sequelae of intubation are presented in Table 1.

## PREDISPOSING FACTORS

### The Patient

#### *Age*

Infants have smaller and more delicate airways than adults so that injury is more likely, especially with an inexperienced operator. It is also easier for malposition [1] and accidental extubation [2] to occur. Infants have a higher incidence of subglottic stenosis following intubation, which is often associated with the use of a tracheal tube of inappropriate size [3]. The development of the palate can be affected by long-term intubation, particularly in the preterm infant [4, 5]. Additionally, sucking efficacy is reduced after oral intubation [6].

Adults, on the other hand, are more prone to develop granulomatous reactions to intubation [7].

Elderly patients have a more easily damaged and less elastic trachea; perforation of the trachea is thus a hazard. The ease of intubation may be influenced by age-related arthritic conditions involving the head and neck. Geriatric patients can suffer a whole range of complications [8].

#### *Sex*

Post intubation sore throat [9], granulomatous lesions [10] and post suxamethonium pains are more common in women. Women have also been shown to be at greater risk than men for malpositioning of tracheal tubes in the emergency situation [11]. The main problem is that the tube lies very close to the carina; presumably a reflection of the shorter trachea in women.

#### *Adverse anatomical features*

Facial or cervical abnormalities as well as short neck, receding chin or obesity make intubation more difficult and are associated with a higher incidence of traumatic complications.

**Table 1** Classification of complications associated with tracheal intubation

**At intubation**
Direct trauma
Fracture and/or subluxation of cervical spine
Haemorrhage
Trauma to the eye
Mediastinal emphysema and pneumothorax
Pharyngeal damage
Aspiration of gastric contents and foreign bodies
Accidental intubation of the oesophagus
Misplacement of the tube

**During intubation**
Obstruction of the airway:
  Outside the tube
  By the tube itself
  Within the tube
Rupture of the trachea and bronchus
Aspiration of stomach contents
Displacement of tube
Ignition of tube

**At extubation**
Difficult or impossible extubation
Tracheal collapse
Airway obstruction
Aspiration of stomach contents

**Following intubation**
*Early* (0–24 h)
Sore throat
Damage to nerves
Glottic oedema:
  Supraglottic
  Retroarytenoid
  Subglottic
Hoarseness and voice changes
Vocal cord paralysis

*Medium* (24–72 h)
Infection

*Late* (72 h +)
Laryngeal ulcer, granuloma and polyp
Synechia of vocal cords
Laryngotracheal membranes and webs
Laryngeal fibrosis
Tracheal stenosis
Stricture of nostril
Mouth and pharyngeal damage
Associated non-airway damage

### *Adverse pathophysiological features*

Upper airway infection may produce difficulty with intubation. Uncomplicated pregnancy can lead to oedema in the upper airway [12], and this may become more serious if the mother has pregnancy-induced hypertension.

## The Operation or Procedure

### Surgery of the neck

Neck surgery is responsible for most cases of laryngeal nerve damage with consequent postoperative hoarseness or respiratory obstruction [13].

### Duration of intubation

There is a direct correlation between the duration of intubation and the extent of laryngotracheal complications. The maximum duration of safe tracheal intubation is not known and many variables are involved (age, tube calibre, underlying pathology). However, the incidence of long-term serious damage increases dramatically after 7 days of intubation [14].

### Route of intubation

Nasal intubation is associated with a higher incidence of injury compared with the oral route; most problems relate to epistaxis [15] although acute airway obstruction may occur from dislodged adenoidal tissue, nasal polyps or inferior turbinate [16]. Intubation by the nasal route is also often associated with paranasal sinusitis [17, 18], which can lead to an unrecognized source of infection in the intubated patient.

## Apparatus

### Size of tube

Placing a tube with an excessively large external diameter in the trachea is associated with a higher incidence of postoperative sore throat, laryngeal damage and tracheal stenosis. This is particularly so in children [3].

### Cuff pressure

A high cuff pressure is a major factor in the occurrence of tracheal wall complications, although the cuff pressure must be sufficient to prevent aspiration. For further details of cuff design and effects see Chapter 3.

### Excessive movement

Allowing excessive movement of the tracheal tube on the vocal cords and tracheal wall increases the risk of sequelae [14]. This is true during both spontaneous and controlled ventilation.

### Tube material

Plastic tubes are preferred to red rubber for both short and long-term intubation; to a large degree the plastic tube has virtually replaced the red rubber tube in routine practice. However, additives used in the manufacture of plastic tubes may act as irritants and produce tissue damage [19]. Vocal cord paralysis has been associated with tubes sterilized with ethylene oxide [20].

### Stylet

This accessory can be useful but a rigid-tipped stylet (including the 'lighted' variety) protruding through the bevel of the tracheal tube is a serious hazard to the larynx [21] and tracheal wall [22].

## COMPLICATIONS AT INTUBATION

### Direct Trauma

Laryngoscopy and intubation inevitably produce an incidence of trauma that depends on the skill of the operator and the difficulties encountered during intubation. These injuries include bruised or lacerated lips and tongue, chipped or inadvertent extraction of teeth, lacerations of the pharynx, submucosal haemorrhage and tears of the vocal cords. With nasal intubation, it is more difficult to avoid trauma and epistaxis is easily produced unless preliminary local application of cocaine or phenylephrine is used to shrink the mucosa. Such damage can be reduced by the use of a 'bubble-tip' to guide the tube [23]. In addition to haemorrhage, dislodgement of nasal polypi has been reported [24].

The incidence and nature of laryngeal trauma after intubation was investigated in 1000 patients by Kambic and Radsel [25]. Laryngoscopy was performed immediately after extubation and revealed a 6.2% incidence of injuries. Haematoma of the vocal cord was the most common (4.5%), while haematoma of the supraglottic region occurred in 0.7% of patients. Injury to the left vocal cord predominated. Haematoma occurred more commonly in patients suffering from allergic laryngitis with local oedema or when the cords were not fully relaxed at intubation, or if intubation was not carefully performed. Laceration of the mucosa of the vocal cord occurred in 0.8% while there was only one case (0.1%) each of deeper laceration of the vocal cord including muscle, and of subluxation of the arytenoid. Most patients suffered no long-term serious disability. A similar pattern of injuries has been confirmed [26] but recovery was generally prompt with conservative management. Dislocation of the arytenoid cartilage (Fig. 1) is an increasingly recognized complication of intubation leading to postoperative hoarseness [21, 27, 28].

Injuries of the laryngeal muscles and suspensory ligaments have been described [29]. They follow severe flexion of the head during intubation when distortion of the whole larynx occurs. If movement of the cricothyroid muscle is affected, serious impairment in singing ability may result.

Injury to teeth upsets the patient and can result in litigation against the anaesthetist. Wright and Manfield [30], officers of a medical defence organization, reported that injuries to teeth most commonly occurred during laryngoscopy for tracheal intubation. The use of an oropharyngeal airway and incorrect use of mouth openers, props and gags also contributed. The incidence of dental complications of tracheal intubation has been quoted as 1 in 1000 [31]. Others have quoted a much higher incidence, depending upon the type of laryngoscope used (Fig. 2) [32]. The risk of injury is greatly increased in the presence of dental disease, crowns, bridges or heavily restored teeth, and in the very young and the elderly. In the young, both deciduous teeth and the permanent teeth (at first) have little support; avoiding damage to the permanent incisors between 5 and 9 years of age is therefore important. With increasing age, teeth become more brittle and are more easily damaged. If a tooth, or part thereof, is lost, its whereabouts must be ascertained by radiology. If it is in the respiratory tract it must be removed. Persisting with instrumentation in difficult cases is more likely to lead to damage.

## Fracture and/or Subluxation of the Cervical Spine

Careless movement of the head may produce serious lesions such as fracture luxation of the cervical spine with spinal cord compression or section [7]. This problem is more likely in the vulnerable

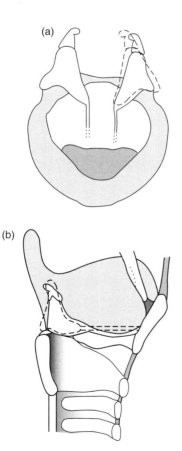

**Figure 1** Anterior and sagittal views of the larynx showing the appearance of a dislocated arytenoid cartilage (solid line) as opposed to the normal position (dotted line). From Szigeti *et al.* [21], with permission.

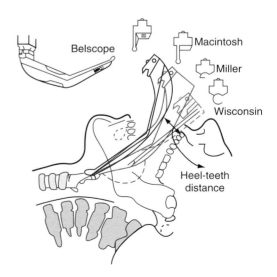

**Figure 2** The distance between the teeth and the blade for different laryngoscopes. From Watanabe *et al.* [32], with permission.

patient whose muscle tone has been abolished by curarizing drugs. Potential cervical cord damage must be particularly borne in mind in patients with existing fractures of the cervical spine, congenital weaknesses or malformations of the cervical spine (Morquio's syndrome), the elderly and those with pathological fragility of the cervical spine (connective tissue disorders, lytic bone tumours and osteoporosis). The act of intubation can be particularly fraught with danger in patients with an acutely injured spine where cervical stabilization must be maintained during intubation [33]. In these circumstances it is advisable to have the head held in a safe position by a colleague during intubation (see Chapter 18).

## Haemorrhage

Minor haemorrhage is common following intubation by the nasal route. This may be reduced in severity by spraying cocaine or phenylephrine in the nose before intubation. Extensive haemorrhage requiring repeated blood transfusion has been reported due to dislocation of the middle turbinate along with a mucosal flap [34]. In addition, laceration to the nasal canal has been caused by the use of aluminium foil wrapped around a tube inserted for laser surgery to the larynx [35].

## Trauma to the Eye

Trauma to the eye may be caused by inadvertently rubbing the cornea with the operator's hand or the catheter mount attached to a tracheal tube. During head and neck surgery, the eyelids should be held closed by tape and the eyes should be covered carefully with soft eyepads to prevent corneal damage by the surgeon or from surrounding sterile covers. Minor corneal abrasions, although painful, usually heal well.

Great care should be taken in patients with penetrating eye injuries not to aggravate the condition by traumatic intubation or the use of depolarizing muscle relaxants. The pathophysiological effects of intubation on the eye are discussed in Chapter 2.

## Mediastinal Emphysema and Pneumothorax

Tearing of the mucosa lining the pyriform fossae may lead to surgical emphysema of the neck and mediastinum when the lungs are inflated before intubation [36, 37]. This injury normally occurs in a patient who is difficult to intubate and several attempts are required to position the tracheal tube. Although this complication usually settles following intubation, it can lead to the development of a tension pneumothorax. It can also cause a persistent fistula and subsequent abscess formation [36]. Although not strictly an intubation problem, in patients with poor lung compliance or with emphysema it is possible to rupture an alveolus, which may lead to pneumothorax [38], subcutaneous emphysema [39], pneumoperitoneum [40] and even a pneumoscrotum [41]!

## Pharyngeal Damage

Nasal intubation may lead to damage and perforation of the nasopharyngeal mucosa with the creation of a false passage. Such injury, in addition to causing haemorrhage, may lead to the formation of a retropharyngeal abscess or mediastinitis. A classical case of retropharyngeal abscess has also been reported [42] that developed one week after a difficult oral intubation using a stylet. Perforation of the pharynx and upper oesophagus have also been described [43, 44].

## Aspiration of Gastric Contents and Foreign Bodies

The risk of aspiration of stomach contents is particularly high in patients with a full stomach, poorly functioning cardiac sphincter or loss of protective reflexes. The pregnant mother is the patient most often requiring the administration of a general anaesthetic with these predisposing factors. Deaths from aspiration of stomach contents during general anaesthesia have been a constant finding in past *Confidential Reports into Maternal Mortality*. Furthermore, a large proportion of the reported cases of aspiration have been associated with difficulty in intubation. It is essential that all anaesthetists have a plan of management for failed intubation in obstetrics. This topic is covered in detail in Chapter 16.

Other patients at risk are those with acute intestinal obstruction. The mainstays of prevention remain the recognition of the risk, preoperative drainage of the full stomach and the use of a smooth rapid sequence induction technique with cricoid pressure applied bimanually.

In addition to stomach contents, the aspiration

of foreign bodies such as teeth and dentures, parts of laryngoscopes [45], and parts of intubation equipment [46, 47] have been reported. If it is suspected that such an item has been inhaled the patient must have a chest radiograph and, if necessary, endoscopic removal of the foreign body.

## Accidental Intubation of the Oesophagus

An anaesthetist may accidentally insert a tracheal tube into the oesophagus. It is obvious that this error must be recognized rapidly and corrected. However, there are reports of accidental oesophageal intubation, even in experienced hands, in which the mistake has remained undetected. This topic is discussed in detail in Chapter 11. The respiratory consequences of accidental intubation of the oesophagus are of paramount importance, but other complications may also result. Excessive distension of the stomach follows vigorous manual inflation while testing for correct placement of the tube. Severe gastric distension can be readily relieved by the passage of a gastric tube. If the cardio-oesophageal sphincter is closed while inflation continues through a tube placed in the oesophagus, gross distension of the oesophagus is a potential hazard. A rare but very serious complication that can be associated with tracheal intubation is rupture of the oesophagus [48].

## Misplacement of the Tube

The most common site for tube misplacement is in a main bronchus, usually the right, although left main bronchus misplacement has been reported [49, 50]. This easily happens if the tube is too long and advanced to its whole length rather than positioned so that the cuff is just through the vocal cords; the use of specific guide marks has been recommended to prevent this complication [51]. If recognized and the tube is resited correctly, there is usually little damage, save a short period of moderate desaturation. The incidence of bronchial intubation seems more common in the emergency situation [52]. Tubes have been misplaced in less obvious sites. One such instance followed attempted nasal intubation in a patient with severe fractures of the face and base of skull where the tube tracted intracranially [53]. Similarly, pneumocephalus has been reported following nasal intubation [54]. However, there is

evidence that nasal intubation does not in itself compound problems associated with a fractured base of the skull [55, 56].

## COMPLICATIONS DURING INTUBATION

### Obstruction of the Airway

Obstruction of the airway must be the most serious complication of tracheal intubation that can occur once the tube has been correctly placed. The possible causes are numerous but can be divided into those circumstances where the tube may be compressed from outside, the tube itself may result in obstruction, or the lumen of the tube can become obstructed.

### *Obstruction from outside the tube*

Biting on the tube by the patient just before extubation is not an uncommon occurrence but inadequate anaesthesia during maintenance may also cause biting. This has been reported even with a wire reinforced tube, which remained pinched when the bite was released [57]. This problem can be prevented either by maintaining an adequate depth of anaesthesia or by the use of an oropharyngeal airway to act as a 'bite-block'.

The distal end of the tracheal tube may become obstructed by abutting against the tracheal wall. The siting of a hole in the tube wall near the tip (a Murphy's eye) helps to prevent this problem. An unusual example of this complication involved the use of an Endotrol tube, which has a tip that can be adjusted by a pull-cord. When such a tube was inserted nasally the loop on the pull-cord abutted against the nares, causing the tip of the tube to bend and obstruct against the tracheal wall. The problem was solved by cutting the pull-cord [58]. Cases have been reported of obstruction of the tracheal tube secondary to intratracheal swellings or displacement [59, 60].

### *Obstruction by the tube*

Kinking of the tube, once a common occurrence with the use of recycled rubber tubes that became old and weakened, is now unusual unless the tube is carelessly inserted so as to cause acute angulation. This can occur when a tube is inserted from the right side of the mouth and transferred to the left side without ensuring that the entire tube has been moved to the left of the tongue. Kinking can also occur if preformed tracheal tubes are not inserted to their full length. If such a tube seems too long, it is best replaced with a different size or type. Armoured latex tubes offer a degree of protection against kinking but this may still occur between the proximal termination of the spiral reinforcement and the non-reinforced section into which the connector is placed. In any type of tube, the cuff may herniate over the distal orifice of the tube causing airway obstruction [61, 62]. This is a well-known hazard. In addition, cuff herniation may occur internally and may not be so obvious when the tube is tested before use [63]. Rare causes of obstruction have been noted due to manufacturing defects in latex armoured tracheal tubes [64, 65].

## Obstruction within the tube

Complete or partial blockage can result from blood clot, tissue [66], dried secretions [67], dried tube lubricants [68], loosened parts of a faulty manufactured tube [69] and foreign bodies (including such unlikely articles as insects and cigarette tips). Acute obstruction of the tube has been reported after aluminium foil covering a tube during carbon dioxide laser surgery broke loose [70] and, in another case, by a nasal turbinate [71].

Another recent report [72] has highlighted the potential hazard of oral premedication where a tablet caused blockage of the tracheal tube.

Airway obstructions may be partial or complete. The signs of tube obstruction are a high inflation pressure and absent or impaired chest excursion. In spontaneously breathing patients, there may be marked inspiratory and expiratory efforts with paradoxical movements, accompanied by cyanosis and venous congestion. Lesser degrees of obstruction may go unnoticed.

If airway obstruction is noticed in the intubated patient:

• Check by direct observation and with a finger in the mouth that there is no kinking of the tube.
• Check the patency of the tube by passing a suction catheter down throughout its length.
• If still in any doubt, change the tube.

## Rupture of Trachea or Bronchus

Rupture of the trachea or a main bronchus is a very rare, but very serious, complication of tra-cheal intubation. Rupture is usually reported in the posterior membranous portion that is unsupported by cartilaginous bands. The membranous portion is more fragile and less elastic in infants, the elderly and in patients suffering from chronic obstructive airway disease [73].

This complication can usually be traced back to a faulty or careless intubation technique. The following factors have been implicated:

• sharply bevelled tubes or sharp-tipped stylets protruding beyond the end of the tube;
• the use of excessive force or repeated attempts at intubation [73];
• overinflation of the cuff [74, 75].

The onset of signs of this complication may be delayed some hours, particularly if the distending force of an overinflated cuff is responsible for airway rupture. Bronchial rupture has been reported in the absence of any trauma or gross airway disease [76]. In one of the few case reports of this complication in neonates, delayed appearance of surgical emphysema resulted in a missed diagnosis and death [77]; more rapid recognition produced a favourable result in another neonate [78]. Particular care is warranted if intubation is to be performed on a patient who has previously undergone pneumonectomy [79]. The use of a guide during the change of a tube has also been reported as the cause of bronchial rupture [22].

The clinical diagnosis may be confirmed by a chest radiograph. Prompt endoscopy should reveal the tracheal or bronchial tear. Conservative management may suffice but chest drainage and open surgical correction may prove necessary [76].

## Aspiration of Stomach Contents

Silent regurgitation occurs in an appreciable proportion of intubated patients [80] and leakage past the cuff may occur particularly during prolonged intubation.

## Displacement of the Tube

The tracheal tube may be displaced downwards into one or other main bronchus or upwards into the hypopharynx. Displacement most commonly occurs when there is movement of the head and neck to accommodate the surgical requirements, although this movement is seldom excessive [51].

Therefore, particular care should be taken in securing tracheal tubes for head and neck surgery.

## Ignition of the Tube

Explosions and fires during anaesthesia have become rare since the diminished use of flammable anaesthetics, although a fire has recently been reported during an electrodissection tonsillectomy [81]. Since the 1970s, the carbon dioxide laser has become increasingly used for laryngeal surgery. The surgical laser may cause ignition of a tracheal tube, whether made of rubber or plastic, leading to serious burns of the airways. There have been several reports of fires being caused in this way [82]. In addition, it is possible for a fire to be started from flaming tissues that are being treated [83].

Several methods have been suggested to avoid this bizarre complication. A ventilating laryngoscope eliminates the need for a tracheal tube [84] but its use is not always convenient or possible. The tube can be wrapped with moistened muslin or with aluminium foil tape [70]. Alternatively, it can be protected by coating the exterior with dental acrylic [85]. However, these precautions have also led to complications; detachment of aluminium foil can lead to airway obstruction [70] and severe epistaxis can result from damage by a sharp edge of a foil cover [35]. A flexible jointed metal tracheal tube has been produced [86, 87], as have non-flammable plastic tubes [82].

Should a fire occur while using a laser, the damage to the patient will be influenced by the material from which the tube is made; PVC tubes cause more damage and red rubber appears to cause less [88]. The use of positive end expiratory pressure (PEEP) seems to lower the risk of laser-induced fires [89].

The problems associated with extubation are dealt with in Chapter 19.

## COMPLICATIONS FOLLOWING INTUBATION

### Early (0–24 h)

#### Sore throat

This is a common and reasonably benign sequel of tracheal intubation, whose incidence has been reported to vary between 6% [90] and 90% [91]. However, it may not be entirely due to intubation,

as Conway [92] reported an incidence of 10.2% in patients who had not even been intubated. The use of lubricant on the tube had no effect on the incidence of sore throat [93]. The type of tube and the intracuff pressure would be expected to be important factors [94, 95], but research has shown no correlations with incidence of sore throat [96]. The use of a pharyngeal pack after nasotracheal intubation is a clear cause of postoperative sore throat [97]. Symptomatic treatment is usually all that is necessary.

### Damage to nerves

Damage to the hypoglossal nerve may be due to pressure from a Macintosh laryngoscope blade in the vallecula region behind the tongue. Lingual nerve damage may occur and is more common on the right side [98], although bilateral injury has been reported [99]; recovery usually occurs over a few months. Neuropraxia of the internal branch of the superior laryngeal nerve can lead to anaesthesia of the upper surface of the larynx and subsequent risk of aspiration [100]. Difficult intubation has also lead to damage of the terminal branches of the trigeminal nerve [101].

### Glottic oedema

Children are the most frequently afflicted by this complication [7]. The oedema may occur in the supraglottic, retroarytenoid or subglottic regions.

#### Supraglottic oedema

Oedema commonly occurs in the loose areolar connective tissue on the anterior surface of the epiglottis and aryepiglottic folds. The epiglottis may be squeezed back by the swelling, blocking the glottic aperture on inspiration and hence causing severe respiratory obstruction.

#### Retroarytenoid oedema

The submucous connective tissue on the vocal cords is dense and therefore not prone to development of oedema, but this may occur in the loose connective tissue just below the cords and behind the arytenoid cartilages. The swelling can limit abduction of the vocal cords on inspiration.

#### Subglottic oedema

This is most serious and frequently requires urgent reintubation or tracheostomy, especially in infants and children. The degree of severity in the young is due to the small internal cross-sectional area of the larynx of the newborn which is no greater than 14 mm$^2$. A 1 mm thick layer of oedema in the subglottis reduces the opening to 5 mm$^2$ (35.7% of normal) and expansion outwards is limited by the cricoid cartilage encircling the subglottic region [7]. Moreover, the subglottic region has fragile respiratory epithelium with loose submucosal connective tissue that is easily traumatized and prone to oedema.

Glottic oedema persisting beyond 24 h is often associated with more serious permanent lesions.

### Hoarseness and voice changes

Hoarseness is quite common after tracheal intubation (32%) but is usually of short duration [102]. The cause of this hoarseness has been attributed to vocal fold trauma but it is more probable that the voice changes are multifactorial in origin [103]. Voice changes are less common if a laryngeal mask airway is used in place of a tracheal tube [104]. If sophisticated acoustic measurements are used, the incidence of hoarseness may be higher than that appreciated clinically [105]. The measured changes usually return to normal in a matter of days.

### Vocal cord paralysis

Vocal cord paralysis following tracheal intubation is not a common finding. One or both cords may be paralysed, usually following head and neck surgery where direct or indirect injury to the recurrent laryngeal nerves has occurred. For instance, 19 of 25 cases followed thyroidectomy [13]. However, vocal cord paralysis has occurred unexpectedly after abdominal and other non-head and neck surgery [106–8]. The proposed cause is compression of the recurrent laryngeal nerve between the inflated tracheal tube cuff and the overlying thyroid cartilage [109].

Unilateral vocal cord paralysis is the more benign condition. Clinical features are limited to hoarseness, usually immediately postoperatively or soon after. Apparent recovery takes place within a few weeks although laryngoscopy has, in some of these cases, revealed that partial unilateral cord paralysis of some degree persists, with compensation by the other vocal cord [107].

Bilateral vocal cord paralysis causes signs of increasing upper airway obstruction that may follow immediately after extubation or be delayed for some hours. The patient has increasing difficulty particularly in vocalizing the letter 'E'. Auscultation over the larynx reveals inspiratory and expiratory vibrations [110]. As the respiratory obstruction progresses, stridor appears together with paradoxical respiration and eventually complete airway obstruction supervenes. The usual methods of relieving respiratory obstruction (extension of the neck, insertion of an oropharyngeal airway or manual protraction of the jaw) do not help. The administration of a steroid, such as dexamethasone, is also ineffective. Obstruction may be relieved by positive pressure ventilation through a facemask. However, the condition is immediately eliminated by reinsertion of a tracheal tube. Laryngoscopy reveals motionless vocal cords which lie adducted with a very narrow glottic chink (2–3 mm). Most cases of bilateral vocal cord paralysis recover but may take up to 34–36 days. Tracheostomy is often required to tide the patient over this period.

## Medium (24–72 h)

### Infection

Infection may occur at any point along the route of the tube. This may be minor and little more than an inconvenience to the patient, or may lead to the development of life-threatening abscess formation. Most severe infections, such as retropharyngeal abscess, follow a difficult intubation with mucosal damage. It is known that nasotracheal intubation can be followed by sinusitis [17, 18]. Infection with the herpes simplex virus has also been associated with tracheal intubation [111].

The treatment of infections following intubation ranges from management of local problems by the use of mouthwashes to the use of parenteral antibiotic therapy.

## Late (72 h+)

### Laryngeal ulcer, granuloma and polyp

Clausen [112] first reported a polypoid growth of granulation tissue on the vocal cord after tracheal intubation. The incidence is low, from about 1:10 000–20 000 [113]. Females are usually affected (80–90%) and the condition is extremely rare in children [114].

Granulomata related to tracheal intubation most commonly lie on the posterior third of the posterior process of the arytenoid cartilages [115] and least commonly on the anterior and middle thirds of the vocal process. Less than half the lesions are bilateral. The aetiology of granulomata is almost certainly due to trauma to a vocal cord. Injury may also result from pressure of the tube when the head and neck are excessively flexed or extended (Fig. 3). This may explain the high incidence of granuloma following surgery of the head and neck [113] or thyroidectomy [116]. Excessive movement of the tube in the larynx or of the larynx against the tube and allergic reaction to the lubricant are also possible contributing factors.

The development of a granuloma does not seem to be related to the type of tube, the route of intubation, or the duration of the intubation [10].

The initial damage is ulceration which usually heals, but if there is excessive granulation tissue then a small granulomatous nodule forms, sessile at first and then pedunculated. Rarely, a pedunculated granuloma can cause acute airway obstruction [115].

Granuloma should be suspected if a patient complains of persistent hoarseness more than 1 week postoperatively. Other symptoms include fullness or discomfort in the throat, the feeling of the presence of a foreign body or even pain radiating to the ear.

Although granulomata occur in spite of prophylactic measures, the avoidance of intubation trauma, excessively large tube, extreme positions of the head and neck and excessive movements during intubation would all seem to be worthwhile preventative measures.

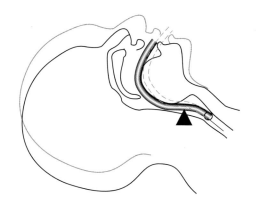

**Figure 3**   The movement of the tracheal tube in the larynx and trachea induced by movement of the head and neck. From Whited [14], with permission.

Treatment is usually by surgical excision or laser ablation, though reoccurrence often happens [117]. There have been reports of successful treatment with low-dose radiotherapy [118].

### Synechia of vocal cords

The posterior third of the vocal cords may stick and fuse together following necrosis of the free edges of the vocal cords. The same may occur with the arytenoid vocal processes, leading to a glottic bar [119]. Clinically, there is aphonia and respiratory obstruction; with early diagnosis, surgical correction is satisfactory [120].

### Laryngotracheal membranes and webs

Laryngeal and subglottic webs were found by Stein in three out of 42 postmortems performed on previously intubated patients [7]. The membrane formed may be extensive and occupy some two-thirds of the glottic opening. These sequelae are particularly dangerous as a portion of the membrane may become detached, leading to sudden respiratory obstruction. Surgical removal of webs can be difficult, as they become covered by laryngotracheal mucosa and form a continuous sheet.

### Laryngeal fibrosis

This is the gravest of the postintubation sequelae since surgical correction is limited. Fibrous tissue formation leads to ankylosis of the cricoarytenoid joints, laryngeal stenosis and hence narrowing of the subglottic region. The result is always respiratory obstruction [121]. Symptoms come late (45–60 days post extubation) and children are more susceptible than adults [120].

### Tracheal stenosis

A minor area of mucosal insult as a result of excessive cuff pressure or tube tip erosion may be followed by spontaneous resolution, or a devastating sequence of events may produce necrosis [122], tracheomalacia or even tracheo-oesophageal fistula [123]. The reported incidence of tracheal stenosis following long-term intubation varies from 1% [124] to 19% where patients were studied with tomography [33].

A number of factors act alone or together to influence the frequency and severity. These include size of tube relative to the size of the trachea, duration of intubation, shape and composition of the tube and cuff, chemical irritants used in cleaning reusable tubes, movement of the tube in the trachea, inflation pressure of the cuff, and intubation trauma. In addition, patient factors such as infection, diabetes, anaemia and hypotension may influence the vulnerability of the mucosa [121].

In severe cases it may be necessary to resect the affected portion of the trachea [125], although this procedure may lead to stitch granuloma formation, especially if non-absorbable suture material is used [126]. This may lead to further stenosis. More recently, the use of self expandable stents has been described [127]. Corticosteroids have also been used with some effect [128].

Further details concerning the cuff and its effect on the trachea may be found in Chapter 3.

### Stricture of nostril

Long-term nasal intubation may lead to damage to the alar rim which is followed by fibrosis and stricture formation. In the extreme case, this can result in a nasal adhesion [129]. Stricture of the nostril may cause airway problems in small children. In addition, necrosis can occur to the nasal septum leading to fistula formation.

### Mouth and pharyngeal damage

Uvula necrosis of unknown origin may cause sore throat and a sensation of foreign body presence some days after intubation [130].

Prolonged orotracheal intubation or tracheostomy may lead to disorders in swallowing [131]; these disorders improve with time and are of uncertain importance.

Long-term changes to the shape of the mouth have been reported in young children who have been intubated, particularly as a neonate [132]. The changes are often a high palate and altered midfacial development. The palatal grooving associated with intubation can be prevented by the use of an intraoral prosthetic appliance [133].

### Other complications

The most serious complications that do not directly affect the airway relate to erosion of blood vessels secondary to prolonged tracheal intubation. Such dramatic, and usually fatal, complications may be associated with other therapy such as chemotherapy for lymphoma [134], or occur after major neck surgery [135], or may be just as a consequence of tracheal intubation [136].

## CONCLUSION

The process of tracheal intubation represents a minefield into which the unwary may wander with potentially disastrous results for the patient. The majority of complications associated with tracheal intubation are minor and self limiting (though a sore throat and hoarseness may be considered as important by the patient!). Other complications can be more serious and on occasion even fatal, either immediately or in the long term. The importance of careful, non-forceful instrumentation and a keen awareness of the possibility of airway damage will go a long way towards the prevention of serious complications.

---

# KEY POINTS

- Minor complications such as sore throat or hoarseness are quite common.

- Most complications are related to forceful attempts at intubation.

- Beware of intubating stylets and other instruments that may protrude from the tip of the tube.

- Haemorrhage from the nose can be reduced by the use of a vasoconstrictor.

- Complications during intubation are almost entirely related to changes in the patency of the tracheal tube.

- Sudden, unexpected appearance of a pneumothorax, or even a pneumoperitoneum, may have resulted from a difficult and traumatic intubation.

- Excessive tube movement may predispose to long-term laryngeal or tracheal damage.

# REFERENCES

1 Black A. E. and Mackersie A. M. Accidental bronchial intubation with RAE tubes. *Anaesthesia* 1991; **46:** 42.

2 Rivera R. and Tibballs J. Complications of endotracheal intubation and mechanical ventilation in infants and children. *Critical Care Medicine* 1992; **20:** 193.

3 Sherman J. M. and Nelson H. Decreased incidence of subglottic stenosis using 'appropriate-sized' endotracheal tube in neonates. *Pediatric Pulmonology* 1989; **6:** 183.

4 Ash S. P. and Moss J. P. An investigation of the features of the pre-term infant palate and the effect of prolonged orotracheal intubation with and without protective appliances. *British Journal of Orthodontics* 1987; **14:** 253.

5 Molteni R. A. and Bumstead D. H. Development and severity of palatal grooves in orally intubated newborns. *American Journal of Diseases of Children* 1986; **140:** 357.

6 Bier J. A., Ferguson A., Cho C., Oh W. and Vohr B. R. The oral motor development of low-birth-weight infants who underwent orotracheal intubation during the neonatal period. *American Journal of Diseases of Children* 1993; **147:** 858.

7 Blanc V. F. and Tremblay N. A. G. The complications of tracheal intubation. A new classification with a review of the literature. *Anesthesia and Analgesia* 1974; **53:** 202.

8 Weymuller E. A. Jr and Bishop M. J. Problems associated with prolonged intubation in the geriatric patient. *Otolaryngology Clinics of America* 1990; **23:** 1057.

9 Wolfson B. Minor laryngeal sequelae from endotracheal intubation. *British Journal of Anaesthesia* 1958; **30:** 326.

10 Howland W. S. and Lewis J. S. Post intubation granulomas of the larynx. *Cancer* 1965; **9:** 1244.

11 Schwarz D. E., Lieberman J. A. and Cohen N. H. Women are at greater risk than men for malpositioning of the endotracheal tube after emergent intubation. *Critical Care Medicine* 1994; **22:** 1127.

12 Mackenzie A. I. Laryngeal oedema complicating obstetric anaesthesia. *Anaesthesia* 1978; **33:** 271.

13 Gorman J. B. and Woodward F. D. Bilateral paralysis of the vocal cords. *Southern Medical Journal* 1965; **58:** 34.

14 Whited R. E. A prospective study of laryngotracheal sequelae in long-term intubation. *Laryngoscope* 1984; **94:** 367.

15 O'Hanlon J. and Harper K. W. Epistaxis and nasotracheal intubation – prevention with vasoconstrictor spray. *Irish Journal of Medical Science* 1994; **163:** 58.

16 Ripley J. F., McAnear J. T and Tilson H. B. Endotracheal tube obstruction due to impaction of the inferior turbinate. *Journal of Oral and Maxillofacial Surgery* 1984; **42:** 687.

17 Deutschman C. S., Wilton P., Sinow J., Dibbell D. Jr, Konstantinides F. N. and Cerra F. B. Paranasal sinusitis associated with nasotracheal intubation: a frequently unrecognized and treatable source of sepsis. *Critical Care Medicine* 1986; **14:** 111.

18 Pedersen J., Schurizek B. A., Melsen N. C. and Juhl B. The effect of nasotracheal intubation on the paranasal sinuses. A prospective study of 434 intensive care patients. *Acta Anaesthesiologica Scandinavica* 1991; **35:** 11.

19 Stetson J. B. and Guess W. L. Causes of damage to tissues by polymers and elastomers used in the fabrication of tracheal devices. *Anesthesiology* 1970; **33:** 635.

20 Jones G. O. M., Hale D. E., Wasmuth C. E., Homi J., Smith E. R. and Biljoen J. A survey of acute complications associated with endotracheal intubation. *Cleveland Clinical Quarterly* 1968; **35:** 23.

21 Szigeti C. L., Baeuerle J. J. and Mongan P. D. Arytenoid dislocation with lighted stylet intubation: case report and retrospective review. *Anesthesia and Analgesia* 1994; **78:** 185.

22 Seitz P. A. and Gravenstein N. Endobronchial rupture from endotracheal reintubation with an endotracheal tube guide. *Journal of Clinical Anesthesiology* 1989; **1:** 214.

23 Watanabe S., Yaguchi Y., Suga A. and Asakura N. A 'bubble-tip' (Airguide) tracheal tube system: its effect on incidence of epistaxis and ease of tube advancement in the subglottic region during nasotracheal intubation. *Anesthesia and Analgesia* 1994; **78:** 1140.

24 Binning R. A hazard of blind nasal intubation. *Anaesthesia* 1974; **29:** 366.

25 Kambic V. and Radsel Z. Intubation lesions of larynx. *British Journal of Anaesthesia* 1978; **50:** 587.

26 Peppard S. B. and Dickens J. H. Laryngeal injury following short-term intubation. *Annals Otology Rhinology and Laryngology* 1983; **92:** 327.

27 Castella X., Gilabert J. and Perez C. Arytenoid dislocation after tracheal intubation: an unusual cause of acute respiratory failure? *Anesthesiology* 1991; **74:** 613.

28 Tolley N. S., Cheesman T. D., Morgan D. and Brookes G. B. Dislocated arytenoid: an intubation-induced injury. *Annals of the Royal College of Surgeons of England* 1990; **72:** 353.

29 Paparella M. M. and Shumrick D. A. *Otolaryngology*. Philadelphia: W. B. Saunders. 1973; vol. 13.

30 Wright R. B. and Manfield F. F. Damage to teeth during the administration of general anaesthesia. *Anesthesia and Analgesia* 1974; **53:** 405.

31  Lockhart P. B., Feldbau E. V., Gabel R. A., Connolly S. F. and Silversin J. B. Dental complications during and after tracheal intubation. *Journal of the American Dental Association* 1986; **112**: 480.

32  Watanabe S., Suga A., Asakura N. *et al.* Determination of the distance between the laryngoscope blade and the upper incisors during direct laryngoscopy: comparisons of a curved, and angulated straight, and two straight blades. *Anesthesia and Analgesia* 1994; **79**: 638.

33  Stauffer J. L., Olson D. E. and Petty T. L. Complications and consequences of endotracheal intubation and tracheostomy: a prospective study of 150 critically ill adult patients. *American Journal of Medicine* 1981; **70**: 65.

34  Scamman F. L. and Babin R. W. An unusual complication of nasotracheal intubation. *Anesthesiology* 1983; **59**: 352.

35  Brightwell A. P. A complication of the use of the laser in ENT surgery. *Journal of Laryngology and Otology* 1983; **97**: 671.

36  Wengen D. F. Pyriform fossa perforation during attempted tracheal intubation. *Anaesthesia* 1987; **42**: 519.

37  Lee T. S. and Jordan J. S. Pyriform sinus perforation secondary to traumatic intubation in a difficult airway patient. *Journal of Clinical Anesthesiology* 1994; **6**: 152.

38  Biswas C., Jana N. and Maitra S. Bilateral pneumothorax following tracheal intubation. *British Journal of Anaesthesia* 1989; **62**: 338.

39  Tan C. S., Tashkin D. P. and Sassoon H. Pneumothorax and subcutaneous emphysema complicating endotracheal intubation. *Southern Medical Journal* 1984; **77**: 253.

40  Ballester E. E., Torres A., Rodriguez-Roisin R. and Agusti-Vidal A. Pneumoperitoneum: an unusual manifestation of improper oral intubation. *Critical Care Medicine* 1985; **13**: 138.

41  Redman J. F. and Pahls W. L. Pneumoscrotum following tracheal intubation. *Journal of Urology* 1985; **133**: 1056.

42  Majumdar B., Stevens R. W. and Obara L. G. Retropharyngeal abscess following tracheal intubation. *Anaesthesia* 1982; **37**: 67.

43  Kras J. F. and Marchmont-Robinson H. Pharyngeal perforation during intubation in a patient with Crohn's disease. *Journal of Oral and Maxillofacial Surgery* 1989; **47**: 405.

44  Tartell P. B., Hoover L. A., Friduss M. E. and Zuckerbraun L. Pharyngoesophageal intubation injuries: three case reports. *American Journal of Otolaryngology* 1990; **11**: 256.

45  Delport S. D. and Gibson B. H. Ingestion of a laryngoscope light bulb during tracheal intubation. *South African Medical Journal* 1992; **81**: 579.

46  McGrath R. B. and Einterz R. M. Aspiration of a nasotracheal tube. A complication of nasotracheal intubation and mechanism for retrieval. *Chest* 1987; **91**: 148.

47  Cook W. P. and Schultetus R. R. Obstruction of an endotracheal tube by the plastic coating sheared from a stylet. *Anesthesiology* 1985; **62**: 803.

48  Norman E. A. and Sosis M. Iatrogenic oesophageal perforation due to tracheal or nasogastric intubation. *Canadian Anaesthetists Society Journal* 1986; **33**: 222.

49  Saunders C. E. and Sedman A. J. Left mainstem bronchus intubation. *American Journal of Emergency Medicine* 1984; **2**: 406.

50  Ribeiro B. J. Inadvertent intubation of the left mainstem bronchus. *American Journal of Emergency Medicine* 1993; **11**: 33.

51  Mehta S. Intubation guide marks for correct tube placement. A clinical study. *Anaesthesia* 1991; **46**: 306.

52  Bissinger U., Lenz G. and Kuhn W. Unrecognised endobronchial intubation of emergency patients. *Annals of Emergency Medicine* 1989; **18**: 853.

53  Horrelou M. F., Mathe D. and Feiss P. A hazard of nasotracheal intubation. *Anaesthesia* 1978; **33**: 73.

54  Conetta R. and Nierman D. M. Pneumocephalus following nasotracheal intubation. *Annals of Emergency Medicine* 1992; **21**: 100.

55  Bahr W. and Stoll P. Nasal intubation in the presence of frontobasal fractures: a retrospective study. *Journal of Oral and Maxillofacial Surgery* 1992; **50**: 445.

56  Rhee K. J., Muntz C. B., Donald P. J. and Yamada J. M. Does nasotracheal intubation increase complications in patients with skull base fractures? *Annals of Emergency Medicine* 1993; **22**: 1145.

57  McTaggart R. A., Shustack A., Noseworthy T. and Johnston R. Another cause of obstruction in an armoured endotracheal tube. *Anesthesiology* 1983; **59**: 164.

58  Glinsman D. and Pavlin E. G. Airway obstruction after nasal tracheal intubation. *Anesthesiology* 1982; **56**: 229.

59  Cone A. M. and Stott S. Intermittent airway obstruction during anaesthesia with an undiagnosed anterior mediastinal mass. *Anaesthesia and Intensive Care* 1994; **22**: 204.

60  Stoen R. and Smith-Erichsen N. Airway obstruction associated with an endotracheal tube. *Intensive Care Medicine* 1987; **13**: 295.

61  Grime P. D. and Tyler C. An obstructed airway: cuff herniation during nasotracheal anaesthesia for a bimaxillary osteotomy. *Bristish Journal of Oral and Maxillofacial Surgery* 1991; **29**: 14.

62  Treffers R. and de Lange J. J. An unusual case of cuff herniation. *Acta Anaesthesiology Belgium* 1989; **40**: 87.

63  Famewo C. E. A not so apparent cause of intralu-

minal tracheal tube obstruction. *Anesthesiology* 1983; **58:** 593.

64 Populaire C., Robard S. and Souron R. An armoured endotracheal tube obstruction in a child. *Canadian Journal of Anaesthesiology* 1989; **36:** 331.

65 Wright P. J., Mundy J. V. and Mansfield C. J. Obstruction of armoured tracheal tubes: case report and discussion. *Canadian Journal of Anaesthesiology* 1988; **35:** 195.

66 Barat G., Ascorve A. and Avello F. Unusual airway obstruction during pneumonectomy. *Anaesthesia* 1976; **31:** 1290.

67 Torres L. E. and Reynolds R. C. A complication of the use of a microlaryngeal surgery endotracheal tube. *Anesthesiology* 1980; **53:** 355.

68 Uehira A., Tanaka A., Oda M. and Sato T. Obstruction of an endotracheal tube by lidocaine jelly. *Anesthesiology* 1981; **55:** 598.

69 Harrington J. F. An unusual cause of endotracheal tube obstruction. *Anesthesiology* 1984; **61:** 116.

70 Kaeder C. S. and Hirshman C. A. Acute airway obstruction: a complication of aluminium tape wrapping of tracheal tubes in laser surgery. *Canadian Anaesthetists Society Journal* 1979; **26:** 138.

71 Sprung J., Bourke D. L., Harrison C. and Barnas G. M. Endotracheal tube and tracheobronchial obstruction as causes of hypoventilation with high inspiratory pressures. *Chest* 1994; **105:** 550.

72 Ehrenpreis M. B. and Oliverio R. M. Endotracheal tube obstruction secondary to oral preoperative medication. *Anesthesia and Analgesia* 1984; **63:** 867.

73 Thompson D. S. and Read R. C. Rupture of the trachea following endotracheal intubation. *Journal of the American Medical Association* 1968; **204:** 995.

74 Tornvall S. S., Jackson K. H. and Oyanedel E. T. Tracheal rupture, complications of cuffed endotracheal tube. *Chest* 1971; **59:** 237.

75 Smith B. A. C. and Hopkinson R. B. Tracheal rupture during anaesthesia. *Anaesthesia* 1984; **39:** 894.

76 Patel K. D., Palmer S. K. and Phillips M. F. Mainstream bronchial rupture during general anaesthesia. *Anesthesia and Analgesia* 1979; **58:** 59.

77 Serlin S. P. and Daily W. J. R. Tracheal perforation in the neonate: a complication of endotrachial intubation. *Journal of Pediatrics* 1975; **86:** 596.

78 Finer N. N. and Stewart A. R. Tracheal perforation in the neonate: treatment with a cuffed endotracheal tube. *Journal of Pediatrics* 1976; **89:** 510.

79 Epstein S. K., Gottlieb D. J. and Faling L. J. Bronchial stump disruption following inadvertent right mainstem intubation 9 years after pneumonectomy. *American Journal of Emergency Medicine* 1993; **11:** 47.

80 Blitt C. D., Gutman H. L., Cohen D. D., Weisman H. and Dillon J. B. 'Silent' regurgitation and aspiration with general anesthesia. *Anesthesia and Analgesia* 1970; **49:** 707.

81 Keller C., Elliott W. and Hubbell R. N. Endotracheal tube safety during electrodissection tonsillectomy. *Archives of Otolaryngology, Head and Neck Surgery* 1992; **118:** 643.

82 Wainwright A. C., Moody R. A. and Carruth J. A. Anaesthetic safety with the carbon dioxide laser. *Anaesthesia* 1981; **36:** 411.

83 Hirshman C. A. and Smith J. Indirect ignition of the endotracheal tube during carbon dioxide laser surgery. *Archives of Otolaryngology* 1980; **106:** 639.

84 Oulton J. L. and Donald M. A ventilating laryngoscope. *Anesthesiology* 1971; **35:** 540.

85 Kumar A. and Frost E. Prevention of fire hazard during laser microsurgery. *Anesthesiology* 1981; **54:** 350.

86 Norton M. L. and Devos P. New endotracheal tube for laser surgery of the larynx. *Annals Otology Rhinology and Laryngology* 1978; **87:** 554.

87 Fried M. P., Mallampati S. R., Liu F. C., Kaplan S., Caminear D. S. and Samonte B. R. Laser resistant stainless steel endotracheal tube: experimental and clinical evaluation. *Lasers in Surgical Medicine* 1991; **11:** 301.

88 Ossoff R. H., Eisenman T. S., Duncavage J. A. and Karlan M. S. Comparison of tracheal damage from laser-ignited endotracheal tube fires. *Annals Otology Rhinology and Laryngology* 1983; **92:** 333.

89 Pashayan A. G., SanGiovanni C. and Davis L. E. Positive end-expiratory pressure lowers the risk of laser-induced polyvinylchloride tracheal-tube fires. *Anesthesiology* 1993; **79:** 83.

90 Hartsell C. J. and Stephen C. R. Incidence of sore throat following endotracheal intubation. *Canadian Anaesthetists Society Journal* 1964; **11:** 307.

91 Loeser E. A., Stanley T. H., Jordan W. and Machin R. Postoperative sore throat: influence of tracheal tube lubrication versus cuff design. *Canadian Anaesthetists Society Journal* 1980; **27:** 156.

92 Conway C. M., Miller J. S. and Sugden F. L. H. Sore throat after anaesthesia. *British Journal of Anaesthesia* 1960; **32:** 219.

93 Stock M. and Downs J. B. Lubrication of tracheal tubes to prevent sore throat from intubation. *Anesthesiology* 1982; **57:** 418.

94 Mandoe H., Nikolajsen L., Lintrup U., Jepsen D. and Molgaard J. Sore throat after endotracheal intubation. *Anesthesia and Analgesia* 1992; **74:** 897.

95 Sprague N. B. and Archer P. L. Magill versus Mallinckrodt tracheal tubes. A comparative study of postoperative sore throat. *Anaesthesia* 1987; **42:** 306.

96 Shah M. V. and Mapleson W. W. Sore throat after intubation of the trachea. *British Journal of Anaesthesia* 1984; **56:** 1337.

97  Fine J., Kaltman S. and Bianco M. Prevention of sore throat after nasotracheal intubation. *Journal of Oral and Maxillofacial Surgery* 1988; **46**: 946.

98  Loughman E. Lingual nerve injury following tracheal intubation. *Anaesthesia and Intensive Care* 1983; **11**: 171.

99  Brimacombe J. Bilateral lingual nerve injury following tracheal intubation. *Anaesthesia and Intensive Care* 1993; **21**: 107.

100  Aucott W., Prinsley P. and Madden G. Laryngeal anaesthesia with aspiration following intubation. *Anaesthesia* 1989; **44**: 230.

101  Faithfull N. S. Injury to terminal branches of the trigeminal nerve following tracheal intubation. *British Journal of Anaesthesia* 1985; **57**: 535.

102  Jones M. W., Catling S., Evans E., Green D. H. and Green J. R. Hoarseness after tracheal intubation. *Anaesthesia* 1992; **47**: 213.

103  Beckford N. S., Mayo R., Wilkinson A. and Tierney M. Effects of short-term endotracheal intubation of vocal function. *Laryngoscope* 1990; **100**: 331.

104  Lee S. K., Hong K. H., Choe H. and Song H. S. Comparison of the effects of the larygeal mask airway and endotracheal intubation on vocal function. *British Journal of Anaesthesia* 1993; **71**: 648.

105  Priebe H. J., Henke W. and Hedley-Whyte J. Effects of tracheal intubation on laryngeal acoustic waveforms. *Anesthesia and Analgesia* 1988; **67**: 219.

106  Yamashita T., Harada Y. and Ueda N. Recurrent laryngeal nerve paralysis associated with endotracheal anesthesia. *Nippon Jibiinkoka Gakkai Kaiho* 1965; **68**: 1452.

107  Hahn F. W., Martin J. T. and Lillie J. C. Vocal cord paralysis with endotracheal intubation. *Archives of Otolaryngology* 1970; **92**: 226.

108  Cox R. H. and Welborn S. G. Vocal cord paralysis after endotracheal anesthesia. *Southern Medical Journal* 1981; **74**: 1258.

109  Cavo J. R. Jr. True vocal cord paralysis following intubation. *Laryngoscope* 1985; **95**: 1352.

110  Holley H. S., Gildea J. E. Vocal cord paralysis after tracheal intubation. *Journal of the American Medical Association* 1971; **215**: 278.

111  Hanley P. J., Conaway M. M., Halstead D. C., Rhodes L. V. and Reed J. Nosocomial herpes simplex virus infection associated with oral endotracheal intubation. *American Journal of Infection Control* 1993; **21**: 310.

112  Clausen R. J. Unusual sequelae of tracheal intubation. *Proceedings of the Royal Society of Medicine* 1932; **25**: 1507.

113  Snow J. C., Harano M. and Balogh K. Post intubation granuloma of the larynx. *Anesthesia and Analgesia* 1966; **45**: 425.

114  Drosnes D. L. and Zwillenberg D. A. Laryngeal granulomatous polyp after short-term intubation of a child. *Annals Otology Rhinology and Laryngology* 1990; **99**: 183.

115  Balestrieri F. and Watson C. B. Intubation granuloma. *Otolaryngology Clinics of North America* 1982; **15**: 567.

116  Campkin V. Postintubation ulcer of the larynx. *British Journal of Anaesthesia* 1959; **31**: 561.

117  Shin T., Watanabe H., Oda M., Umezaki T. and Nahm I. Contact granulomas of the larynx. *European Archives of Otorhinolaryngology* 1994; **251**: 67.

118  Harari P. M., Blatchford S. J., Coulthard S. W. and Cassady J. R. Intubation granuloma of the larynx: successful eradication with low-dose radiotherapy. *Head and Neck* 1991; **13**: 230.

119  McCombe A. W., Philips D. E. and Rogers J. H. Inter-arytenoid glottic bar following intubation. *Journal of Laryngology and Otology* 1990; **104**: 727.

120  Debain J. J., LeBrigand H. and Binet J. B. Quelques incidents et accidents de l'intubation tracheale prolongue. *Annals de Otolaryngologie Chirurgie Cervicofaciale* 1986; **85**: 379.

121  Keane W. M., Denneny J. C., Rowe L. D. and Atkins J. P. Complications of intubation. *Annals Otology Rhinology and Laryngology* 1982; **91**: 584.

122  Abbey N. C., Green D. E. and Cicale M. J. Massive tracheal necrosis complicating endotracheal intubation. *Chest* 1989; **95**: 459.

123  Tan K. K., Lee J. K., Tan I. and Sarvesvaran R. Acquired tracheo-oesophageal fistula following tracheal intubation in a burned patient. *Burns* 1992; **19**: 360.

124  Lindholm C.-E. Prolonged endotracheal intubation (a clinical investigation with specific reference to its consequences for the larynx and the trachea and to its place as an alternative to intubation through a tracheostomy). *Acta Anaesthesiologica Scandinavica* 1969; **33** (suppl.): 1.

125  Kossowska E., Korycki Z., Walkiewicz W. and Marcinski A. Treatment of post-intubation laryngotracheal stenosis. *International Journal of Pediatric Otorhinolaryngology* 1980; **2**: 301.

126  Grillo H. C. Surgical treatment of postintubation tracheal injuries. *Journal of Thoracic and Cardiovascular Surgergy* 1979; **78**: 860.

127  Santhosh J., Mandalam K. R., Rao V. R. *et al*. Self-expandable stents for tracheal stenosis: experience in two patients. *Australasian Radiology* 1994; **38**: 78.

128  Braidy J., Breton G. and Clement L. Effect of corticosteroids on post-intubation tracheal stenosis. *Thorax* 1989; **44**: 753.

129  Sherry K. M., Murday A. A nasal adhesion following prolonged nasotracheal intubation. *Anaesthesia* 1987; **42**: 651.

130  Krantz M. A., Soloman D. L. and Poulos J. G.

Uvular necrosis following endotracheal intubation. *Journal of Clinical Anesthesiology* 1994; **6:** 139.

131 DeVita M. A. and Spierer-Rundback L. Swallowing disorders in patients with prolonged orotracheal intubation or tracheostomy tubes. *Critical Care Medicine* 1990; **18:** 1328.

132 Rotschild A., Dison P. J., Chitayat D. and Solimano A. (1990) Midfacial hypoplasia associated with long-term intubation for bronchopulmonary dysplasia. *American Journal of Diseases of Children* 1990; **144:** 1302.

133 Fadavi S., Punwani I. C., Vidyasagar D. and Adeni S. Intraoral prosthetic appliance for the prevention of palatal grooving in premature intubated infants. *Clinical Preventive Dentistry* 1990; **12:** 9.

134 Dikman P. S., Nussbaum E. and Finkelstein J. Z. Arteriotracheal fistula in patients treated for lymphoma. *Pediatric Pathology* 1989; **9:** 329.

135 Mika H., Bumb P. and Fries J. Rupture of supra-aortic neck arteries due to lesions caused by tracheal tubes. *Journal of Laryngology and Otology* 1984; **98:** 509.

136 LoCicero J. Tracheo-carotid artery erosion following endotracheal intubation. *Journal of Trauma* 1984; **24:** 907.

# 16

# Difficult and Failed Intubation in Obstetrics

*Michael Harmer*

---

---

## INTRODUCTION

In past decades, difficulties with tracheal intubation have accounted for a large percentage of the deaths reported in the triennial *Confidential Enquiries into Maternal Deaths* as directly due to anaesthesia [1, 2]. In the triennial report for the years 1976–78, there were 27 deaths classified as avoidable and associated with anaesthesia [1]. Of these, 16 were associated with difficulty in tracheal intubation; in seven, the main cause of death was inhalation of stomach contents. The report of 1982–84 classified 18 deaths as being directly associated with anaesthesia with 10 being judged as due to intubation difficulties. Eight of the reported deaths associated with intubation difficulties were due to cerebral hypoxia, with the remaining two being due to aspiration of stomach contents. The two most recent triennial reports [3, 4] have shown an encouraging reduction in the number of deaths directly due to anaesthesia (eight in 1985–87, and five in 1988–90). However,

of the eight deaths reported for 1985–87, seven were in some aspect associated with intubation problems; in only one of those reported for 1988–90 was there a proven association with intubation problems.

It would seem, therefore, that there has been an encouraging decrease in the number of deaths associated with tracheal intubation difficulties (from 16 to one over a 15-year period). Does this mean that there is no longer a problem regarding intubation in obstetrics? The past decade has seen a number of changes in obstetric anaesthetic practice that may account for some, if not all, of this improvement. There has been a general appreciation of the inadequacy and possible hazards of particulate antacids [5] and the subsequent change to non-particulate substances, with gastric secretions being further altered by the regular use of $H_2$-receptor blocking agents [6]. This has significantly reduced the risk of death due to aspiration of stomach contents. The increased ability of modern intensive therapy to treat iatrogenically induced insults has further reduced mortality. However, this may be at the expense of long-term significant morbidity. The triennial reports of 1985–87 and 1988–90 both detail deaths that occurred some time after delivery following a prolonged period of intensive therapy; these deaths may represent but the tip of a morbidity iceberg. The widespread availability of patient monitoring devices and recommendations on minimum monitoring [7] has allowed early recognition and rectification of many problems long before they become life-threatening. Finally, the change from general to regional anaesthesia has obviously led to a reduction in intubation problems, but this could be at the expense of fatal complications of local anaesthesia [4].

Despite the reducing number of deaths associated with difficult and failed intubation in obstetrics, there is no place for complacency and it is as important as ever to ensure that proper guidelines are available for the recognition and management of intubation problems.

## INCIDENCE OF FAILED INTUBATION IN OBSTETRICS

It has been estimated that failed intubation occurs in about 1 in 300 general anaesthetics given in obstetrics [8, 9]. This figure was derived at a time when the majority of operative procedures in obstetrics were performed under general anaesthesia and staff involved had greater familiarity with the technique. There is a current trend towards the increased, and in some centres almost exclusive, use of regional techniques in obstetrics. This may mean that staff, especially trainees, while competent to deal with the complications of regional techniques may, owing to unfamiliarity, be unable to cope with problems arising during general anaesthesia, particularly those involving the airway.

While failed intubation in obstetrics is not uncommon, the incidence of failed intubation among the non-obstetric population is considerably lower at about 1 in 2230 [9]. It is not immediately obvious why there should be such a difference between these two populations but a number of factors may play a part. On anatomical grounds there is no change in bony structure between the pregnant and comparable non-pregnant patient, so it must be postulated that

any changes occur in the soft tissues. During pregnancy, total body water increases, there is a generalized deposition of fat [10], and even in an uncomplicated pregnancy, the mucosa around the upper airway can become swollen [11]. Oedema occurring during normal pregnancy is probably as a result of oestrogens acting on connective tissues and is of limited significance compared with the oedema that can be associated with pregnancy-induced hypertension (pre-eclampsia), and may lead to extensive laryngeal swelling and subsequent intubation problems [12]. Similar swelling has been seen in patients without pre-eclampsia when a hypothesis of oedema secondary to venous engorgement of the head and neck associated with strenuous efforts in labour has been put forward [13].

There are also technical reasons for intubation being more difficult in the pregnant woman: poor head positioning, engorged breasts preventing correct laryngoscope placement, full dentition, overenthusiastic or misplaced cricoid pressure. In addition, there is a psychological element that may make the anaesthetist more anxious than would be the case in a non-pregnant patient. This may increase the difficulty of intubation. There is nearly always an implied or implicit element of haste in the provision of general anaesthesia in obstetrics and this, combined with the added responsibility of caring for more than one patient, is also likely to cause further anxiety. As an illustration, consider the stress involved in anaesthetizing a 25-year-old woman with twins. Assuming a life expectancy of 70 years, a drastic error in the anaesthetic may eliminate nearly 200 years of useful life! There are few times in anaesthetic practice when such responsibility is so apparent. It is, therefore, hardly surprising that anxiety may play a major part in the inability to intubate the trachea.

However, despite these quite understandable reasons for the difference in the incidence of failed intubation between the pregnant and non-pregnant woman, it may purely be due to the fact that failed intubation drills are a well-recognized feature of obstetric anaesthetic practice and, with the serious consequences of not ensuring oxygenation, are more readily followed than in non-obstetric practice.

## ORGANIZATIONAL ASPECTS OF AN OBSTETRIC ANAESTHETIC SERVICE

Prevention is always preferable to treatment. Thus, the proper organization of an obstetric anaesthetic service will go far to limit the incidence of intubation problems. The staffing and managerial requirements are outlined in Table 1. It is important that trainees who work on the maternity unit have at least one year's anaesthetic experience and that they are adequately supported by consultant cover. The recommendation of the Obstetric Anaesthetists' Association is that there should be a minimum of one consultant anaesthetist daytime session for every 500 deliveries performed per year, with full cover provided if there are more than 3500 deliveries per year. In addition, consultant advice and cover must be available 24 hours per day. There should be trained assistance for the anaesthetist; this will vary between units to include operating department practitioners, anaesthetic nurses and trained midwives. A training programme for all staff will, in addition to providing education, help to develop a close liaison between staff that will encourage co-operation and reduce the danger of any misunderstanding occurring.

In addition to staffing, there is a need for adequate equipment to be readily available in the maternity theatre. A minimum list is shown in Table 2. This equipment must be kept close at hand as it may be required in an emergency and its function should be checked regularly. The role and importance of each piece of equipment is discussed later in the text.

**Table 1**  Staffing and managerial requirements for the maternity unit.

Staff-in-training with at least 1 year of anaesthetic experience

Trained assistance for the anaesthetist (anaesthetic nurse, ODP, trained midwife)

Consultant anaesthetist daytime sessions (a minimum of 1 session per 500 deliveries)

Consultant anaesthetist cover available 24 hours per day

In-service training programmes for all staff – anaesthetic and midwifery

Close liaison between anaesthetists, obstetricians, paediatricians and midwives

**Table 2**  Equipment that should be readily available in the maternity operating theatre for any general anaesthetic.

Two Macintosh laryngoscopes (one standard blade, one long blade)

Short-handled Macintosh laryngoscope (or Polio blade laryngoscope)

McCoy levering laryngoscope (optional)

Gum elastic bougie

Wide selection of tracheal tubes

Selection of oral and nasal airways

Laryngeal mask airway (size 3)

Percutaneous cricothyrotomy kit

Standard monitoring equipment (ECG, non-invasive blood pressure, carbon dioxide analyser, oxygen monitor, pulse oximeter, ventilator alarm). Volatile agent analyser (optional)

## PREOPERATIVE ASSESSMENT OF THE AIRWAY

An overall assessment of the mother should be made before any anaesthetic, but particular attention should be paid to the assessment of the airway in an attempt to predict the difficult or impossible intubation. The tests described to assess the airway are multitude and are covered in Chapter 4. As obstetric procedures are often undertaken on an emergency basis, there is insufficient time for elaborate tests to be performed and it is more appropriate to use a set of simple, reliable observations. Although such a set of tests may not be perfect, they should alert the anaesthetist to any major anatomical abnormality. A suitable list of simple tests is shown in Table 3. These tests are based on the work of Mallampati et al. [14] and Wilson et al. [15], but other tests can be used. Rather than use the extended scoring originally proposed for each test, these modified tests depend upon a simple 'yes/no' observation. If one test is abnormal, this should act as a cautionary sign (unless it is so abnormal as to contraindicate general anaesthesia, e.g. gross restriction of mouth opening). If two or more are abnormal, general anaesthesia should be avoided and a regional technique should be used. If regional anaesthesia is contraindicated (e.g. due to a coagulopathy), consideration should be given to performing an awake intubation prior to induction of general anaesthesia. These simple tests can

**Table 3** List of simple tests that may be used to assess the airway in obstetric patients.

---

1 Mouth opening – should have an interincisor gap of at least 5 cm (three fingers breadth)

2 Pharyngeal view – should be able to see the posterior pharyngeal wall

3 Temporomandibular joint mobility – should be able to move lower incisors anterior to the upper incisors

4 Neck mobility – should be able to achieve 90° of movement of the head on the neck with particular reference to atlanto-occipital movement

5 Weight – should not be > 90 kg 'booking' weight

6 Risk of airway oedema – a history of pregnancy-induced hypertension, upper respiratory tract infection, stridor, voice change

---

be performed very quickly, with the patient either sitting or lying [16].

## INDUCTION OF ANAESTHESIA

Unlike many other operations, induction of anaesthesia in obstetrics is usually performed with the mother on the operating table in the theatre. This has some advantages (adjustable working height, ease of table tilt) and some disadvantages (narrow table, anxious patient). Patient positioning is important in reducing the possible difficulties that may arise during intubation. The mother should be placed supine with the table tilted to the left (or a wedge placed under the right buttock) to ensure uterine displacement. The head should be supported on a single pillow and marked neck flexion should be avoided.

Before induction of anaesthesia, a period of preoxygenation should be performed. This should consist of the mother breathing 100% oxygen via an anaesthetic breathing system and a tight-fitting facemask for a minimum of 3 min. Other methods of preoxygenation utilizing different percentages of oxygen, equipment or duration [17, 18] are unacceptable for the pregnant patient on two grounds: first, there is a high oxygen demand from the maternal/fetal unit, and second, the functional residual capacity is diminished in pregnancy, so reducing the lung 'reservoir' for oxygen [19]. The objective of proper preoxygenation is to 'buy' time should a problem arise in the delivery of oxygen to the mother.

After preoxygenation, induction of anaesthesia may commence. Cricoid pressure should be applied gently as the induction agent is given with the applied force increasing as consciousness is lost. The optimum force applied should be 40 newtons; if applied correctly, this should not distort the laryngeal anatomy [20]. Cricoid pressure can be applied with either one or two hands. The two-handed application, with one hand applying force to the cricoid cartilage and the other hand providing counterforce on the back of the neck, is the preferred method as it provides the better intubating position [21]. One-handed cricoid pressure tends to cause marked flexion of the neck (and hence possible increased difficulty in intubation) unless the neck is supported on a firm block [22]. When cricoid pressure has been applied, suxamethonium is given to facilitate tracheal intubation.

The problems that may be encountered during the intubation process are dealt with in a chronological order.

## INSERTION OF THE LARYNGOSCOPE

It is surprising that the simple procedure of inserting a laryngoscope can cause such difficulty in the pregnant woman (Fig. 1). However, a number of factors may combine in the pregnant woman to make this simple procedure much more difficult to perform. The most common cause relates to incorrect positioning of the patient and can be avoided if care is taken to ensure a correct head and neck position before induction of anaesthesia.

One major change associated with pregnancy is the enlargement of breast tissue. This can easily limit the ability to position the laryngoscope by restricting the space available in which to manoeuvre the handle. This limitation can be further compounded if the mother's arms are folded across her chest, forcing the breasts towards the mid line, just where the laryngoscope handle needs to be to allow insertion of the laryngoscope blade into the mouth. This latter situation is readily prevented by having the mother's arms either by her side or on 'arm boards' during the induction of anaesthesia. If, despite proper positioning, difficulty is encountered in manoeuvring the standard Macintosh laryngoscope into place, a short-handled version or a Polio blade laryngoscope may be used with good effect (see Chapter 6, Fig. 21). An alternative approach is to separate the handle and the blade of the laryngoscope, insert the blade into the mouth and then reattach the handle.

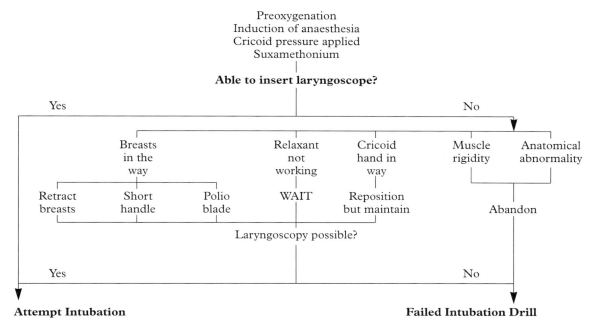

Preoxygenation
Induction of anaesthesia
Cricoid pressure applied
Suxamethonium

**Able to insert laryngoscope?**

Yes                                                                                     No

| Breasts in the way | | Relaxant not working | Cricoid hand in way | Muscle rigidity | Anatomical abnormality |

| Retract breasts | Short handle | Polio blade | WAIT | Reposition but maintain | | Abandon |

Laryngoscopy possible?

Yes                                                                                     No

**Attempt Intubation**                                        **Failed Intubation Drill**

**Figure 1**   Problems associated with insertion of the laryngoscope.

Another source of obstruction is the position of the assistant's hand as cricoid pressure is applied. This is rarely a problem with a skilled assistant but can be so if inexperienced help is all that is available (a situation that is unacceptable in a properly staffed maternity unit). Should the 'cricoid hand' be a problem, it can be overcome by gentle repositioning while, at the same time, maintaining the cricoid pressure.

Anxiety associated with obstetric anaesthesia can lead the relatively inexperienced anaesthetist to attempt intubation before full muscle relaxation has occurred; it is important to witness fasciculation before attempting laryngoscopy.

Perhaps the most feared problem after induction of anaesthesia is that it is found to be impossible to open the mother's mouth. This may be due to either an anatomical abnormality or muscle rigidity. The former should not present as an unexpected feature as it should have been recognized in the preoperative assessment of the airway. Muscle rigidity has a sinister connotation to most anaesthetists as it can be first warning sign of malignant hyperthermia [23]. However, it is also the case that muscle rigidity can occur in some patients given suxamethonium chloride. Whatever the cause of the inability to open the mouth, there is no place for persistent attempts at laryngoscopy.

Attempts at intubation should be abandoned and a failed intubation drill followed.

## LARYNGOSCOPY AND INTUBATION

After successful insertion of the laryngoscope, the next difficulties centre around the view obtained of the glottic opening (Fig. 2). The classification of Cormack and Lehane [24] divides the view at laryngoscopy according to how much of the glottis or epiglottis is visible. In general, grade 1 and 2 views do not pose great difficulty in intubation, while grades 3 and 4 often do. Intubation in a grade 3 situation can usually be achieved with the help of a gum elastic bougie, taking great care to check the tracheal tube position after intubation as the insertion may have been largely a blind procedure. A grade 4 view with a standard Macintosh laryngoscope may be improved if a longer blade is used. The McCoy levering laryngoscope has the theoretical potential to improve a grade 3 or 4 view into a more easily managed grade 2 view [25] (see Chapter 6, Fig. 27). Recent work in normal and in simulated cervical spine injured patients supports this supposition [26, 27]. This potential benefit may make this the laryngoscope of choice for obstetric general anaesthetic practice.

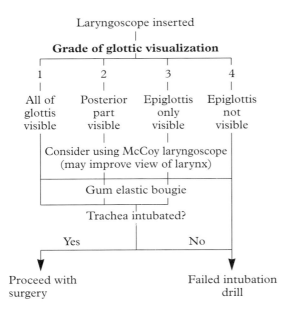

**Figure 2**   Visualization of the glottis.

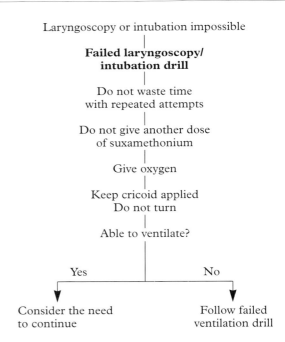

**Figure 3**   Initial drill for failed laryngoscopy or intubation.

In general, if the epiglottis is visible with any laryngoscope, it should be possible to pass a gum elastic bougie and use it to 'railroad' a tube into the trachea. There is, however, one further potential complicating factor of laryngeal oedema in the pregnant woman, especially if she has pregnancy-induced hypertension [12]. For this reason it is always important to have a wide range of tracheal tubes readily available. Severe laryngeal oedema is often associated with voice changes or the development of stridor [28]. Any such evidence should not be taken lightly as failure to appreciate and deal with this very serious condition may lead to a life-threatening situation.

## INITIAL FAILED LARYNGOSCOPY/ INTUBATION DRILL

If laryngoscopy or intubation are deemed impossible, it is important to institute a failed intubation drill without delay (Fig. 3). It is acceptable to consider one change of technique (head position, change of laryngoscope/blade) in an effort to perform intubation but time should not be wasted with repeated attempts as these are seldom beneficial and, more usually, are detrimental. Equally, there is no benefit in giving a second dose of suxamethonium as it is unlikely to produce better intubation conditions. In fact, the administration

of a second dose of suxamethonium has, in past reports [2], heralded impending disaster.

Cricoid pressure should be maintained and the mother left in the supine position with left lateral uterine displacement. The original failed intubation drill of Tunstall [29] included turning the mother into the lateral position; however, current thinking has questioned the advisability of this procedure.

The first problem is the pure physical difficulty of turning the mother into the lateral position while keeping her safely on the narrow operating table; the situation becomes virtually impossible if the mother is large (> 100 kg) and the anaesthetist is small (< 60 kg).

The next problem relates to the maintenance of cricoid pressure during and after this move. If one-handed cricoid pressure is employed initially, it must be changed to two-handed prior to and after the change to the lateral position.

In the lateral position, it is very difficult to ventilate the lungs using a 'bag and mask' as there is no support for the occiput. This means that the anaesthetist must hold the mask on the face with one hand and provide counterpressure on the occiput with the other hand – one must then wonder how to squeeze the reservoir bag!

Finally, it is not easy for the surgeon to perform

the operation with the mother in the lateral position. Provided that uterine displacement is ensured, and hence the risk of aortocaval compression minimized, there can be little detriment and definite benefits to keeping the mother in the supine position.

The prime objective in any emergency airway problem, including failed intubation, must be to ensure adequate oxygenation. Proper preoxygenation before induction of anaesthesia will 'buy' some time should a problem arise, but with high oxygen demands, the pregnant woman rapidly becomes desaturated. It is therefore important to attempt to ventilate the lungs with 100% oxygen as soon as possible in the management of failed intubation. In Tunstall's original failed intubation drill [29], it was assumed that ventilation would always be possible. However, experience from past *Confidential Enquiries into Maternal Deaths* [1, 2] has shown this not to be the case. This inability to ventilate the lungs adds further support for maintaining the mother in the more familiar supine position and not turning her into the lateral position. Even with optimal positioning, it may still prove difficult to ventilate the mother's lungs and hence a failed ventilation drill should be available (Fig. 4).

# FAILED VENTILATION DRILL

The importance of adequate maternal oxygenation cannot be overstressed and should take preference over all other considerations (e.g. fetal well-being, risk of regurgitation).

If ventilation of the lungs is impossible with 'bag and mask', the simplest initial procedure is to 'ease' the cricoid pressure. If applied with the correct force in the correct position [20], cricoid pressure should not cause airway embarrassment. However, there is evidence that if excessive force is applied, cricoid pressure can obstruct the airway, even causing collapse of the cricoid cartilage [30]. The simple expediency of easing the cricoid pressure may make ventilation possible without increasing the risk of regurgitation.

If reduction in the force applied to the cricoid cartilage is ineffective, it is likely that the reason for the difficulty in ventilation lies in the pharyngeal region and is probably related to the anatomy causing the difficulty in intubation. In this situation, it may be sufficient to insert an oral or nasal

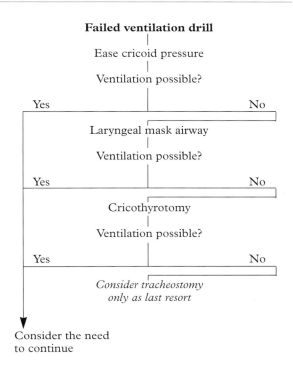

Figure 4   Failed ventilation drill.

airway to overcome any obstruction. However, if a nasal airway is used, care must be taken not to damage the nasal mucosa as that may lead to significant haemorrhage. As an alternative, the laryngeal mask airway (LMA), even though designed with normal anatomy in mind, has been shown to be of value [31, 32]. There is some controversy as to whether it is possible to place the LMA in its correct position with cricoid pressure still applied [33, 34]. It would seem logical that the tip of the LMA will only reach its proper position if cricoid pressure is released [34]. The risk of regurgitation may be increased by the release of the cricoid pressure but when oxygenation is the prime objective of management, it should take preference over everything else. The somewhat complicated protocol of Brimacombe and Berry [35] for the use of the LMA in failed intubation in obstetrics is perhaps too elaborate for what is an emergency situation. A fuller discussion of this aspect of LMA insertion may be found in Chapter 8.

If ventilation is still impossible, a direct route into the airway must be established; perhaps the easiest method is by cricothyrotomy. The passage of a tube through the cricothyroid membrane is not without risk [36] but the modern disposable cricothyrotomy kits (see chapter 13, Fig. 9), utilizing a guidewire technique, are simple and safe to use and carry the added advantage that once inserted they allow attachment to a standard 15 mm tapered connector. An alternative to a formal cricothyrotomy and insertion of a tube is the use of a cannula inserted through the cricothyroid membrane with oxygen at high pressure being delivered through it. If such a system is to be used, it is vitally important that its correct position in the airway is confirmed before the application of high pressure, otherwise extensive surgical emphysema of the neck will ensue, making any further procedure, such as tracheostomy, impossible. With the availability of disposable cricothyrotomy kits, and the increased experience on the intensive care unit with the similar percutaneous tracheostomy technique, the use of high pressure ventilation through a cannula, with its inherent danger, should be discouraged.

The final option, if all these methods fail to allow ventilation, is to perform a tracheostomy. This must be reserved as the last resort, as attempting to perform a tracheostomy on a grossly hypoxic woman would present a considerable challenge to even the most skilled ENT surgeon and certainly it is probably far beyond the scope of the majority of obstetricians and anaesthetists. The major problem with performing an emergency tracheostomy under such conditions is uncontrollable haemorrhage. This has been responsible in the past for a number of deaths where the mother has 'drowned' in her own blood [2].

The use of other ventilation aids such as the oesophageal gastric tube airway have been used with effect in obstetrics [37]. There has been, however, concern as to the damage that the oesophageal component can cause and the advent of the laryngeal mask airway has largely led to the demise of the oesophageal gastric tube airway. The Combitube is another combined tracheal/oesophageal tube that has been advocated for use with difficult intubations [38], but, as yet, there has been no experience in obstetrics (see Chapter 14).

Once it is possible to ventilate the lungs and maternal oxygenation is ensured, consideration can be given to the degree of urgency of the procedure.

## ASSESSMENT OF THE URGENCY OF THE PROCEDURE

The degree of urgency is an important consideration in the further management of a failed intubation. There are occasions when delivery of the fetus is not an intention of the procedure (e.g. insertion of a Shirodker suture) and clearly, there is no immediate urgency necessitating continuation of anaesthesia. However, the majority of problems with intubation in obstetric practice centre around procedures for the operative delivery of the fetus. Consideration must be given as to the urgency of that delivery. The usual scenario of a failed intubation is that it arises with no warning and there is confusion over the need for immediate delivery as opposed to the option of a short delay while an alternative technique is employed. As a consequence, the anaesthetist, often a trainee, is under an inordinate degree of stress and an error of judgement is possible.

The concept of preoperative scoring is well recognized for the assessment of a patient's general condition or airway. It would seem sensible to consider the development of a similar system to aid the anaesthetist in making a decision between the continuation of a general anaesthetic without the protection of a tracheal tube and the use of an alternative technique requiring an element of delay. Such a possible scoring system is presented in Table 4. This division into grades allows all staff to appreciate the potential problem and what actions might be taken by the anaesthetist should laryngoscopy or intubation prove impossible. The decision as to whether anaesthesia must be continued is fairly clear for the extremes of the grades. In grade 1, there is no alternative but to continue general anaesthesia as evacuation of uterine contents is fundamental to a successful outcome [39]. Conversely, in grade 5 there is no indication to risk the mother's life by continuing with general anaesthesia without a tracheal tube. The other grades will require some discussion between all interested parties to agree a management guideline. Whilst it may be acceptable to continue with a general anaesthetic in a grade 2 mother, it could also be argued that an awake intubation is an acceptable alternative. Long-standing fetal distress showing good recovery between contractions hardly warrants the continuation of general anaesthesia and experience has shown that the vast majority of these fetuses can be delivered without

**Table 4**   A proposed scoring system to aid the management of failed intubation in obstetrics.

| | |
|---|---|
| Grade 1 | The mother's life depends upon the completion of the surgery (e.g. cardiac arrest, massive antepartum haemorrhage) |
| Grade 2 | There is a degree of maternal pathology that makes alternative regional techniques unsuitable (e.g. decompensated heart disease, coagulopathy) |
| Grade 3 | Sudden and severe fetal distress not recovering between contractions (e.g. sudden placental abruption, prolapsed cord) |
| Grade 4 | Long-standing fetal distress of varying severity showing good recovery between contractions |
| Grade 5 | Elective procedure or maternal distress |

detriment under regional anaesthesia. The situation of grade 3 does, however, pose a dilemma. Some consider that to abandon general anaesthesia in favour of a regional technique is likely to lead to fetal death. Others may argue that maternal well-being is paramount and a regional technique is still appropriate despite any delay. Although not a widely recognized scoring system, in the current climate of relative inexperience in general anaesthesia for obstetrics, this system may act as a helpful aid to the trainee.

The decision, therefore, for each case of failed intubation, is either to wake up the mother and use an alternative technique or to continue with general anaesthesia in less than favourable circumstances. The fact that ventilation is possible, either without or by using ancillary techniques (see the failed ventilation drill), should not influence the decision regarding the urgency of the procedure. There seems little merit in continuing with surgery using a laryngeal mask airway for an elective caesarean section. There is no guaranteed protection of the airway [40] and hence there is an unacceptable risk.

## MANAGEMENT OF THE 'WOKEN UP' MOTHER

Ventilation should be continued until such time as the mother resumes spontaneous ventilation. If the decision has been made to wake her up, the mother is turned into the lateral position and allowed to recover while receiving continuous oxygen therapy.

Thereafter, consideration needs to be given as to the preferred method of providing alternative anaesthesia (Fig. 5). The choice of regional anaesthesia lies between a spinal or an epidural technique. If there is an element of fetal distress, spinal may be preferable as it provides suitable operating conditions more rapidly. However, if there is any cardiovascular instability, spinal block is best avoided for fear of producing precipitous falls in blood pressure. It has been said that spinal is an inappropriate method following failed intubation as a high block may develop which may necessitate resuscitative measures (including tracheal intubation) [41]. However, the majority consider that with an appropriate regimen, spinal anaesthesia is perfectly acceptable [42]. If an epidural anaesthetic is to be used, it must be administered extremely carefully. The danger is that if a large dose of local anaesthetic is inadvertently injected into the subarachnoid space, a 'total spinal' block will occur and with a known inability to achieve intubation is likely to be fatal. Such an occurrence has been reported in the *Confidential Enquiries into Maternal Deaths* [3].

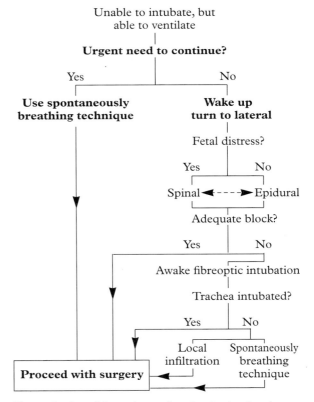

**Figure 5**   Possible options when intubation has been abandoned.

Given slowly in fractionated doses, an epidural can be safely used following a failed intubation. If for some reason the regional technique of choice is ineffective, it is possible to attempt the alternative, but great care is necessary as there may be an exaggerated response to the second technique leading to an unexpectedly high block [43].

If all attempts at regional anaesthesia fail, or such techniques are contraindicated, an alternative approach must be used. If the equipment and suitably experienced staff are available, awake intubation using a fibreoptic technique is a simple, safe and reliable technique [44]. Alternatively, a 'retrograde' technique is possible using a minimum of equipment [45]. For either method, anaesthesia is induced once the airway has been secured.

A final alternative utilizing local anaesthesia is the infiltration of the surgical site and gentle dissection with continuing infiltration [46]. Whilst this is a feasible method of providing anaesthesia, it is seldom used on grounds of unfamiliarity and availability of alternative techniques.

If all attempts at alternative techniques to general anaesthesia have failed, the only remaining option, after taking action to ensure that gastric contents have been reduced to a minimum, is to resort to a general anaesthetic with the mother unintubated and breathing spontaneously. Such a technique under controlled circumstances is an entirely different situation to that encountered when a failed intubation is converted to a spontaneously breathing anaesthetic (see later).

## EMERGENCY SPONTANEOUSLY BREATHING ANAESTHETIC TECHNIQUE IN THE UNINTUBATED MOTHER

If there is an urgent need to continue with surgery and it is impossible to intubate the mother, it is important that action is taken rapidly to convert to a spontaneously breathing anaesthetic technique (Fig. 6). It should be possible to ventilate the lungs by some route (see failed ventilation drill) and it is important that the depth of anaesthesia is increased as rapidly as possible to ensure that safe surgical anaesthesia is achieved before the start of surgical stimulation. The problem in this respect is illustrated in Fig. 7 where there is a delay in the delivery of the volatile anaesthetic owing to the attempts at laryngoscopy or intubation. This means that anaesthesia produced by the induction

agent will be wearing off before sufficient volatile agent has been delivered. The result is that the depth of anaesthesia encroaches on the potentially dangerous level associated with excitation and increased incidence of vomiting. The difference when a volatile agent is given from the moment of induction is clearly illustrated and explains the relative safety of an elective spontaneously breathing technique (as routinely used for obstetric procedures before the advent of muscle relaxants).

In order to overcome the problem of delayed volatile agent administration, a high percentage of agent should be delivered in the early part of the emergency anaesthetic technique. Something in the order of 3× minimum alveolar concentration (MAC) of whichever volatile agent is readily available delivered in 100% oxygen will rapidly deepen anaesthesia to a level sufficient for surgery. The choice of volatile agent will depend upon availability. Volatile agents, especially halothane, are known to reduce uterine contractility and may lead to excessive bleeding [47]. However, haemorrhage

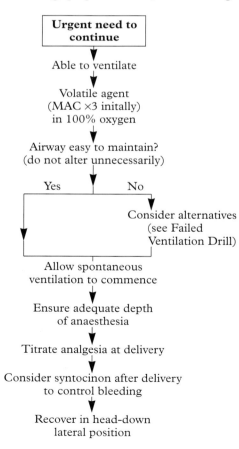

**Figure 6**   Spontaneously breathing technique.

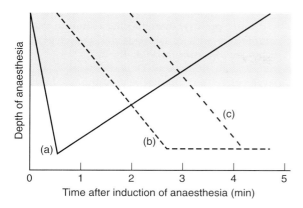

**Figure 7**  Schematic diagram to show the relationship between depth of anaesthesia and time for elective and 'failed intubation' cases. (a) Intravenous induction agent; (b) volatile agent (elective); (c) volatile agent (failed intubation). The shaded area represents the 'light' plane of anaesthesia.

## CONCLUSIONS

Difficult and failed intubation in obstetrics has been responsible for a number of deaths over the years. The majority of them can be attributed to a combination of poor organization, poor judgement and failure to ensure maternal oxygenation. The development of failed intubation and ventilation drills has gone a long way to making such disastrous occurrences much rarer. It is essential that every anaesthetist working in obstetrics ensures that if they are confronted with a difficult or impossible intubation, they are able to overcome each problem logically and never take a route of action from which there is no escape.

should be a secondary consideration to an agent's ability to allow a rapid and smooth induction of anaesthesia. If at any stage the airway becomes difficult to maintain, any of the methods discussed earlier for the management of 'failed ventilation' should be employed.

Once an adequate level of anaesthesia has been attained, surgery may commence. At delivery of the fetus, analgesia can be titrated and bleeding can be controlled by an infusion of syntocinon. Care must be taken to balance the adequacy of analgesia against the risk of respiratory depression. During general anaesthesia, it has been recommended that a large bore nasogastric tube should be passed to allow stomach contents to be aspirated [4]. However, such advice relates to the intubated situation; in the unintubated emergency situation; it is inadvisable to perform any kind of instrumentation in the pharyngeal region as this may stimulate vomiting or embarrass the airway. At completion of surgery, the mother should be turned into the lateral position and the anaesthetist should remain with her throughout the recovery period.

Postoperative management should include counselling the mother about the difficult intubation and advice regarding any future anaesthetics. Often, though, the woman who is difficult or impossible to intubate when pregnant presents no problems when not pregnant.

## KEY POINTS

- Proper organization of an obstetric anaesthetic service should ensure adequate staffing at all levels

- Preoperative assessment of the airway is mandatory before any obstetric anaesthetic is administered

- If problems are encountered at any time during the process of intubation, do not delay or waste time with repeated attempts but quickly adopt an agreed failed intubation drill

- Oxygenation is the prime objective of any failed intubation drill. Always be prepared for the inability to ventilate and have the necessary equipment readily available

- Give consideration to the urgency of the procedure

- Do not use complicated or unfamiliar techniques to manage a failed intubation. Keep things as simple as possible

- Never embark on a method of management from which there is no alternative if it should prove impossible

# REFERENCES

1 Department of Health and Social Security. *Report on Confidential Enquiries into Maternal Deaths in England and Wales 1976–78*. London: HMSO.

2 Department of Health. *Report on Confidential Enquiries into Maternal Deaths in England and Wales 1982–84*. London: HMSO.

3 Department of Health, Welsh Office, Scottish Home and Health Department, Department of Health and Social Services, Northern Ireland. *Report on Confidential Enquiries into Maternal Deaths in the United Kingdom 1985–87*. London: HMSO.

4 Department of Health, Welsh Office, Scottish Home and Health Department, Department of Health and Social Services, Northern Ireland. *Report on Confidential Enquiries into Maternal Deaths in the United Kingdom 1988–90*. London: HMSO.

5 Gibbs C. P., Schwartz D. J., Wynne J. W., Hood C. and Kuck E. J. Antacid pulmonary aspiration in the dog. *Anesthesiology* 1979; **51:** 380.

6 McAuley D. M., Moore J., McCaughey W., Donnelly B. D. and Dundee J. W. Ranitidine as an antacid before elective Caesarean section. *Anaesthesia* 1983; **38:** 108.

7 Association of Anaesthetists of Great Britian and Ireland. *Recommendations for Standards of Monitoring during Anaesthesia and Recovery*. 1988.

8 Lyons G. Failed intubation. Six years' experience in a teaching maternity unit. *Anaesthesia* 1985; **40:** 759.

9 Samsoon G. L. T. and Young J. R. B. Difficult tracheal intubation: a retrospective study. *Anaesthesia* 1987; **42:** 487.

10 Hytten F. E. Weight gain in pregnancy. In: Hytten F. and Chamberlain G. (eds) *Clinical Physiology in Obstetrics*. Oxford: Blackwell Scientific Publications. 1980; 193.

11 Mackenzie A. I. Laryngeal oedema complicating obstetric anaesthesia. *Anaesthesia* 1978; **33:** 271.

12 Brock-Utne J. G., Downing J. W. and Seedat F. Laryngeal oedema associated with pre-eclamptic toxaemia. *Anaesthesia* 1977; **32:** 556.

13 Jouppila R., Jouppila P. and Hollmén A. Laryngeal oedema as an obstetric anaesthesia complication. *Acta Anaesthesiologica Scandinavica* 1980; **24:** 97.

14 Mallampati S. R., Gatt S. P., Gugino L. D. *et al.* A clinical sign to predict difficult intubation: a prospective study. *Canadian Anaesthetists Society Journal* 1985; **32:** 429.

15 Wilson M. E., Spiegelhalter D., Robertson J. A. and Lesser P. Predicting difficult intubation. *British Journal of Anaesthesia* 1988; **61:** 211.

16 Tham E. J., Gildersleve C. D., Sanders L. D., Mapleson W. W. and Vaughan R. S. Effects of posture, phonation and observer on Mallampati classification. *British Journal of Anaesthesia* 1992; **68:** 32.

17 Hett D. A., Geraghty I. F., Radford R. and House J. R. Routine pre-oxygenation using a Hudson mask. A comparison with a conventional pre-oxygenation technique. *Anaesthesia* 1994; **49:** 157.

18 Maurette P., O'Flaherty D. and Adams A. P. Pre-oxygenation: an alternative technique. *European Journal of Anaesthesiology* 1993; **10:** 147.

19 Moir D. D. and Thorburn J. *Obstetric Anaesthesia and Analgesia* 3rd edn. Eastbourne: Baillière Tindall. 1986; p. 24.

20 Vanner R. G., O'Dwyer J. P., Pryle B. J. and Reynolds F. Upper oesophageal sphincter pressure and the effect of cricoid pressure. *Anaesthesia* 1992; **47:** 95.

21 King T. A. and Adams A. P. Failed tracheal intubation. *British Journal of Anaesthesia* 1990; **65:** 400.

22 Crawford J. S. The 'contra cricoid' cuboid aid to tracheal intubation. *Anaesthesia* 1982; **37:** 345.

23 Ellis F. R. and Hallsall P. J. Suxamethonium spasm. *British Journal of Anaesthesia* 1984; **56:** 381.

24 Cormack R. S. and Lehane J. Difficult tracheal intubation in obstetrics. *Anaesthesia* 1984; **39:** 1105.

25 McCoy E. P. and Mirakhur R. K. The levering laryngoscope. *Anaesthesia* 1993; **48:** 516.

26 Tuckey J. P., Cook T. M. and Render C. A. An evaluation of the levering laryngoscope. *Anaesthesia* 1996; **51:** (in press).

27 Laurent S. C., deMelo A. E. and Alexander-Williams J. M. The use of the McCoy laryngoscope in patients with potential cervical spine injuries. *Anaesthesia* 1996; **51:** (in press).

28 Heller P. J., Scheider E. P. and Marx G. F. Pharyngolaryngeal edema as a presenting symptom in preeclampsia. *Obstetrics and Gynecology* 1983; **62:** 523.

29 Tunstall M. E. Failed intubation drill. *Anaesthesia* 1976; **31:** 850.

30 Vanner R. G. Tolerance of cricoid pressure by conscious volunteers. *International Journal of Obstetric Anesthesia* 1992; **1:** 195.

31 Chadwick I. S. and Vohra A. Anaesthesia for emergency Caesarean section using the Brain laryngeal airway. *Anaesthesia* 1989; **44:** 261.

32 McClune S., Regan M. and Moore J. Laryngeal mask airway for Caesarean section. *Anaesthesia* 1990; **45:** 227.

33 Ansermino J. M. and Blogg C. E. Cricoid pressure may prevent insertion of the laryngeal mask airway. *British Journal of Anaesthesia* 1992; **69:** 465.

34 Asai T., Barclay K., Power I. and Vaughan R. S. Cricoid pressure impedes placement of the laryngeal mask airway and subsequent tracheal intubation through the mask. *British Journal of Anaesthesia* 1994; **72:** 47.

35 Brimacombe J. and Berry A. The laryngeal mask airway for obstetric anaesthesia and neonatal resuscitation. *International Journal of Obstetric Anesthesia* 1994; **3:** 211.

36 Cobley M. and Vaughan R. S. (1992) Recognition and management of difficult airway problems. *British Journal of Anaesthesia* 1992; **68:** 90.

37 Tunstall M. E. and Geddes C. 'Failed Intubation' in obstetric anaesthesia: an indication for use of the 'Esophageal Gastric Tube Airway'. *British Journal of Anaesthesia* 1984; **56:** 659.

38 Frass M., Frenzer R., Zdrahal F., Hoflehner G., Porges P. and Lackner F. The esophageal tracheal Combitube: preliminary results with a new airway for CPR. *Annals of Emergency Medicine* 1987; **16:** 768.

39 Rees G. A. D. and Willis B. A. Resuscitation in late pregnancy. *Anaesthesia* 1988; **43:** 347.

40 Griffin R. M. and Hatcher I. S. Aspiration pneumonia and the laryngeal mask airway. *Anaesthesia* 1990; **45:** 1039.

41 Bembridge M., MacDonald R. and Lyons G. Spinal anaesthesia with hyperbaric lignocaine for elective Caesarean section. *Anaesthesia* 1986; **41:** 906–909.

42 Russell I. F. Inadvertent total spinal for Caesarean section. *Anaesthesia* 1985; **40:** 199.

43 Stone P. A., Thorburn J. and Lamb K. S. R. Complications of spinal anaesthesia following extradural block for Caesarean section. *British Journal of Anaesthesia* 1989; **62:** 335.

44 Edwards R. M. Fibreoptic Intubation: a solution to failed intubation in a parturient? *Anaesthesia and Intensive Care* 1994; **22:** 718.

45 Harmer M. and Vaughan R. S. Guided blind oral intubation. *Anaesthesia* 1980; **35:** 921.

46 Ranney B. and Stanage W. F. Advantages of local anesthesia for Caesarean section. *Obstetrics and Gynecology* 1975; **45:** 163.

47 Naftalin N. J., McKay D. M., Phear W. P. C and Goldberg A. H. The effects of halothane on pregnant and non-pregnant human myometrium. *Anesthesiology* 1977; **46:** 15.

# 17

# Endobronchial Intubation

*Ralph S. Vaughan*

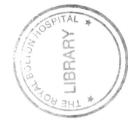

## INTRODUCTION

The history and evolution of thoracic anaesthesia, and endobronchial intubation in particular, have been elegantly reviewed by White [1] and Rendall-Baker [2]. Both articles deal with various influences that eventually led to the development of present day skills, techniques and equipment.

The practice of endobronchial intubation in the UK was last reviewed by Pappin in 1979 [3]. He showed that the use of double lumen endobronchial tubes (DLT) had increased. The most popular double lumen tube was the Robertshaw [4], used by 72% of anaesthetists practising thoracic anaesthesia. This percentage has probably continued to rise.

The use of single lumen endobronchial tubes, however, has decreased. Indeed, the 'majority of anaesthetists never use single lumen endobronchial tubes' [3]. The most popular single lumen endobronchial tubes used were the Gordon Green [5] and the Brompton Pallister [6]. The use of these tubes was limited to cases in which there were secretions, a 'wet lung', or when a bronchopleural fistula was present. This continuing decline in use has been associated with improved living conditions, advances in antibiotic therapy and a decline in the incidence of tuberculosis. The

preoperative condition of patients presenting for pulmonary surgery has therefore improved.

Bronchial blockers are 'rarely to never' used. The Magill and Vernon–Thompson blockers are of historical interest. The only 'bronchial blockers' that are occasionally used are Fogarty and Foley catheters. With the decline in the use of bronchial blockers there has been little need for intubating bronchoscopes so that the uses of the Magill and the modified Mansfield are no longer taught. The increasing use of both rigid and flexible fibreoptic instruments has completely replaced these traditional intubating bronchoscopes.

Thus, endobronchial intubation in advanced countries is achieved with double lumen tubes. Single lumen tubes and bronchus blockers are used only very occasionally [7].

This review of endobronchial intubation concentrates on the indications for use, equipment available in current practice, methods of intubation and possible complications [7].

## INDICATIONS FOR USE OF DOUBLE LUMEN TUBES

In adults, the indications can be classified in conjunction with the surgical pathology. There are no double lumen tubes designed for children.

*Cardiac*

- Closure of patent ductus arteriosus;
- Repair of coarctation of the aorta;
- Resection of intrathoracic aneurysm;
- Closed mitral valvotomy;
- Pericardectomy;
- Insertion of cardiac pacemakers.

*Pulmonary*

- Pulmonary resection;
- Pleurectomy;
- Pleuropneumonectomy [8];
- Surgical correction of unilateral pneumothorax;
- Surgery associated with the diaphragm.

*Oesophageal*

- Repair of hiatus hernia;
- Repair of oesophageal pouches;
- Heller's operation;
- Resection of tumours.

*Others*

- Chest wall surgery;
- Gastric and hepatic surgery;
- Correction of vertebral column deformities.

In all these surgical conditions, the anaesthetist could use a tracheal tube. Most anaesthetists and surgeons prefer to use a DLT, which enables greater control of the lung and increased safety, particularly in the presence of pus or a broncho-pleural fistula.

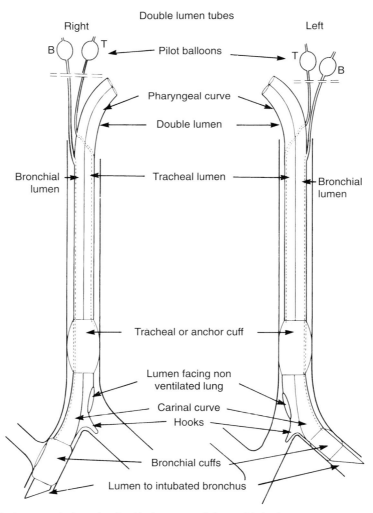

Double lumen tubes

Right                                                                    Left

B    T  ——— Pilot balloons ———  T    B

——— Pharyngeal curve ———

——— Double lumen ———

Bronchial lumen  ——— Tracheal lumen ——— Bronchial lumen

——— Tracheal or anchor cuff ———

Lumen facing non ventilated lung

——— Carinal curve ———
——— Hooks ———

——— Bronchial cuffs ———
Lumen to intubated bronchus

**Figure 1**    Structural characteristics of a double lumen endobronchial tube.

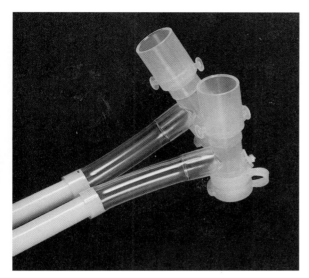

**Figure 2** Purpose-designed catheter mount.

# EQUIPMENT

## Endobronchial tubes

Endobronchial tubes currently available are divided into double and single lumen tubes. Recent developments include the Univent and Nazari tubes.

## *Double lumen tubes*

The tubes available are usually named after their designer (e.g. Robertshaw [4]). Regardless of type of tube, there are fundamental design characteristics common to all. These are illustrated in Fig. 1 and described below.

### Pilot balloons

There are two pilot balloons linked either with the tracheal or the bronchial cuffs. The linkage is either colour coded or each pilot balloon has a capital T (tracheal) or B (bronchial) marked on it. These balloons indicate that the cuffs have been inflated. They do not indicate the volume of gas required to create a seal or record the pressure necessary for an airtight fit. Excessive inflating pressure may cause rupture of the balloon or bronchus.

### Curves

All double lumen tubes have two curves. The proximal curve follows the shape of the pharynx and the distal curve is designed to assist entry into the appropriate bronchus.

### Double lumen

Each lumen is hemispherical (D) in shape and can be separately connected to a purpose-designed catheter mount (Fig. 2). Each lumen can also be labelled as the tracheal or bronchial component of the DLT (Fig. 3). These individual catheter mountings assist with the correct placing of the tube, permit individual lung ventilation and suction if required.

### Tracheal cuff

The tracheal cuff not only seals off the trachea, but also acts as the 'anchor cuff', fixing the endobronchial tube in the trachea.

### Lumen to the non-intubated bronchus

This is nearly always placed 'blind'. Ideally, it

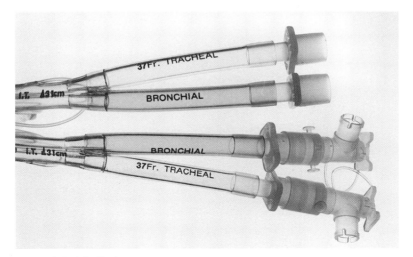

**Figure 3** Each lumen separately labelled.

should completely face the bronchus of the lung that requires surgery, the 'non-dependent lung'.

### Hooks

The first endobronchial DLT was introduced by Carlens [9] for differential bronchospirometry. It had a hook attached so that the tube would arrest at the carina. However, in newer versions of endobronchial tubes there are no hooks, as they have caused difficulty with intubation, extubation and, occasionally, trauma.

### Bronchial cuff

This cuff is inflated to obtain an airtight seal in the appropriate main bronchus so that one lung ventilation can be maintained, if required, during surgery. Excessive inflating pressure may rupture the cuff, damage the bronchus, or cause the cuff to herniate and block the open end of the distal lumen. In addition, the design of this cuff has altered significantly in a right-sided tube. The cuff is set at an angle to the main lumen so that the chance of obstructing the right upper lobe bronchus is much reduced (Fig. 4). Double cuffs, one proximal and one distal to the right upper lobe bronchus, are also used in some varieties of DLTs.

### Lumen in the intubated bronchus

This lumen allows ventilation of the isolated lung. This lung usually, but not always, is the lower lung during surgery and is known as the 'dependent lung'.

### Slit for the right upper lobe bronchus

The anatomy of the bronchi differ (Chapter 1). The bronchus to the right upper lobe usually arises about 2.5 cm from the carina. It is essential that the position of this bronchus is noted initially at bronchoscopy. After right-sided endobronchial intubation, the position of the slit relative to the bronchus is checked by auscultation over the right upper lobe. Increasingly, the position of the right upper lobe bronchus relevant to the slit in the right-sided tube is checked using fibreoptic techniques [7].

## Single lumen tubes

Although ordinary tracheal tubes can enter either the right or left main bronchus, they are not used as endobronchial tubes. Indeed, on the right side, they could be positively dangerous since there is no slit for the upper lobe bronchial orifice. Some single lumen tubes are designed to be introduced blindly into the appropriate bronchus while others have a curve similar to a tracheal tube so that they may be placed over an intubating bronchoscope [10]. There are fundamental characteristics in design regardless of the type of tube; these are illustrated in Fig. 5.

### Pilot balloons

There are always a minimum of two balloons, one each for the tracheal and bronchial cuffs. Each is marked T or B as appropriate or they can be colour coded. However, with left-sided tubes there

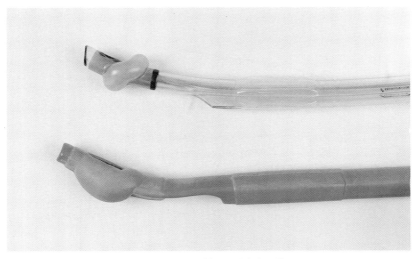

**Figure 4**   Lateral view of the two different right-sided bronchial cuffs.

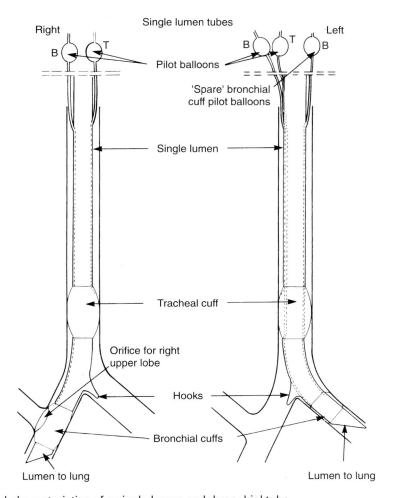

**Figure 5**   Structural characteristics of a single lumen endobronchial tube.

is a 'spare' pilot balloon for the 'spare' cuff. This is placed underneath the bronchial cuff. This concept was originally introduced by Pallister [6]. If one bronchial cuff was surgically damaged and collapsed, the second cuff could be inflated.

**Single lumen**
This lumen runs the length of the endobronchial tube and may vary in shape from above down.

**Tracheal cuff**
This is generally longer but otherwise similar to the cuff of tracheal and double lumen endobronchial tubes.

**Hooks**
These were designed to fit over the carina but are no longer included.

**Bronchial cuff**
This is usually shorter than the tracheal cuff and isolates the lung distal to the intubated bronchus. Single and double lumen right-sided endobronchial tubes have similar cuffs with a special slit for the right upper lobe bronchus.

No double or single lumen tubes similar to adult tubes are available for children. In rare circumstances where an endobronchial tube is required, small tracheal tubes have been adapted for selective main bronchus intubation. They are placed using auscultation, fibreoptic methods and radiological techniques.

**Recent developments**

Over the last decade, the Univent [11] and Nazari [12] tubes have been introduced into clinical practice.

## The Univent tube

The Univent tube is illustrated in Fig. 6. It is shaped like a normal tracheal tube but is made of silastic. Contained in the concavity of the anterior wall is a small passage that enables a small 'bronchus blocker' to pass through the distal tip of the tube into the relevant bronchus. In order to accomplish endobronchial intubation, it is recommended that the concavity of the tracheal tube should face the same direction as the bronchus to be intubated. The blocker can extend around 8 cm from the end of the tip of the main tube. It is about 2.0 mm in diameter and can therefore allow both insufflation or suction to the distal bronchial lumen. The cuff is small but has high volume and low pressure characteristics.

## The Nazari tube

The Nazari tube is illustrated in Fig. 7. It is similar to a coaxial system with the inner section capable of being advanced into either bronchus. However, there are two different inner sections which can be used depending on which bronchus is to be intubated. In contrast to the Univent tube, the sections that are advanced can be used to ventilate selectively either the right or left lung. When the inner tube has been correctly placed, both lungs can be ventilated simultaneously.

## Bronchoscopes

Three types of bronchoscopes are used by anaesthetists: the straight Negus/Storz, the intubating and fibreoptic varieties.

### *Negus/Storz bronchoscopes*

These are widely available for diagnostic purposes. The anaesthetist should use them to examine the larynx, the trachea and main bronchi to see if there is an obstruction that would prevent endobronchial intubation. The position of the right upper lobe bronchus must be identified when the right lung is to be electively ventilated. The Storz bronchoscope utilizes a fibreoptic light source and has quite excellent optics. Artificial ventilation can be performed with the Storz bronchoscope using either a Sanders injector [13] (Fig. 8) or an adaptation of a standard breathing circuit (Fig. 9).

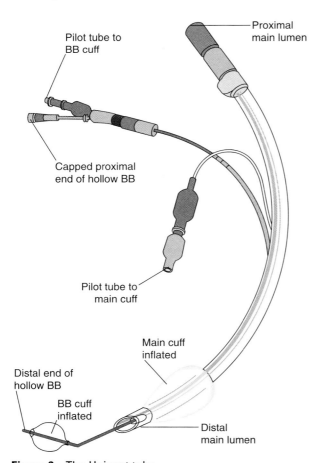

Pilot tube to BB cuff

Proximal main lumen

Capped proximal end of hollow BB

Pilot tube to main cuff

Main cuff inflated

Distal end of hollow BB

BB cuff inflated

Distal main lumen

**Figure 6**   The Univent tube.

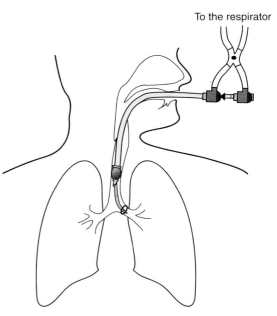

To the respirator

**Figure 7**   The Nazari tube.

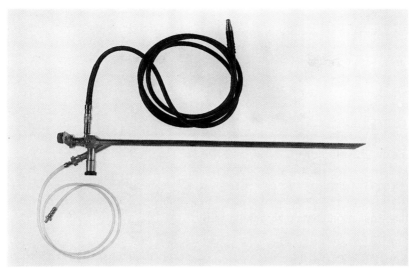

**Figure 8**   The Storz bronchoscope with the Sanders injector.

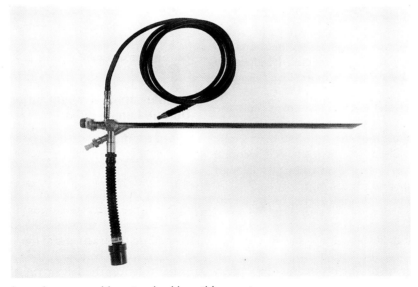

**Figure 9**   The Storz bronchoscope with a standard breathing system.

## Intubating bronchoscopes

The traditional Magill and Mansfield varieties have disappeared from clinical use. The main replacement, the Storz Hopkins intubating bronchoscope, is illustrated in Fig. 10. This bronchoscope consists of two parts:

- a stainless steel sheath. The sheath serves two purposes, first to protect the telescope, and second to support a tracheal or endobronchial tube;
- a rigid fibreoptic telescope. The eyepiece pro-

duces a clear and enlarged view of the respiratory tract.

## Fibreoptic bronchoscopes

These are increasingly used for diagnostic purposes, as an aid for the introduction of both tracheal and endobronchial tubes, and for the confirmation of correct placement of such tubes (Chapter 10). The superb optical system and flexibility enhance all these uses.

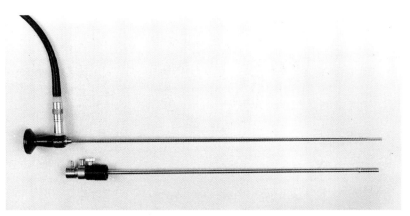

**Figure 10**   The Storz Hopkins intubating bronchoscope.

## METHODS OF ENDOBRONCHIAL INTUBATION

Before endobronchial intubation is attempted, the anaesthetist should perform a preliminary bronchoscopy. This is usually carried out under general anaesthesia or occasionally, local analgesia. Bronchoscopy must be practised before an anaesthetist can become an expert. The following are instructions in this skill.

The patient's neck is partially flexed and the head extended. A rigid bronchoscope is introduced into the mouth in the mid line or laterally through a suitable gap in the teeth. A fibreoptic bronchoscope can also be introduced through either the nasal or oral routes.

There are two possible approaches to the laryngeal aperture:

- The fibreoptic bronchoscope is passed through the nose or over the tongue until the tip of the epiglottis is seen. The bronchoscope is then eased over the posterior surface of the epiglottis and the cords visualized.
- The rigid bronchoscope is 'dropped' onto the posterior wall of the pharynx and moved slowly anteriorly. It may be useful to look for transillumination through the anterior aspect of the neck at this point. As the bronchoscope is brought forward, the larynx appears and the vocal cords are visualized.

The bronchoscope is passed through the vocal cords into the trachea, which appears as a series of glistening whitish ridges in between red troughs. The bronchoscope is advanced to the carina. The angle of the carina is noted and the bronchoscope 'tapped' against the carina to give some indication as to the texture (e.g. rigid or soft). The orifice of the right upper lobe bronchus should be noted, particularly if the right lung is to be electively ventilated. Any abnormality seen is noted, especially those that may cause difficulty during intubation, for example external compression causing bronchial narrowing.

## Endobronchial Intubation with a Double Lumen Tube

### Blind method

The patient's head should be correctly positioned for laryngoscopy. The DLT, occasionally with its connectors attached, is held so that the protruding tip is in the anteroposterior plane (Fig. 11). The tube is passed through the cords under direct vision into the trachea and the laryngoscope is usually removed. The tube is then rotated through 90° either to enter the left or right main bronchus, as appropriate. It may be helpful to turn the head and neck to the opposite side (Fig. 12). The tube is then advanced until it enters the appropriate bronchus. This is usually recognized by an increased resistance as the main part of the tube abuts against the carina.

### Fibreoptic method

The blind method has been associated with a 25% failure rate while attempting to place a DLT correctly [14]. To achieve a more accurate placement percentage, a flexible fibreoptic bronchoscope has been used [15, 16].

After the DLT has been introduced into the

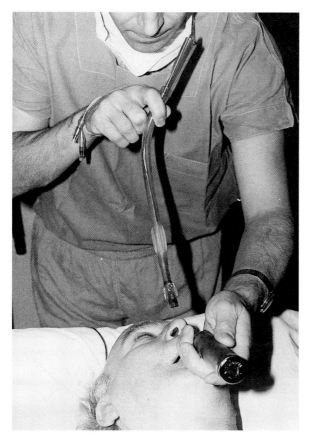

**Figure 11** A double lumen tube just before it is passed into the mouth.

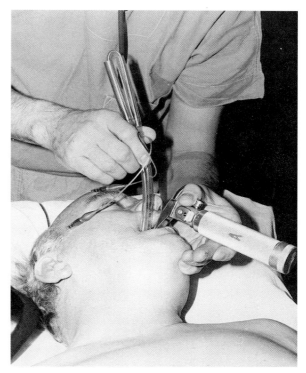

**Figure 12** Insertion of a right double lumen tube. The patient's head is turned away from the bronchus that is to be intubated.

trachea and the ventilation checked, the flexible bronchoscope is passed through the bronchial lumen of the endobronchial tube. The broncho-scope is advanced into the appropriate bronchus and the endobronchial tube guided over the bronchoscope into the same bronchus.

The same bronchoscope can be passed through the tracheal lumen to check the positions of both the bronchial cuff and the opening of the tracheal lumen relative to the main bronchus leading to the non-dependent lung. It is recommended that teaching this use of the flexible fibreoptic bron-choscope should be incorporated into all training programmes [17].

### Checking that the DLT is properly positioned

The tracheal cuff is gradually inflated until no air leak is audible and the air entry to both lungs checked. A capnograph will confirm adequate ventilation of both lungs. The bronchial cuff is usually inflated after the tracheal cuff.

There are several methods used to inflate the bronchial cuff. An example of one such method is as follows:

- The connector to the 'tracheal limb' of the DLT is clamped, i.e. that part of the tube facing the non-dependent lung (Fig. 13).
- This limb is opened to the atmosphere.
- Gas inflating the dependent lung can only enter the non-dependent lung by 'leaking' around the bronchial cuff. This leak results in an audible gas flow to the atmosphere through the open-ended tube 'the tracheal limb'. The bronchial cuff is gradually inflated until this audible leak disappears and an airtight seal achieved.

Traditionally, confirmation was accomplished by the triad of 'looks good, feels good and sounds good'. It is essential to check air entry to the iso-lated lung with a stethoscope, particularly when the right side is intubated. Increasingly, a fibre-optic bronchoscope is used to check that the DLT is correctly placed [18]. In addition, a new method

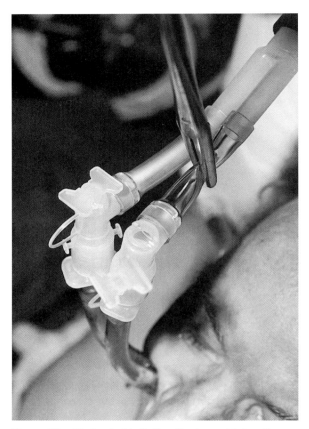

**Figure 13**    Method of inflating the bronchial cuff.

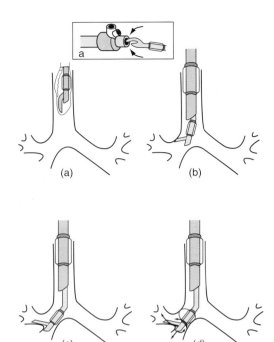

**Figure 14**    The Nazari tube – technique for insertion into the right main bronchus.

has been described to confirm the correct position of the DLT using pressure volume loops [19]. When the position of the tube is satisfactory, the bung is replaced, the clamp removed and the tube firmly secured with bandage or adhesive tape.

The position of the tube is checked once more after the patient has been moved from the supine to the lateral position. Some anaesthetists also check that selective one-lung ventilation (OLV) is possible in the lateral position before surgery commences.

## Endobronchial Intubation with a Nazari Tube

The following technique is recommended for the insertion of the Nazari tube [12]. The tube is inserted into the trachea using a standard technique. The cuff is inflated and the ventilation of both lungs checked. Both the inside of the tracheal tube and the outside of the inner tube are well lubricated. The inner tube is then passed through the main tracheal tube. There is a special mark on both right and left inner tubes which indicates the length of the tracheal tube so that the operator knows that the end of the inner tube is inserted to the same distance as the outer tube.

The tube to the right main bronchus is advanced until the inverted Y shaped piece at the end halts at the carina between the right intermediate and the right upper lobe bronchi (Fig. 14). The cuff of the inner tube is then inflated.

The technique on the left side is somewhat different. A guide is inserted into the left main bronchus. The tube is then advanced over the guide (Fig. 15). Once both tubes are confirmed to be in the correct position, they are fixed with external movable plastic rings to maintain the correct position of the inner tube. Again, the ventilation to both lungs is confirmed.

## Endobronchial Intubation with a Single Lumen Tube

There are two methods which can be used.

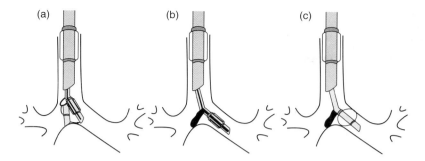

**Figure 15**   The Nazari tube – technique for insertion into the left main bronchus.

## The use of a rigid intubating bronchoscope

The endobronchial tube with its catheter mount attached is slipped over the intubating broncho-scope. The external surface of the bronchoscope is lightly lubricated. The optical system is checked and the patient's head placed in the classic intu-bating position [10].

The bronchoscope and endobronchial tube can be introduced into the larynx either by exposing the laryngeal aperture with a laryngoscope or in a similar fashion to conventional bronchoscopy. The head may also be moved to the opposite side similar to the technique described earlier for double lumen intubation. When the carina is seen, the bronchoscope is advanced into the appropriate bronchus. The tube is held firmly with the left hand and the bronchoscope smoothly withdrawn with the right hand. It may be difficult to withdraw the bronchoscope without moving the endo-bronchial tube unless the external surface of the bronchoscope has been well lubricated. Special attention must be paid to the relationship between a right-sided endobronchial tube and the origin of the right upper lobe bronchus.

## The use of a fibreoptic bronchoscope

There are two main methods. In the first method, the fibreoptic bronchoscope is passed through an endobronchial tube until the end just protrudes. The combination is then introduced together. In the second method, the endobronchial tube is passed into the trachea followed by the broncho-scope. In both methods the fibrescope is passed into the appropriate bronchus and the endo-bronchial tube passed over it.

The tracheal and bronchial cuffs are inflated to achieve an airtight seal. Confirmation of the cor-rect position is achieved with both stethoscope and fibreoptic bronchoscope. The tracheal cuff anchors the endobronchial tube in the trachea. The endobronchial tube can easily be converted into a tracheal tube by deflating the bronchial cuff. Both cuffs remain inflated while the patient is turned into lateral position and the checking process repeated. Excessive inflation pressures must be avoided as the bronchial cuff may herni-ate over the lumen of the tube, become displaced or even rupture the bronchus.

Malalignment and kinking are strong possi-bilities at the carina and can present as 'bron-chospasm'. This can be corrected by adjusting the tube and firmly anchoring the tube with the tracheal cuff. At the pharyngeal curve, kinking of the tube may occur if the neck is allowed to flex excessively, particularly in the lateral position. Excessive neck flexion may also cause kinking in the roof and angle of the mouth.

When a single lumen tube has been correctly placed and anchored at a tracheal level, it should be firmly secured. This prevents the tube slipping or being pulled out either accidentally or by the weight of the breathing system connections. When the patient is placed in the lateral position, the neck should be slightly extended and the position of the tube rechecked.

## Univent tube

The Univent tube is introduced into the trachea in conventional manner. The cuff is inflated and ventilation to both lungs confirmed [11]. The 'blocker' is introduced through the wall of the tra-cheal tube into the trachea. The proximal end of the blocker is rotated so that the cuff will be guided towards either the right or left main bronchus. When the bronchus blocker is thought to be in the correct position, the cuff is inflated and ventilation checked using a stethoscope. However, experience has shown that it is very difficult to enter the appropriate bronchus selectively. Currently, it is recommended that the bronchus blocker is introduced into the respective bronchus under direct vision using a fibreoptic bronchoscope [20].

Regardless of which variety of tube is used, checks have to be made to confirm that the tube is in the correct position. Confirmation depends on auscultation and fibreoptic inspection. When a patient is turned to a new position, the tubes have to be rechecked.

## Extubation

Before extubation, 100% oxygen is administered for several minutes before suction is applied to the bronchi. The patient should remain in the lateral and head down position. Provided that the spontaneous ventilation is adequate, some anaesthetists will extubate the patient. Others extubate the patient with the suction catheter sticking out beyond the end of the tube. This allows secretions to be removed when the endobronchial tubes are removed [21].

## ENDOBRONCHIAL INTUBATION IN INFANTS AND CHILDREN

This is a difficult procedure but can be accomplished either blindly or under direct vision.

## Blind Method

A technique using a suitably sized Portex plain tracheal tube was originally described by Cullum et al. [22]. A lateral chest X-ray is taken and the distance from the mouth to the carina measured against the film. One centimetre is added to that length so that the tube, when correctly placed, will enter either main bronchus. If the right side is to be intubated, the bevel of the Portex tube must be lengthened under sterile conditions (Fig. 16).

The tube is introduced into the trachea with the open bevel pointing to the side to be intubated (Fig. 17). The tracheal tube is then rotated through 180° and the head of the infant is moved away from the side where intubation is planned.

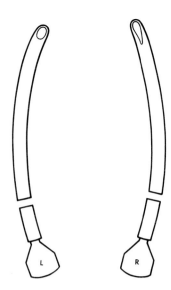

**Figure 16**  A plain Portex tube with the bevel lengthened. From Cullum et al. [22], with permission.

As the anaesthetist advances the tube, the tip passes along the lateral tracheal wall towards the appropriate main brochus. When the full extent of the tube is in place with the connector at the mouth, the tube is rotated back through 180° so that the bevel now faces the lateral wall of the appropriate bronchus. The position is confirmed with a stethoscope and, if possible, with a fibreoptic bronchoscope.

## Direct Vision Methods
### Rigid bronchoscopic method

A Fogerty catheter [23] can be passed through a suitably sized bronchoscope into the main bronchus to block off the diseased lung or lobe bronchus. It is inflated under direct vision to just fill the bronchial lumen. Excessive pressure may cause damage to the bronchus and force the balloon proximally. The bronchoscope is carefully removed so that the catheter is not displaced. A tracheal tube is inserted (cuffed or uncuffed, depending on the age of the child) and the lungs inflated.

### Fibreoptic method

Flexible paediatric fibreoptic bronchoscopes have been used to achieve both intubation and selective endobronchial blocking.

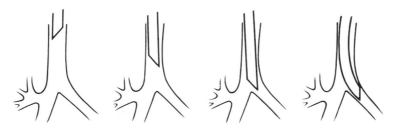

**Figure 17**   Insertion of a plain tube into a bronchus using a rotational technique. From Cullum *et al.* [22], with permission.

### Other methods

In one report [24], a Swan–Ganz catheter was introduced into the trachea under direct vision. The tip was guided into the diseased pulmonary lobe using the bronchoscope. When the tip was in the correct place, the balloon was inflated. A tracheal tube was introduced and the chest auscultated to confirm that both the balloon and tracheal tube were correctly placed.

Others have used both flexible [25] and rigid [26] fibreoptic bronchoscopes to place suitably sized tracheal tubes accurately in the appropriate bronchus to act as endobronchial tubes. These methods have also found a place in the management of critical care patients [27].

Correct placement should always be carefully confirmed clinically by auscultation, fibreoptic inspection and occasionally with chest radiography.

### Extubation

Before extubation, 100% oxygen is administered, the operating table is tilted into the head down position and secretions sucked out. If the child's spontaneous breathing is adequate, the tube is removed. If suction is not possible, the child should be placed in a steep head down position so that secretions can run down the trachea. These will be removed by suction from the pharynx or expectorated. A postextubation bronchoscopy may be performed if required.

## COMPLICATIONS

Complications associated with endobronchial tubes are predominantly traumatic, positional and physiological [28].

### Traumatic

An endobronchial tube is both longer and thicker than a tracheal tube. Most double lumen tubes are still passed 'blind' and can cause trauma to the respiratory tract. It is sometimes forgotten that such tubes can also cause damage at extubation. The trauma varies from mild ecchymosis of mucous membranes to arytenoid dislocation. Vocal cords and tracheal mucosa have also been torn by these tubes [21].

The most serious complication, however, is tracheobronchial rupture [28–30]. Such injuries are usually associated with a large tube which has been forcefully passed. The tip of the tube may pass into the mediastinum or the bronchus may rupture following the very rapid over inflation of the cuffs. There is evidence that most cuffs are inflated to a pressure higher than is required [31]. High pressures generated in this way could increase the chance of bronchial rupture.

A clinical diagnosis of bronchial rupture is made if unusual haemorrhage occurs or if a pneumothorax and surgical emphysema present unexpectedly as the 'Michelin man syndrome'. There may also be inadequate gas exchange. The diagnosis should be confirmed by rapid bronchoscopy. Any laceration found should be repaired immediately.

Modern double lumen tubes, made from polyvinyl chloride (PVC), have a much smoother surface and come with specific introducers. It has been shown that the PVC tubes were easier to pass, with a higher percentage of 'first time' correct placements [32, 33]. In addition, the time taken from beginning of intubation to correct placing was much reduced (3 min for PVC as against 10 min for red rubber). Furthermore when the respiratory tract was compared before intubation and after extubation, there was considerably less damage following the use of PVC endobronchial tubes. These results and cost effectiveness of PVC tubes are likely to result in the red rubber tubes being used less commonly [34].

## Positional

Difficulty in correct positioning of endobronchial tube is usually due to the tube being too large. Reduction in size usually overcomes the problem. However, an extensive tumour causing anatomical abnormality may prevent any endobronchial tube being correctly placed. Bronchoscopy performed before intubation should alert the anaesthetist to this difficulty.

Any endobronchial tube incorrectly placed will cause impaired ventilation. Sometimes neither lung can be isolated nor ventilated. This is usually associated with the endobronchial tube failing to pass beyond the carina and subsequent inflation of the bronchial cuff obstructing the distal lumen of the tube. Further, an incorrectly placed tube with an inflated cuff can also cause serious problems as some of the inflating volume remains in the lung at the end of each respiratory cycle. This will eventually increase the intra-alveolar pressure, cause lung rupture and a pneumothorax. If unrecognized, a tension pneumothorax may occur.

Occasionally, the lung may not deflate after the chest is opened. If the surgeon is unable to proceed easily, deflating the appropriate cuff may deal with the problem. Adjustments can also be achieved by advancing or withdrawing the tube and reinflating the cuffs. During these manoeuvres, the ventilation of the upper lung can be observed through the thoracotomy wound but the ventilation of the dependent lung needs to be checked by auscultation. Occasionally a fibreoptic bronchoscope is used.

Another method [35] has been described to help overcome difficulties in positioning when the non-dependent lung will not collapse during the operation. A Foley catheter was introduced 'blindly' into the appropriate bronchus and its balloon inflated. The balloon then acts as a bronchus blocker and the distal lung collapses as alveolar gas passes through the catheter to the atmosphere. The position of the balloon is confirmed by observing the lung collapse, the movements of the mediastinum and auscultation over the dependent lung.

A major danger exists if malposition occurs when the right lung is the dependent lung, as it is imperative that the right upper lobe remains ventilated. This lobe should be checked after intubation, turning and at frequent intervals during the procedure. Failure to ensure right upper lobe ventilation can lead to severe hypoxaemia as the total gas exchange will have to occur within the right middle and lower lobes. This type of problem can occur on the left side if the tip of endobronchial tube passes beyond the orifice of the upper lobe bronchus.

It is important to remember that lung operations were successfully performed before endobroncheal tubes were available. Lung operation can still be performed with the use of ordinary tracheal tubes.

## Physiological

The most common and dangerous complication associated with endobronchial intubation is hypoxaemia. There are several reasons for the hypoxaemia [36–38].

### Ventilation perfusion defects

The blood continues to flow through both pulmonary arteries after one lung has collapsed. Volatile anaesthetic agents and continuous infusion of some induction agents will increase this shunt due to pulmonary vasodilation. There is also increased shunting in the dependent lung which receives the total minute volume. There is therefore a considerable increase in venous admixture.

### Pressure

When only one lung is ventilated and the tidal volume delivered remains the same as it was originally for both lungs, the intra-alveolar pressure in that lung inevitably increases. This increase in pressure decreases both venous return and cardiac output and increases the resistance to blood flow through the dependent lung. More of the cardiac output is then diverted through the collapsed lung, thereby increasing venous shunting.

## Treatment

Before commencing one-lung ventilation, the following parameters should have been recorded:

1 respiratory rate;
2 tidal volume;
3 inspired oxygen concentration ($FiO_2$);
4 inflation pressures;
5 pulse oximetry reading;
6 end tidal carbon dioxide level.

Hypoxia, suspected or measured, associated with one-lung anaesthesia should be treated as follows:

- Increase the inspired oxygen concentration to at least 0.5 and, if necessary, to 1.0.
- The intra-alveolar pressure in the dependent lung should be kept as low as possible. The minute volume should remain the same but the respiratory rate increased and the tidal volume decreased. High frequency ventilation may be valuable in achieving such a pattern of ventilation.
- The use of volatile agents may have to be discontinued if severe hypoxia or hypotension develop. However, this can lead to awareness and haemodynamic stimulation so that additional intravenous analgesia and anaesthesia will be required. This may lead to delay in the onset of spontaneous ventilation at the end of the operation. Alfentanil or propofol may be useful in such circumstances.
- Surgical clamping of the pulmonary artery to the non-ventilated lung will help but this manoeuvre is only performed preceding pneumonectomy. Snaring the arterial supply to the non-dependent lung may be useful temporarily in difficult circumstances.
- Ensure that carbon dioxide tension remains within normal limits.
- Decrease oxygen consumption by total muscle relaxation and profound analgesia.
- Constantly observe the pulse oximetry reading. Arterial blood gases should also be measured to monitor progress. Occasionally a metabolic acidosis will develop which may need treatment.
- Finally, two-lung anaesthesia may be reintroduced and surgery performed on a moving target and not on a 'quiet' lung. Patient safety must always come before surgical convenience.

## KEY POINTS

- Always check that the two cuffs on the single and double lumen tubes are intact.

- Perform a bronchoscopy before introducing any endobronchial tube. The origin of the right upper lobe bronchus can be variable.

- Always check that the endobronchial tube is in the correct position using alternate clamping and auscultation. Correct positioning can also be confirmed with a fibreoptic bronchoscope.

- Always check that the position of the endobronchial tube has not altered after turning the patient.

- Before extubation, ensure all secretions are removed.

- The main complications are endobronchial movement with increase in the percentage shunt.

- The treatment is readjustment of the tube and prevention of hypoxia.

## REFERENCES

1 White G. M. J. Evolution of endotracheal and endobronchial intubation. *British Journal of Anaesthesia* 1960; **32:** 235.
2 Rendall-Baker L. History of thoracic anaesthesia. In: Mushin W. W. (ed.) *Thoracic Anasthesia.* Oxford: Blackwell Scientific Publications. 1963; Ch. 20.
3 Pappin J. C. The current practice of endobronchial intubation. *Anaesthesia* 1979; **34:** 57.
4 Robertshaw F. L. Low resistance double lumen endobronchial tubes. *British Journal of Anaesthesia* 1962; **34:** 576.
5 Green R. and Gordon W. Right lung anaesthesia. Anaesthesia for left lung surgery using a new right endobronchial tube. *Anaesthesia* 1957; **12:** 86.
6 Pallister W. K. A new endobronchial tube for left lung surgery with specific reference to reconstructive pulmonary surgery. *Thorax* 1959; **14:** 55.
7 Vaughan R. S. Double lumen tubes [editorial]. *British Journal of Anaesthesia* 1993; **70:** 497.
8 Butchart E. G., Ashcroft T., Barnsley W. C. and Holden M. P. The role of surgery in diffuse malig-

nant mesothelioma of the pleura. *Seminars in Oncology* 1981; **8**: 321.

9 Bjork V. O., Carlens E. and Freiberg O. Endobronchial anaesthesia. *Journal of Thoracic and Cardiovascular Surgergy* 1953; **14**: 60.

10 Buchanan C. C. R., Vaughan R. S. and Verdi I. Right upper lobectomy in a patient with an iatrogenic tracheo-oesophageal fistula after laryngectomy. *British Journal of Anaesthesia* 1995; **74**: 461.

11 Gayes J. M. The Univent tube is the best technique for providing one lung ventilation. *Journal of Cardiothoracic and Vascular Anaesthesia* 1993; **17**: 103.

12 Nazari S., Trazzi R., Moncaluo F. *et al.* Selective bronchial intubation for one lung anaesthesia in thoracic surgery. *Anaesthesia* 1986; **41**: 519.

13 Sanders R. D. Two ventilating attachments for bronchoscopes. *Del Medical Journal* 1967; **39**: 170.

14 Read R. C., Friday C. D. and Eason C. N. Prospective study of the Robertshaw endobronchial catheter in thoracic surgery. *Annals of Thoracic Surgery* 1977; **24**: 156.

15 Ovassapian A., Braunschweig R. and Joshi C. W. Endobronchial intubation using a flexible fiberoptic bronchoscope. *Anesthesiology* 1983; **59**: 501.

16 Shinnick J. P. and Freedman A. P. Bronchofiberscopic placement of a double-lumen endotracheal tube. *Critical Care Medicine* 1982; **10**: 544.

17 Ovassapian A. Fiberoptic bronchoscope and double-lumen tracheal tubes. *Anaesthesia* 1983; **38**: 1104.

18 Ovassapian A. Fiberoptic aided bronchial intubation. In: *Fiberoptic Airway Endoscopy in Anesthesia and Critical Care.* New York: Raven Press. 1990.

19 Bardoczky G. I., Levarlet M., Engelman E. and de Francquen P. Continuous spirometry for detection of endobronchial tube displacement. *British Journal of Anaesthesia* 1993; **70**: 499.

20 MacGillivray R. G. Evaluation of a new tracheal tube with a moveable bronchus blocker. *Anaesthesia* **43**: 687.

21 Hartley M. and Vaughan R. S. Problems with extubation. A review. *British Journal of Anaesthesia* 1993; **71**: 561.

22 Cullum A. R., English I. C. W. and Branthwaite M. A. Endobronchial intubation in infancy. *Anaesthesia* 1973; **28**: 66.

23 Vale R. Selective bronchial blocking in a small child. Case report. *British Journal of Anaesthesia* 1969; **41**: 453.

24 Dalers E., Labbe A. and Haberer J. P. Selective endobronchial blocking vs selective intubation. *Anesthesiology* 1982; **57**: 55.

25 Watson C. B., Bowe E. A. and Bunk W. One lung anesthesia for pediatric thoracic surgery: a new use for the fiberoptic bronchoscope. *Anesthesiology* 1982; **56**: 314.

26 Rao C. C., Krishna P. and Grosfeild J. L. One lung pediatric anesthesia. *Anesthesia and Analgesia* 1981; **60**: 450.

27 Cay D. L., Csenderitz L. E., Lines V., Lomaz J. P. and Overton J. H. Selective bronchial blocking in children. *Anaesthesia and Intensive Care* 1975; **3**: 127.

28 Brodsky J. B. Complications of double lumen tubes In: Bishop M. H. (ed.) *Problems in Anesthesia: Physiology and Consequences of Tracheal Intubation.* Philadelphia: J. B. Lippincott. 1989; 292.

29 Guernelli N., Bragagha R. B., Briccoli A *et al.* Tracheobronchial ruptures due to cuffed Carlens tubes. *Annals of Thoracic Surgery* 1979; **28**: 66.

30 Heiser M., Steinberg J. J., Macvaugh H. *et al.* Bronchial rupture, a complication of use of the Robertshaw double lumen tube. *Anaesthesia* 1979; **51**: 88.

31 Cobley M., Kidd J. F., Willis B. A. and Vaughan R. S. Endobronchial cuff pressures. *British Journal of Anaesthesia* 1993; **70**: 576.

32 Clapham M. C. and Vaughan R. S. Endobronchial intubation. A comparison between polyvinyl chloride and red rubber double lumen tubes. *Anaesthesia* 1985; **40**: 1111.

33 Watson C. B., Kasik L. R., Battaglini J. *et al.* A functional comparison of polyvinyl chloride and red rubber double lumen endobronchial tubes. *Abstract from Society of Cardiovascular Anesthesiologists,* Massachussetts: Boston. May 1984.

34 Linter S. P. K. Disposable double lumen bronchial tubes. *Anaesthesia* 1985; **40**.

35 Conacher I. D. The urinary catheter as a bronchial blocker. *Anaesthesia* 1983; **38**: 475.

36 Benumof J. Special respiratory physiology of the lateral decubitus position, the open chest and one lung ventilation. In: *Anesthesia for Thoracic Surgery,* 2nd edn. Philadelphia: W. B. Saunders. 1995.

37 Gothard J. W. W. *Anaesthesia for Thoracic Surgery,* 2nd edn. Oxford: Blackwell Scientific Publications. 1994.

38 Respiratory physiology and pharmacology section. In: Kaplan J. A. (ed.) *Thoracic Anaesthesia,* 2nd edn. New York: Churchill Livingstone. 1991.

# 18

# Intubation of Patients with Cervical Spine Injuries

*Jeremy Nolan*

## INTRODUCTION

The incidence of cervical spine injury following major trauma is approximately 1.5–3% [1–3]. This figure varies depending on the precise definition and cause of the major trauma. Motor vehicle accidents (cars and motorcycles) cause approximately half of cervical injuries and a major proportion of these are in men between 15 and 35 years of age [1]. Following frontal collisions at greater than 35 mph, 10% of drivers and 6% of passengers will sustain cervical spine injuries [4]. In the UK, falls, diving accidents and sports injuries are the main causes for the remainder of cervical spine injuries. In the USA, gunshot wounds are a significant cause of cervical spine injury.

The proportion of spinal injuries thought to be unstable ranges from 24–75% [5]. Approximately 30% of patients with cervical spine injury will have some degree of neurological deficit [6]. The early recognition of a cervical spine injury is vitally important in preventing iatrogenic creation or extension of a neurological (cord) injury. In a series of 740 patients with cervical spine injury the diagnosis was missed in 34 (4.6%) cases and 10 of these developed permanent neurological sequelae as a result of these delays [7]. A considerable proportion of patients with cervical spine injuries will require tracheal intubation at some stage during their management. Of 393 patients with cervical spine injuries admitted to the Maryland Institute for Emergency Medical Services Systems (MIEMSS) Shock Trauma Center, 104 (26%) required intubation within the first 24 h of admission [6]. Inappropriate airway management of the patient with a cervical spine injury can result in the disaster of permanent cord injury [8].

## ANATOMY

Stability of the cervical spine can be defined as the maintenance of vertebral alignment throughout the normal range of movement [9]. Displacement of one cervical vertebra relative to another risks injury to the spinal cord. The structures contributing to the stability of the cervical spine may be grouped into the anterior and posterior columns (Fig. 1). Theoretically, the cervical spine will be unstable if all the elements of one column are disrupted. Following a hyperextension injury, e.g. a blow to the forehead or whiplash, the anterior elements tend to be disrupted and the spine is likely to be more stable in flexion. Hyperflexion injuries (Figs 2 and 3) usually result from blows to the back of the head, or from forceful deceleration (e.g. motor vehicle accidents); this mechanism of injury will tend to cause disruption of the elements in the posterior column and will be more stable with slight extension. In practice, 'pure' flexion and hyperextension injuries are uncommon; there are usually elements of shear and rotation. In very severe cervical spine injuries both columns may be disrupted; this causes gross instability and any movement of the cervical spine is unacceptable. Compression of the spine in the axial plane will result in burst fractures. These fractures are technically stable but depending on the extent of the forces involved, posterior displacement of comminuted fragments may have produced cord injury.

## ASSESSMENT

Following significant blunt trauma, the cervical spine cannot be deemed undamaged until the patient has been examined by an experienced clinician *and* appropriate radiological procedures have been completed. A reliable clinical examination

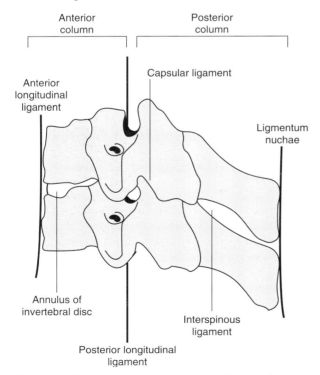

**Figure 1**   The anterior and posterior columns of the cervical spine.

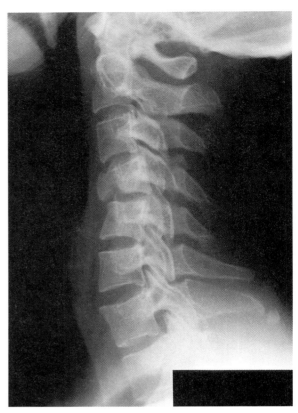

**Figure 2**   A hyperflexion injury. Teardrop fracture of C4. Note widening of the facet joints of C4–C5. X-ray courtesy of Mr Maurice Paterson, Consultant Orthopaedic Surgeon, Royal United Hospital, Bath, UK.

cannot be obtained if the patient has sustained a significant closed head injury, is intoxicated, or has a reduced conscious level from any other cause. In a recent review of 216 patients with cervical spine injuries, 28 (13%) were initially asymptomatic with no neurological deficit; of these 28 patients, 17 were intoxicated or had mild closed head injuries [10]. All patients who have sustained major, blunt trauma should have routine cervical spine X-rays [11]. It is generally accepted that at least three views of the cervical spine are required: lateral, anteroposterior, and open-mouth view of the odontoid [10]. If the cervical spine cannot be seen clearly, down to the junction of the seventh cervical (C7) and first thoracic (T1) vertebrae, a swimmer's view (lateral oblique with one arm raised) will be required. If these fail to show the C7–T1 junction, computerized tomography (CT) scanning should be used [10].

Interpretation of cervical spine X-rays is notori-

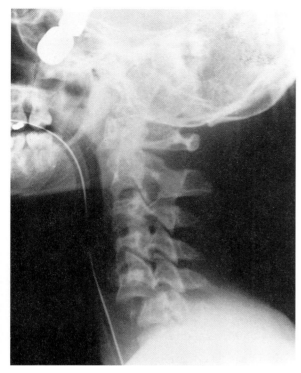

**Figure 3**   Bilateral facet dislocation at C5–C6.

ously difficult and relatively few anaesthetists have the experience to exclude confidently radiological evidence of significant injury. Alignment can be checked by identifying the four lordotic curves on the lateral X-ray: the anterior vertebral line, the anterior spinal canal, the posterior spinal canal, and the spinous process tips (Fig. 4). Widening of the prevertebral space may be another indication of cervical spine injury. Remember, X-rays show the resting position and not the dynamics of the injury.

It must be emphasized that apparently normal cervical X-rays *per se* do not 'clear' the cervical spine; they must be accompanied by a reliable clinical examination. Thus, a sensible approach to the airway management of patients with known mechanisms of injury is to initially treat all of them as if they had an unstable cervical spine injury, even if the initial plain films are normal [12].

## IMMOBILIZATION

Any patient who has sustained significant blunt trauma should have their cervical spine immobi-

lized at the accident scene. The most effective method comprises a combination of an appropriately sized semirigid cervical collar (e.g. Stiffneck or Philadelphia), and bilateral sandbags joined with 3" (7.5 cm) cloth tape across the forehead [13]. This combination will virtually eliminate neck flexion, although 30% of normal extension is still possible. Soft collars do nothing to prevent cervical spine movement.

A study of the effect of basic and advanced airway manoeuvres on the unstable neck of a fresh cadaver showed significant subluxation of the cervical spine during aggressive chin lift or jaw thrust despite the presence of a Philadelphia collar [14]. Mask ventilation can produce at least as much displacement of the cervical spine as that produced by oral intubation [15]. Manual in-line stabilization of the neck will minimize movement of the cervical spine during oral intubation [16], but care must be taken to avoid excessive traction which may distract a cervical fracture [17, 18].

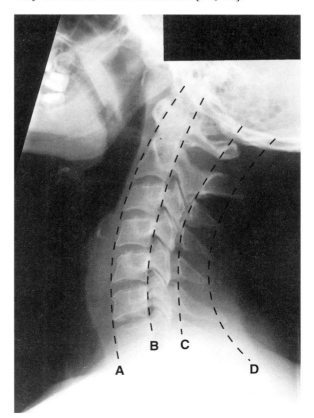

**Figure 4**   The four lordotic curves seen on the lateral view of the cervical spine. A = anterior vertebral bodies; B = anterior spinal canal; C = posterior spinal canal; D = spinous process tips.

## INTUBATION

The choice of technique for intubating a patient with a suspected or confirmed cervical spine injury will depend on the indication and on the skill and experience of the individual clinician. There is increasing evidence that, if performed with care, tracheal intubation of a patient with a cervical spine injury carries relatively little risk [19]. There are perhaps three common scenarios dictating the need for a definitive airway in a patient with a cervical spine injury:

- urgent intubation during resuscitation;
- intubation as a component of general anaesthesia for surgery to related injuries;
- intubation before definitive surgery to stabilize the cervical spine.

## Urgent Intubation During Resuscitation of the Injured Patient

The first priority during the resuscitation of any severely injured patient is to ensure a clear airway and maintain adequate oxygenation. If the airway is obstructed, immediate basic manoeuvres may temporarily clear it. In the unconscious patient, or in the presence of haemorrhage from maxillofacial injuries, for example, the airway must be secured by placing a cuffed tube in the trachea. Other reasons for intubating the trauma patient during the resuscitation phase are to optimize oxygen delivery and to allow appropriate procedures to be performed on unco-operative patients. At this early stage, for the reasons discussed previously, the patient who has sustained injuries as a result of blunt trauma must be assumed to have a cervical spine injury. A number of techniques have been described for intubating a patient with a potential cervical spine injury (Table 1).

Clinicians who are not experienced in direct laryngoscopy and oral intubation, and who are not familiar with the use of neuromuscular blocking drugs, may prefer the nasotracheal route for intubation. This route is preferred by emergency physicians in the USA and, until recently, was the technique recommended in the Advanced Trauma Life Support Manual [11]. Advocates of the nasotracheal technique [20] claim that it results in less movement of the cervical spine in comparison with orotracheal intubation, but the majority of

**Table 1** Techniques for intubating the patient with a potential cervical spine injury.

| |
|---|
| Awake blind nasal intubation |
| Awake oral intubation under direct laryngoscopy |
| Digital blind oral intubation |
| Awake fibreoptic assisted intubation via oral or nasal routes |
| Retrograde catheter technique (awake) |
| Blind oral intubation aided by the Augustine Guide |
| Fibreoptic techniques under general anaesthesia |
| Rapid sequence induction of general anaesthesia and muscle paralysis, with cricoid pressure, manual in-line stabilization of the cervical spine, direct laryngoscopy and oral intubation. |

UK anaesthetists would disagree [21]. Nasal intubation is contraindicated in the presence of a basal skull fracture because of the risk of accidental intracranial placement! Other disadvantages of awake blind nasal intubation are:

- bleeding is a common complication;
- unrecognized oesophageal intubation is a significant risk;
- coughing, bronchospasm and/or laryngospasm may be provoked;
- sinusitis is a significant risk with long-term nasal intubation;
- this technique is not as successful as direct laryngoscopy and oral intubation [22].

Awake oral intubation is favoured by some clinicians. Advocates of this technique claim that awake patients will tend to protect their own cervical spines by splinting the injury site with muscle spasm [20]; however, there is no evidence to support this hypothesis.

Digital blind oral intubation is rarely used and cannot be recommended for use by anaesthetists. Enthusiasts claim that, with practice, the majority of deeply unconscious patients can be intubated by the digital (or tactile) method with minimal movement of the head and neck. It has been used in North America, particularly in the prehospital environment [23].

The retrograde technique (using a wire or epidural catheter passed up through the cricothyroid membrane) has been described elsewhere (p.148). Although it certainly is a method of intubating a patient with minimal movement of the cervical spine, it takes too long to be practical in the emergency setting. Blind oral intubation with the aid of an Augustine Guide™ minimizes movement of the cervical spine, but again takes significantly longer than direct laryngoscopy [24]. It has yet to be proven as an ideal technique for urgent intubation.

The awake fibreoptic technique, via either the oral or the nasal route, is regarded by many anaesthetists as the safest method for intubating a patient with a potential cervical spine injury. However, it is not normally appropriate for urgent intubation of a patient during resuscitation; any blood in the airway will completely obscure the view ('red out') and even in skilled hands awake fibreoptic intubation takes a few minutes to perform.

The Bullard laryngoscope (CIRCON ACMI, Stamford, Connecticut, USA) allows oral intubation without the need to move the cervical spine [25, 26], but it utilizes fibreoptics which would be obscured by blood in the airway. The time to intubation is significantly longer than that for direct laryngoscopy and oral intubation with the aid of a bougie [26, 27].

Oral or nasal intubation using a lighted stylet would be another option but this technique carries a higher failure rate than intubation under direct vision.

In the author's opinion, the technique of choice for emergency intubation of a patient with a potential cervical spine injury is direct laryngoscopy and oral intubation with manual in-line stabilization of the cervical spine, following a period of preoxygenation, intravenous induction of anaesthesia, paralysis with suxamethonium, and application of cricoid pressure. This will rapidly secure the patient's airway and it is undoubtedly the method favoured by anaesthetists in the UK [6].

### Recommended method of intubating under anaesthesia

The patient lies supine with the head in the neutral position; an assistant applies manual in-line stabilization by grasping the mastoid processes, whereupon the semirigid collar can be removed safely. The collar will impede mouth opening [28], does not contribute significantly to neck stabilization during laryngoscopy [14, 16], and will be an obstruction if a surgical airway is required. In the case of a two-piece collar the anterior portion

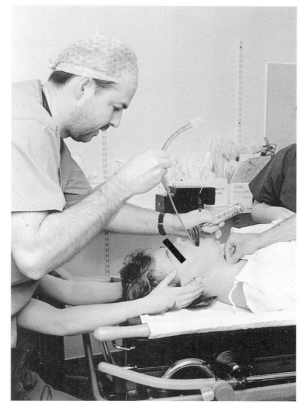

**Figure 5** Orotracheal intubation with cricoid pressure and manual in-line cervical stabilization. Note the use of the gum elastic bougie.

alone may be removed. Manual in-line stabilization reduces neck movement during intubation [16, 29], but care must be taken to avoid excessive axial traction.

This technique of emergency airway management involves a minimum of three, but ideally four individuals (Fig. 5): the first person is needed to preoxygenate and intubate the patient's trachea, the second to apply cricoid pressure, the third to maintain manual in-line stabilization of the head and neck, and the fourth to give intravenous drugs and assist. Placing the patient's head and neck in neutral alignment will tend to make the view at laryngoscopy worse; in this position one can expect the view of the larynx to be grade 3 or worse in approximately 20% of patients [27, 28].

Intubation will be aided greatly by the use of a gum elastic bougie. Another very useful instrument to use in these circumstances is the McCoy levering laryngoscope; a recent study has shown that it reduces the incidence of grade 3 or worse views to 5% [30]. A further refinement has been to use a surgeon (standing at the patient's left side) to apply the cricoid pressure. The surgeon has one hand free to perform an immediate cricothyroidotomy if required.

There are now considerable data supporting the safety of this technique (Table 2), and when performed properly there have been no reported cases of neurological deterioration in patients with cervical spine injuries. Indeed, one group have reported that in four patients with cervical spine injuries peripheral neurological deficits actually improved following oral intubation [31].

In an emergency, and in the event of failure to intubate a patient with suspected cervical spine injury, options include insertion of a laryngeal mask [35, 36] or Combitube to provide a temporary airway, or cricothyroidotomy.

## Intubation as a Component of General Anaesthesia for Surgery to Related Injuries

### Under general anaesthesia

It is not uncommon for a patient with a known cervical spine injury to require surgery for other injuries (e.g. limb fractures or intra-abdominal injury) very soon after admission to hospital. In most cases general anaesthesia will be required and, as these patients are assumed to have full stomachs, a definitive airway is necessary. In contrast to the scenario above, in which intubation is required immediately, the anaesthetist has more time and can select one of many intubation techniques.

**Table 2** Data supporting the safety of direct laryngoscopy and oral intubation in patients with cervical spine injuries.

| Author | Patients with cervical spine injuries intubated orally (n) | Unstable (n) | Neurological deterioration (n) |
|---|---|---|---|
| Criswell et al., 1994 [6] | 73 | N/A | 0 |
| Scannell et al., 1993 [31] | 81 | 58 | 0 |
| Wright et al., 1992 [32] | 26 | 26 | 0* |
| Suderman et al., 1991 [33] | 91 | 91 | 0 |
| Rhee et al., 1990 [34] | 17 | N/A | 0 |

* One of the other patients in this study, who had undergone nasal intubation, did sustain neurological deterioration.

N/A = not available.

Manual in-line stabilization followed by rapid sequence induction, cricoid pressure, and direct laryngoscopy and oral intubation, is still a very reasonable option. Depending on the urgency for surgery, many patients with unstable cervical spine injuries would have had skull traction tongs (e.g. Gardner–Wells, Crutchfield's) applied, under local anaesthesia, before coming to the operating theatre. Clearly, if cervical traction has been established by the surgeons, it should be maintained during intubation attempts.

### Awake intubation

Awake intubation with the aid of a fibreoptic scope, via either the nasal or oral route, is a possibility, though not if there is blood in the airway. Some anaesthetists are concerned about applying local anaesthetic agents to the airway of a patient with a potentially full stomach. The theoretical risk of aspiration does not seem to be a problem in practice, particularly if sedation is minimized, thus preserving patient co-operation and lower oesophageal tone [37, 38]. Techniques for locally anaesthetizing the airway and fibreoptic intubation have been described elsewhere (Chapters 7 and 10). Normally, the optimal position for fibreoptic laryngoscopy is provided by extension of the cervical spine. However, patients with cervical spine injuries must have their head and neck maintained in neutral alignment throughout the procedure. One advantage of awake intubation under these circumstances is that, following successful intubation, the neurological status of the patient can be sought and documented; this has significant medicolegal implications if the patient subsequently suffers any neurological deterioration.

The retrograde technique would be another option. It is an awake technique, with the advantage of postintubation assessment, and under these non-urgent circumstances, a little time is available to the intubator. The retrograde technique is uninfluenced by blood in the airway; indeed a very good success rate has been reported in patients with maxillofacial trauma [39].

The Bullard laryngoscope and Augustine Guide could be used for awake intubation of patients with cervical spine injuries; however, with the exception that the Augustine Guide is uninfluenced by blood in the airway, it is hard to see how they have an advantage over the fibreoptic scope. If intubation is being attempted during rapid sequence induction of general anaesthesia, use of these instruments is likely to prolong the intubation time (in comparison with direct laryngoscopy), and thus would be unwise in the patient who has a potentially full stomach.

## Intubation Before Definitive Surgery to Stabilize the Cervical Spine

Unless the spinal cord is at immediate risk, definitive surgery to the cervical spine is usually deferred for a few days, by which time the patient's general condition should be stable. Most of these patients will have had skull traction applied from the time of diagnosis and this is ideally maintained during intubation. These patients will have been starved before surgery and will generally not be at risk of regurgitation and aspiration of gastric contents.

Many anaesthetists would elect to intubate these patients awake and with the aid of a fibreoptic scope. In experienced hands this technique will result in minimal movement of the cervical spine. For what is effectively an elective procedure, there is time to prepare the patient properly by giving a full explanation of the technique and prescribing an antisialogogue premedication. In the anaesthetic room, once full monitoring has been applied, the patient can be sedated safely with a combination of fentanyl and midazolam. The airway can be anaesthetized with local anaesthetic as described previously (Chapter 7) and fibreoptic intubation performed via the nasal or oral routes. A technique utilizing a laryngeal mask as an aid to fibreoptic intubation of a patient with a cervical spine injury has been described recently [40]. During fibreoptic intubation, skull traction can remain throughout the procedure and once the patient is positioned on the operating table, a final neurological examination can be made before inducing general anaesthesia. This has advantages from a medicolegal viewpoint and is therefore a particularly popular technique in the USA.

In this elective setting other awake techniques for intubating the patient would be perfectly reasonable and would carry similar advantages to the fibreoptic scope. The Bullard laryngoscope or Augustine Guide are reputedly easy to use in the anaesthestized patient and, assuming that the patient is easy to ventilate by facemask, there should be plenty of time available to complete the intubation; use of either of these devices should result in minimal cervical spine movement.

In the UK, even in the elective setting, many anaesthetists would still prefer first to induce general anaesthesia and then use direct laryngoscopy and oral intubation with manual in-line stabilization of the cervical spine. The main disadvantage of this technique is that the patient cannot then be neurologically examined directly after intubation and positioning for surgery.

## SUMMARY

The best method for intubating the patient with a known or suspected cervical spine injury will depend on the experience and skills of the intubator and the exact circumstances surrounding the need for intubation. In the hypoxic patient an airway must be established quickly and this is no place for lengthy, complex techniques.

In reality, based on published data, it would appear that if performed carefully, tracheal intubation is relatively safe in the patient with a cervical spine injury. Indeed, despite this author's preference for direct laryngoscopy and oral intubation with manual in-line stabilization, there are in fact relatively few data supporting one mode of intubation over another. However, the occasional report of neurological deterioration after tracheal intubation [8] prompts the anaesthetist to be aware that the danger exists.

---

## KEY POINTS

- Any patient who has sustained significant blunt trauma has a cervical spine injury until proven otherwise.

- If intubation is required urgently, the technique of choice is preoxygenation, intravenous induction of anaesthesia, cricoid pressure, manual in-line cervical stablization, direct laryngoscopy, and oral intubation.

- A gum elastic bougie is very useful.

- Awake fibreoptic intubation is a good option for the elective patient with cervical spine injury.

## REFERENCES

1 Hastings R. H. and Marks J. D. Airway management for trauma patients with potential cervical spine injuries. *Anesthesia and Analgesia* 1991; **73**: 471.

2 Roberge R. J., Wears R. C., Kelly M. *et al.* Selective application of cervical spine radiography in alert victims of blunt trauma: a prospective study. *Journal of Trauma* 1988; **28**: 874.

3 Kreipke D. I., Gillespie K. R., McCarthy M. C., Mail J. T., Lappas J. C. and Broadie T. A. Reliability of indications for cervical spine films in trauma patients. *Journal of Trauma* 1989; **29**: 1438.

4 Daffner R., Deeb Z., Lupetin A. and Rothfus W. Patterns of high speed impact injuries in motor vehicle occupants. *Journal of Trauma* 1988; **28**: 498.

5 Crosby E. T. and Lui A. The adult cervical spine: implications for airway management. *Canadian Journal of Anaesthesiology* 1990; **37**: 77.

6 Criswell J. C., Parr M. J. A. and Nolan J. P. Emergency airway management in patients with cervical spine injury. *Anaesthesia* 1994; **49**: 900.

7 Davis J. W., Phreaner D. L., Hoyt D. B. and Mackersie R. C. The etiology of missed cervical spine injuries. *Journal of Trauma* 1993; **34**: 342.

8 Hastings R. H. and Kelley S. D. Neurologic deterioration associated with airway management in a cervical spine-injured patient. *Anesthesiology* 1993; **78**: 580.

9 Jeffreys E. Applied anatomy. In: Jeffrey E. (ed.) *Disorders of the Cervical Spine*, 2nd edn. Oxford: Butterworth-Heinemann. 1993; p. 1.

10 Woodring J. H. and Lee C. Limitations of cervical radiography in the evaluation of acute cervical trauma. *Journal of Trauma* 1993; **34**: 32.

11 The American College of Surgeons Committee on Trauma *Advanced Trauma Life Support Program For Physicians: Instructor Manual.* Chicago: American College of Surgeons. 1993.

12 Stemp L. I. A normal cervical spine X-ray does not 'clear' the patient with suspected cervical spine injury. *Anesthesiology* 1993; **79**: 619.

13 Podolsky S., Baraff L. J., Simon R. R., Hoffman J. R., Larmon B. and Ablon W. Efficacy of cervical spine immobilisation methods. *Journal of Trauma* 1983; **23**: 461.

14 Aprahamian C., Thompson B. M., Finger W. A. and Darin J. C. Experimental cervical spine injury model: Evaluation of airway management and splinting techniques. *Annals of Emergency Medicine* 1984; **13**: 584.

15 Hauswald M., Sklar D. P., Tandberg D. and Garcia J. F. Cervical spine movement during airway management: cinefluroscopic appraisal in human cadavers. *American Journal of Emergency Medicine* 1991; **9**: 535.

16 Majernick T. G., Bieniek R., Houston J. B. and Hughes H. G. Cervical spine movement during orotracheal intubation. *Annals of Emergency Medicine* 1986; **15**: 417.

17 Bivins H. G., Ford S., Bezmalinovic Z., Price H. M. and Williams J. L. The effect of axial traction during orotracheal intubation of the trauma victim with an unstable cervical spine. *Annals of Emergency Medicine* 1988; **17**: 25.

18 Turner L. M. Cervical spine immobilization with axial traction: a practice to be discouraged. *Journal of Emergency Medicine* 1989; **7**: 385.

19 Crosby E. T. Tracheal intubation in the cervical spine-injured patient. *Canadian Journal of Anaesthesiology* 1992; **39**: 105.

20 Meschino A., Devitt J. H., Koch J. P., Szalai J. P. and Schwartz M. L. The safety of awake tracheal intubation in cervical spine injury. *Canadian Journal of Anaesthesiology* 1992; **39**: 114.

21 Wood P. R. and Lawler P. G. P. Managing the airway in cervical spine injury. A review of the Advanced Trauma Life Support protocol. *Anaesthesia* 1992; **47**: 792.

22 Dronen S. C., Merigian K. S., Hedges K. R., Hoekstra J. W. and Borron S. W A comparison of blind nasotracheal and succinylcholine assisted intubation in the poisoned patient. *Annals of Emergency Medicine* 1987; **16**: 650.

23 Stewart R. D. Tactile orotracheal intubation. *Annals of Emergency Medicine* 1984; **13**: 175.

24 Fitzgerald R. D., Krafft P., Skrbensky G. *et al.* Excursions of the cervical spine during tracheal intubation: blind oral intubation compared with direct laryngoscopy. *Anaesthesia* 1994; **49**: 111.

25 Abrams K. J., Desai N. and Katsnelson T. Bullard laryngoscopy for trauma airway management in suspected cervical spine injuries. *Anesthesia and Analgesia* 1992; **74**: 623.

26 Cooper S. D., Benumof J. L. and Ozaki G. T. Evaluation of the Bullard laryngoscope using the new intubating stylet: comparison with conventional laryngoscopy. *Anesthesia and Analgesia* 1994; **79**: 965.

27 Nolan J. P. and Wilson M. E. Orotracheal intubation in patients with potential cervical spine injuries. An indication for the gum elastic bougie. *Anaesthesia* 1993; **48**: 630.

28 Heath K. J. The effect on laryngoscopy of different cervical spine immobilisation techniques. *Anaesthesia* 1994; **49**: 843.

29 Hastings R. H. and Wood P. R. Head extension and laryngeal view during laryngoscopy with cervical spine stabilization maneuvers. *Anesthesiology* 1994; **80**: 825.

30 Laurent S. C., de Melo A. E. and Alexander-Williams J. M. The McCoy laryngoscope is superior to the Macintosh laryngoscope for laryngoscopy in

patients with potential cervical spine injuries. *Anaesthesia* 1996; **51:** 74.

31 Scannell G., Waxman K., Tominaga G., Barker S. and Annas C. Orotracheal intubation in trauma patients with cervical fractures. *Archives of Surgery* 1993; **128:** 903.

32 Wright S. W., Robinson G. G. and Wright M. B. Cervical spine injuries in blunt trauma patients requiring emergency intubation. *American Journal of Emergency Medicine* 1992; **10:** 104.

33 Suderman V. S., Crosby E. T. and Lui A. Elective oral intubation in cervical spine-injured adults. *Canadian Journal of Anaesthesiology* 1991; **38:** 785.

34 Rhee K. J., Green W., Holcroft J. W. and Mangili J. A. A. Oral intubation in the multiply injured patient: the risk of exacerbating spinal cord damage. *Annals of Emergency Medicine* 1990; **19:** 511.

35 Greene M. K., Roden R. and Hinchley G. The laryngeal mask airway. Two cases of pre-hospital trauma care. *Anaesthesia* 1992; **47:** 688.

36 Pennant J. H., Pace N. A. and Gajraj N. M. Role of the laryngeal mask airway in the immobile cervical spine. *Journal of Clinical Anesthesiology* 1993; **5:** 226.

37 Benumof J. L. Management of the difficult adult airway with special emphasis on awake tracheal intubation. *Anesthesiology* 1991; **75:** 1087.

38 Morris I. R. Fibreoptic intubation. *Canadian Journal of Anaesthesiology* 1994; **41:** 996.

39 Barriot P. and Riou B. Retrograde technique for tracheal intubation in trauma patients. *Critical Care Medicine* 1988; **16:** 712.

40 Asai T. Fibreoptic intubation through the laryngeal mask in an awake patient with cervical spine injury. *Anesthesia and Analgesia* 1993; **77:** 404.

# 19

# Difficulties at Tracheal Extubation

*Michael Hartley*

## INTRODUCTION

The major part of this book is devoted to the techniques used to achieve tracheal intubation and their associated problems. Tracheal extubation also produces well-defined pathophysiological responses and is associated with its own specific problems [1]. Indeed, while data comparing the incidence of problems at extubation to problems at intubation are lacking, the evidence of the *Survey of Anaesthetic Practice* [2], in which the anaesthetic details of over 10 000 patients from centres throughout the UK and Ireland were reviewed, suggests that the frequency of major airway problems at or after tracheal extubation may exceed the frequency of such problems relating to tracheal intubation. It was found that 2.4% of intubated patients developed signs of upper airway obstruction and/or cyanosis after extubation. Emergency reintubation in the immediate postextubation period was required in 0.8% of patients. This chapter therefore considers the pathophysiological responses and the problems associated with tracheal extubation. Proposed guidelines for the management of extubation and its associated problems are also discussed.

## PATHOPHYSIOLOGICAL RESPONSES TO EXTUBATION

Tracheal extubation may produce a variety of responses (Table 1). These responses are comparable to those that may result from tracheal intubation in the lightly anaesthetized patient. They range from local airway responses to systemic responses involving the cardiovascular and other organ systems. They are tolerated by the majority of patients, but may occasionally have significant consequences, especially in those with coexisting medical problems.

### Clinical Significance

Tracheal extubation sometimes precipitates upper airway obstruction due to a variety of causes (Table 2).

In the majority of cases, the cause of the upper

**Table 1** Pathophysiological effects of tracheal extubation.

Airway
  Obstruction
  Coughing
  Breathholding
Cardiovascular system
  Tachycardia
  Increased systemic arterial pressure
  Increased pulmonary arterial pressure
Central nervous system
  Increased intracranial pressure
Eye
  Increased intraocular pressure

**Table 2** Causes of upper airway obstruction after tracheal extubation.

Upper airway muscle relaxation
Foreign body aspiration
Surgical causes
  Haemorrhage
  Tracheomalacia
Laryngospasm
Laryngeal oedema
Vocal cord dysfunction

airway obstruction is reduced tone in the musculature supporting the upper airway due to the residual effects of general anaesthetic agents and muscle relaxants. Such airway obstruction is easily and rapidly corrected by manoeuvres such as head tilt and jaw support, or by the use of devices such as oropharyngeal and nasopharyngeal airways. However, if not treated immediately, it may become life-threatening as hypoxaemia and hypercarbia develop.

The airway responses to extubation include coughing and breathholding. These responses may also contribute to the development of hypoxaemia and hypercarbia. Sometimes they also compromise the surgical procedure, for example when extubation induces coughing in a patient who has undergone delicate upper airway or aural surgery.

The cardiovascular responses to extubation include significant increases in heart rate and systemic arterial pressure [3–6]. Pulmonary arterial pressure and pulmonary arterial occlusion pressure may also increase significantly at extubation [6]. The mechanism underlying these cardiovascular responses is almost certainly identical to that occurring at tracheal intubation, with an increase in sympathoadrenal activity producing increases in heart rate, myocardial contractility, systemic and pulmonary vascular resistances [7].

In patients with coronary artery disease, the haemodynamic responses to extubation may upset the balance between myocardial oxygen supply and demand and produce myocardial ischaemia. Biochemical and electrocardiographic evidence of myocardial ischaemia have been documented in some patients after extubation [8–10]. While such a response may have no adverse effect in the majority of patients, there will be a small number with coronary artery disease in whom a single ischaemic myocardial episode may be life-threatening.

In hypertensive patients, an exaggerated haemodynamic response to awakening and tracheal extubation has been described [11]. In the parturient with a severe hypertensive disorder of pregnancy, the cardiovascular response to extubation is as dramatic as the response to intubation [12]. Such hypertensive surges may result in acute left ventricular failure and pulmonary oedema, or in cerebral haemorrhage.

The secondary effects of the local and systemic responses to extubation include increases in intraocular and intracranial pressures. Significant increases in these variables have been recorded at extubation in patients who have undergone intraocular [13, 14] or intracranial [15] surgery. They are a consequence of the increase in systemic arterial pressure that may occur at extubation, as well as of the coughing and breathholding that often accompany extubation. These responses can lead to increases in intrathoracic and central venous pressures and reduced drainage from the ocular and cranial venous systems. In patients with pre-existing raised intraocular or intracranial pressure, further increases in pressure may precipitate organ ischaemia or oedema.

It is therefore appropriate, in some patients, to attempt to prevent or suppress these responses to extubation.

## Prevention

In some circumstances, the pathophysiological responses might best be prevented by avoiding tracheal intubation and hence extubation altogether. Consideration should always be given to the use of general anaesthetic techniques not requiring a tracheal tube, and to local or regional anaesthetic techniques (Table 3).

The use of the laryngeal mask airway (LMA),

**Table 3** Prevention of pathophysiological effects of tracheal extubation.

Avoid tracheal intubation/extubation
    Local or regional anaesthesia
    Laryngeal mask airway
Deep anaesthesia
Opioids
Lignocaine
Agents acting directly on cardiovascular system

when compared with the tracheal tube, is associated with reduced local and cardiovascular responses at both insertion and removal [16]. In patients undergoing intraocular surgery, the use of the LMA has been shown to minimize the intraocular pressure changes both at insertion and removal [13, 14]. Furthermore, it has been suggested that in patients who have undergone a surgical procedure that has required tracheal intubation, the LMA might be substituted for the tracheal tube, with the patient in a deep plane of anaesthesia or before the reversal of neuromuscular blockade, in order to reduce the local airway and cardiovascular responses to extubation [17]. Such use of the LMA cannot be recommended in those patients at risk of regurgitation and aspiration of gastric contents.

The pathophysiological responses may also be avoided by extubating the patient in a deep plane of anaesthesia achieved by the continued administration of inhalational or intravenous anaesthetic agents. However, these agents do produce depression of the protective laryngeal reflexes and, occasionally, difficulty in the management of the upper airway. Again, such an approach is not appropriate where there is an increased risk of aspiration of gastric contents or in the presence of a known difficult upper airway.

Opioids may be administered to minimize the responses to awakening and extubation. Alfentanil has been shown to minimize the cardiovascular responses to awakening, but prolongs the time to extubation, at which point it is no longer cardioprotective [18].

Lignocaine, administered by both the intravenous and intratracheal routes, has been used successfully to suppress the local airway and the cardiovascular responses to extubation in patients in a light plane of anaesthesia [3, 4, 19]. Evidence from other studies does not, however, support the ability of intravenous or intratracheal lignocaine to suppress these responses [5, 6].

Finally, the cardiovascular responses to extubation can be obtunded by pharmacological agents acting directly on the cardiovascular system. The cardioselective β-adrenoceptor antagonist esmolol, administered intravenously in a dose of 1.5 mg kg$^{-1}$ 2–5 mins before extubation, is particularly effective in attenuating the short-lived increases in heart rate and arterial pressure that occur at extubation, without producing bradycardia or hypotension in the recovery period [20].

## ASPIRATION OF GASTRIC CONTENTS AFTER EXTUBATION

Pulmonary aspiration of gastric contents, or other foreign bodies, at or immediately after extubation, may occur for several reasons. The residual effects of anaesthetic agents, opioids and muscle relaxants may all obtund the protective laryngeal reflexes. Furthermore, even in alert patients, there is evidence that the protective function of the larynx is impaired for at least 4 h after extubation [21].

In the light of these findings, the safest protection against aspiration in the extubation period must be to reduce the chances of gastric contents entering the larynx. This is best achieved by extubation with the patient placed in the lateral position with a head down tilt.

## DIFFICULT EXTUBATION

Difficulty in removing a tracheal tube at the end of a procedure is a rare, but dangerous, complication of tracheal intubation. Such difficulty may be attributed to one of three basic mechanisms:

- a failure to deflate the cuff;
- an excessively large cuff catching on the vocal cords;
- transfixion of the tube by a suture or a wire to an adjacent structure.

In the majority of cases the cause of difficulty is a failure to deflate the cuff. This may occur when a patient suddenly awakens and makes vigorous attempts to remove the tracheal tube. On other occasions, there may be a failure of the cuff deflating mechanism. This may occur after the tube inflating the cuff of the tracheal tube has been clipped off by a pair of artery forceps. The walls of the inflating tube remain stuck together and the cuff remains inflated, thus making extubation difficult. A similar mechanism has been reported where the inflating tube was kinked by the retaining bandage attached to the tracheal tube [22]. Other case reports have described the inadvertent separation of the pilot balloon and valve assembly from the tracheal tube cuff at various points along the inflating tube [23, 24]. The cuff remains inflated and extubation is impossible (Fig. 1a). In this situation, deflation of the cuff may be achieved by performing direct laryngoscopy and withdrawing the tracheal tube until the cuff rests against the vocal cords. It may then be possible to insert a syringe and needle into the stump of the

inflating tube under direct vision, deflate the cuff and remove the tracheal tube (Fig. 1b). If this approach fails, it may be possible to deflate the cuff by puncturing it with a needle passed through the cricothyroid membrane, before removing the tracheal tube [23].

Difficult tracheal extubation may also follow forceful intubation with an inappropriately large tracheal tube [25], or may follow uneventful intubation with an appropriately sized tracheal tube in patients with a laryngeal or tracheal abnormality [26, 27]. In such circumstances, rotation of the tracheal tube [25] or manipulation of the larynx and tracheal tube under direct vision [26] may allow successful extubation.

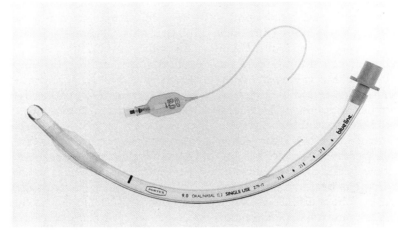

**Figure 1**    (a) The cuff inflating tube has become disconnected from the tracheal tube. The cuff remains inflated and tracheal extubation is impossible.

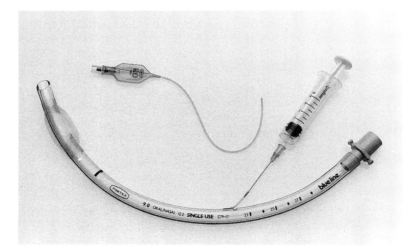

**Figure 1**    (b) The cuff is deflated by inserting a needle attached to a syringe into the stump of the cuff inflating tube under direct vision.

Several instances of difficult extubation have been recorded as a result of sleeve formation by the cuffs of tracheal tubes [28–31]. The sleeve is formed after the tracheal tube cuff is deflated and folds on itself during attempted extubation. The increase in the external diameter becomes too great for easy passage through the vocal cords. Should this occur, reinsertion, rotation and traction on the tracheal tube may allow successful extubation. If not, reinsertion and inflation of the cuff may smooth out the fold in the cuff and allow extubation after further deflation [28]. Other techniques using skin hooks [29] or forceps [30] to reduce the cuff fold have also been described.

Most reports of difficult extubation are due to fixation of the tracheal tube to adjacent structures, and are associated particularly with orofacial surgery. Surgical perforation and fixation of a nasotracheal tube has been described with both surgical wires [32, 33, 84] and screws [34]. It has been recommended that when the possibility of external fixation of the tube during surgery exists, the tube should be moved up and down slightly to ensure that it has not been accidentally fixed [32]. Others have suggested the routine passage of a suction catheter down the tracheal tube when wires or screws have been inserted in a blind fashion [33]. More recently, the use of the flexible fibreoptic bronchoscope has been recommended to confirm the integrity of the tracheal tube [34]. However, a case has been reported where a nasotracheal tube could not be removed despite these recommendations and manoeuvres [35]. The tube

was subsequently removed without difficulty after the cuff inflating port was cut. After extubation, it was discovered that a Kirschner wire had passed between the nasotracheal tube and the cuff inflating port, thus preventing extubation. A similar case has also been recorded when a nasogastric tube became entangled with the same port in the nasopharynx [36]. Extubation was prevented by tightening of a loop which wedged the inflating tube adaptor between the walls of the nose and the nasotracheal tube. Extubation was only possible after the inflating port was cut just behind the adaptor.

A further report describes a nasotracheal tube being partially severed during a maxillary osteotomy procedure [37]. The partially cut tube formed a 'barb' that caught on the posterior aspect of the hard palate when extubation was attempted (Fig. 2). Tracheal extubation was only possible after the removal of the surgical sutures and wires.

Trauma to the larynx is particularly likely after a difficult extubation. It has been suggested that direct laryngoscopy should be performed in order to determine the extent of laryngeal damage if attempts to remove a tracheal tube have been forceful or prolonged [28].

Endobronchial tubes may also be fixed by the surgeon during thoracic surgery. A case of fatal circulatory collapse has been described after the removal of a Carlens double lumen tube which had been accidentally sutured to the pulmonary artery [38]. It was subsequently recommended

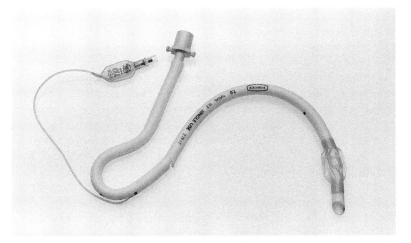

**Figure 2**  A nasotracheal tube partially severed during a maxillary osteotomy procedure. The tube formed a 'barb' that caught on the posterior aspect of the hard palate when extubation was attempted.

that when endobronchial extubation proves difficult, fibreoptic bronchoscopy should be performed to inspect the tube for a tethering suture. More recently, a similar case presented as an impossible extubation of a left-sided double lumen tube [39]. Fibreoptic bronchoscopy revealed adequate cuff deflation and no apparent cause of tube fixation, although the presence of blood in the left lumen was noted. A further vigorous attempt at extubation resulted in fresh bleeding from the left lumen and surgical fixation of the tube was strongly suspected. The surgical wound was reopened and the tube freed after the removal of some sutures. Subsequent endobronchial extubation was uneventful.

## UPPER AIRWAY OBSTRUCTION AFTER EXTUBATION

The majority of problems presenting at or immediately after extubation are characterized by the development of upper airway obstruction (Table 2). The immediate management of such problems involves the recovery and maintenance of an adequate airway, while the longer-term management varies according to the particular cause of the upper airway obstruction. It is always essential, however, to consider and exclude causes of airway obstruction relating to foreign bodies such as throat packs, dentures and blood clots. All require immediate removal.

In some patients, the airway obstruction occurs as a consequence of the surgical procedure as, for example, haemorrhage complicating thyroid surgery [40] or other procedures in and around the neck [41, 42]. The upper airway obstruction in such cases probably results from laryngeal and pharyngeal oedema secondary to venous and lymphatic congestion rather than compression of the trachea by haematoma [43]. In the case of post-thyroidectomy bleeding, immediate release of the wound sutures may produce dramatic improvement. Definitive treatment always requires tracheal intubation followed by surgical decompression and control of the source of bleeding.

In other patients, the airway obstruction may occur as a consequence of tracheomalacia, a weakening of the supporting structures in the trachea. A case of tracheomalacia has been described in a 14-year-old boy with tuberculous disease of the cervical spine [44]. Respiratory obstruction only occurred while attempting extubation after retracting the tracheal tube 4–5 cm from the carina. It was corrected by reinserting the tracheal tube to within 1–2 cm of the carina. It was recommended that, in such cases, tracheal extubation should be performed slowly. If respiratory obstruction should occur, the tracheal tube should be repositioned and retained until surgical correction of the lesion is possible. Tracheomalacia may more commonly result from prolonged compression by an expanding thyroid goitre, particularly within the confines of the thoracic inlet. The cartilaginous rings supporting the trachea may be weakened or even destroyed, compromising the structural integrity of the upper airway after the extrinsic compression is relieved. Tracheal collapse usually occurs after extubation and requires emergency reintubation. The subsequent options include surgical resection of the affected segment of the trachea, internal or external tracheal support, and/or airway diversion below the affected trachea through a tracheostomy [45].

However, the cause of upper airway obstruction after tracheal extubation in the majority of patients is laryngospasm. Laryngeal oedema or vocal cord paralysis occur only rarely.

## LARYNGOSPASM

Laryngospasm has been defined as the occlusion of the glottis by the action of the intrinsic laryngeal muscles [46]. It is the result of a protective reflex, mediated by the vagus nerves, which exists to prevent foreign material entering the tracheobronchial tree.

Laryngospasm is the commonest cause of postextubation upper airway obstruction. It is particularly common in children after upper airway surgery, for example after adenotonsillectomy, where the incidence is approximately 20% [47, 48]. It is precipitated by local irritation of the vocal cords by secretions or blood, when the plane of anaesthesia is insufficient to prevent the laryngospasm reflex but too deep to allow co-ordinated coughing. Thus, it is more likely to occur when a patient is extubated in a plane of anaesthesia somewhere between an awake and a deeply anaesthetized state.

The evidence relating the incidence of laryngospasm and arterial oxygen desaturation to tracheal extubation performed in awake compared with deeply anaesthetized patients is conflicting. One study suggests that in children undergoing minor surgery not involving the airway, awake extubation is associated with a greater likelihood of arterial oxygen desaturation than is extubation while deeply anaesthetized [49]. There is no significant difference in the incidence of airway-related complications between the various agents if the trachea is extubated while the children are deeply anaesthetized. However, isoflurane is associated with more airway-related complications compared with halothane in children who are extubated awake. Another study, however, did not demonstrate any significant difference in the incidence of such complications between awake and anaesthetized extubations after either upper airway or other surgery in a similar group of children [50].

The technique used to achieve extubation may also influence the incidence of laryngospasm. It is common practice to deflate the tracheal tube cuff and perform extubation after maximal inflation of the lungs with oxygen. This manoeuvre fills the lungs to their total capacity, producing a forceful expiration immediately after extubation which clears the vocal cords and upper airway of blood and other debris which might precipitate laryngospasm.

Lignocaine has been used successfully in both children and adults to prevent extubation laryngospasm after upper airway surgery [47, 51]. In one study, lignocaine was administered intravenously before extubation, which subsequently took place at a consistent depth of anaesthesia, namely when signs of swallowing activity developed. No beneficial effects could be demonstrated [48]. It seems likely that any benefits of lignocaine result from a central increase in the depth of anaesthesia. Therefore, if lignocaine is to be used to prevent laryngospasm associated with extubation, it should be given before signs of swallowing activity occur.

Laryngospasm presents clinically as a spectrum ranging from mild inspiratory stridor to complete upper airway obstruction. Although the former is not life-threatening it may rapidly progress to the latter if incorrectly managed. The development of complete upper airway obstruction results in loss of the inspiratory stridor and it is of paramount importance that this 'silence' is not mistaken for an improvement in the clinical state.

## Management of Laryngospasm

Any precipitating cause should be identified and removed by performing direct laryngoscopy and suctioning of the laryngopharynx. Subsequently:

- 100% oxygen must be administered, with continuous positive airway pressure, until the laryngospasm disappears; or
- the plane of anaesthesia may be deepened by using intravenous or inhalational anaesthetic agents until the laryngospasm reflex is abolished.

However, as neither method is successful on every occasion, it may be necessary to administer a short acting neuromuscular blocking agent to improve oxygenation or to facilitate tracheal intubation. A very small dose of suxamethonium (0.1 mg kg$^{-1}$) has been recommended as a reliable treatment of laryngospasm, while having little effect on spontaneous ventilatory effort [52]. Other anaesthetists administer a larger dose of suxamethonium (1 mg kg$^{-1}$), often preceded by intravenous atropine if repeated doses are required or if there is hypoxia. The indication to establish muscle paralysis and ventilation should be guided by the arterial oxyhaemoglobin saturation level indicated by pulse oximetry (Table 4).

Other measures that have been used to suppress the laryngospasm reflex after extubation include lignocaine [47] and diazepam [53] by intravenous injection. Doxapram (1.5 mg kg$^{-1}$) has also been successfully used to treat postextubation laryngospasm [54]. In this author's experience, the administration of intravenous doxapram by increments of 0.2 mg kg$^{-1}$ to a maximum dose of 1 mg kg$^{-1}$ has proved a reliable treatment. The increased

**Table 4** Guidelines for management of postextubation laryngospasm.

| |
|---|
| Direct laryngoscopy and suctioning of pharyngeal debris |
| Administer 100% oxygen with continuous positive airway pressure |
| Administer doxapram by increments of 0.2 mg kg$^{-1}$ to a maximum dose of 1 mg kg$^{-1}$ |
| If SaO$_2$ < 95% and falling, administer general anaesthetic agent ± suxamethonium 0.1 mg kg$^{-1}$ |
| If SaO$_2$ < 85% and falling, administer general anaesthetic agent + suxamethonium 1 mg kg$^{-1}$, intubate and ventilate. |

*Note*: Intravenous atropine 10–20 µg kg$^{-1}$ is recommended before suxamethonium in children, and in adults if repeated doses are required or there is hypoxia.

respiratory drive produced by doxapram appears to be sufficient to overcome the laryngospasm reflex. Doxapram may also have a role, therefore, in the prevention of laryngospasm.

## LARYNGEAL OEDEMA

Laryngeal oedema is an important cause of post-extubation upper airway obstruction in children, particularly in neonates and infants. The oedema may be localized to the supraglottic, retroarytenoidal or subglottic regions [44].

- *Supraglottic oedema.* Oedema occurs in the loose connective tissue on the anterior surface of the epiglottis and in the aryepiglottic folds. The epiglottis may be displaced posteriorly by the swelling, blocking the glottic aperture on inspiration and resulting in severe acute upper airway obstruction.
- *Retroarytenoidal oedema.* Oedema occurs in the loose connective tissue just below the vocal cords and behind the arytenoid cartilages. Movement of the arytenoid cartilages is thus restricted and this limits abduction of the vocal cords on inspiration.
- *Subglottic oedema.* The subglottic region has fragile respiratory epithelium with loose submucosal connective tissue that is easily traumatized and prone to oedema. The non-expandable cricoid cartilage, which encircles the subglottic region, is the narrowest part of the airway in children and limits the outwards expansion of the oedema.

Subglottic oedema is therefore a particular problem in neonates and infants as a minor degree of oedema may produce a significant reduction in the internal laryngeal cross-sectional area. This area in the newborn is no greater than 14 mm$^2$ and a 1 mm thick layer of oedema in the subglottic region will reduce this area to 5 mm$^2$, which significantly compromises the upper airway [55]. In an older child or an adult, a similar degree of oedema would not cause such significant upper airway obstruction.

Laryngeal oedema after extubation occurs in approximately 1% of patients under the age of 17; children under the age of four are particularly susceptible [56]. The use of a tight-fitting tracheal tube, the occurrence of trauma at intubation, a duration of intubation of greater than 1 h, coughing or bucking on the tracheal tube or a change in position of the patient's head and neck during surgery are all positive risk factors [56].

Laryngeal oedema presents as inspiratory stridor, usually within 6 h of extubation. In patients who develop laryngeal oedema, diminishing stridor may represent impending complete upper airway obstruction rather than resolving oedema.

## Management of Laryngeal Oedema

Management of laryngeal oedema after extubation depends upon the degree of airway obstruction (Table 5).

Mild cases may respond to conservative measures with inhalation of a warmed, humidified and oxygen-enriched gas mixture. Nebulized adrenaline 1:1000 has also been successfully employed [57–59]. Relief is dramatic but short-lived and further nebulized adrenaline may be required at regular intervals. The value of systemic steroids is less clear. Intravenous dexamethasone (0.25 mg kg$^{-1}$ immediately followed by 0.1 mg kg$^{-1}$ 6-hourly for 24 h) has been recommended for the treatment of postextubation laryngeal oedema [60], although studies in both children and adults indicate that dexamethasone is ineffective in the prevention of postextubation laryngeal oedema [61–63].

More severe cases of postextubation oedema, or cases which fail to respond to the above measures, may require a period of reintubation with a smaller tracheal tube.

In the older patient who unexpectedly develops laryngeal oedema after extubation, it is important to consider the possibility of dislocation of the arytenoid cartilages, which may occur as a consequence of trauma at any stage of the intubation/extubation processes [64–66]. Management requires immediate reintubation. The subsequent treatment involves either early reduction of the

**Table 5** Guidelines for management of postextubation laryngeal oedema.

| |
| --- |
| Direct laryngoscopy to confirm diagnosis |
| Management dependent upon severity |
|    Humidified and warmed oxygen-enriched air |
|    Nebulized adrenaline 1:1000 0.5 ml kg$^{-1}$ (repeat at 1–4 hourly intervals) |
|    Intravenous dexamethasone 0.25 mg kg$^{-1}$ stat followed by 0.1 mg kg$^{-1}$ 6-hourly for 24 h |
| Reintubation with a smaller tracheal tube |

arytenoids by application of gentle pressure with a laryngeal spatula or prolonged tracheal intubation, or even tracheostomy. These measures prevent arytenoid movement and enable healing of the dislocated joint [64].

## VOCAL CORD DYSFUNCTION

Vocal cord paralysis, following trauma to the vagus nerves or their branches, is a rare cause of upper airway obstruction after extubation. It is usually described after surgical procedures involving the head and neck, the thyroid gland or the thoracic cavity. However, it has also occurred unexpectedly where surgery was remote from the head and neck [67, 68]. It has been suggested that tracheal intubation itself may result in nerve damage leading to vocal cord paralysis [69]. The tracheal tube cuff may compress the anterior branch of the recurrent laryngeal nerve where it lies beneath the mucosa and immediately medial to the lamina of the thyroid cartilage [70].

Unilateral vocal cord paralysis is usually a benign condition. Bilateral vocal cord paralysis, however, is a more serious condition which may present as upper airway obstruction immediately after extubation. The usual methods of relieving upper airway obstruction are not effective, although assisted ventilation with a facemask or LMA may overcome the upper airway obstruction. Laryngoscopy reveals motionless vocal cords which lie adducted with a very narrow glottic aperture. Immediate insertion of a tracheal tube eliminates the upper airway obstruction. Recovery is usual but often delayed, and a tracheostomy may be required until vocal cord function is restored.

## PULMONARY OEDEMA AFTER UPPER AIRWAY OBSTRUCTION

Pulmonary oedema may follow acute upper airway obstruction after tracheal extubation [71–80]. The pathogenesis of the pulmonary oedema is multifactorial, although the markedly negative intrathoracic pressure generated during an episode of acute upper airway obstruction is probably the dominant mechanism [77].

The onset of the pulmonary oedema is usually within minutes of either the development of acute upper airway obstruction or following the relief of the obstruction. Spontaneous resolution is usual over a period of a few hours. The essentials of management are the maintenance of the airway by tracheal intubation, administration of supplementary oxygen with continuous positive airway pressure and, if necessary, institution of positive pressure ventilation until the condition resolves. The majority of cases do not require either aggressive haemodynamic monitoring or drug therapy.

## GUIDELINES FOR MANAGEMENT OF EXTUBATION

Major problems can occur after tracheal extubation. In particular, extubation may precipitate major difficulties in the management of the upper airway. A number of other pathophysiological changes associated with anaesthesia and surgery may, at the same time, have significant adverse effects on respiratory function, resulting in a tendency to develop significant hypoxaemia [81]. It is essential, therefore, that all anaesthetists adopt a logical approach to guide patients through this vulnerable period.

The following factors warrant attention whenever extubation is contemplated:

- pulse oximetry and capnography should be continued throughout the extubation period;
- suppression of the pathophysiological responses to extubation should always be considered;
- recovery from neuromuscular blockade should be confirmed, preferably by an assessment of the response to peripheral nerve stimulation, before performing extubation;
- extubation should be performed with the patient either awake or deeply anaesthetized. Extubation in intermediate planes of anaesthesia should be avoided to minimize the likelihood of developing postextubation laryngospasm.

In many clinical situations, the anaesthetist is able to choose between an 'awake' and a 'deep' extubation. Suggested guidelines for the management of extubation in the awake patient and in the deeply anaesthetized patient are presented in Tables 6 and 7.

Extubation of the deeply anaesthetized patient affords some protection against the pathophysiological responses to extubation and their harmful consequences. However, it is contraindicated in

**Table 6** Guidelines for management of awake extubation after artificial ventilation.

---

100% oxygen for 2–5 min
Direct laryngoscopy and suction
Discontinue anaesthetic agents and reverse residual
    effects of muscle relaxants
Lateral position with head down tilt
Demonstrate return of consciousness and adequate
    spontaneous ventilation
Consider stimulation of the respiratory centre with
    doxapram
Deflate cuff and extubate at end of inspiration
Transfer to recovery area breathing oxygen-enriched air

---

**Table 7** Guidelines for management of 'deep' extubation after artificial and spontaneous ventilation.

---

100% oxygen for 2–5 min
Maintain adminstration of anaesthetic agent
Direct laryngoscopy and suction
Reverse residual effects of muscle relaxants
Lateral position and head down tilt
Demonstrate adequate spontaneous ventilation
Deflate cuff and extubate at end of inspiration
Consider insertion of laryngeal mask airway
Discontinue anaesthetic agent
Transfer to recovery area breathing oxygen-enriched air
Patient remains in recovery area until awake

---

**Table 8** Contraindications to 'deep' extubation.

---

Increased risk of aspiration of gastric contents
Known difficult airway
Known difficult intubation
The obese patient

---

those patients with an increased risk of aspiration of gastric contents or with a potential difficulty in airway management (Table 8). Such patients should generally be extubated awake and, if necessary, the pathophysiological responses to extubation controlled pharmacologically.

It is also important that the anaesthetist should formulate an airway management plan to be implemented if it is not possible to maintain an adequate airway or achieve adequate ventilation and oxygenation after extubation. A range of drugs and equipment identical to that required at intubation should be immediately available at the time of extubation.

In the majority of patients reintubation, if necessary, can be accomplished with direct laryngoscopy. In those patients who are known to be difficult to intubate however, an alternative

strategy is indicated. In these patients, consideration should be given to the use of a stylet, for example, a gum elastic bougie inserted through the lumen of the tracheal tube into the trachea before extubation to serve as a guide for speedy reintubation [82]. Such stylets must be rigid enough to facilitate intubation. In addition, they may be hollow, thereby enabling oxygenation by insufflation or jet ventilation. The use of such a device allows a gradual, reversible withdrawal of airway support [83].

---

## KEY POINTS

- Difficulty with the management of the airway may develop at or immediately after tracheal extubation. The incidence of major airway problems at this time probably exceeds the incidence of similar problems relating to tracheal intubation.

- Drugs and equipment to facilitate reintubation should always be available when extubation is to be performed.

- Tracheal extubation should always be preceded by the administration of 100% oxygen for a period of 2–5 min to minimize the occurrence of hypoxaemia in the immediate postextubation period.

- Complete recovery from neuromuscular blockade should be established before extubation is performed.

- Tracheal extubation of the patient who is known to be difficult to intubate should be performed awake, and consideration given to the use of a bougie to facilitate reintubation, if this should prove to be necessary.

- In other patients, the choice between an 'awake' and a 'deep' extubation must be made. Extubation of a deeply anaesthetized patient minimizes the pathophysiological responses to extubation, but may result in the development of upper airway obstruction or the aspiration of regurgitated gastric contents.

# KEY POINTS (CONTINUED)

- Laryngospasm is the commonest cause of postextubation upper airway obstruction and may result in significant hypoxaemia. The incidence can be minimized by avoiding extubation during intermediate planes of anaesthesia. Management should follow a graded approach, guided by the continuous measurement of arterial oxygen saturation.

- Laryngeal oedema and vocal cord dysfunction are rarer causes of postextubation upper airway obstruction.

- Pulmonary oedema may follow upper airway obstruction after extubation, whatever its aetiology. Management is supportive until spontaneous recovery occurs.

- Tracheal extubation may occasionally prove difficult. Forceful attempts at extubation may result in significant laryngeal trauma.

# REFERENCES

1 Hartley M. and Vaughan R. S. Problems associated with tracheal extubation. *British Journal of Anaesthesia* 1993; **71:** 561.
2 Association of Anaesthetists of Great Britain and Ireland. *Survey of Anaesthetic Practice.* 1988.
3 Bidwai A. V., Bidwai V. A., Rogers C. R. and Stanley T. H. Blood pressure and pulse rate responses to endotracheal extubation with and without prior injection of lidocaine. *Anesthesiology* 1979; **51:** 171.
4 Bidwai A. V., Stanley T. H. and Bidwai V. A. Blood pressure and pulse rate responses to extubation with and without prior topical tracheal anaesthesia. *Canadian Anaesthetists Society Journal* 1978; **25:** 416.
5 Edde R. R. Cardiovascular responses to extubation. *Anesthesiology* 1979; **51:** S195.
6 Wohlner E. C., Usubiaga L. J., Jacoby R. M. and Hill G. E. Cardiovascular effects of extubation. *Anesthesiology* 1979; **51:** S194.
7 Lowrie A., Johnston P. L., Fell D. and Robinson S. L. Cardiovascular and plasma catecholamine responses at tracheal extubation. *British Journal of Anaesthesia* 1992; **68:** 261.
8 Elia S., Liu P., Chrusciel C., Hilgenberg A., Skourtis C. and Lappas D. Effects of tracheal extubation on coronary blood flow, myocardial metabolism and systemic haemodynamic responses. *Canadian Journal of Anaesthesiology* 1989; **36:** 2.
9 Wellwood M., Aylmer A., Teasdale S. *et al.* Extubation and myocardial ischemia. *Anesthesiology* 1984; **61:** A132.
10 Edwards N. D., Alford A. M., Dobson P. M. S., Peacock J. E. and Reilly C. S. Myocardial ischaemia during tracheal intubation and extubation. *British Journal of Anaesthesia* 1994; **73:** 537.
11 Stone J. G., Foex P., Sear J. W., Johnson L. L., Khambatta H. J. and Triner L. Risk of myocardial ischaemia during anaesthesia in treated and untreated hypertensive patients. *British Journal of Anaesthesia* 1988; **61:** 675.
12 Hodgkinson P., Husain F. J. and Hayashi R. H. Systemic and pulmonary blood pressure during Caesarean section in parturients with gestational hypertension. *Canadian Anaesthetists Society Journal* 1980; **27:** 389.
13 Lamb K., James M. F. M. and Janicki P. K. The laryngeal mask airway for intraocular surgery: effects on intraocular pressure and stress responses. *British Journal of Anaesthesia* 1992; **69:** 143.
14 Holden R., Morsman C. D. G., Butler J., Clark G. S., Hughes D. S. and Bacon P. J. Intra-ocular pressure changes using the laryngeal mask airway and tracheal tube. *Anaesthesia* 1991; **46:** 922.
15 Leech P., Barker J. and Fitch W. Changes in intracranial pressure and systemic arterial pressure during the termination of anaesthesia. *British Journal of Anaesthesia* 1974; **46:** 315.
16 Cork R. C., Depa R. M. and Standen J. R. Prospective comparison of use of the laryngeal mask and endotracheal tube for ambulatory surgery. *Anesthesia and Analgesia* 1994; **79:** 719.
17 George S. L. and Blogg C. E. Role of the LMA in tracheal extubation? *British Journal of Anaesthesia* 1994; **72:** 610.
18 Fuhrman T. M., Ewell C. L., Pippin W. D. and Weaver J. M. Comparison of the efficacy of esmolol and alfentanil to attenuate the haemodynamic responses to emergence and extubation. *Journal of Clinical Anaesthesia* 1992; **4:** 444.
19 Wallin G., Cassuto J., Hogstrom S. *et al.* Effects of lidocaine infusion on the sympathetic response to abdominal surgery. *Anesthesia and Analgesia* 1987; **66:** 1008.
20 Dyson A., Isaac P. A., Pennant J. H., Giesecke A. H. and Lipton J. M. Esmolol attenuates cardiovascular responses to extubation. *Anesthesia and Analgesia* 1990; **71:** 675.
21 Burgess G. E., Cooper J. R., Marino R. J., Peuler M. J. and Warriner R. A. Laryngeal competence after tracheal extubation. *Anesthesiology* 1979; **51:** 73.
22 Tanski J. and James R. H. Difficult extubation due to a kinked pilot tube. *Anaesthesia* 1986; **41:** 1060.
23 Tavakoli M. and Corssen G. An unusual case of dif-

ficult extubation. *Anesthesiology* 1976; **45:** 552.

24 Brock-Utne J. G., Jaffe R. A., Robins B. and Ratner E. Difficulty in extubation. A cause for concern. *Anaesthesia* 1992; **47:** 229.

25 Tashayod M. and Oskoui B. A case of difficult extubation. *Anesthesiology* 1973; **39:** 337.

26 Sprung J., Conley S. F. and Brown M. Unusual cause of difficulty extubation. *Anesthesiology* 1991; **74:** 796.

27 Asai T. Difficult tracheal extubation in a patient with an unsuspected congenital subglottic stenosis. *Anaesthesia* 1995; **50:** 243.

28 Lall N. G. Difficult extubation. A fold in the endotracheal cuff. *Anaesthesia* 1980; **35:** 500.

29 Grover V. K. Difficulty in extubation. *Anaesthesia* 1985; **40:** 198.

30 Khan R. M., Khan T. Z., Ali M. and Khan M. S. A. Difficult extubation. *Anaesthesia* 1988; **43:** 515.

31 Mishra P. and Scott D. L. Difficulty at extubation of the trachea. *Anaesthesia* 1983; **38:** 811.

32 Lee C., Schwartz S. and Mok M. S. Difficult extubation due to transfixation of a nasotracheal tube by a Kirschner wire. *Anesthesiology* 1977; **46:** 427.

33 Bhaskar P. B., Scheffer R. B. and Drummond J. N. Bilateral fixation of a nasotracheal tube by transfacial Kirschner wires. *Journal of Oral and Maxillofacial Surgery* 1987; **45:** 805.

34 Lang S., Johnson D. H., Lanigan D. T. and Ha H. Difficult tracheal extubation. *Canadian Journal of Anaesthesiology* 1989; **36:** 340.

35 Hilley M. D., Henderson R. B. and Giesecke A. H. Difficult extubation of the trachea. *Anesthesiology* 1983; **59:** 149.

36 Fagraeus L. Difficult extubation following nasotracheal intubation. *Anesthesiology* 1978; **49:** 43.

37 Schwartz L. B., Sordill W. C., Liebers R. M. and Schwab W. Difficulty in removal of accidentally cut endotracheal tube. *Journal of Oral and Maxillofacial Surgery* 1982; **40:** 518.

38 Dryden G. E. Circulatory collapse after pneumonectomy (an unusual complication from the use of a Carlens catheter): case report. *Anesthesia and Analgesia* 1977; **56:** 451.

39 Akers J. A. and Riley R. H. Failed extubation due to 'sutured' double-lumen tube. *Anaesthesia and Intensive Care* 1990; **18:** 577.

40 Wade J. S. Cecil Joll Lecture, 1979. Respiratory obstruction in thyroid surgery. *Annals of the Royal College of Surgeons of England* 1980; **62:** 15.

41 Bukht D. and Langford R. M. Airway obstruction after surgery in the neck. *Anaesthesia* 1983; **38:** 389.

42 Cook L. B. and Varley S. Fatal tracheal compression after haemorrhage into the axilla. *British Journal of Anaesthesia* 1992; **69:** 322.

43 Hare R. M. Respiratory obstruction after thyroidectomy. *Anaesthesia* 1982; **37:** 1136.

44 Blanc V. F. and Tremblay N. A. G. The complications of tracheal intubation: A new classification with a review of the literature. *Anesthesia and Analgesia* 1974; **53:** 202.

45 Geelhoed G. W. Tracheomalacia from compressing goiter: management after thyroidectomy. *Surgery* 1988; **104:** 1100.

46 Rex M. A. E. A review of the structural and functional basis of laryngospasm and a discussion of the nerve pathways involved in the reflex and its clinical significance in man and animals. *British Journal of Anaesthesia* 1970; **42:** 891.

47 Baraka A. Intravenous lidocaine controls extubation laryngospasm in children. *Anesthesia and Analgesia* 1978; **57:** 506.

48 Leicht P., Wisborg T. and Chraemmer-Jorgensen B. Does intravenous lidocaine prevent laryngospasm after extubation in children? *Anesthesia and Analgesia* 1985; **64:** 1193.

49 Pounder D. R., Blackstock D. and Steward D. J. Tracheal extubation in children: halothane versus isoflurane, anesthetized versus awake. *Anesthesiology* 1991; **74:** 653.

50 Patel R. I., Hannallah R. S., Norden J., Casey W. F. and Verghese S. T. Emergency airway complications in children: a comparison of tracheal extubution in awake and deeply anesthetized patients. *Anesthesia and Analgesia* 1991; **73:** 266.

51 Gefke K., Andersen L. W. and Friesel E. Lidocaine given intravenously as a suppressant of cough and laryngospasm in connection with extubation after tonsillectomy. *Acta Anaesthesiologica Scandinavica* 1983; **27:** 111.

52 Chung D. C. and Rowbottom S. J. A very small dose of suxamethonium relieves laryngospasm. *Anaesthesia* 1993; **48:** 229.

53 Gilbertson A. A. Laryngeal spasm. *British Journal of Anaesthesia* 1993; **71:** 168.

54 Owen H. Postextubation laryngospasm abolished by doxapram. *Anaesthesia* 1982; **37:** 1112.

55 Sumner E. Respiration. In: Dickson J. A. S. (ed.) *Clinical Paediatric Anatomy.* London: Blackwell. 1984.

56 Kota B. V., Jeon I. S., Andre J. M., MacKay I. and Smith R. M. Postintubation croup in children. *Anesthesia and Analgesia* 1977; **56:** 501.

57 Child C. S. B. Nebulised adrenaline. *Anaesthesia* 1987; **42:** 322.

58 Choudhry A. K. Nebulised adrenaline. *Anaesthesia* 1987; **42:** 321.

59 Gwinnutt C. L. and Lord W. D. Nebulised adrenaline. *Anaesthesia* 1987; **42:** 320.

60 Hatch D. J. Acute upper airway obstruction in children. In: Atkinson R. S., Adams A. P. (eds) *Recent Advances in Anaesthesia and Analgesia.* Edinburgh: Churchill Livingstone. 1985; vol. 15, p. 133.

61 Darmon J. Y., Rauss A., Dreyfuss D. *et al.* Evaluation of risk factors for laryngeal edema after tracheal

extubation in adults and its prevention by dexamethasone. *Anesthesiology* 1992; **77:** 245.

62 Ferrara T. B., Georgieff M. K., Ebert J. and Fisher J. B. Routine use of dexamethasone for the prevention of postextubation respiratory distress. *Journal of Perinatology* 1989; **9:** 287.

63 Tellez D. W., Galvis A. G., Storgion S. A., Amer H. N., Hoseyni M. and Deakers T. W. Dexamethasone in the prevention of postextubation stridor in children. *Journal of Pediatrics* 1991; **118:** 289.

64 Castella X., Gilabert J. and Perez C. Arytenoid dislocation after tracheal intubation: an unusual cause of acute respiratory failure? *Anesthesiology* 1991; **74:** 613.

65 Tolley N. S., Cheesman T. D., Morgan D. and Brookes G. B. Dislocated arytenoid: an intubation induced injury. *Annals of the Royal College of Surgeons of England* 1990; **72:** 353.

66 Chatterji S., Gupta N. R. and Mishra T. R. Valvular glottic obstruction following extubation. *Anaesthesia* 1984; **39:** 246.

67 Gibbin K. P. and Egginton M. J. Bilateral vocal cord paralysis following endotracheal intubation. *British Journal of Anaesthesia* 1981; **53:** 1091.

68 Holley H. S. and Gildea J. E. Vocal cord paralysis after tracheal intubation. *Journal of the American Medical Association* 1971; **215:** 281.

69 Cavo J. W. True vocal cord paralysis following intubation. *Laryngoscope* 1985; **95:** 1352.

70 Ellis P. D. M. and Pallister W. K. Recurrent laryngeal nerve palsy and endotracheal intubation. *Journal of Laryngology and Otology* 1975; **89:** 823.

71 Barin E. S., Stevenson I. F. and Donnelly G. L. Pulmonary oedema following acute upper airway obstruction. *Anaesthesia and Intensive Care* 1986; **14:** 54.

72 Cozanitis D. A., Leijala M., Pesonen E. and Zaki H. A. Acute pulmonary oedema due to laryngeal spasm. *Anaesthesia* 1982; **37:** 1198.

73 Dohi S., Okubo N. and Kondo Y. Pulmonary oedema after airway obstruction due to bilateral vocal cord paralysis. *Canadian Journal of Anaesthesiology* 1991; **38:** 492.

74 Frank L. P. and Schreiber G. C. Pulmonary edema following acute upper airway obstruction. *Anesthesiology* 1986; **65:** 106.

75 Jenkins J. G. Pulmonary edema following laryngospasm. *Anesthesiology* 1984; **60:** 611.

76 Kamal R. S. and Agha S. Acute pulmonary oedema. A complication of upper airway obstruction. *Anaesthesia* 1984; **39:** 464.

77 Lang S. A., Duncan P. G., Shephard D. A. E. and Ha H. C. Pulmonary oedema associated with airway obstruction. *Canadian Journal of Anaesthesiology* 1990; **37:** 210.

78 Lee K. W. T. and Downes J. J. Pulmonary edema secondary to laryngospasm in children. *Anesthesiology* 1983; **59:** 347.

79 Melnick B. M. Postlaryngospasm pulmonary edema in adults. *Anesthesiology* 1984; **60:** 516.

80 Scherer R., Dreyer P. and Jorch G. Pulmonary edema due to partial upper airway obstruction in a child. *Intensive Care Medicine* 1988; **14:** 661.

81 Miller K. A., Harkin C. P. and Bailey P. L. Postoperative tracheal extubation. *Anesthesia and Analgesia* 1995; **80:** 149.

82 Caplan R. A., Benumof J. L. and Berry F. A. Practice guidelines for management of the difficult airway. *Anesthesiology* 1993; **78:** 597.

83 Benumof J. L. Management of the difficult adult airway. *Anesthesiology* 1991; **75:** 1087.

84 Munro F. J., Makin A. P. and Reid, J. Airway problems after carotoid endarterectomy. *British Journal of Anaesthesia* 1996; **76:** 156.

# 20

# Teaching Intubation

*Michael Harmer and Peter Latto*

## INTRODUCTION

All practising anaesthetists will at some time have been taught how to perform laryngoscopy and intubation. The methods used may have been largely trial and error, or if they were lucky some form of organized teaching programme may have been employed. In general terms, there are three groups to whom intubation is taught; each will require a slightly different approach as each will be expected to utilize the learned skills in different ways. Teaching of intubation to medical students is an important part of general medical training and should be designed to generate an awareness of airway management in all fields of practice. Teaching of anaesthetists should aim to allow skills to develop in order that complex intubation problems may be overcome with confidence. Finally, the paramedical group require sound training in airway management, stressing the problems of performing intubation outside the hospital environment and guidelines on its usage.

## MEDICAL STUDENTS

### Aims of Teaching

Medical students are seldom seconded to anaes-thetic departments for very long, the normal attachment being for 1–2 weeks only. It is widely accepted that this does not allow enough time to teach the subject of anaesthesia in any depth, if at all. Faced with this short attachment period it is best to highlight certain aspects of anaesthetic practice that will be of value to the student after qualification irrespective of the speciality he/she chooses to follow. In Cardiff, the teaching has been towards an understanding of basic applied physi-ology, perioperative management of the patient, the technique of intravenous cannulation, airway management and cardiopulmonary resuscitation.

Although intubation is a part of cardiopul-monary resuscitation in the hospital situation, it is important to point out to undergraduates that intubation is not absolutely essential in order to perform adequate ventilation of the lungs. Airway management and lung inflation by means of mask and self inflating bag are simple and important techniques that should ideally be mastered before intubation training is introduced. It must also be made quite clear that attempts at tracheal intuba-tion by inexperienced personnel may cause more harm than good by imposing unnecessary delays in the implementation of adequate ventilation and oxygenation.

Once students have mastered the technique of artificial ventilation of the lungs using a mask and bag, the teaching of tracheal intubation should proceed in a gradual and ordered manner. The process of teaching might be divided into lectures, films, demonstrations and practice on teaching aids and finally experience in the operating theatre.

## Initial Methods

### Lectures

Preliminary lectures should be used to point out the indications for intubation both electively and in emergencies, to introduce the equipment used, and to describe its mode of usage. The relevant anatomy needs to be emphasized: particular reference should be made to positioning of the head and neck prior to intubation. However, regional anatomy is often difficult to illustrate as the three-dimensional structure of the larynx is hard to visualize with simple drawings.

### Films

Short films are very useful to illustrate the anatomical considerations of intubation. It can clearly demonstrate the position in which to place the head and neck for optimal intubating conditions. In addition, most of these films give a view of the larynx as seen by the operating anaesthetist. They should also highlight the importance of checking the tube position following intubation.

### Demonstration and practice with teaching aids

Teaching aids for intubation have been available for some time. The various models have different features and, while not always being lifelike either in look or feel, they do provide a valuable method of allowing the student to get early manual experience at intubation without the fear of causing any damage.

To obtain the best from such aids it is important to allow plenty of time for practice. The instructor should demonstrate the technique of laryngoscopy, first to the group, and then to individuals. This is usually the hardest part to master, and is followed by the more easily performed act of intubation. The control of the laryngoscope and minimization of trauma should be stressed. Students should then be allowed to practise on the teaching aid with no restriction on the time taken to achieve intubation. Once they are able to

intubate with a degree of confidence, a time limit should be imposed, of say 30 s, and the students allowed to practise again.

Safar [1] recommends the use of a checklist with strict criteria of intubation competence as in Fig. 1. The advantage of using training aids was realized by Hilary Howells and colleagues in 1973 [2]. They pointed out that such aids allow unlimited time to acquire manipulative expertise, which enables subsequent experience on the human subject to be gained confidently, safely and quickly.

## Practice in the Operating Theatre

Once students are confident in their ability to intubate a teaching aid they may be allowed to intubate patients in the operating theatre. However, this must be done under the direct supervision of a qualified anaesthetist. It is important to point out the delicacy of pharyngeal and laryngeal tissues and the possibility of causing injuries to eyes by careless technique and hand positioning. Laryngoscopy and demonstration of the anatomy is difficult for students to master quickly; this is often related to a hurried approach to laryngoscope placement. Tube placement is usually simple once the larynx has been clearly displayed. Another common mistake made by students is to place their eyes too close to the mouth, thus preventing binocular vision. If the operator's head is approximately 1 foot (30 cm) from the mouth this problem should be avoided. All students should aim to perform 10 intubations in the operating theatre during their attachment.

## Assessment of Competence

The degree to which medical student training in tracheal intubation is successful is hard to assess. One article evaluating medical students' practical experience upon qualification showed that in a group of 89 students studied, 7% had never performed tracheal intubation, while a further 40% had done so on only one occasion. The remaining 53% had performed intubation on more than three occasions. Of the whole group, only 30% perceived themselves competent at tracheal intubation [3].

A more recent study has shown that in only 33% of first attempts was the tracheal tube correctly placed. The success increased with repeated attempts, reaching a figure of 93% by the third

Student's name                    Date                Evaluator's name

☐ Passed

☐ Failed

| Measures | Technique | Time |
|---|---|---|
| | ☑ Check if correct performance | ☑ Check if within correct time lapse |
| Tracheal intubation of *adult* manikin | ☐ Checked laryngoscope light before use<br>☐ Checked tube patency before use<br>☐ Held laryngoscope correctly<br>☐ Used no grossly traumatic manoeuvre during intubation attempt<br>☐ Inserted tube into trachea rapidly...................<br>☐ Gave first lung inflation rapidly via tube by bag-valve or mouth......................<br>☐ Inflated cuff of tube correctly (with helper)<br>☐ Used bite-block, secured tube and connected ventilation device correctly<br>☐ Checked to rule out bronchial intubation | sec.<br><br><br><br>☐ <30<br>☐ <60 |
| Tracheal intubation of *infant* manikin | ☐ Checked laryngoscope light before use<br>☐ Checked tube patency before use<br>☐ Held laryngoscope correctly<br>☐ Used no grossly traumatic manoeuvre during intubation attempt<br>☐ Inserted tube into trachea rapidly...................<br>☐ Gave first lung inflation rapidly via tube (by mouth)........................................<br>☐ Used bite-block, secured tube and connected ventilation device correctly<br>☐ Checked to rule out bronchial intubation | ☐ <30<br>☐ <60 |
| Tracheal suctioning (curved-tipped catheter) | ☐ Used correct technique to suction each lung separately................................................ | ☐ <60 |

**Figure 1**   A checklist for intubation competence (as recommended by Safar [1]).

attempt [4]. The method of teaching intubation to students does not seem to have a major effect. From *et al.* compared the outcome of teaching using either a self learning mannikin system with didactic instruction. They found that there was no difference in the success rate for intubation in patients between the two methods [5].

A very short introduction to the technique of tracheal intubation does not, however, make the medical student an expert. Further exposure to intubation may occur during appointment as a house officer. A survey of preregistration house officers has shown that all those interviewed had performed tracheal intubation on more than three occasions and 89% of them considered themselves competent at the skill, though this was not tested [6].

It is probable that there is a difference between perceived and actual competence in an emergency situation. This has been highlighted by Casey [7], who tested junior hospital doctors' theoretical and practical skills at single-handed cardiopulmonary resuscitation using a mannikin. Only 8% were able to manage a cardiopulmonary arrest adequately. Similar disappointing findings were reported by Skinner [8] where intubation skills of house officers were assessed on training mannikins. Only 34% were able to intubate the mannikin at all and none were able to intubate in less than 35 s (the upper limit of time allowed for pass grade in advanced cardiac life support examination in the USA). There must be a need for organized programmes of training for all medical staff. This may include the appointment of permanent resuscitation training officers and the availability of adequate resuscitation training areas as described by Baskett *et al.* [9].

## ANAESTHETISTS

### Initial Training

Intubation is normally performed by the anaesthetist to facilitate the management of general anaesthesia rather than for cardiopulmonary resuscitation. Trainees undergo an initial induction period during which they are taught the principles governing the running of the department. When starting clinical duties, the trainee works closely with one consultant for at least a month. The consultant demonstrates the techniques and teaches the principles of intubation both for elective and emergency anaesthesia. The trainee then learns to intubate under close supervision. He or she is first taught to demonstrate the anatomy at laryngoscopy and second, to insert the tracheal tube. At a later stage, which varies widely between departments and trainees, the trainee is allowed to undertake the management of anaesthesia without direct supervision. Help should be readily and immediately available at this transition stage as difficult intubations and other problems can present unexpectedly and quickly. Every trainee should have been taught a simple, efficient method of dealing with a difficult intubation. The transition can be stressful to trainees and potentially harmful to patients. Acute airway problems, difficult or failed intubation and aspiration of gastric contents are hazards that may trap the unprepared trainee. The Obstetric Anaesthetists' Association, mindful of the occurrence in obstetric practice of the unexpectedly difficult intubation with accompanying airway problems, has recommended that trainees should have at least 1 year's anaesthetic experience before working without direct supervision in this area.

The time taken for the trainee to achieve competence depends on the number of intubations he or she is able to perform. There may, in addition, be variations in the speed of learning and manual dexterity between individuals. It is therefore not appropriate to have rigid rules indicating when the trainee should be allowed to work without supervision for the first time.

The trainee needs 'hands on' experience and it is important that he or she be allowed to attempt intubation when difficult cases occur. The duration of the attempt must be a matter for the judgement of the teacher. Some clinicians find delegation difficult under these circumstances and may take over the procedure too hastily.

The apprentice system in operation in the UK means that the types of intubation procedures taught may vary widely. This will depend on the number of difficult cases encountered, the common techniques chosen to facilitate the procedure, and the experience the teacher has with complex techniques. Techniques taught should include rapid sequence induction and intubation together with preoxygenation and cricoid pressure; the management of a difficult intubation with a gum elastic bougie or stylet; simulated difficult intubation (see p.126) to gain experience and confidence for the unexpected case when the cords cannot be visualized. A failed intubation drill for obstetric anaesthesia, which is also applicable in any patient with a full stomach, should also be rehearsed.

The UK system of training is in marked contrast to that in the USA, where all residents are supervised during the induction of anaesthesia and intubation for the duration of their residency. This has the advantage of offering extra protection for the patient but has the disadvantage that the trainee is never put in a position where he or she has unexpectedly to manage single-handed a problem airway or difficult intubation. The adoption of such a staffing pattern in the UK clearly would have major implications on the deployment of medical manpower. However, the implementation of the Calman report is intended to make the trainee supernumary in nature and therefore more likely to be supervised.

### Teaching Fibreoptic Intubation

Although fibreoptic instruments have been available for many years, only a small proportion of anaesthetists are trained in their use. Many try, but abandon the technique after a few unsuccessful attempts. In one survey, only 16.5% of anaesthetists had tried the technique more than 25 times [10] (Table 1) and in another survey, only 9% had tried more than 30 times [11]. Sia and Edens recommended that at least 30 successful elective fibreoptic intubations in conscious and anaesthetized patients should be undertaken before attempting a difficult intubation [12]. All agree that it takes a great deal of practice to become skilled with fibreoptic equipment. However, others have suggested that as few as 10 intubations are sufficient to demonstrate competence [13].

## Training programmes

In an attempt to improve training methods Ovassapian *et al.* have developed a training programme [14–16]. After a careful demonstration of the instrument the programme was divided into three parts:

*Part 1: Practice on a training model*
Trainees were given unlimited time to familiarize themselves with the anatomy and the manipulation and visual characteristics of the fibrescope.

*Part 2: Exposure of the epiglottis and vocal cords in six patients*
Written consent was obtained and the epiglottis and cords subsequently demonstrated in six patients recovering from anaesthesia. The trainee learned to identify the appearance of live, moving laryngeal structures and how to recognize and correct problems caused by secretions. The fibrescope was inserted through a nasopharyngeal airway. The instrument was kept well clear of the vocal cords in order to avoid the risk of laryngospasm. The trainee was formally evaluated on all six attempts. The mean time to demonstrate the epiglottis and cords by 12 trainees was reported as 1.4 min (range 0.75–4.0 min) [15].

*Part 3: Intubation in six awake sedated patients*
Verbal consent was obtained and the procedure explained to patients requiring nasotracheal intubation for elective operations. Patients were premedicated with atropine and morphine. Further sedation was provided with approximately 0.15 mg kg$^{-1}$ i.v. of diazepam and 1.5 µg kg$^{-1}$ i.v. of fentanyl. Topical anaesthesia was achieved with 3 ml of 4% lignocaine injected by the translaryngeal route and application of 6% cocaine to the nasal mucosa. The trainee followed a written step-by-step guide to the procedure. An 8 mm nasotracheal tube was inserted through the chosen nostril into the pharynx and after removal of pharyngeal secretions by suctioning, the fibrescope was passed through the tube into the pharynx. The epiglottis and cords were identified and the fibrescope passed into the trachea.

All intubations were closely supervised but advice was given regarding sedation and topical

**Table 1** Survey of number of fibreoptic intubations performed by a group of clinicians. From Ovassapian and Dykes [10], with kind permission of the authors, the editor of *Anesthesiology*, and the publishers, J. B. Lippincott Co.

| No. of intubations | No. of clinicians performing intubations | % |
|---|---|---|
| None | 51 | 30 |
| 1–5 | 55 | 32.4 |
| 6–10 | 22 | 12.9 |
| 11–25 | 13 | 7.6 |
| >25 | 28 | 16.5 |
| Not answered | 1 | 0.6 |
| Total | 170 | 100 |

anaesthesia only for the first case unless difficulty occurred in subsequent cases. The trainee was formally evaluated on the sixth attempt. The total time for intubation, that is from the start of application of the local anaesthetic, the actual time for intubation and the number of attempts (each removal of scope from nasal tube) were recorded. The mean total time was 17.7 min (range 9–25 min). The mean intubation time was 3.3 min (range 1–8 min) and only one trainee required two attempts at intubation [15].

The results of the formal training programme were compared with results obtained using the traditional approach in which the instrument was demonstrated and then one intubation was observed [14]. The formal programme yielded significantly better results: 88.9% of patients were successfully intubated compared with 54.2% in the control group (*P*< 0.001) and a shorter mean time was required for intubation, 2.8 min and 4.5 min respectively.

Only nine out of 371 patients (1.6%) indicated at a postoperative interview that they would not like to have an awake intubation again. Furthermore, 27 patients (7.3%) remembered the procedure as being mildly unpleasant, while 205 patients (55.3%) did not remember the procedure at all [16].

In the patient with a full stomach, topical anaesthesia was applied to the vocal cords through the suction channel of the scope just before intubation. Translaryngeal injection of local anaesthetic was avoided to minimize the risk of aspiration.

The technique can be performed under general

anaesthesia. In some cases, however, the procedure will take a considerable time. It is important, therefore, to be able to ventilate during the attempts and this can be accomplished in a number of different ways [17] (Fig. 2). Experience with fibreoptic equipment can be gained in patients ventilated by mask, oropharyngeal or nasopharyngeal airways and in spontaneously breathing patients through ports in the face mask. Most difficult cases should be intubated under local anaesthesia.

## Problems in Training in Fibreoptic Intubation in the UK

There have been two recent articles on training in fibreoptic intubation [18, 19]. Vaughan teaches intubation under general anaesthesia on a gynaecology list [18]. He stresses the importance of assessing the distance between the tragus of the ear and the angle of the mouth; this is approximately the same as the distance from the lips to the rima glottidis. The advantage of this method is that there is always a steady supply of patients available. In the absence of teaching programmes on awake patients, such an approach is invaluable.

However, Ball contends that a teaching programme should be designed to prepare the anaesthetist for intubation of a patient in whom difficulty is anticipated [20]. He recommended that this should ideally be achieved by gaining competence in awake fibreoptic intubation. Clinicians need to gain expertise both in application of local anaesthesia for an awake intubation and in the use of the fibreoptic laryngoscope. It appears, however, that there are very few centres in the UK where awake intubation on patients undergoing elective procedures is considered ethically acceptable. However,

(a)　　　　　　　　　　(b)

(c)　　　　　　　　　　(d)

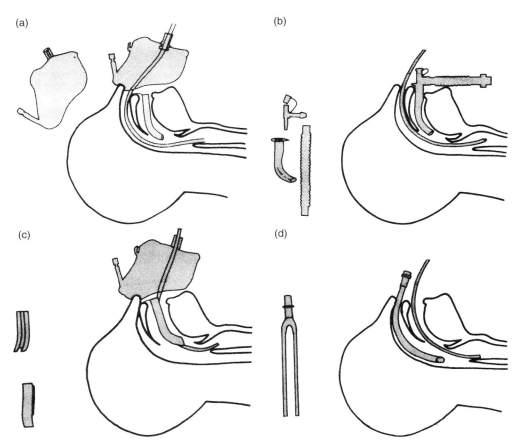

**Figure 2**    Methods to facilitate ventilation during fibreoptic intubation: (a) mask with endoscopic port; (b) oral airway with Rowbotham connector and corrugated tubing; (c) oral airway with central groove for passage of endoscope and side ports for suction catheter; (d) binasal airway. From Patil *et al.* [17], with kind permission of the authors, the editor of *Anesthesiology*, and the publishers, J. B. Lippincott Co.

in many centres in the USA, awake fibreoptic intubations are carried out on all patients requiring intubation by the nasal route.

Mason runs a teaching programme using patients who are electively scheduled for a fibreoptic bronchoscopy [19]. The teaching programme is structured; topics include handling of the bronchoscope, practice on a model, application of local anaesthesia and, only then, practice under supervision with patients. It is very clear that once the trainees have mastered these techniques on patients with normal anatomy, they can use them in patients where there is an indication for an awake intubation. Mason stresses the need for every department to run a structured training programme on awake fibreoptic intubation. It is clearly necessary to have the co-operation of a chest physician when setting up such a programme. Mason considers that awake intubation is essential and states:

> None of the approaches under anaesthesia permit the unhurried sequential identification of the nasal, pharyngeal and laryngeal structures which is possible in the awake subject and essential when patients with abnormal anatomy or pathology are subsequently encountered. In addition, techniques performed under general anaesthesia do not prepare the trainee adequately to perform an awake fibreoptic intubation in a patient with a difficult airway.

The use of closed circuit television enables the instructor to observe clearly attempts at intubation [21]. This enables instructors, if required, to give practical advice and assistance to the trainee. This technique was used as part of a structured training programme. The structured programme included: introduction to the fibreoptic scope, practice on the model, endoscopy in patients with a tracheal tube *in situ*, and finally, intubation. The use of closed circuit television in this way resulted in fewer failures in achieving intubation and shorter intubation times.

There is still much to be done in the UK to improve training in fibreoptic intubation. Ideally, each department should have a consultant with special responsibilities in this area. However, since training is frequently inadequate, a number of departments have set up specialized programmes for anaesthetists from other areas wishing to gain expertise in fibreoptic intubation.

## Other Techniques

There are a number of important techniques that should be taught to all anaesthetists in training. These include optimum use of the bougie, use of the stylet, simulated difficult intubation using the bougie, intubation through the laryngeal mask, retrograde intubation and transtracheal ventilation. In addition, failed intubation and ventilation drills need to be discussed. These topics are dealt with in other chapters. There appears to be a need for the expansion of departmental teaching programmes to encompass the above topics and thereby to improve the clinical skills of anaesthetists.

The major weakness of the system in operation in the UK is that advanced techniques are rarely taught on a formal basis. In many centres, skills in fibreoptic and retrograde techniques for intubation are not available. It is clear that these techniques are not required on a regular basis and that many clinicians seem able to manage the majority of cases without them. In larger teaching centres, however, it is important that trainees are thoroughly taught the principles and practice of such techniques.

Since suitable cases present only rarely, and it is not ethical to practise retrograde techniques electively on normal patients, 'hands on' experience in patients is difficult to achieve. This difficulty may be solved to some extent by a combination of theoretical teaching, practice on cadavers or models and training films. The technique is usually quick and easy to perform. It is certainly ethical to perform this technique electively in the patient judged preoperatively to have a very difficult airway or in a patient with a previous failed intubation.

## PARAMEDICAL STAFF

### The Need for Paramedical Training

Although there can be little doubt that the technique of tracheal intubation is an important part of every medical person's training, there has been some controversy as to the value of teaching this technique to paramedical staff. Safar [1] suggested that intubation should be taught to intensive care unit staff and a selected group of paramedics. In the UK, the majority of health authorities have trained groups of paramedical staff to be proficient in the insertion of intravenous cannulae and tracheal intubation, in addition to basic airway management. However, what evidence is there that such training is beneficial to the patient?

There is a good deal of information on the effect that such trained staff have on survival following cardiac arrest in the non-hospital situation. Vertesi [22] reported the experience of using 'paramedic' ambulances over a 27-month period. There were 227 cases of cardiac arrest of which 198 (87.2%) were intubated. The number surviving to hospital admission was 58 (25.6% of cases) but of these only 21 (9.25%) were discharged alive. The authors concluded from this experience that 'sudden death from cardiac disease can be prevented in a considerable proportion of instances and that early circulatory and ventilatory support may prevent deterioration in a variety of other disorders'. However, set alongside this is the fact that survival figures following cardiac arrest can be greatly improved by widespread training in basic resuscitation. Lund and Skulberg [23] showed that 36% of cardiac arrest victims who were given prompt attention by bystanders survived and were subsequently discharged from hospital. The ideal situation would seem to be a combination of widespread education of the general public in the basic skills of resuscitation (expired air ventilation and external cardiac massage) in combination with a small group of highly trained 'paramedics' skilled at more complex resuscitation techniques.

## Indications for 'Field' Intubation

The main occasion when intubation by paramedical staff may be deemed necessary is at cardiac arrest following myocardial infarction. Comatose patients and those with extensive trauma where intubation may be necessary to provide an adequate airway are further examples.

If the management of cardiac arrest is considered, it is clear that intubation is not an essential part of resuscitation. The lungs can be adequately ventilated using a bag and mask but, if intubation can be performed rapidly and correctly, this aids both lung inflation and protects the airway from soiling. There is very little literature available to evaluate the performance of intubation by 'paramedics'. Stewart et al. [24] presented the results of attempted intubation by paramedics in 779 patients. A total of 701 (90%) were successfully intubated. The majority of these (57.9%) were intu-

bated at the first attempt, while 26.1% and 5.3% were intubated at the second and third attempts, respectively. There was a complication rate of 9.5%, the major part of these being due to prolonged attempts at intubation (> 45 s). However, perhaps of greater concern were three unrecognized oesophageal intubations. Of the patients intubated, 224 (28.8%) were reported to have vomited before attempts at intubation while seven (0.9%) vomited during intubation. Intubation in these situations would be advantageous in protecting the airway.

The value of early 'field' intubation following major trauma is even harder to assess. The type of case where this is likely to be most beneficial, apart from trauma-induced cardiac arrest, would be in head and neck and chest injuries. However, it is these very cases that can pose intubation problems even for the most skilled of anaesthetists. In addition, unless intubation is performed with great care, it may aggravate the injuries. Unlike the situation of managing cardiac arrest following myocardial infarction there may not be such a strong argument for 'paramedics' performing tracheal intubation on trauma victims.

One major problem would seem to be that while it is not difficult to train a group of people to be proficient at intubation, it can be difficult to identify when not to intubate patients. Guidelines for training should include the categories of patients where intubation should be attempted, the number and duration of attempts, the route to be utilized and a list of conditions in which intubation is contraindicated.

## Training Programmes

The method of training such personnel varies between the UK and North America. From experience in Brighton, where a coronary ambulance service has been in existence since 1969, the training of ambulancemen for such duties is extensive. The main course is hospital based and comprises over 24 lectures of 90 min each, plus 1 month full time attachment to the Cardiac Care Unit. After passing the course examination, a further 6 months on-the-road experience is completed before a further week's training in airway management is undertaken. A 5-day refresher course is taken annually covering all areas of resuscitation and emergency care [25]. Similar schemes are used throughout the UK and follow a recognized paramedic training programme. Training in the

USA is even more extensive and a typical programme would be similar to that employed in Seattle. Training consists of intensive theoretical and clinical training covering all aspects of resuscitation as well as emergency operative procedures such as tracheostomy and thoracotomy [26].

In so far as tracheal intubation is part of this extensive training programme for paramedics, some thought must be given to how best to train these people. It is reasonable to set about teaching in a similar manner to that advocated for medical students. As there is no substitute for 'hands on' practice, as much time as possible should be spent under supervision in the operating theatre with anaesthetized patients. However, two studies have questioned the importance of operating theatre training for paramedics and have shown that such a component may not be so important in the success of intubation [27, 28].

## CONCLUSION

It is unfortunate that intubation is frequently not well taught. If a structured training programme is not employed, this is hardly surprising. Even if such a programme is used and the initial training is of good quality with a high degree of success in skill acquisition, the skills learned will soon deteriorate to a dangerous level. It is essential that all medical and paramedical staff who may be called upon to perform intubation have regular reinforcement of their initial training.

The major shortcomings of training are different in each group. The medical student training is normally somewhat fundamental but the aim should be to impress the value of the skill in their future career, especially if this is in hospital practice. The anaesthetist's training may be deficient in the ability to cope with problems or utilize complex techniques. The shortcoming for the paramedic is in the need for patient selection, as intubation may be dangerous in certain circumstances.

Although in the hospital situation emergency intubations are usually performed by an anaesthetist, it is important that other staff should be able to perform ventilation and intubation if the anaesthetist is unavailable. For this reason, intubation should be one of the skills acquired and regularly practised by all medical staff involved in the acute hospital care of patients.

## KEY POINTS

- For all type of staff in training, the importance of airway maintenance and simple ventilation without the need for intubation should be stressed.

- The use of mannikins can be very useful to allow the trainee to gain confidence in the use of equipment.

- Training programmes are needed for the teaching of specific techniques such as fibreoptic intubation.

- In the training of paramedics, it is important to stress the indications for intubation.

- In all fields of practice, it is not sufficient just to teach a technique, it must be also be used regularly to maintain a level of expertise.

## REFERENCES

1 Safar P. *Cardiopulmonary Cerebral Resuscitation*. Philadelphia: W. B. Saunders. 1981.

2 Hilary Howells T., Emery F. M. and Twentyman J. E. C. Endotracheal intubation training using a simulator. *British Journal of Anaesthesia* 1973; **45**: 400.

3 Wakeford R. and Roberts S. An evaluation of medical students' practical experience upon qualification. *Medical Teacher* 1983; **4**: 140.

4 O'Flaherty D. and Adams A. P. Endotracheal intubation skills of medical students. *Journal of the Royal Society of Medicine* 1992; **85**: 603.

5 From R. P., Pearson K. S., Albanese M. A., Moyers J. R., Sigurdsson S. S. and Dull D. L. Assessment of an interactive learning system with 'sensorized' manikin head for airway management instruction. *Anesthesia and Analgesia* 1994; **79**: 136.

6 Evans I. and Wakeford R. House officers' perceptions of their experience and competence. *Medical Teacher* 1983; **5**: 68.

7 Casey W. F. Cardiopulmonary resuscitation: a survey of standards among junior hospital doctors. *Journal of the Royal Society of Medicine* 1984; **77**: 921.

8 Skinner D. V., Camm A. J. and Miles S. Cardiopulmonary resuscitation skills of preregistration house officers. *British Medical Journal* 1985; **290**: 1549.

9 Baskett P. J. F., Lawler P. G. P., Hudson R. B. S., Makepeace A. P. W. and Cooper C. Resuscitation

teaching room in a district general hospital: concept and practice. *British Medical Journal* 1976; **i:** 568.

10 Ovassapian A. and Dykes M. H. Difficult pediatric intubation – an indication for the fibreoptic bronchoscope. *Anesthesiology* 1982; **56:** 412.

11 James W. and Latto I. P. *Retrospective Intubation Survey.* Unpublished data presented to Welsh Society of Anaesthetists. 1982.

12 Sia R. L. and Edens E. T. How to avoid problems when using fibreoptic bronchoscope for difficult intubations. *Anaesthesia* 1981; **36:** 74.

13 Johnson C. and Roberts J. T. Clinical competence in the performance of fibreoptic laryngoscopy and endotracheal intubation: a study of resident instruction. *Journal of Clinical Anesthesia* 1989; **1:** 344.

14 Ovassapian A., Yelich S., Dykes M. H. M. and Golman M. E. Fibreoptic nasotracheal intubation: stepwise training versus traditional teaching. *Anesthesiology* 1981; **55:** A347.

15 Ovassapian A., Yelich S. J., Dykes M. H. M. and Golman M. E. A training program for fibeoptic nasotracheal intubation. Use of a model and live patients. *Anaesthesia* 1983; **38:** 795.

16 Ovassapian A., Yelich S. J., Dykes M. H. M. and Brunner E. E. Fibreoptic nasotracheal intubation – incidence and causes of failure. *Anesthesia and Analgesia* 1983; **62:** 692.

17 Patil V., Stehling L. C., Zauder H. L. and Koch J. P. Mechanical aids for fibreoptic endoscopy. *Anesthesiology* 1982; **57:** 69.

18 Hartley M., Morris S. and Vaughan R. S. Teaching fibreoptic intubation. Effect of alfentanil on the haemodynamic response. *Anaesthesia* 1994; **49:** 335.

19 Mason R. A. Learning fibreoptic intubation: fundamental problems. *Anaesthesia* 1992; **47:** 729.

20 Ball D. R. Awake versus asleep fibreoptic intubation. *Anaesthesia* 1994; **49:** 921.

21 Smith J. E., Fenner S. G. and King M. J. Teaching fibreoptic nasotracheal intubation with and without closed circuit television. *British Journal of Anaesthesia* 1993; **71:** 206.

22 Vertesi L. The paramedic ambulance: a Canadian experience. *Journal of Canadian Medical Association* 1978; **119:** 25.

23 Lund I. and Skulberg A. Cardiopulmonary resuscitation by lay people. *Lancet* 1976; **ii:** 702.

24 Stewart R. D., Paris P. M., Winter P. M., Pelton G. H. and Cannon G. M. Field endotracheal intubation by paramedical personnel. *Chest* 1984; **85:** 341.

25 Studd C. Abstract from International Conference on Cardiac Arrest and Resuscitation. 1982.

26 Mayer J. D. Seattle's paramedic programme: geographical distribution, response times and mortality. *Society of Science and Medicine* 1979; **13D:** 45.

27 Stratton S. J., Kane G., Gunter C. S., Wheeler N. S., Ableson-Ward C., Reich E., Pratt F. D., Ogata G. and Gallaher C. Prospective study of manikin-only versus manikin and human subject endotracheal intubation training of paramedics. *Annals of Emergency Medicine* 1991; **20:** 1314.

28 Stewart R. D., Paris P. M., Peton G. H. and Garreson D. Effect of varied training techniques on field endotracheal intubation success rates. *Annals of Emergency Medicine* 1984; **13:** 1032.

# 21

# Legal Implications of Difficult Intubation

*Keith R. Murrin*

## GENERAL LEGAL PRINCIPLES

A brief explanation of general legal principles precedes their application to problems related to tracheal intubation.

## Negligence

### Definition

Negligence is the omission to do something which a reasonable man would do, or doing something which a prudent and reasonable man would not do. To succeed in action for negligence, the plaintiff must prove three things:

- the defendant owed a duty of care to avoid causing injury;
- there was a breach of that duty of care by the defendant;
- in consequence the plaintiff suffered injury, damage or, in some cases, financial loss.

Medical negligence is sometimes called malpractice; these terms are not strictly synonymous as professional misconduct may also be described as professional malpractice.

Every individual has a duty not to injure another member of the public. Failure to observe this duty of care, negligence, is a civil wrong known as a tort.

When a plaintiff sues in tort he* must normally prove his loss, but the necessary basis of his claim is that he has actually suffered a wrong. If there is no wrong (injuria) for which the law gives a remedy, no amount of loss (damnum) caused by the defendant can make him liable. Damnum sine injuria (loss not caused by wrong) is not actionable.

Most torts are wrongful *acts*. There can, however, be liability for *omission* or *failure to act* in circumstances where there is a duty to do so.

### Breach of duty of care

The question asked is whether the standard of treatment given by the defendant fell below the standard expected of him by the law and whether there was any fault in the legal sense. Except in relatively special circumstances, the burden of proving fault lies with the plaintiff. The standard of proof required is the normal civil standard 'on the balance of probabilities', which contrasts with the criminal standard of 'beyond reasonable doubt'.

Increasingly, the Crown Prosecution Service is pressing for criminal proceedings when the death of the patient is totally predictable as a result of negligent medical behaviour. There is little excuse for leaving an unconscious patient to fend for themselves in an operating theatre.

### Standard of care

Patients have a right to assume that they will be looked after by a competent and caring doctor.

As early as 1838, Judge C. Tindall [1] ruled that a professional should exhibit a reasonable degree of care and skill. This does not mean that cure is guaranteed or that the highest possible degree of skill will be employed. Therefore, juries should neither expect the highest or very high standard nor should it be content with a very low standard. The Bolam principle [2] is the test which is most commonly applied. It is the standard of the ordinary skilled man exercising and professing to have that special skill. A charge of negligence cannot be made if the defendant did not practise with the highest expert skill. It is well established in law that it is sufficient if he exercises the ordinary skill of an ordinary man exercising that particular art. Therefore, the degree of competence expected is that which would not be disapproved of by a responsible opinion within the profession.

*Here 'he' is used to mean both 'he' and 'she'.

However, if a doctor specializes, or even subspecializes, his actions will be judged against a reasonable body of practitioners from that specialty or subspecialty.

A doctor should have a reasonably *sound grasp of medical techniques* and should be *informed of new medical developments* as the average competent doctor would expect to be.

Therefore, three facts require to be established to prove negligence:

- there is a usual and normal practice;
- the offender has not adopted that practice;
- the course the doctor adopted is not that which a professional of ordinary skill would have taken if he had been acting with ordinary care.

However, if there are two schools of thought involved in any procedure, then the doctor would not be negligent if he merely practised one school of thought which existed at the time of injury. However, the *body of responsible medical practitioners* must be rightly so regarded before their opinion is acceptable to the court.

The duty to keep abreast of medical development does not involve reading every single article, but certainly includes heeding a preceding series of warnings given in the medical press that were subsequently ignored by the defendant.

An error of judgement is not necessarily negligence but it could be negligent if it is an error which would not have been made by a reasonably competent professional acting with ordinary care.

## Standards of Medical Care

For an effective medical audit to be established, there must be an agreed minimal standard of care. By definition, conduct that meets this standard is usually not considered to be negligence. As indicated in the discussion on legal principles of negligence, excellence is not expected. If this were to be the case, the majority of practitioners would always be seen as failures in their standards of care.

A standard of care is a corporate agreement from a reasonable body of practitioners to ensure patient safety. Obviously, problems arise when there are alternative means of achieving the same end.

Standards are established in two ways. They may arise from previous legal disputes or from central governing bodies or societies. The content of standards is also influenced by the reports of confidential enquiries such as the *Confidential Enquiry into Perioperative Deaths* (CEPOD) [3] and *Confidential Enquiry into Maternal Mortality* (CEMM) [4]. In the USA, it is possible to study the outcome of closed claims from the records of insurance companies.

The conclusions from these studies tend to be a potent deciding factor with any legal claim and also determine future clinical standards, i.e. they become the acceptable majority opinion. There may be a knock-on effect with clinical freedom being eroded as legal pressures increase, and this can reduce the doctor to the level of a medical technician [5].

### *Functions of standards*

Standards serve various different functions:

- mark of minimal acceptable practice;
- yardstick for comparison;
- argument for expenditure on equipment and personnel;
- compulsion for colleagues to adhere to safe practice.

Regular audit, including critical incidence reporting, is essential to establish policies which in turn can be subjected to reaudit. If practice falls below an established standard, it is difficult to justify in the court of law. A review of closed malpractice claims in the USA, i.e. those which have been settled, revealed that 80% of care was substandard, yet payment was made in 40% of cases where care reached and exceeded the required standard [6].

## Causation

It must be demonstrated that the damage the plaintiff has suffered was actually caused by, and was directly attributable to, the act of negligence and would not have occurred in any case.

## Staff in Training

The law insists that the public are entitled to expect a reasonable standard of competence in their medical attendants. The acceptable standard of care provided by staff in training is based on a medical practitioner of similar experience irrespective of the post in which he is employed. Therefore, a senior house officer with 10 years experience would not be judged as a senior house officer who has come straight from his house appointments.

## Delegation

Improper delegation of responsibility can result in negligence if it is carried out in the knowledge that the person receiving the responsibility was incapable of performing the duties proposed. The junior, therefore, should try to carry out his duties as instructed by his superior in order to avoid liability. However, obedience should not be adhered to if improper instructions would result in damage and obvious negligence.

## Vicarious Liability

An employer is normally responsible for all the actions of his employees. Previous to the recent changes in the structure of the National Health Service (NHS), the State was responsible for the actions of all its employees. Currently, in the case of Trust hospitals, the hospital is now liable for the actions of its employees. However, it should be realized that when doctors perform a service in a private hospital, they become an independent contractor and, as such, their medical insurance company assumes liability.

At present, in the UK, the distinction between independent contractor and employee is unambiguous for medical and nursing staff. There may be confusion, however, when a doctor acts as a 'good Samaritan' or performs sessional duties in a Trust Hospital for single payments. In the USA, the distinction is not always so clear and the principles of status – employee or independent contractor – are sometimes questioned in order to clarify the true defendant and the avenue for financial recompense [7].

## Locality Rule

All hospitals in the UK are seen to be equal in the legal sense. It is therefore incumbent on all medical practitioners to provide satisfactory service irrespective of the location and size of the hospital. Standards of care refer to national standards and not to the local hospital policy.

### *Res Ipsa Loquitur*

The strict translation of the Latin is 'the thing

speaks for itself'. This doctrine is occasionally invoked when it is almost impossible to establish negligence because of the intricacy of events or the fact that the plaintiff was unconscious at the time. This then shifts the burden of proof on to the defendant, who has to explain how the accident could have occurred without negligence.

In the UK the use of this principle is rare but there is a tendency to follow practices acceptable in the USA. However, even in the USA, before instruction for the use of *res ipsa loquitur*, the plaintiff has to demonstrate that the event in question must be of a kind which does not ordinarily occur in the absence of negligence and the agency or instrumentality causing the harm must have been in the exclusive control of the defendant.

## Medical Ability

It is not a defence if the doctor acted in good faith to the best of his ability but failed to reach the objective standard of the ordinary competent and careful doctor.

## LEGAL IMPLICATIONS OF DIFFICULT TRACHEAL INTUBATION

The salient preceding legal points can now be considered in relation to the various aspects of tracheal intubation.

## Magnitude of the Risk

Consecutive studies of Utting [8] and Aitkenhead [9] in the UK have demonstrated that the greatest percentage of claims associated with anaesthesia are as a result of brain and spinal cord damage. In a 13-year period of reports to the Medical Defence Union, there were 326 cases of death and cerebral damage thought to be the results of errors in anaesthetic technique. Errors associated with tracheal intubation accounted for 31% and this was the most important group.

Data from the Committee on Professional Liability of American Society of Anesthesiologists (ASA) [10] has demonstrated that adverse outcomes associated with respiratory events constituted the largest single class of injury in their study. Death or brain damage occurred in 85% of the cases. Most outcomes (72%) were considered preventable with better monitoring. Three mecha-

nisms of injury accounted for the majority of these cases:

- inadequate ventilation;
- oesophageal intubation;
- difficult tracheal intubation.

Medical care was judged to be substandard in 76% of the claims for adverse respiratory events. This differed significantly from non-respiratory claims. Anaesthetic care was rarely considered appropriate in cases of inadequate ventilation or oesophageal intubation but in the case of difficult intubation, there was considerable improvement in the figures. Almost all (greater than 90%) of claims for inadequate ventilation and oesophageal intubation were considered preventable with better monitoring as opposed to 36% of claims for difficult tracheal intubation. The reviewers in the survey stressed the importance of pulse oximetry and capnometry or both as the most efficient means of detecting problems. *Only 23% of the oesophageal placements were due to, or occurred with, difficult intubation*. The remaining 77% contained no indication that intubation was difficult.

Cheyney *et al.* [6] utilized a peer review system in a closed claim study, i.e. those claims, which had been settled. The panel of experts found a greater incidence of negligence in the claims, for severe injuries and death than in claims for lesser nerve injuries. Of the successful claims, 46% involved cases where negligence was not involved in the anaesthetic management. This study demonstrates that while the current tort-based insurance system in the USA favoured the injured patient, there were inequalities in the system for both the anaesthetist and the patient.

Holland *et al.* [11] demonstrated that errors of judgement were a common cause of anaesthetic catastrophic misadventures in Australia. Again, the same pattern emerged, i.e. the two most common causes of death were inhalation of gastric contents and airway complications.

Lunn and Mushin [12], in the precursor to the CEPOD studies, prepared a report involving all the hospitals in five regions. This was equivalent to about one-third of all the hospitals in the UK. Once more, the conclusion reached was that 70% of anaesthetic deaths were due to an error of judgement by the anaesthetist. Another major cause was lack of clinical expertise.

Although the studies mentioned are likely to be important in formulating future policy documents, data from Medical Protection Societies adds a further dimension. From 1990 onwards, however, the records of the Societies are incomplete because of the advent of the NHS indemnity. In 1989, 759 medical claims were settled. Of these 9.7% were for negligence in anaesthetics, 2.3% for dental damage, 1.8% for awareness under anaesthesia and 2.5% were for brain damage or postoperative death. These were associated with a low inspired oxygen concentration as a result of human error; and inappropriate gas flows or inadequate ventilation as a result either of disconnection of a ventilator or the tracheal tube being placed in the oesophagus rather than the trachea [13].

## Anatomy of Accidents

Charles Perow [14] has hypothesized that certain systems in accidents involve multiple and unexpected interactions; failures are inevitable since although single events may be prevented by fail safe devices, these are inadequate to cope with a multifactorial situation.

Some processes are complex with rapidly changing, closely dependent interacting component functions. The propensity for an overwhelming crisis is so great that it is unavoidable. Such a process or system produces 'system accidents'. Two variables that are associated with system accidents are complexity of interactions and tightness of coupling between the components. Because of tight coupling of all the factors associated with the anatomy and physiology of the patients together with the complexity of anaesthesia, a simple incident may easily become critical through a chain of events. The whole process is therefore one of passage from incident to accident precipitated by the speed of events.

The majority of potential accidents are effectively dealt with by a combination of prevention and recovery. Such planning can make the difference between an incident and an accident. The detection of possible problems with difficult airways will be increased if anaesthetists examine the patient carefully preoperatively. Recovery from a potential disaster is ensured by exercises in simulation and adherence to agreed protocols.

Because of the tight integration of the factors involved in safety of anaesthesia, most anaesthetists develop a mental map of these variables. Accidents involving faulty mental maps may be insidious. Many believe that experience improves mental mapping as much as it does vigilance.

Mental maps can be established with the assistance of anaesthesia simulation models. These teach the individual to differentiate critical from non-critical events and enable the trainee to switch from routine management to intervention to avoid incident becoming accident.

In summary, whenever possible, the equilibrium of the tightly coupled variables associated with anaesthesia is maintained by keeping changes to a minimum. In the case of difficult intubation, techniques utilized in the conscious state (awake intubation and regional anaesthesia) attempt to maintain coupling mechanisms as close to equilibrium as possible.

## Safety Strategies

Elements that constitute an overall strategy for avoiding mishaps have been proposed [15]:

- train, educate and supervise;
- use appropriate monitoring instrumentation and vigilance aids;
- minimize factors that limit individual performance;
- establish and follow preparation inspection protocols;
- assure equipment performance;
- design and organize the workspace;
- act on incident reports – eliminate the pitfalls.

## Risk Management

The *definition* of risk management in relation to healthcare is:

> The process of applying sound management techniques to identification, assessment and resolution of problems to prevent medical mishaps and to minimize the adverse effects of injury and loss to patients, employees, visitors and the hospital corporation [16].

The term risk management was coined by the insurance industry in 1963 and related primarily to the funding and control of predictable losses in business activity. Essentially, risk management involves the planning, organizing, directing, controlling of resources and activities so that accidental losses in terms of financing are kept at the least possible amount [17].

The approach to both *quality assurance* and *risk management* is essentially the same and consists of the following steps:

- identification of the problem;
- assessment of the problem;
- resolution of the problem;
- re-evaluation of the problem.

These steps have a familiar ring about them and there is a risk of such management programmes reinventing the wheel.

## Clinical Application of Risk Management

The following steps must be taken for successful outcome [18].

### Recognize and define the risk

If there is any doubt that the airway will be lost and ventilation cannot be maintained by any means, it is mandatory that the patient remains awake during intubation. The importance of thorough documentation and dissemination of critical information as part of an in-hospital computerized difficult airway/intubation registry has been emphasized [19]. This should include the use of a patient wristband while in hospital combined with enrolment with the Medi-alert Foundation.

### Define the severity of the risk

This requires careful assessment of anatomical factors predisposing to difficult airway management.

### Identify all possible alternatives of management

This involves careful theatre preparation, availability of a variety of equipment and the presence of trained staff.

### Select and apply the correct strategy to minimize the risk

A preconceived plan must be constructed to minimise the risk and maximise the success of the attempt.

### Be prepared to change course at any time

Repetition of one strategy which is leading to failure should be changed before trauma and irrevocable damage is done. *The cardinal lesson is that patients die from failure to oxygenate rather than failure to intubate.* If it is possible to ventilate via a laryngeal mask, surgery can commence, provided that a full stomach is not a possibility and no

extreme positions are required for surgery, e.g. prone position.

*If cyanosis occurs in a patient who had a normal oxygen saturation preoperatively and there is the smallest doubt regarding tracheal placement, the tube should be withdrawn and the facemask and oxygen applied.*

The key points for safe clinical practice associated with airway management have been described [20]:

- Preventing crisis airway management by avoiding the obvious pitfalls must be the prime objective.
- Preoperative airway assessment and preoxygenation should be routine.
- All anaesthetists should aim to be competent in fiberoptic intubation.
- A thorough understanding of simple changes in the position of the jaw and head to maintain a clear airway is mandatory.
- Skilled use of the gum elastic bougie will enable success with many difficult intubations.
- The role of the laryngeal mask airway in obstetric anaesthesia has become more clearly defined. The recommendation of the report *Confidential Enquiries into Maternity Mortality in the UK* (1985–87) is that the use of the laryngeal mask airway (LMA) in obstetric patients must be accompanied by the continued application of cricoid pressure. Cricoid pressure may well have to be released temporarily to allow the insertion of the LMA. The report also advises that the LMA should be available for dealing with a difficult intubation.
- An appropriate technique of transtracheal ventilation should be immediately available wherever anaesthetics are being administered.

## Recognition of Difficult Intubation

There is little doubt that an anaesthetist is negligent if he fails to perform an adequate medical assessment of a patient in an elective situation. Two aspects of the assessment of the patient regarding difficult intubation need to be explored. These are the reliability of the predictive tests and measurements and the influence of a positive recognition in relation to the final outcome.

## Preoperative assessment

Preoperative assessment is essential and should include assessment of the airway and related problems. It has been recommended that the preoperative anaesthetic assessment, with emphasis on airway examination, is made before the patient arrives in theatre [21]. With the pressures in day surgery, this is not always possible. Airway examination refers specifically to problems of receding mandible, limited mouth opening, limited cervical movement, short, thick neck, and dental problems. These may have a profound effect on the course of the subsequent anaesthetic.

Although a variety of clinical and radiological tests have been proposed to predict difficult intubation, none are 100% reliable. However, a reasonable group of practitioners would agree that if there was gross limitation of cervical extension, i.e. less than 30°, a grossly anterior larynx, or extremely limited mouth opening, difficulties could be anticipated and plans drawn up well in advance.

The following three tests should be employed routinely to evaluate the airway and identify patients who are at risk of entry into life-threatening situations when unconscious:

- tongue and pharyngeal inlet size (Mallampati test [22]);
- atlanto-occipital extension;
- anterior mandibular space (thyromental distance) or horizontal length of the mandible.

They only take a short time to perform and should be a routine part of preoperative assessment.

## Recognition of known medical syndromes

Failure to recognize a known medical syndrome that can result in difficult intubation could be regarded as negligence, especially if the diagnosis has been recorded in the notes. However, it would have to be subsequently proven that this factor resulted in the consequent damage to the patient. It is negligent not to make adequate inquiry into the patient's medical history. If a patient has been reported as difficult to intubate in the past, then guidelines outlined elsewhere in this book should be followed.

## Radiological tests

Radiological tests should be reserved for the patients who suffer from diseases known to cause difficult intubation or those patients who fail the three clinical tests: Mallampati [22], cervical extension and thyromental distance.

## Intubation clinics

The importance of preoperative assessment of the airway is demonstrated by the establishment of special 'intubation clinics'. Their role can only be considered advisory since the final responsibility for this assessment lies with the patient's anaesthetist.

## Consent

The patient may sue in battery if no consent at all is obtained. Alternatively, if the quality of the consent obtained was not good enough, i.e. the patient did not really know what was being proposed, action in negligence can be brought. Consent does not necessarily need to be in writing although a written consent acts as evidence that consent was sought. However, a signed consent form does not necessarily mean that the patient had all the details of the procedure explained and freely consented knowing all the risks of that procedure. Provided that the defendant can produce evidence that the procedure was explained thoroughly, that is all that is required in law.

If a patient was informed that there was a slightly increased risk to his/her life with a non-essential procedure, then he may wish to opt out of the proposed procedure. Alternately, he/she may well accept a local anaesthetic technique. Consent to a procedure must not be exceeded. If a patient is informed that an intubation may be difficult and for safety's sake will have to be carried out in the awake state, then the patient may very well refuse to have a general anaesthetic should the attempt at awake intubation fail. Under those circumstances, if a general anaesthetic is given against the patient's wishes, the anaesthetist might be guilty of battery.

## Content of consent

For consent to treatment to be effective, three criteria must be met:

- The patient must be legally competent (capacity), i.e. capable of consenting.
- The person consenting must be suitably informed.
- The consent must be freely given.

A patient is capable of consenting (or refusing) if he/she understands the procedure proposed, in terms of both short-term and longer-term consequences. Capacity depends on understanding, not age or status.

The patient should be warned of possible airway difficulties. If the surgery is not life-threatening, he/she may wish to refuse surgery. The possibility and reality of 'awake intubation' or alternative local anaesthetic techniques should be fully explored, detailing the risks associated with general anaesthesia. The patient must be in a position to make a free and informed choice. A balance between dissuading the patient from an essential surgical procedure and neglecting to provide information of an appreciable risk is a matter of clinical judgement.

In regard to airway problems that are recognized preoperatively, the wise physician will make adequate written records of the problem to avoid subsequent legal problems.

## Common Practice

The mere fact that shortcuts may have become common practice is no defence in law. In other words, the court may occasionally condemn even a universally followed practice as negligent. Thus because many anaesthetists do not immediately utilize capnography following intubation, is not to say that such action is not negligent.

A slight departure from the standard textbook treatment may not necessarily be negligent. Otherwise, no advances would be made in medicine.

With patients presenting with difficult intubation, each case has to be judged on its own merits and sometimes slightly irregular actions are taken to circumvent the problem. However, in each instance the departure from the common practice will have to be justified.

Regimens followed in other countries to deal with the problem of difficult intubation are not necessarily evidence of the appropriate standard in the UK. Therefore, superior devices or drugs which may be available for use with difficult intubation may not necessarily be available in the UK. Failure to use these devices is not negligence.

Foreseeability and reasonableness are two aspects or common threads that are found in many issues within the legal system. Therefore, problems which occurred 5 years ago should not be judged against the modern day knowledge.

This might be of particular reference in terms of late claims for brain damage as a result of difficult intubation some years ago before the advent of the fiberoptic bronchoscope and laryngoscope. However, a specialist will be judged by the ordinary competent specialist and not by the ordinary competent doctor. Therefore, if a consultant is involved in cases of difficult intubation, his/her actions will be judged by the ordinary consultant dealing with that problem.

## Experience

There is a definite correlation between inexperience and problems during and after anaesthesia. Inexperience is not a defence for negligent actions. The patient is entitled to receive all the care and skill which a fully qualified and an experienced anaesthetist would possess and use. Undertaking work beyond one's competence constitutes negligence.

## Delegation

A consultant or head of department can only shift responsibility to members of staff if he/she can prove that:

- He/she has ensured that the staff are properly trained, qualified and experienced.
- He/she has devised a safe system for working.
- He/she has made staff fully aware of this system, preferably by written orders.

## Emergency Situations

The law will make due allowance for emergency situations, but again, the comparison is with a reasonably competent doctor in the same situation. Where an emergency is foreseeable appropriate action must be taken. With regard to difficult intubation, it may be negligent to have an inadequate system for dealing with known risks this is likely to create, e.g. failing to have an essential piece of equipment readily available, failing to have an assistant, or failing to check the safety of the equipment.

## Tiredness

Should an employing authority or trust hospital fail to abide with the agreed hours of work for junior staff, the employer will be held responsible for a doctor's negligence due to tiredness.

## Personal Services for the Anaesthetist

Rest periods must be assured during a busy working period. Counselling should be provided for anaesthetists who undergoing critical periods in their lives.

## Training

An editorial in the *Lancet* [23] emphasized the importance of good training and thorough knowledge of failed intubation drill in averting disasters associated with patients who are difficult to intubate. It also emphasized the importance of skill in the use of the fibreoptic laryngoscope. At that time there was inadequate training in the use of the instrument owing to lack of interest by senior anaesthetists and underfunding of anaesthetic departments. The editorial stipulated that instruction in the use of the fibreoptic laryngoscope or bronchoscope was an essential component in the training programme of junior anaesthetic staff. A fibreoptic technique should be learned under unhurried controlled conditions and not reserved for difficult emergency situations. It is also advisable to use a fibreoptic instrument with an incorporated a suction facility.

## Roadside Care

Knight [24] states that a duty to exercise skill and care may not be obvious when a person acts as a good Samaritan, e.g. in a road traffic accident. The converse is not true in that a doctor is not negligent if he does not offer his services in an emergency to a person who is not his patient. Therefore, there may be a tendency for medical practitioners purposely to avoid rushing to the scene of an accident. In the case of a paramedic, a duty of care will exist when the paramedic becomes involved with the patient but the level of skill and care expected would be that of a reasonable body of people of the same standing.

## Chronology

There is a well-worn legal maxim in the respect of negligence stating that 'the categories of negligence are never closed', indicating that as medical technology advances, so claims of negligence will follow this trend. However, the facts of each case will be judged against the medical opinion prevailing at the time of the alleged breach.

# CONDUCT OF INTUBATION

## Equipment

Preoperative check of the anaesthetic equipment is essential. Maintenance, recognition of obsolescence and subsequent replacement of equipment should be routine.

## Difficult Intubation Trolley

An emergency cricothyrotomy set, emergency tracheostomy set and a fibreoptic intubating bronchoscope are regarded as essential components of the equipment on the 'difficult intubation trolley' [21]. These must be accompanied by the presence of trained staff. The fibreoptic scope is the method of choice – not a last resort. It is the opinion of the authors of this textbook that *all anaesthetists should be familiar with, and trained in, the use of the fibreoptic scope.*

This statement implies that all consultants should be versed in the use of the apparatus and programmes should be drawn up to teach all the staff in training. Proficiency in the use of this equipment can only be assumed if 30 successful intubations have been performed under supervision [25].

## Confirmation of Tracheal Placement

Confirmation of the correct position of the tracheal tube is made by the following methods:

- direct vision – the tube is seen to pass through the cords;
- auscultation;
- capnography;
- direct vision with fibreoptic scope;
- aspiration of gas.

Capnography is the most reliable of these methods and should be available in all areas where tracheal intubation is practised on a regular basis [26].

## Oesophageal Intubation

Although this sometimes occurs in patients where there does not seem to be any difficulty with direct laryngoscopy, inability to visualize the larynx denies the anaesthetist a very important confirmatory sign of successful tracheal placement. It is therefore imperative that the following points are emphasized.

- Auscultation of the chest and epigastrium is unreliable and may even lead to a false sense of security.
- A fall in the oxygen saturation after attempted tracheal intubation should lead to removal of the tube and subsequent manual ventilation with a facemask.
- The patients at the greatest risk of unrecognized oesophageal intubation are those with melanotic skin.

Twenty-five cases where death ensued over the 5-year period between 1982 and 1986 were studied following a computer search of the records of the Medical Protection Society. The commonest cause of death was failed intubation in patients such as those suffering from Hurler's syndrome or those with obesity or short, thick necks; some deaths were caused by undetected oesophageal intubation [27].

These cases differed from those of the CEPOD study in that only one-quarter of the patients were above age 60 and the majority of deaths occurred during elective procedures.

Criticisms were also made about inadequate preoperative assessment. In several cases the patient was seen by the anaesthetist for the first time in the anaesthetic room and this may have an important bearing on the prediction of a difficult airway. Again, failed intubation is an accepted hazard but the failure to detect oesophageal placement is a matter of great concern. In one case, three consultant anaesthetists failed to recognize that the tracheal tube was in the oesophagus. Problems occurred in patients with pigmented skin.

Standardized protocols need to be established regarding important details in the past medical history, assessment of patients before anaesthesia and dissemination of information prior to discharge of patients following surgery.

In summary, it is alarming to see the same factors consistently emerging in series of anaesthetic problems from different studies. The same factors seem to be repeatedly identified yet they keep recurring. The answer to this problem may well be lack of adequate training.

*This fails to explain why experienced anaesthetists reject the hypothesis that the tracheal tube is in the oesophagus and attempt instead to identify other problems while the patients is becoming hypoxic.*

## Auscultation of Breath Sounds

In 48% of the oesophageal misplacements [27], auscultation led to the erroneous conclusion that the tracheal tube was located in the trachea when it was actually in the oesophagus. The haemodynamic changes which occurred, mainly asystole and hypotension, were late occurrences in the chain of events and at that stage, organ damage had already occurred to some degree.

Prompt detection of oesophageal intubation is a primary concern in anaesthetic practice. A disturbing feature of the above study was that detection of oesophageal intubation required 5 min or more in the majority of cases. This delay could be attributed to the incidence of preoxygenation prior to induction.

Since the reliability of auscultation is in great doubt, and may even adversely affect the final outcome, *it is mandatory that all hospitals in the UK provide capnography and oximetry in all anaesthetic areas* [26]. It is also incumbent on all the anaesthetists to utilise this equipment in all cases.

## Use of Muscle Relaxants

Whenever there is doubt about the ease of intubation, there is a golden rule that muscle relaxants should not be employed. The choice between local anaesthesia (awake intubation) and general anaesthesia is still open to opinion. Therefore, there are two schools of thought. However, in the emergency situation, the reasonable anaesthetist would not render a patient unconscious with a full stomach knowing that the airway could not be secured with a tracheal tube. The risks of aspiration with 'awake intubation' utilizing local anaesthesia and judicious sedation is not associated with a greater risk of aspiration of gastric contents [28].

## Post Mortem Placement

Despite the apparent advisability of leaving the tracheal tube *in situ* to verify initial correct placement following a subsequent unexplained anaesthetic death [29], objections to this opinion were provided in subsequent correspondence [30, 31].

## Local Anaesthetic Solutions

Toxic reactions to local anaesthetic solutions used for 'awake intubation' are uncommon. A nerve block to prevent conduction from the mucosal surfaces of the upper airway should be used whenever possible as this results in lower levels of local anaesthetic agent in the blood. It is indefensible to perform this procedure in the absence of an indwelling intravenous cannula, i.v. anticonvulsant drugs, antagonists to the sedation and full cardiopulmonary resuscitation equipment.

Regarding the use of all drugs, reference to the manufacturer's data sheet is essential. However, the opinion of a reasonable body of experts in this field would recommend an upper limit of at least 4 mg kg$^{-1}$ of lignocaine for topical use [32]. The risk of overdose is reduced by the inevitable passage of some of the administered drug and its subsequent degradation in the liver (first pass effect).

## Teaching

It is very difficult to teach the various techniques used on patients with difficult intubation and most anaesthetists agree that teaching intubation on a manikin without subsequent training on the human is insufficient. Despite the condemnation of cadaveric practice by the British Medical Association and the Royal College of Nurses, Brattebo *et al.* [33] performed a public poll and found an overwhelming response in favour of this practice in Norway.

The training of paramedics in the art of intubation raises several legal issues. The standard of care expected is that of a reasonable group of similarly qualified practitioners. Allowance would have to be made for the increased difficulties of the emergency situation in a non-clinical environment.

## Effect of Litigation on the Conduct of Anaesthesia

Another important aspect is the effect of negligence claims on the clinical practice of the anaesthetist. An attempt to assess this was made in Canada [34].

This survey demonstrated that 48.7% of the respondents had changed their practice patterns as a result of liability concerns. Around 94% had increased the amount of monitoring used as a result of Society recommendations or as a result of the annual report issued by their malpractice insurers. The authors also stated that the physician–patient relationship had suffered in recent years and many of the senior anaesthetists were considering leaving medicine.

In the USA, the adoption of minimum standards of monitoring has reduced the cost of malpractice claims in the last 10 years by 60%. The medical staff have subsequently benefited by a reduction in premiums of 40%.

## Risk to Provider

A disturbing result was found when Solazzi and Ward [35] assessed claims on the basis of a reasonable, prudent approach to the care given. The plaintiff was successful in 50% of cases where care was above this standard. In fact, three of the anaesthetists in this study who were sued for alleged malpractice committed suicide. The ratio of suicides and attempted suicides in this series thus became one in every 45 anaesthesiologists who were sued. The logical conclusion from these findings is that the anaesthesiologist should receive counselling both before and after the settlement of a case.

## KEY POINTS

King and Adams [36] have outlined the pitfalls in airway management:

- inadequate preoperative assessment of the airway;

- inexperience of the anaesthetist;

- lack of skilled and dedicated assistants;

- persistent attempts at intubation;

- failure to recognize oesophageal intubation by routine use of the capnograph;

- aspiration of gastric contents with difficult or failed intubation;

- failure to follow a failed intubation drill;

- failure to recognize cyanosis in dark skinned patients;

- inappropriate anaesthetic technique;

- attempting tracheostomy when cricothyrotomy would be more appropriate;

- failure to recognize that preoxygenation should be an essential part of the induction of anaesthesia for all patients except those who adamantly refuse.

- The idea of a mask being placed on the face in the conscious state in a small group of patients could theoretically make the anaesthetists liable for action in battery, although this is highly unlikely. The problem can be circumvented even with these patients by suggesting that a cupped hand is placed around the mouth and the oxygen fed to produce a micro-climate around this area. Although this is not as efficient as the application of the mask in performing a nitrogen washout, it is certainly better than nothing.

King and Adams [36] suggest that when performing an 'awake intubation' on patients

who are at risk of vomiting and subsequent aspiration, the following steps should be followed:

- avoidance of sedation;

- avoidance of cricothyroid puncture (only applying topical anaesthesia below the cords just prior to intubation);

- intubate in the sitting position;

- take precautions beforehand to reduce the volume and acidity of gastric contents and to increase the lower oesophageal sphincter tone.

## REFERENCES

1 Lanphier v. Phipos (1838) 8 C&P 475.
2 Bolam v. Friern Hospital Management Committee. (1957). 1 WLR 582.
3 Buck N., Devlin H. B. and Lunn J. N. *The report of a confidential enquiry into perioperative deaths*. The Nuffield Provincial Hospitals Trust and the King's Fund, London. 1988.
4 Hibbard B. M., Anderson M. M., Drife J. *et al*. *Report on confidential enquiries into maternal deaths in the United Kingdom 1988–1990*. London: HMSO. 1994.
5 Feldman S. Standards of care in anaesthesia. In: Taylor T. H. and Goldhill D. R. (eds) Oxford: Butterworth-Heinemann.
6 Cheyney F. W., Posner K., Caplan R. A. and Ward R. J. Standard of care and anaesthetic liability. *Journal of the American Medical Association* 1989; **261:** 1599.
7 Thomas v. Raleigh General Hospital 358S.E. 2d 222- WV. In: Tamelleo A. D. *Regan Reports Nursing Law* 1987; **28:** 4.
8 Utting J. E. Pitfalls in anaesthetic practice. *British Journal of Anaesthesia* 1987; **59:** 877.
9 Aitkenhead A. R. Risk management in anaesthesia. *International Journal of Risk Safety of Medicine* 1991; **2:** 113.
10 American Society of Anesthesiologists Committee on Professional Liability: Preliminary Study of Closed Claims. *American Society of Anesthesiologists Newsletter* 1988; **52:** 8.
11 Holland R., Webb R. K. and Runciman W. B. Oesophageal intubation: an analysis of 2000 incident reports. *Anaesthesia and Intensive Care* 1993; **21:** 608.
12 Lunn J. N. and Mushin W. W. *Mortality associated with anaesthesia*. London: Nuffield Provincial Hospitals Trust. 1982.

13 Hoyte P. Personal communication. Medical Defence Union. 1994.

14 Perow C. *Normal Accidents*. New York: Basic Books Inc. 1984.

15 Pearce C. E. and Cooper J. B. Analysis of anaesthetic mishaps. *International Anesthesiology Clinics* 1984; **22**.

16 Holzer J. F. Analysis of anaesthetic mishaps. Current concepts in risk management. *International Anesthesiology Clinics* 1984; **22**: 91.

17 Orlikoff J. E., Fifer W. R. and Greeley H. P. *Malpractice Prevention and Liability Control for Hospitals*. Chicago: American Hospital Association. 1981: 28.

18 Strauss E. J., Poplak T. M. and Braude B. M. Anaesthetic management of a difficult intubation. *South African Medical Journal* 1985; **68**: 414.

19 Mark L. J., Beattie C., Ferrell C. L., Trempy G., Dorman T. and Schauble J. F. The difficult airway: mechanisms for effective dissemination of critical information. *Journal of Clinical Anesthesiology* 1992; **4**: 247.

20 King T. A. Emergency control of the airway. In: Atkinson R. S. and Adams A. P. (eds) *Recent Advances in Anaesthesia and Analgesia*. Edinburgh: Churchill Livingstone. 1994.

21 Taylor T. H. and Goldhill D. R. *Standards of Care in Anaesthesia*. Oxford: Butterworth-Heinemann. 1992.

22 Mallampati S. R., Gatt S. P., Gugino L. D. *et al.* A clinical sign to predict difficult intubation: a prospective study. *Canadian Anaesthetists Society Journal* 1985; **32**: 429.

23 Editorial. Difficult intubation. *Lancet* 1987; **2**: 778.

24 Knight B. *Legal Aspects of Medical Practice*, 5th edn. Edinburgh: Churchill Livingstone. 1992.

25 Ovassapian A., Dykes M. H. M. and Golmon M. Fiberoptic nasotracheal intubation: a training programme. *Anesthesiology* 1980; **53**: 352.

26 Eickhhorn J. H., Cooper J. B., Allen D. S. *et al.* Standards for patient monitoring during anaesthesia at Harvard Medical School. *Journal of the American Medical Association* 1986; **256**: 1017.

27 Gannon K. Mortality associated with anaesthesia: a case review study. *Anaesthesia* 1991; **46**: 962.

28 Ovassapian A., Krejcie T., Yelich S. and Dykes M. Awake fiberoptic intubation in the patient at a high risk of aspiration. *British Journal of Anaesthesia* 1989; **62**: 13.

29 Knight B. H. and Addicott L. S. Postmortem removal of tracheal tube [letter]. *Anaesthesia* 1987; **42**: 554.

30 Johnson K. R. Postmortem removal of tracheal tube [letter]. *Anaesthesia* 1987; **42**: 1242.

31 Charteris P. Postmortem removal of the tracheal tube [letter]. *Anaesthesia* 1987; **42**: 1243.

32 Taylor T. H. and Major E. *Hazards and Complications of Anaesthesia*. Singapore: Longmans Pte Ltd, 1993.

33 Brattebo G., Wisborg T., Solheim K. and Oyen N. Public opinion on different approaches to teaching intubation techniques. *British Medical Journal* 1993; **307**: 1256.

34 Cohen M. M., Wade J. and Woodward C. Medical–legal concerns among Canadian anaesthetists. *Canadian Journal of Anaesthesiology* 1990; **37**: 102.

35 Solazzi R. W. and Ward R. J. Analysis of anaesthetic mishaps. The spectrum of medical liability cases. *International Anesthesiology Clinics* 1984; **22**: 43.

36 King T. A. and Adams A. P. Failed tracheal intubation. *British Journal of Anaesthesia* 1990; **65**: 400.

# Index

Note - Page numbers in *italic* refer to illustrations; **bold** page numbers refer to tables.

40t